# The Infectious Diseases Manual

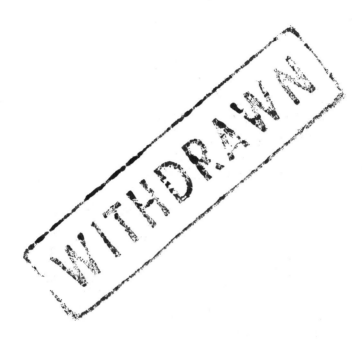

# The Infectious Diseases Manual

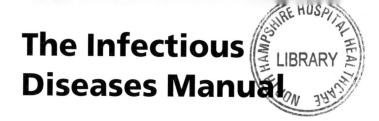

## David Wilks
MA, MD, FRCP, DTM&H
*Consultant Physician*
*Regional Infectious Diseases Unit*
*Western General Hospital*
*Edinburgh*

## Mark Farrington
MA, MB, BChir, FRCPath
*Consultant Microbiologist*
*Clinical Microbiology Laboratory*
*Addenbrooke's Hospital*
*Cambridge*

## David Rubenstein
MA, MD, FRCP
*Department of Medicine*
*Addenbrooke's Hospital*
*Cambridge*

SECOND EDITION

**Blackwell**
Science

© 2003 by Blackwell Science Ltd
a Blackwell Publishing company
Blackwell Science, Inc., 350 Main Street, Malden, Massachusetts 02148-5018, USA
Blackwell Science Ltd, 9600 Garsington Road, Oxford OX4 2DQ, UK
Blackwell Science Asia Pty Ltd, 550 Swanston Street, Carlton, South Victoria 3053, Australia
Blackwell Wissenschafts Verlag, Kurfürstendamm 57, 10707 Berlin, Germany

First published 1995
Second edition 2003

Library of Congress Cataloging-in-Publication Data
Wilks, David.
    The infectious diseases manual / David Wilks, Mark Farrington, David Rubenstein. — 2nd ed.
        p. ; cm.
Includes index.
    ISBN 0-632-06417-X
    1. Communicable diseases—Handbooks, manuals, etc.   2. Infection—Handbooks, manuals, etc.
3. Medical microbiology—Handbooks, manuals, etc.
    [DNLM:   1. Communicable Diseases—Handbooks. WC 39 W688i 2003]   I. Farrington, Mark.
II. Rubenstein, David.   III. Title.

RC111 .W68   2003
616.9—dc21

                                                                                              2002013472
ISBN 0-632-06417-X

A catalogue record for this title is available from the British Library

Set in 9/11pt Minion by SNP Best-set Typesetter Ltd., Hong Kong
Printed and bound in Great Britain by MPG Books Ltd, Bodmin, Cornwall

Commissioning Editor: Maria Khan
Editorial Assistant: Elizabeth Callaghan
Production Editor: Nick Morgan
Production Controller: Kate Charman

For further information on Blackwell Publishing, visit our website:
http://www.blackwellpublishing.com

# Contents

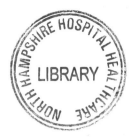

# Section I

# Introduction

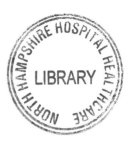

# Chapter 1

# Introduction

There have been many changes in the practice of microbiology and clinical infectious diseases since the first edition of this manual was published in 1995. Molecular techniques, which had only recently been discovered, are now in routine use. New antivirals and a new understanding of viral kinetics have revolutionized HIV care, and clinical guidelines, which were few and far between then, are now available in almost every area. Antibiotic-resistant organisms become more prevalent month by month, and for the first time in decades drugs from totally novel classes of antibiotics have been licensed. We were very encouraged by the positive response given to the first edition of the *Manual* by working clinicians, and we believe that there is even more need now for a convenient and portable source of detailed and practical information on all aspects of infectious diseases and microbiology.

For the second edition, the entire text of the manual has been carefully revised. Some sections, such as the chapter about HIV infection, have been completely rewritten. Our aim has been to produce a handbook that every SpR in infectious diseases will want in their white-coat pocket for consultant ward rounds, and every SpR in microbiology will keep by the telephone in the reporting room. As before, common conditions are described in detail. The clinical presentation of rarely seen and usually tropical conditions is described in sufficient detail to allow their recognition, whereas their treatment, which would always be a matter for specialist referral, is described in outline only.

Some areas have been given a more detailed treatment than their frequency might suggest, either because of their potential significance, or because we think they are interesting. Some areas of specialist interest have been described in more detail, because patients with neutropenia or HIV may present outside their usual units, and specialist help may not always be immediately available.

We have not attempted to reference the manual comprehensively, but we have tried to demonstrate its evidence base by including key references such as national guidelines, recent authoritative reviews, or unique papers that have significantly changed practice. We have also included many useful website addresses which satisfy the same criteria and which are likely to remain accessible during the life of this edition (in general we have omitted the prefix http:// to save space).

To make the best use of space, we have used symbols and abbreviations, defined on the following pages. Throughout the text, the symbol (➤000) indicates that further information is available on that particular page.

Tables of antibiotics, doses and side effects are located in section IV. Whilst every care has been taken to ensure that these tables contain no errors, we cannot accept responsibility for any that have occurred. We regard it as good practice for prescribers to check the dose of any drug with which they are unfamiliar by reference to the manufacturer's data sheet or the *British National Formulary*.

🖥 bnf.vhn.net/home/

## Abbreviations

Abbreviations which are used only within one or two sections of the manual are defined therein. Abbreviations listed here are those that are used many times throughout the manual.

| | |
|---|---|
| AFB | acid-fast bacillus |
| AIDS | acquired immune deficiency syndrome |
| ARDS | adult respiratory distress syndrome |
| ASOT | anti-streptolysin O titre |
| BAL | broncho-alveolar lavage |
| BT | bioterrorism |
| CAPD | chronic ambulatory peritoneal dialysis |
| CCDC | Consultant in Communicable Disease Control |
| CDSC | Communicable Disease Surveillance Centre (Colindale) |
| CF | cystic fibrosis |
| CMI | cell-mediated immunity |
| CMV | cytomegalovirus |
| CNS | central nervous system |
| CNSt | coagulase-negative staphylococcus |
| COAD | chronic obstructive airways disease |
| CSF | cerebrospinal fluid |
| CT | computed tomography (scan) |
| CXR | chest X-ray |
| DIC | disseminated intravascular coagulation |
| EBV | Epstein–Barr virus |
| ECHO | echocardiogram |
| ELISA | enzyme-linked immunosorbent assay |
| ENT | ear, nose and throat |
| ERCP | endoscopic retrograde cholecystopancreatogram |
| FBC | full blood count |
| G6PD | glucose-6-phosphate dehydrogenase |
| GAS | group A β-haemolytic streptococcus |
| GI | gastrointestinal |
| GN | glomerulonephritis |
| h | hour |
| HAV | hepatitis A virus |
| HBV | hepatitis B virus |
| HCV | hepatitis C virus |

| | |
|---|---|
| HD | % drug removed by haemodialysis |
| HDV | hepatitis D virus |
| HEPA | high-efficiency particulate arrester |
| HHV-6 | human herpes virus type 6 |
| Hib | *Haemophilus influenzae* type b |
| HIG | normal human immunoglobulin |
| HIV | human immunodeficiency virus |
| HLGR | high-level gentamicin-resistant |
| HSV | herpes simplex virus |
| IA | invasive aspergillosis |
| ICU | intensive-care unit |
| id | intradermal |
| IE | infective endocarditis |
| IFAT | indirect fluorescent antibody test |
| im/IM | intramuscular |
| ip | intraperitoneal |
| IUD | intrauterine device |
| iv/IV | intravenous |
| IVDU | intravenous drug use(r) |
| LP | lumbar puncture |
| LRTI | lower respiratory tract infection |
| MAI | *Mycobacterium avium-intracellulare* |
| MBC | minimum bactericidal concentration |
| MDa | megadalton |
| MIC | minimum inhibitory concentration |
| min | minute |
| MOSF | multi-organ system failure |
| MRI | magnetic resonance imaging |
| MRSA | methicillin-resistant *Staphylococcus aureus* |
| MSU | mid-stream urine |
| MW | molecular weight |
| NSAID | non-steroidal anti-inflammatory drug |
| PCP | *Pneumocystis carinii* pneumonia |
| PD | % drug removed by peritoneal dialysis |
| PHLS | Public Health Laboratory Service |
| PID | pelvic inflammatory disease |
| po | orally (per os) |
| PUO | pyrexia of unknown origin |
| PVE | prosthetic valve endocarditis |
| RSV | respiratory syncytial virus |
| RUQ | right upper quadrant |
| SBC | serum bactericidal concentration |
| sc | subcutaneous |
| SLE | systemic lupus erythematosus |
| SRSV | small round structured virus |
| STD | sexually transmitted disease |

| | | | |
|---|---|---|---|
| TB | tuberculosis | VDRL | Venereal Disease Research Laboratory (syphilis) |
| TPHA | *Treponema pallidum* haemagglutination assay | VHF | viral haemorrhagic fever |
| TSS(T) | toxic shock syndrome (toxin) | VZV | varicella zoster virus |
| URTI | upper respiratory tract infection | WBC | white blood cell (count) |
| USS | ultrasound scan | WHO | World Health Organization |
| UTI | urinary tract infection | ZN | Ziehl–Nielsen |

# Symbols

| Symbol | Meaning | Further details |
|---|---|---|
| ➤ | Refer to page number | |
| ☎ | Discussion with microbiology/specialist referral recommended | |
| 🛎 | Antibiotic level assay required | ➤388 |
| Σ | Cases per annum reported in England and Wales | |
| ✈ | Test performed by a reference laboratory | |
| ⊠ | Notifiable disease | ➤7 |
| ① | Standard isolation | ➤8 |
| ② | Body fluids isolation | ➤8 |
| ③ | Infection risk from blood isolation | ➤8 |
| ④ | Strict isolation | ➤8 |
| ✓ | Antibiotic penetrates this fluid (e.g. CSF✓) | |
| ✗ | Antibiotic does **not** penetrate this fluid (e.g. CSF✗) | |
| 🖳 | Internet resource—usually a website address (the prefix http:// is omitted to save space) | |
| ⊢ | Key reference. Usually a national guideline, a recent authoritative review, or a unique paper that has significantly changed practice | |
| ☠ | Organisms which are a hazard to laboratory staff | |
| 📄 | See manufacturer's data sheet | |

## ✉ Notifiable diseases

In England and Wales, the following diseases must be notified to the local authority, via the local consultant in communicable disease control (CCDC).

| | | | |
|---|---|---|---|
| Acute encephalitis | (➤101) | Paratyphoid fever | (➤280) |
| Acute poliomyelitis | (➤348) | Plague | (➤305) |
| Anthrax | (➤263) | Rabies | (➤357) |
| Cholera | (➤285) | Relapsing fever | (➤326) |
| Diphtheria | (➤268) | Rubella | (➤127) |
| Dysentery (amoebic or bacillary) | (➤209) | Scarlet fever | (➤135) |
| Food poisoning | (➤57) | Smallpox | (➤341) |
| Leprosy | (➤46) | Tetanus | (➤315) |
| Leptospirosis | (➤327) | Tuberculosis | (➤38) |
| Malaria | (➤211) | Typhoid fever | (➤280) |
| Measles | (➤126) | Typhus | (➤329) |
| Meningitis | (➤96) | Viral haemorrhagic fever | (➤206) |
| Meningococcaemia | (➤185) | Viral hepatitis | (➤70) |
| Mumps | (➤128) | Whooping cough | (➤136) |
| Ophthalmia neonatorum | (➤107) | Yellow fever | (➤352) |

Chickenpox (➤130) is a notifiable disease in Scotland. Certain other diseases may be made **locally** notifiable.

# Isolation

Isolation is a key technique for preventing spread of infectious diseases in hospitals. It can be physically and emotionally disturbing, and disruptive of clinical care, and therefore should only be used where there is proven or likely benefit. Strong evidence of efficacy is available for some infections including MRSA, tuberculosis and multiply-resistant coliforms. Isolation policies are made at individual hospitals, and local protocols should always be consulted. If these are not available, consult your microbiologists ☎ and infection control team. We have not included detailed instructions for medical and nursing procedures for the surveillance, control and prevention of infection in hospital; we refer readers searching for this information to the excellent handbooks and comprehensive reference texts that cover nosocomial infection control. Systematic reviews of the evidence for infection control interventions are being published, e.g.

💻 www.epic.tvu.ac.uk

💻 www.cdc.gov/ncidod/hip

**Source isolation** is designed to prevent infected patients from transmitting their disease to others. It may generally be considered in four categories:

| Level of isolation | Examples | Route | Main suggested precautions |
|---|---|---|---|
| SUP (standard universal precautions) | All patients | | Aprons, gloves and handwashing, but no need for separate room. Aprons and gloves should be used whenever there is the possibility of contact with patients' body fluids, and hands should be cleaned after every patient contact, irrespective of the diagnosis. These simple measures form the backbone of infection control in hospital |
| ① Standard | *Neisseria meningitidis*, Group A β-haemolytic streptococci | Airborne or direct contact | Separate room. Negative pressure ventilation if available. Aprons, gloves ± masks for all entering room |
| ② Body fluids | *Salmonella* spp., *Shigella* spp., multiply-resistant *Acinetobacter* spp. | Contact with urine, faeces and secretions | Separate room. Aprons and gloves for patient contact |
| ③ Infection risk from blood | Hepatitis B, HIV | Contact with blood or blood-stained body fluids* | Separate room only required if patients are bleeding, likely to bleed, undergoing major invasive procedure, incontinent or confused. Plastic aprons, gloves (±visors) for procedures where contact with body fluids is possible |
| ④ Strict | Lassa fever | Airborne or direct contact | Strict isolation in specialist unit—usually regional infectious diseases centre. **Do not send any specimens without discussion with lab** |

*Including CSF, pleural fluid, vaginal secretions, peritoneal fluid, synovial fluid, semen, pericardial fluid, amniotic fluid and breast milk.

Throughout text, recommended levels of isolation are indicated by the use of symbols (e.g. ④).

**Protective isolation** is used to prevent immunocompromised patients from acquiring infection. It is of less certain value, particularly as most infections in neutropenic patients are endogenous (➤174). Most units concentrate on protecting against specific organisms, e.g. nursing in HEPA-filtered air (vs. aspergillosis), antibiotic prophylaxis and microbiologically clean food (to avoid colonization with new strains of Gram-negative bacteria).

# Recommendations for isolation

For category codes ➤8.

| Disease | Category | See | Disease | Category | See |
|---|---|---|---|---|---|
| Anthrax ⊠ | SUP | 263 | Hepatitis ?cause ⊠ | ② | |
| *Bordetella pertussis*[1] ⊠ | ① | 136 | Hepatitis A | ② | 70 |
| *Borrelia recurrentis*[2] ⊠ | ① | 326 | Hepatitis B, fulminant liver | ③ | 70 |
| Bronchiolitis (RSV)[24] | ① | 23 | failure of undetermined | | |
| *Campylobacter jejuni*[3] | ② | 288 | cause | | |
| *Candida* spp.[4] | ② | 367 | Hepatitis C | ③ | 73 |
| Chickenpox ⊠[6] | ① | 130 | Herpes simplex[17] | ① | 334 |
| *Chlamydia trachomatis*[5] | ② | 329 | Herpes zoster[6] | ① | 130 |
| (ophthalmia neonatorum⊠, | | | HIV | ③ | 143 |
| conjunctivitis, genital | | | Impetigo[10] | ① | 111 |
| infection) | | | Lassa fever ⊠ | ④ | 206 |
| Cholera[7] ⊠ | ② | 285 | Leprosy ⊠ | | 46 |
| *Clostridium difficile*[8] | ② | 63 | Smear negative | — | |
| Coxsackievirus[9] | ② | 349 | Smear positive | ① | |
| *Cryptosporidium parvum* | ② | 230 | Leptospirosis[1] ⊠ | ② | 327 |
| Dermatitis[10] (severely | ① | 111 | Lice, fleas[1] | ② | 94 |
| infected) | | | Listeriosis[18] | ② | 267 |
| Diarrhoea of unknown cause[12] | ② | 57 | Marburg virus disease ⊠ | ④ | 206 |
| Diphtheria[11] ⊠ | ① | 268 | Measles[19] ⊠ | ① | 126 |
| Dysentery ⊠ | | | Melioidosis[15] | ① | 293 |
| Amoebic[13] or bacillary[14] | ② | 209 | Meningitis ⊠ | | |
| Ebola virus ⊠ | ④ | 206 | *Neisseria meningitidis*[1] | ① | 96 |
| Eczema[10] (severely | ① | 111 | (including | | |
| infected) | | | meningococcal | | |
| Encephalitis ?cause ⊠ | ① | 101 | septicaemia/other | | |
| Erysipelas[10] | ① | 113 | invasive meningococcal | | |
| Erythema infectiosum | ① | 135 | infections) | | |
| *Escherichia coli* diarrhoea, | ② | 275 | Neonatal | ② | 139 |
| travellers' diarrhoea, | | | Viral[9] | ① | 100 |
| haemolytic uraemic syndrome | | | Meningoencephalitis, | ① | 348 |
| (O157, VTEC, EIEC, EPEC, | | | acute (acute | | |
| EAggEC, ETEC, etc.) | | | poliomyelitis) ⊠ | | |
| Exanthem subitum | ① | 134 | MRSA[20] | ① | 251 |
| Food poisoning ⊠ | | | Multiply-resistant Gram- | ② | |
| Undiagnosed cause[12] | ② | 57 | negative bacteria[20] | | |
| *Campylobacter jejuni*[3] | ② | | Mumps[9] ⊠ | ① | 128 |
| Salmonella[15] | ② | | Ophthalmia neonatorum[1] ⊠ | ② | 107 |
| *Francisella tularensis*[15] | ① | 307 | Parvovirus B19 | ① | 135 |
| Gastroenteritis, viral | ② | 350 | Penicillin-resistant *Streptococcus* | ① | 261 |
| Giardiasis | ② | 218 | *pneumoniae*[11] | | |
| Gonococcal conjunctivitis[1] | ② | 86 | Pertussis[1] ⊠ | ① | 136 |
| Haemolytic streptococcus[10] | ① | 254 | Plague ⊠ | ④ | 305 |
| Lancefield group A, B[3], C or | | | Poliomyelitis, acute ⊠ | ① | 348 |
| G (*Streptococcus pyogenes*) | | | *Pseudomonas pseudomallei*[15] | ① | 293 |

(continued...)

| Disease | Category | See | Disease | Category | See |
|---|---|---|---|---|---|
| Psittacosis | ① | 329 | Tuberculosis[23] (open pulmonary, wound, urinary) ✉ | ① | 38 |
| PUO[21] | ① | 179 | Tularaemia[15] | ① | 307 |
| Rabies ✉ | ④ | 357 | Typhoid, paratyphoid and carriers[7] ✉ | ② | 280 |
| Ratbite fever[1] | ② | 306 | | | |
| Relapsing fever[2] ✉ | ① | 326 | Typhus[2] ✉ | ① | 329 |
| Respiratory syncytial virus[24] | ① | 23 | Vaccinia, generalized | ④ | 341 |
| Rotavirus | ② | 350 | Vancomycin-resistant Gram-positive organisms[20] (usually *Enterococcus faecalis* or *faecium*) | ① | 262 |
| Rubella[16] ✉ | ① | 127 | | | |
| Salmonellosis[15] (excluding typhoid and paratyphoid) | ② | 57 | | | |
| Scabies[1] | ① | 95 | Varicella ✉[6] | ① | 130 |
| Scarlet fever[10] ✉ | ① | 135 | *Vibrio parahaemolyticus*[15] | ② | 287 |
| Smallpox[22] ✉ | ④ | 341 | Viral haemorrhagic fever ✉ | ④ | 206 |
| *Streptococcus pyogenes*—see Haemolytic streptococcus | | | Whooping cough[1] ✉ | ① | 136 |
| Syphilis (1° or 2° only)[1] | ② | 89 | *Yersinia enterocolitica* and *pseudotuberculosis*[15] | ② | 284 |
| Tapeworms | ② | 237 | | | |

[1] For first 24 h of treatment.   [2] Until patient and contacts deloused.   [3] Neonates only.   [4] If part of proven outbreak.   [5] For first 48 h of treatment.   [6] Until vesicles are crusted and dry. Staff in contact should be immune. Notifiable in Scotland.   [7] Until asymptomatic with three negative stool cultures.   [8] Until asymptomatic for 3 days.   [9] For 10 days after onset.   [10] Until cultures known to be negative for β-haemolytic streptococci.   [11] Until culture negative.   [12] Until transmissible pathogens excluded.   [13] Until asymptomatic and treated for cyst carriage.   [14] Until asymptomatic and one negative stool culture.   [15] Until asymptomatic.   [16] Until 7 days after onset of rash.   [17] Only for infants with disseminated infection.   [18] Infants and mothers only.   [19] Until 4 days after onset of rash.   [20] Until agreed by microbiologist.   [21] If outside Europe and N. America within 4 weeks.   [22] Even if only suspected.   [23] For first 14 days of therapy.   [24] Cohorting on children's ward whilst symptomatic.

# Microbiological specimens

Details of **sample collection** and transport vary from laboratory to laboratory, but a general summary of principles follows. Laboratories differ (based on local prevalence) on whether they routinely perform certain tests on particular specimens (e.g. *Clostridium difficile* toxin on all faeces). The importance of listing **full clinical details** has been emphasized throughout this book. **Always** give details of recent hospital in-patient stays and travel, and also occupation if the patient has diarrhoea or skin infection and works in catering, school or hospital. Similarly, **details of past, current and intended antibiotic therapy** are valuable for interpretation of many culture results. **Virus culture** is usually only worth attempting early in the course of infection. Specimens for **culture of bacteria and fungi** should always be taken **before antibiotic therapy is commenced**; sputum, mucosae and open wounds become colonized particularly rapidly with resistant bacteria.

• **Screening of contacts, or of cases for clearance**, is only occasionally useful for any pathogen out of hospital, and should always be done only according to locally written policies or after discussion with a microbiologist, ID physician or CCDC.

• Specimens are always best transported immediately to the laboratory. If delay is necessary, **in general all samples should be refrigerated at 4°C**, except inoculated blood culture bottles, which should be incubated at 37°C.

## Swabs, tissue and pus

Send pus, if available, in a sterile universal container, because additional rapid tests can be performed (e.g. HPLC for short-chain fatty acids from anaerobes); a swab is an inferior substitute upon which delicate organisms die. Use firm pressure when taking swabs and always use the appropriate swab transport medium (bacterial, viral, chlamydial). Inclusion of charcoal in transport media or swab tips increases recovery of many bacteria, especially *Neisseria gonorrhoeae*. Use special **pernasal swabs** for *Bordetella pertussis*. Gonococcal culture plates are best inoculated at the bedside. Surface swabs of deeply infected lesions (e.g. sinus tracks from osteomyelitis) usually grow surface contaminants (e.g. coliforms and pseudomonads) and rarely grow the causative organism. Only isolation of *Staphylococcus aureus* from this type of specimen correlates with true deep infection. Culture of bone marrow, liver biopsies etc. is occasionally useful, but should be discussed in advance with a microbiologist. Samples from drainage bags (e.g. biliary, wound, nephrostomy) are not representative of the microbial population within the patient; cultures are frequently overgrown with commensal bacteria, especially *Bacillus* spp. Take samples of freshly drained fluid from close to the patient.

## Medical devices

The tips of iv catheters suspected of being infected should be cut off with alcohol-wiped scissors and sent in a sterile universal container for semiquantitative culture. Growth of >15–20 colonies of coagulase-negative staphylococci or diphtheroids suggests infection, and any growth of other bacteria or fungi is likely to be significant. Small infected prostheses (e.g. heart valves) can be sent entire, but it is best to scrape adherent material from larger prostheses and send that.

## Urine

Prepuce and labia should be held away from the urine stream, but periurethral cleaning does not additionally reduce contamination of MSUs from adults as long as the initial stream is discarded. Most laboratories supply universal containers with borate preservative, or dip-slides for urine collection in domiciliary practice. The former preserves both host and bacterial cells for 48 h. Dip-slides should be only dipped into urine, and the transport container should not be filled with it. Catheter urine specimens should be taken by aseptic puncture of the sampling area close to the patient. Culturing urinary catheter tips is a waste of time. Paediatric bag collection systems are often contaminated, but this is reduced by cleaning the perineum with antiseptic; a negative culture is useful, but positive results must be interpreted with care. Suprapubic aspiration is the gold standard for detecting bladder urine infection. Early morning urine (EMU) specimens for AFB microscopy and culture should be ≈150 mL volumes, and taken on different days.

## Sputum

Efforts, such as vigorous physiotherapy, to obtain expectorated sputum before antibiotics have been given improve the isolation rate of pneumococci and other significant pathogens. Three samples on successive days are needed to exclude open pulmonary tuberculosis. Broncho-alveolar lavage is the most sensitive diagnostic procedure, but induced sputum is simpler, with adequate sensitivity for *Pneumocystis carinii* diagnosis. In ventilated patients, non-directed lavage allows recognition of significant isolates by quantitative culture ($>10^5$/mL).

## Faeces

A walnut-sized sample is needed; this is most easily collected by passing stool onto folded toilet paper in the lavatory bowl, and scooping the sample into a universal container with a spatula attached to the inside of the lid. The best chance of isolating causative agents of acute diarrhoea is on the first sample, and only if it is taken early in the course of illness. Many pathogens are only transiently excreted (e.g. *Escherichia coli* O157), so multiple samples are only required for exclusion of some parasites (e.g. *Giardia*) and to detect carriage of typhoid bacilli in food handlers (➤63). 'Hot' stool samples for visualization of trophozoites of *Entamoeba histolytica* are only useful if the patient has dysentery, i.e. bloody diarrhoea.

## Blood cultures

Blood cultures should be taken from any patient who is systemically ill in whom an in-

fective diagnosis is being considered. Before venepuncture, the skin should be carefully disinfected with an alcoholic antiseptic, which is allowed to dry. Most laboratories now use automated blood culture systems, which come with instruction sheets and should be inoculated with the specified volumes of blood (both over- and under-inoculation impair performance). Check the expiry date on the bottles and do not use if cloudy. Modern systems have greatly improved efficiency, and 2–3 cultures are sufficient for all indications, except when the patient has received antibiotics recently. In this case, when IE is suspected, it is worth taking two cultures on day 1, and daily cultures for the next 3–4 days. It is not necessary to change needles before injecting the culture bottles. It is often recommended to inoculate small volumes of normally sterile fluids (e.g. CAPD, ascitic, joint) to blood culture bottles. Unfortunately, blood culture broths are optimized for bacterial recovery only when blood is included, and other laboratory procedures become impossible (e.g. microscopy, incubation at different temperatures and atmospheres, mycobacterial culture). Always also send some fluid in a sterile universal container or capped syringe if blood culture broths are inoculated.

## CSF

Best taken in three consecutively labelled bottles, and transported immediately to the laboratory. Take simultaneous blood glucose. For a reasonable chance of detecting AFB, 10 mL or more CSF is required.

## Serum

Listing the **times of doses and samples** is important for interpretation of antibiotic assays. Specifying the **date of onset of illness** is vital for choosing and interpreting serological tests; acute and convalescent (10–14 days later) sera are often needed to prove recent infection. Most laboratories will store many such sera, issue a request for a convalescent sample, and only perform the assays (in parallel) if a later serum is received. IgM assay diagnosis on single acute sera is possible for some infections (e.g. *Mycoplasma*, *Rubella*, hepatitis viruses, *Toxoplasma*), and very high single titres are diagnostic for others (e.g. *Legionella*, respiratory *Chlamydia*, *Coxiella*). **Exposure history** and **date of leaving the endemic area** are essential for performance of tests for many geographically-restricted infections (e.g. brucellosis, schistosomiasis).

## Molecular tests

Local protocols for sampling and transport should always be followed. Care with these stages is as important as for conventional diagnostic testing if potential cross-reactions and inhibition of PCRs are to be avoided. Details of construction of the swab and of the composition of the transport medium may affect the sensitivity and specificity of the result. EDTA blood samples are preferred by many laboratories, but these bottles are frequently contaminated with pseudomonads.

# Clinical Infectious Diseases

# Chapter 2

# Upper respiratory tract infections

## Sinusitis

Most often affects the maxillary sinuses. May be acute or chronic and recurrent. Complications are due to the proximity of the orbits and intracranial structures.

**Risk factors:** Frequently secondary to: acute viral URTI, complicating ≈0.5% of childhood URTIs. Dental sepsis or procedures, nasal polyps or deviated septum. Rarely, immunodeficiency (AIDS, IgG, IgA deficiency), cystic fibrosis, immotile cilia syndrome.

**Clinical features:** Facial pain, fever and purulent nasal discharge. Headache, nasal obstruction, halitosis, toothache and anosmia may occur. Cough is frequent in children.

**Organisms: Acute:** *Streptococcus pneumoniae*, *Haemophilus influenzae*, viruses, *Moraxella catarrhalis*, rarely *Staphylococcus aureus*. **Chronic:** *Streptococcus pneumoniae*, *Haemophilus influenzae*, *Streptococcus 'milleri'*, mixed oral anaerobes, *Staphylococcus aureus*.

**Microbiological investigations:** Nasal swabs are **not** helpful. Sinus aspiration to obtain material for Gram staining and culture for persistent or recurrent infections.

**Other investigations:** Severe or persistent infection merits sinus X-rays. Fluid level or opacity suggest acute infection. Complete opacity or mucosal thickening alone may be seen in chronic infection. CT, MRI are more sensitive.

**Differential diagnosis:** Consider immunodeficiency, rare non-infectious causes (Wegener's, carcinoma, lymphoma) unusual infections (TB, leprosy, syphilis).

**Antibiotic management:** Amoxicillin or co-amoxiclav or cefuroxime, but dubious clinical efficacy.

**Supportive management:** Nasal decongestants: oxymetazoline hydrochloride nasal spray, 0.05%, 1–2 sprays each nostril 8hly, or pseudoephedrine hydrochloride, 60 mg 8hly, po. ENT referral for persistent or recurrent infection.

**Complications:** Rare but serious. Orbital cellulitis (➤109), osteomyelitis of facial bones (➤123), intracranial abscess (➤103), meningitis (➤96), cavernous and superior sagittal sinus thrombosis, orbital fissure syndrome (sphenoid sinus).

**Comments:** Chronic recurrent sinusitis reflects impaired drainage from the sinuses and merits ENT referral. Infection is usually due to mixed aerobic and anaerobic oral flora and responds poorly to antibiotic therapy alone. Immunocompromised patients may develop fungal sinusitis (*Aspergillus* spp., *Mucor* spp. and relatives ➤369). Urgent ENT referral is required.

## Otitis media (OM)

**Risk factors:** Frequently follows URTI. Common in children because of short, straight Eustachian tubes and blockage secondary to lymphoid hyperplasia.

**Clinical features:** Fever and earache. Otorrhoea if perforation has occurred. Presentation may be non-specific in infants. Tenderness over the mastoid process and redness and bulging of the tympanic membrane, which may have perforated.

**Organisms:** *Streptococcus pneumoniae*, non-capsulate *Haemophilus influenzae*, *Moraxella catarrhalis*; ≈30% are viral, frequently due to respiratory syncytial virus. *Staphylococcus aureus*, *Mycoplasma pneumoniae*, and GAS are seen rarely. Chronic infection may proceed to cholesteatoma with involvement of *Proteus* spp. and pseudomonads.

**Microbiological investigations:** In uncompli-cated cases, none.

**Antibiotic management:** Role of antibiotics controversial. Distinguish between acute OM with fever, otalgia and erythema of tympanic membrane, which may merit antibiotics, and chronic OM with effusion, which does not. Chronic suppurative OM with perforation has a different microbial aetiology and requires ENT referral.

   Goal of therapy in acute OM is to reduce the duration of pain and to prevent complica-tions (mastoiditis, meningitis, intracranial abscess) In the pre-antibiotic era, these affected up to 40%, but they are now very rare. Spontaneous recovery occurs in ≈80% of acute OM without antibiotics. Systematic review suggests small benefit from antibio-tics, especially in prevention of complications. We recommend giving antibiotics for acute OM; they can be withheld in patients over 2 years, who are not systemically unwell, have normal host defences and who are likely to return for follow-up assessment at 48 h. If not improved at 48 h, commence antibiotics. All authorities agree that children under 6 months should receive antibiotics. Amoxicillin is the drug of choice (erythromycin if allergic).

**Supportive management:** Analgesia.
↦   Schloss MD, Can Respir J 1999; 6 (Suppl. A): 51A

### Otitis externa

A hypersensitivity reaction of the skin lining the external auditory canal. Symptoms include itching, pain and a feeling of fullness. On otoscopy, oedema and redness of the walls of the meatus. Often responds to careful cleansing and topical steroids. If infection is present, it is usually mixed due to diphtheroids, pseudomonads and coliforms. Neomycin and hydrocortisone drops may be used. If there is evidence of local skin infection, such as a boil, flucloxacillin is given. Perforation must be excluded before drops are prescribed. *Aspergillus* and other fungal infections are best treated with clotrimazole drops.

   **Malignant otitis externa** is a rare infection usually with *Pseudomonas aeruginosa* which affects diabetics and the immunocompro-mised. It has a significant mortality, due to infection of adjacent bone and soft tissue, and requires aggressive systemic treatment with anti-pseudomonal antibiotics and surgical debridement. Urgent ENT referral is essential.

## Dental and oral infections

Dental caries is related to acid production from fermentation of dietary carbohydrates by bac-teria, including *Streptococcus mutans* and lacto-bacilli. Its significance for the physician lies in its effects on nutrition and as a risk factor for gingival disease, dental abscesses and Vincent's angina.

### Vincent's angina

**Risk factors:** Poor oral hygiene, poor nutrition, smoking and severe intercurrent illness.

**Clinical features:** Oral pain, gingival bleed-ing, halitosis, fever and anorexia. On exami-nation there is necrosis and pseudomem-brane formation on tonsils and gums. There may be local lymphadenopathy and excess salivation.

**Organisms:** Mixed infection due to *Leptotrichia* spp., *Bacteroides* spp. and *Fusobacterium* spp.

**Differential diagnosis:** Candidiasis (➤367), herpes simplex stomatitis (➤129), diphtheria (➤268).

**Microbiological investigations:** Gram stain of scrapings from the affected area. Throat swab for *Candida albicans* and *Corynebacterium diphtheriae* if suspected.

**Antibiotic management:** Penicillin V/amoxi-cillin + metronidazole **or** co-amoxiclav.

**Supportive management:** Attention to oral and dental hygiene.

**Complications:** In the severely malnourished or immunocompromised patient progression to noma, a severe gangrenous stomatitis, may occur rarely.

> **Practice point**
>
> Patients with agranulocytosis may present with severe oral and pharyngeal ulceration due to *Candida* spp., herpes simplex or *Capnocytophaga* spp. infection, which may subsequently act as a portal of entry for oral streptococcal bacteraemia.

## Dental abscess

**Risk factors:** Poor dental hygiene, pregnancy.

**Clinical features:** Fever, toothache, facial pain and swelling.

**Organisms:** Mixed oral aerobes and anaerobes.

**Antibiotic management:** Penicillin V/ amoxicillin + metronidazole **or** co-amoxiclav.

> *Ludwig's angina* refers to a severe cellulitis of the floor of the mouth, almost always arising from the second or third mandibular molars. Infection is polymicrobial and may become extensive.

## Parapharyngeal abscess

May complicate quinsy (➤21), but usually arises from dental abscess. Infection by mixed oral flora in lateral pharyngeal space displaces tonsil towards midline and causes lateral neck swelling below mandible. Severe **trismus** is characteristic; may progress rapidly to systemic sepsis and local suppurative complications, including involvement of jugular vein and carotid artery (see also Lemierre's disease ➤20).

# Pharyngitis

Infection of the posterior oral cavity, often involving the lymphoid tissue of Waldeyer's ring. Most cases are viral; management is aimed at relieving symptoms. Differential diagnosis includes acute bacterial epiglottitis and, rarely, diphtheria.

**Clinical features:** Fever, malaise, sore throat and myalgia. On examination, erythema and oedema of the tonsils and pharyngeal mucosa. It is usually impossible to determine the cause clinically, although some features are suggestive of particular organisms. Cough and coryza suggest influenza or rhinoviruses, whereas conjunctivitis suggests adenovirus. Vesicles and ulceration affecting both the pharynx and mouth are seen in herpes simplex stomatitis; in Coxsackie A herpangina (➤135), small vesicles and ulcers are usually confined to the posterior pharynx. Purulent tonsillar exudate suggests streptococcal infection or EBV; the latter is often accompanied by generalized lymphadenopathy and/or hepatosplenomegaly. Purulent tonsillar exudate is rare in influenza or rhinovirus infection.

**Organisms:** Rhinovirus, coronavirus, adenovirus, influenza A and B, parainfluenza, herpes simplex virus, coxsackievirus A, EBV, and CMV infection. Group A β-haemolytic streptococci (GAS), less often groups C or G. Rarely, *Arcanobacterium haemolyticum*, *Neisseria gonorrhoeae*. Very rarely, *Corynebacterium diphtheriae*.

**Microbiological investigations:** A rise in ASOT may give retrospective confirmation of streptococcal infection. Throat swab is often sent. Latex agglutination tests for the rapid diagnosis of GAS antigens in throat swabs are widely used in USA, and are specific and quite sensitive when compared to throat swab. However, neither antigen tests nor throat swabs are sensitive or specific for GAS infection when compared to ASOT, due to asymptomatic GAS carriage. Flora recovered from the surface of the tonsil correlates poorly with that of tonsillar crypt but quantitative culture may predict true infection. Viral culture may be positive, particularly in HSV infection. Viral serology may be useful in retrospect.

🖥 med.mssm.edu/ebm/cpr/strep_cpr.html

**Differential diagnosis:** Diphtheria is extremely rare in the developed world, but has recently become endemic in parts of the former Soviet Union and should be suspected in an unimmunized patient who is unwell, particularly if there is a grey tonsillar exudate spreading from the tonsils to involve the uvula, palate or posterior pharyngeal wall (➤268). If diphtheria is suspected, liaison with the microbiology department is essential ☎.

**Antibiotic management:** As most cases are viral, the value of antibiotics for sore throat has been questioned. Trial of penicillin vs. no treatment vs. delayed treatment showed no benefit, although patients who were unwell, had recurrent tonsillitis or suspected rheumatic fever were excluded. Immunological sequelae of GAS infection (➤256) are now very rare in the UK, so value of antibiotics in preventing them is unquantifiable. There is some evidence to suggest that antibiotic therapy prevents local suppurative complications such as quinsy. For a full discussion see:

> 💻 www.sign.ac.uk/guidelines/fulltext/34/
> ↪ Zwart S, BMJ 2000; 320: 150

If patients are unwell, give penicillin V for 10 days. For **recurrent tonsillitis**, cefuroxime and clindamycin have been shown to be superior to penicillin V. Consider ENT referral.

---

**Practice point**

Patients with 1° EBV infection develop a widespread maculopapular rash after treatment with ampicillin or amoxicillin. These antibiotics should be avoided in sore throat unless the diagnosis of bacterial infection has been firmly established.

---

**Complications:** Lower respiratory tract infection, peritonsillar (➤21) and retropharyngeal abscess (➤21).

**Comments: Scarlet fever** ✉, now rare in the UK, is caused by streptococcal erythrodermic toxin, which may be produced in streptococcal infection at any site (➤254).

## Lemierre's disease
**'Anaerobic tonsillitis':** Severe pharyngitis associated with fever, septicaemia, metastatic pulmonary infection and jugular vein thrombosis is rarely seen in young adults and is caused by *Fusobacterium necrophorum* (➤321).

## Laryngitis
In addition to the symptoms of pharyngitis, some patients with URTI may develop hoarseness and odynophagia. Laryngitis is usually viral in aetiology, although it may accompany infection by streptococci or *Mycoplasma pneumoniae*. Persistent hoarseness is usually due to non-infectious causes, but may indicate chronic granulomatous laryngitis. Causes include *Candida albicans* and herpes simplex virus; diagnosed on biopsy.

---

**Croup (acute laryngotracheobronchitis)**

Croup typically affects children from a few months old to the age of 3 years, and occurs in epidemics in autumn and early spring. During the course of a viral URTI, inspiratory stridor and a distinctive 'seal's bark' cough develop. Cyanosis and intercostal recession indicate more severe airway obstruction. Antibiotics, steroids and mist inhalation have not been shown to be of value. Hypoxia is common. Careful observation is needed, with a view to timely intubation or tracheotomy should airway obstruction progress. The important differential diagnosis is acute epiglottitis (➤21).

---

## Bacterial tracheitis
Retrosternal discomfort commonly accompanies viral URTI. Rarely, bacterial tracheitis may follow with fever, dyspnoea and stridor with purulent sputum. Gram stain and culture of sputum and blood culture are required if severe. Infection is most often due to *Staphylococcus aureus*, GAS and *Haemophilus influenzae* type b. Lateral soft-tissue X-ray of neck may show subglottic narrowing with a normal epiglottis ('pencil sign'). Bacterial tracheitis may follow intubation and trauma.

**Antibiotic management:** Flucloxacillin **or** co-amoxiclav **or** parenteral cephalosporin—to be guided by the results of sputum culture.

## Quinsy

Quinsy (peritonsillar abscess) usually follows bacterial pharyngitis. It is usually polymicrobial in origin, with oral anaerobes and GAS predominating. Patients present with abrupt increase in pain and dysphagia. On examination, there is asymmetrical tonsillar enlargement with swelling in the neck and often a palpable fluctuant mass. Management consists of ENT referral for consideration of surgical drainage and benzylpenicillin or co-amoxiclav, given parenterally.

## Retropharyngeal abscess

Unusual but important complication of bacterial pharyngitis and pharyngeal trauma (e.g. fishbone). Retropharyngeal space lies posterior to pharynx, anterior to cervical vertebrae and contains lymphatic tissue. Commoner in children.

**Clinical features:** Sore throat, dysphagia and neck pain. Bulging of the posterior pharyngeal wall may only be visible with indirect laryngoscopy. Lateral soft tissue X-ray of neck shows widening of pre-vertebral tissue, ±gas in tissues. Airway obstruction may occur.

**Organisms:** GAS and mixed oral flora.

**Differential diagnosis:** Cervical osteomyelitis, meningitis.

**Antibiotic management:** Benzylpenicillin **plus** clindamycin *or* parenteral cephalosporin **plus** metronidazole.

**Supportive management:** Urgent ENT referral for incision and drainage; ≈30% require tracheostomy.

**Comments:** Consider the diagnosis in the patient with neck stiffness and fever who has a normal lumbar puncture.

## Acute epiglottitis

Inflammation, oedema and obstruction of the supraglottic structures including the epiglottis due to *Haemophilus influenzae* type b (rarely other capsular types) typically affecting children aged 3 to 7 yrs.

**Clinical features:** Abrupt onset, over hours, of severe sore throat and fever. Children are unwell, with stridor, drooling and dysphagia. They may adopt a typical posture, sitting up and leaning forward. The swollen, cherry red epiglottis may be visible, but attempts to use a tongue depressor should be avoided, as this may precipitate fatal acute total obstruction.

**Antibiotic management:** Parenteral cephalosporin **or** amoxicillin plus chloramphenicol should be given. Rifampicin prophylaxis should be given to the patient and all household and nursery/day-care contacts including adults if there are other susceptible children in the family (➤100).

**Supportive management:** Management of the airway is paramount. **Elective intubation is associated with reduced mortality, as emergency intubation may be very difficult.** Throat examination and iv cannulation should be delayed until arrival of suitably experienced anaesthetist.

**Other investigations:** Lateral soft-tissue neck X-ray may show the engorged epiglottis (the 'thumb sign').

**Differential diagnosis:** It is essential to distinguish between viral croup and epiglottitis. Salient features are the abrupt onset, toxic appearance, dysphagia and drooling associated with epiglottitis. Diphtheria and inhaled foreign body may also need to be considered.

**Complications:** Systemic spread, bacteraemia, meningitis, arthritis and cellulitis.

**Comments:** This condition has been reported rarely in adults. All forms of invasive *Haemophilus influenzae* type b are less common with the introduction of the Hib vaccine.

## Thyroiditis

Sudden onset of pain, tenderness and swelling in the thyroid may be due to infection by *Staphylococcus aureus, Streptococcus pneumoniae* or mixed oral anaerobes. ENT referral for consideration of needle aspiration (send for culture). Acute suppurative thyroiditis is rare. Often associated with a persistent thyroglossal duct, or a third or fourth branchial arch anomaly with a congenital fistula from the pyriform fossa to the thyroid. Confirmation by barium swallow. Inflammation is more often subacute, sometimes related to recent viral infection (e.g. mumps, measles, influenza and EBV).

# Chapter 3

# Lower respiratory tract infections

## Acute bronchiolitis/viral pneumonia in children ①

Viral URTI may progress to acute bronchiolitis and pneumonia in children under 5 yrs. Pneumonia is most often viral in this age group. Acute bronchiolitis is seen most often under the age of 24 months. There is inflammation of bronchioles 75–300 μm in diameter, with loss of cilia and oedema, leading to obstruction of the lumen by cellular debris and secretions. It occurs in epidemics, usually in winter, and is frequently accompanied by viral pneumonia.

**Clinical features:** After symptoms of URTI, cough, dyspnoea and wheeze develop. Very young children may present with refusal to feed and apnoeic attacks. On examination, there is fever, tachycardia, tachypnoea and sometimes cyanosis. Hyperinflation and intercostal recession suggest bronchiolitis. On auscultation, there are widespread crepitations and wheezes.

**Organisms:** Respiratory syncytial virus (RSV, ①) accounts for the majority of cases. Parainfluenza, adenoviruses and influenza are less common. Some cases may be due to rhinoviruses and coronaviruses. Cytomegalovirus has been reported as a cause of viral pneumonia in very young children.

**Microbiological investigations:** Nasopharyngeal secretions for viral culture and rapid diagnostic tests for RSV and influenza ☎. Serology may be positive in retrospect.

**Other investigations:** Chest X-ray may show hyperinflation, characteristic of acute bronchiolitis, with or without infiltrates, which may be due to concomitant pneumonia or atelectasis.

**Differential diagnosis:** Asthma, inhaled foreign body, bacterial pneumonia.

**Antimicrobial management:** In severe cases, inhaled nebulized ribavarin may be used. This is active against RSV, but has little action against other viruses listed. The benefit of ribavarin is not well established, and its use is controversial. Most recover without specific antiviral therapy. Steroids do not improve the prognosis. Systemic antibiotics (e.g. cefotaxime) are often given, but are of uncertain benefit and should be stopped as soon as possible after bacterial superinfection has been excluded.

**Supportive management:** Oxygen may be needed for hypoxia and bronchodilators for bronchospasm.

**Complications:** Infection may be particularly severe in children with pre-existing cardiopulmonary disease or immunosuppression. Infection may be prevented in children at risk by immunotherapy (➤346).

## Viral pneumonia in adults

**Risk factors:** Viral pneumonia is uncommon in adults (estimated ≈3% of cases of influenza in the community), although viral URTI commonly precedes bacterial pneumonia. Commoner in pregnancy or with pre-existing cardiovascular disease.

**Clinical features:** After symptoms of URTI, cough and alterations in pulmonary function tests are common, but frank pneumonia occurs less often. On examination, there is tachycardia, tachypnoea and sometimes cyanosis. Auscultation reveals crepitations and wheezes. Hypoxia may be severe and difficult to reverse. Infection may be particularly severe if there is pre-existing cardiopulmonary disease. Chest X-ray may show diffuse patchy shadowing.

**Organisms:** Influenza A virus accounts for almost all cases. Pneumonia is occasionally seen as part of other specific viral syndromes, including infectious mononucleosis and chickenpox (➤130).

**Microbiological investigations:** Nasopharyngeal secretions for viral culture and rapid diagnostic tests for RSV and influenza. Serology may be positive in retrospect. Suspected chickenpox may be confirmed by examination of vesicle fluid (➤130). Sputum and blood cultures are essential to exclude a secondary bacterial pneumonia, which is much more likely.

**Antimicrobial management:** As it is impossible to exclude secondary bacterial pneumonia, patients will receive antibiotics (➤31). Antiviral agents (zanamivir and amantadine ➤345) can prevent influenza if given after exposure. For treatment, they must be given within 48 h of onset. Neither has been studied systematically in the treatment of complications such as pneumonia, and their efficacy in this setting is unproven.

**Complications:** Bacterial pneumonia often follows viral URTI, and can complicate viral pneumonia. Commonest organisms are *Streptococcus pneumoniae, Haemophilus influenzae* and *Staphylococcus aureus.*

**Comments:** Annual vaccination against influenza is recommended for all elderly patients and those with cardiac or pulmonary disease (➤345).

# Acute exacerbation of chronic obstructive pulmonary disease

Chronic obstructive pulmonary disease (COPD) is a chronic, slowly progressive disorder characterized by airflow obstruction. COPD incorporates a number of less preferred clinical labels, including chronic bronchitis (defined clinically as a productive cough for greater than 3 months of at least two consecutive years) and emphysema (defined pathologically as distension of the air spaces distal to the terminal bronchioles with destruction of alveolar septa). The long-term management of COPD is outwith the scope of this text. Acute infective exacerbation of COPD is a very common cause of hospital admission in the UK.

The British Thoracic Society has published detailed guidelines:

> 🖳 www.brit-thoracic.org.uk/pdf/copd.pdf
> ↦ Thorax 1997; 52: Suppl. V

**Risk factors:** Mainly smoking. Environmental pollution, occupational exposure to dust and noxious gases make a minor contribution. $\alpha_1$-antitrypsin deficiency causes emphysema in non-smokers, but risks are much greater in enzyme-deficient smokers. Infective exacerbation often follows viral URTI. Post-operative exacerbations are common.

**Clinical features:** Patients have pre-existing features of COPD with persistent productive cough, dyspnoea on exercise and physical signs of hyperexpansion. During infective exacerbations, sputum increases in volume and becomes purulent and dyspnoea becomes more severe. Pleurisy and haemoptysis may occur. On examination, the following are often present: fever, tachycardia, cyanosis, tachypnoea, signs of hyperexpansion (reduced cricothyroid distance, barrel chest), signs of airways obstruction (pursed lips breathing, poor chest movement, reduced air entry with added crepitations and wheezes) and changes in mental state, ranging from agitation to toxic confusional state. Signs of secondary pneumonia or of heart failure (congestive cardiac failure or cor pulmonale) may also be seen. Signs of hypercapnia (confusion, bounding pulse and peripheral vasodilatation, flap) may be present, although high $Paco_2$ may be present without these signs in chronic stable COPD.

**Organisms:** Often mixed. *Haemophilus influenzae* (non capsulate) *Streptococcus pneumoniae, Moraxella catarrhalis.* Many less severe cases may be viral. 'Atypical' pathogens (➤26) are unusual.

**Microbiological investigations:** Gram stain and culture of sputum if purulent. Blood culture if pneumonia suspected.

**Other investigations:** Unwell patients will require full blood count, urea, electrolytes, blood glucose and ECG. Chest X-ray usually shows evidence of COPD without obvious consolidation. Arterial blood gas analysis (ABG) should be performed in all patients as a baseline and repeated if the clinical situation changes. May have hypoxia and hypercapnia. Patients with chronic hypercapnia may depend on hypoxia for ventilatory drive. Uncontrolled oxygen therapy may abolish this 'hypoxic drive', resulting in hypoventilation, worsening $CO_2$ retention and progressive respiratory acidosis.

**Differential diagnosis:** Bacterial and viral pneumonia. Pneumothorax, LVF, pulmonary embolism, upper airway obstruction.

**Antibiotic management:** Antibiotics have been shown to be effective only if patient has at least two of the following:

- Increased dyspnoea.
- Increased sputum volume.
- Purulent sputum.

Oral therapy with amoxicillin or tetracycline is usually sufficient unless used with poor response prior to admission. Co-amoxiclav, cefaclor and trimethoprim are also used. For more severe exacerbations, give parenteral cephalosporin or clarithromycin. If pneumonia is present, treat as such (➤29).

**Supportive management:** Nebulized **bronchodilators**: salbutamol 2.5–5 mg neb. q4h, ± ipatropium bromide 100 to 500 μg neb. q4h. Nebulizers should be driven by air to avoid excess inspired oxygen (see above). **Controlled oxygen therapy:** Aim to achieve a $Pao_2 \geq 6.6$ kPa without a fall in pH < 7.26. In patients over 50 years, give no more than 28% oxygen by Venturi mask (2 L/min by nasal cannulae if mask not tolerated). Measure ABG; if acidotic or hypercapnic repeat within 1 h. If $Pao_2$ stable or improved and no deterioration in pH, increase $Fio_2$ and recheck until $Pao_2 \geq 7.5$ kPa. Oximetry may be sufficient if ABG shows normal $Paco_2$

and pH and clinical condition stable. Intravenous **aminophylline** 0.5 mg/kg/h may be given ⚠. **Steroids,** typically prednisolone 30 mg od, po, are usually given, but their efficacy in this situation is disputed. Avoid sedation. Respiratory stimulants (e.g. doxapram 1.5–4 mg/min iv) may be used in patients who are likely to progress to ventilation.

Respiratory referral is indicated for optimization of maintenance therapy and expert guidance on rehabilitation/smoking cessation.

**Complications:** Patients who fail to respond may require intubation and ventilation. If they have severe pre-existing disease, the decision to ventilate must be made by an experienced practitioner. Non-invasive ventilation techniques (using masks rather than endotracheal tubes) are becoming available in some units ☎.

> **Practice point**
>
> It is vital to ascertain the patient's exercise tolerance and lung function when well. Many patients with COAD live close to end-stage respiratory failure, and their pre-morbid condition is an important factor when deciding about intubation and ventilation.
>
> Patients with COAD should receive pneumococcal vaccine and annual influenza vaccine, and be encouraged to start antibiotic therapy at the first signs of an infective exacerbation.

## Pneumonia

It is helpful to distinguish community-acquired pneumonia (CAP) from hospital-acquired pneumonia (HAP), defined as pneumonia occurring >48 h after admission, since different organisms and risk factors are involved.

### Community-acquired pneumonia

The British Thoracic Society (BTS) published guidelines for management of CAP in 1993. It is widely believed that these guidelines have been applied too widely, leading to overtreatment of many cases, with associated side effects including *Clostridium difficile*-associated diarrhoea (➤63). Current BTS guidelines published in 2001, upon which the advice which follows is based, specifically apply to CAP, and not to exacerbation of COPD or 'chest infection' without evidence of pneumonia. Two definitions of CAP are provided, depending on the availability of CXR. **CAP diagnosed in the community** is defined as

- Acute lower respiratory symptoms.
- New focal chest signs.
- ≥1 systemic feature (fever, shivers, aches and pains or temperature ≥38°C).
- No other explanation for illness.

**CAP diagnosed in hospital** is defined as

- Symptoms and signs consistent with an acute lower respiratory infection.
- New radiographic changes for which there is no other explanation.

🖳 www.brit-thoracic.org.uk/pdf/cap.pdf
🕿 Thorax 2001; 56: Suppl. IV

**Epidemiology:** Incidence 0.5–1/100 p.a., of which 20–40% require admission. There are an estimated 10–20 times as many 'chest infections' treated with antibiotics that do not satisfy the criteria; 5–10% mortality depending on age/group studied. Overall, 5–10% require ITU admission, among whom mortality is ≈50%.

**Risk factors:** Common in the elderly and very young, in alcoholics and during any severe intercurrent illness. Other factors include recent URTI, recent anaesthetic, particularly if intubated, HIV, COAD and/or smoking and heart failure. *Streptococcus pneumoniae* is classically described as causing lobar pneumonia in young adults with no previous ill health, but in general, infection by this organism is more often associated with bronchopneumonia in patients with one of the risk factors listed above.

**Organisms:** Results of studies of microbial aetiology of CAP vary depending on country, setting and study design. Representative figures from UK studies are given in Table 3.1, but similar results have been reported from Europe, Australia, New Zealand and the USA. Rate for *Mycoplasma pneumoniae* will vary depending on whether it is an epidemic year (➤329). No clinical features accurately distinguish microbial aetiology. Among elderly patients, *Haemophilus influenzae* is more common and

*Mycoplasma* and *Legionella* are less common. In patients with COPD, *Haemophilus influenzae* and *Moraxella catarrhalis* are more common.

The term '**atypical pneumonia**' was initially coined to describe pneumonia which failed to respond to penicillin or sulpha- drugs and in which bacteriology failed to provide a diagnosis. Prospective studies have shown that it is not possible to distinguish pneumococcal from 'atypical' pneumonias by clinical features or investigations at presentation, and this term is no longer recommended. The term '**atypical pathogens**' (referring to *Mycoplasma pneumoniae, Coxiella burnetii, Chlamydia* spp.) retains some usefulness because these agents:

- Are not respiratory tract colonizers.
- Affect previously healthy individuals.
- Are transmitted by person-to-person droplet spread.
- Occur in epidemics.
- Affect all age groups, although they are commoner in young adults.
- Do not respond to penicillin.

*Mycoplasma pneumoniae* occurs with increased frequency during epidemics, which typically occur every 3–4 yrs.

*Klebsiella pneumoniae* ('Friedländer's bacillus'), typically affects elderly men with diabetes, alcoholism or pre-existing cardiac or pulmonary disease. Often rapid onset, with blood-stained and gelatinous sputum. CXR is said to show bulging of fissures due to expansion in volume of affected lobe with cavitation, but these were not seen in one recent series. Other extremely rare causes of pneumonia include anthrax (➤263), plague (➤305), tularaemia (➤307) and melioidosis (➤293).

---

**Practice point**

The low frequency of legionella, staphylococcal, *C. psittaci* and *C. burnetii* CAP, together with the high frequency of relevant risk factors (e.g. travel, recent flu) suggests that *routine* enquiry about such factors may be misleading. In patients with *severe* illness, in whom legionella and staphylococcal infection are more likely, presence of such risk factors may be more predictive.

**Table 3.1** Organisms responsible for community-acquired pneumonia in UK studies. Modified from British Thoracic Society guidelines (Thorax 2001; 56: Suppl. IV). See original reference for sources of data

| Organism | Percentage of cases in: | | | Epidemiology | Comments | |
| --- | --- | --- | --- | --- | --- | --- |
| | Community | Hospital | ITU | | | |
| *Streptococcus pneumoniae* | 36 | 39 | 22 | Commoner in winter | | (►260) |
| *Haemophilus influenzae* | 10 | 5 | 3.8 | | | (►296) |
| *Legionella pneumophila* | <1 | 3.6 | 18 | Commonest September/October. 50% UK cases are travel-related. 23% occur in clusters, often linked to Mediterranean resorts | Epidemics occur related to water-containing systems in buildings | (►301) |
| *Staphylococcus aureus* | <1 | 1.9 | 9 | Commoner in winter; influenza predisposes to *S. aureus* pneumonia | Septic pulmonary emboli occur in IVDUs (often with endocarditis) | (►249) |
| *Moraxella catarrhalis* | n/a | 1.9 | n/a | | | (►302) |
| Coliforms | 1.3 | 1 | 1.6 | | | (►273) |
| *Mycoplasma pneumoniae* | 1.3 | 11 | 2.7 | Epidemics spanning 3 winters occur every 4 years in UK | | (►329) |
| *Chlamydia pneumoniae* | n/a | 13 | n/a | | Direct role as cause of CAP not established | (►329) |
| *Chlamydia psittaci* | 1.3 | 2.6 | 2.2 | Acquired from birds and animals, but case-to-case spread also occurs. Only 20% of UK cases have history of bird contact. Epidemics may occur in poultry workers | Can be mild flu-like illness or a severe pneumonia. Grossly underdiagnosed | (►329) |
| *Coxiella burnetii* | <1 | 1.2 | <1 | Commonest April–June. Epidemics occur in relation to animal sources (usually sheep), but occupational history in <8% | | (►332) |
| Viruses | 13 | 13 | 10 | Annual winter epidemics of influenza. Pneumonia complicates ≈3% | | (►23) |
| Mixed | 11 | 14 | 6 | | | |
| None | 45 | 30 | 32 | | | |

CAP, community-acquired pneumonia; n/a, data not available; ITU, intensive therapy unit; IVDUs, intravenous drug users.

**Clinical features:** Relatively rapid onset of fever and rigors, often accompanied by a dry cough and pleuritic chest pain. Tachycardia and tachypnoea. As the disease progresses, sputum volume and purulence increase and there may be haemoptysis. On examination, there may be signs of consolidation with bronchial breathing, dull percussion note and crepitations. Auscultation may be normal, even in patients who are unwell or have definite chest X-ray changes. Pleural effusion is present in up to 50% of cases. Elderly patients may be afebrile and present with a toxic confusional state. In severe cases, signs of severe systemic sepsis may supervene with confusion progressing to multi-organ system failure. In the pre-antibiotic era, recovery from classical lobar pneumonia occurred rapidly after the illness had reached its 'crisis'.

**Microbiological investigations:** Gram stain and culture of **sputum** may be helpful; Gram stain is poorly predictive, but culture is useful to assess antibiotic sensitivity. It is much more useful in patients who have not yet received antibiotics. *Staphylococcus aureus* commonly colonizes the upper airways and is regularly grown from sputum; it **rarely** causes pneumonia. **Blood cultures** should be sent, as they are diagnostic if positive ($\approx$25% in pneumococcal pneumonia). **Thoracocentesis** if pleural effusion is large or persistent. In severe infection which fails to respond to antibiotic therapy, bronchoscopy with **broncho-alveolar lavage** and bronchial brushings may provide material for microscopy, culture and histology.

Serum from all patients should initially be stored. In patients who are severely ill and who have had symptoms for more than 7 days, this initial specimen should be tested for antibodies to *Legionella* and atypical pathogens. If patients deteriorate or fail to respond to β-lactam, then a subsequent specimen at 7–10 days can be tested

**Aspiration pneumonia**

Aspiration pneumonia describes the pulmonary consequences of 'macroaspiration' of larger quantities of oral and gastric contents and/or water from the environment. This may result in chemical damage and/or infection with oral flora, particularly anaerobes.

**Risk factors:** Reduced level of consciousness and depressed gag reflex, dysphagia due to local oesophageal or neurological disease, intubation and nasogastric feeding, oesophageal dysmotility and reflux, persistent vomiting. Alcoholics and those severely obtunded by intercurrent illness are at particular risk.

**Clinical features:** Aspiration of gastric contents may cause acute chemical injury to the lungs. Patients may present immediately after an aspiration event, particularly if it occurs in hospital, for example perioperatively. More often, a patient with one or more risk factors presents several days after the event with symptoms and signs suggestive of pulmonary infection. Severe cases may proceed to lung abscess, empyema and bronchopleural fistula. Inhalation of small foreign bodies (typically peanuts) can cause localized bronchial obstruction with distal abscess formation.

**Organisms:** Mixed oral flora including anaerobic streptococci, *Fusobacterium nucleatum* and *Bacteroides* spp. Almost any organism can be involved if it was previously colonizing the upper airways.

**Microbiological investigations:** Gram stain and culture of sputum and blood culture to exclude other organisms. Thoracocentesis if pleural effusion is large or persistent. Bronchoscopy may be required to provide material for microscopy and culture and to exclude an inhaled foreign body.

in parallel with the admission serum. In many cases, it will not be necessary to perform serology.

In **severely ill patients**, the following tests may be diagnostic: pneumococcal antigen testing (blood, sputum, urine), legionella antigen (urine), sputum culture for legionella, immunofluorescence for respiratory viruses and *Chlamydia* spp.

*Mycoplasma pneumoniae* infection is accompanied in ≈25% of cases by the formation of **cold agglutinins**, which are present in serum from early in the illness; this test is rarely requested nowadays. *Mycoplasma*-specific IgM is sensitive and specific.

Detailed prospective studies identify a cause in ≤60% of cases; the rate is much lower in routine practice. Molecular diagnostic methods (e.g. PCR) will become available in this area.

**Other investigations:** Patients usually have a neutrophil leucocytosis, but with overwhelming infection, patients may be neutropenic initially. Mild renal failure is common in the elderly; many have hyponatraemia, which may occur in pneumonia from any cause. Arterial blood gas analysis may show hypoxia. In patients with COPD there may be hypercapnia. C-reactive protein (CRP) is a helpful indicator of likelihood of pneumonia, particularly in patients with COPD, and also provides evidence of a response to therapy.

Chest X-ray may show classical lobar infiltration, but usually shows bronchopneumonia, with patchy shadowing and air bronchograms indicating consolidation. There may be evidence of complications such as lung abscess or empyema, or of underlying disease. CXR features do not confidently predict a likely pathogen. Multilobe involvement and pleural effusions are commoner in bacteraemic pneumococcal infection than in non-bacteraemic pneumococcal pneumonia or legionellosis. CXR changes may take several months to resolve. BTS guidelines recommend a follow-up film at 6 weeks for patients with persistent symptoms or signs, or who are at increased risk of lung cancer (smokers, >50 yrs old).

---

**Practice point**

Cavitation on the chest X-ray suggests lung abscess, a cavitating neoplasm, *Staphylococcus aureus*, *Klebsiella pneumoniae* or *Mycobacterium tuberculosis*.

---

**Complications:** Empyema, metastatic infection (meningitis, arthritis, endocarditis), severe sepsis, ARDS and multi-organ system failure. *Mycoplasma pneumoniae* infection is very rarely associated with acute neurological complications, including meningoencephalitis, acute cerebellar ataxia, mononeuritis multiplex affecting the cranial nerves and brachial plexus, or Guillain–Barré syndrome. Cold agglutinin-mediated haemolytic anaemia, pericarditis, Stevens–Johnson syndrome and erythema nodosum may occur.

**Severity assessment:** The causative agent is usually unknown when therapy is commenced and a definite microbiological diagnosis is only made in a minority. Management depends on a careful assessment of severity to identify those most at risk of death, and those who can safely be managed at home.

Factors associated with increased mortality include:

- Confusion, defined as an abbreviated mental test (AMT) ≤8 (see box).
- Urea >7 mmol/L.
- Respiratory rate >30/min.
- BP low (diastolic <60 mmHg, systolic <90 mmHg).
- Age.
- Co-existing chronic illness (e.g. heart failure, diabetes).
- Atrial fibrillation.
- $Po_2 < 8\,kPa$
- WBC $< 4 \times 10^9/L$ or $>20 \times 10^9/L$.
- Positive blood cultures.
- Bilateral or multilobar CXR changes.

The first four of these are regarded as 'core' factors for severity assessment, often referred to by the acronym **CURB** (*c*onfusion, *u*rea, *r*espiratory rate, *b*lood pressure). Blood urea level and CXR are not usually available for patients assessed in the community, so algorithm for severity assessment at home differs slightly from in hospital (Fig. 3.1).

---

**Abbreviated mental test**

Score 1 for each correct answer:

- Age
- Date of birth

*(continued...)*

- Time
- Year
- Hospital name
- Recognition of two persons (e.g. doctor, nurse)
- Recall address
- Dates of World War 1
- Name of monarch
- Count backwards 20 → 1

Score of 8 or less is defined as confusion for the purposes of severity assessment.

**Antibiotic management:** Choice of initial empirical antibiotic depends on severity assess-ment. See Table 3.2. **Intravenous antibiotics should be switched to oral therapy** as soon as possible, preferably within 24–48 h. Patients on parenteral cephalosporin should be switched to oral co-amoxiclav rather than oral cephalosporins. Switch to oral therapy may take place once there is evidence of a clinical response (resolution of fever, tachycardia, tachypnoea, hypotension, hypoxia) but should be delayed if there is microbiological evidence of legionella, staphylococcal or Gram-negative enteric bacillus infection.

The **duration of treatment** is poorly evi-denced (➤385). For uncomplicated non-severe

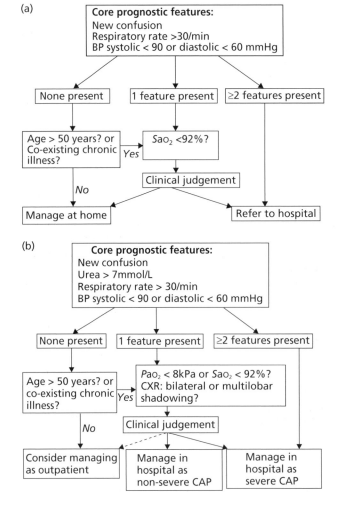

**Figure 3.1** Severity assessment in community-acquired pneumonia. (a) For assessment in the com-munity; (b) for assessment in hospital. Social circumstances and wishes of the patient should also be considered. From BTS guide-lines—Thorax 2001; 56: Suppl. IV.

**Table 3.2** Preferred regimens for empirical treatment of community-acquired pneumonia are based on severity assessment

| Severity | Preferred | Alternative |
|---|---|---|
| **Home-treated, not severe** or **Hospital-treated, admitted for non-clinical reasons** | Amoxicillin 500 mg – 1 g q8h oral | Erythromycin 500 mg q6h oral *or* clarithromycin 500 mg q12h oral |
| **Hospital-treated, not severe** | | |
| Oral | Amoxicillin 500 mg – 1 g q8h oral **plus** erythromycin 500 mg q6h oral *or* clarithromycin 500 mg q12h oral | Levofloxacin 500 mg q24h oral |
| If intravenous therapy needed (e.g. intolerant of oral therapy because of vomiting) | Ampicillin 500 mg q6h iv *or* benzylpenicillin 1.2 g q6h iv **plus** erythromycin 500 mg q6h iv *or* clarithromycin 500 mg q12h iv | Levofloxacin 500 mg q24h iv |
| **Hospital-treated, severe** | Co-amoxiclav 1.2 g q8h *or* parenteral cephalosporin **plus** erythromycin 500 mg q6h iv *or* clarithromycin 500 mg q12h iv. Consider adding rifampicin 600 mg q12h iv | Levofloxacin 500 mg q12h iv **plus** benzylpenicillin 1.2 g q6h iv |

From BTS guidelines – Thorax 2001; 56: Suppl. IV.

CAP or uncomplicated proven pneumococcal CAP, 7 days is usually sufficient. For severe disease or for legionella or Gram-negative enteric bacillus infection, 14–21 days is recommended. For any severe invasive staphylococcal infection we recommend 28 days, therapy (➤250).

If there is microbiological confirmation of aetiology, the regimen can be adjusted. See Table 3.3.

---

**Practice point**

Ciprofloxacin is not recommended for empirical treatment of CAP, because it has relatively poor activity against *Streptococcus pneumoniae*. This is not true of **newer fluoroquinolones**, including levofloxacin and moxifloxacin, which are licensed for this indication.

---

**Supportive management:** Patients should stop smoking and rest. Give adequate analgesia for pleuritic pain, to promote expansion. Oxygen therapy should be given to all unwell patients — unless there is evidence of severe COPD with ventilatory failure, ≥35% $O_2$ should be administered. Careful attention should be paid to adequate fluid intake and fluid balance. Pleural effusion should be drained promptly and effectively.

**Failure to respond to treatment** may be due to complications such as pleural effusion (➤36) or lung abscess (➤35) or to infection by an organism resistant to the drug regimen chosen. In non-severe CAP, addition of a macrolide or changing to levofloxacin should be considered. In the severely ill patient already receiving a β-lactam/macrolide combination, consider adding rifampicin and respiratory referral for possible bronchoscopic sampling. Knowledge of local prevalence of penicillin resistance in pneumococci is useful. Also consider β-lactam allergy (➤401), iv catheter infection and antibiotic-associated diarrhoea (➤63) as causes of prolonged fever.

### Legionellosis (Legionnaire's disease)

Initially described after a dramatic outbreak of pulmonary disease in Philadelphia in 1976 at a meeting of American war veterans. Infection due to *Legionella pneumophila* has been implicated in 1–20% of community-acquired pneumonias. **Pontiac fever** is a self-limiting non-pulmonary febrile illness caused by *Legionella pneumophila* or *Legionella feeleii*.

*Legionella pneumophila* (➢301) colonizes water piping systems, including wet areas within air conditioning. Infection is acquired by inhalation and there is an incubation period of 2–10 days. Human-to-human transmission does not occur.

**Risk factors:** Host factors are important predictors of infection, including male sex, smoking, COPD, travel, immunosuppressive drugs and recent anaesthetics (particularly if intubated).

**Clinical features:** Presents as severe community-acquired pneumonia with fever, rigors, headache, myalgia and a non-productive cough. Chest pain, dyspnoea, purulent sputum and haemoptysis may follow. Up to 50% have abdominal pain, nausea and diarrhoea. Toxic confusional state and more rarely focal neurological deficits may occur. Renal and hepatic dysfunction are common in legionellosis. This may reflect the severity of infection rather than a specific effect. May progress to fulminant respiratory failure, accompanied by other features of multi-organ system failure.

**Microbiological investigations** (➢301): Detection of *Legionella pneumophila* serogroup 1 antigens in urine and respiratory secretions is available (✈). The urinary antigen test is extremely valuable in the assessment of the acutely unwell patient, with a sensitivity of >80% and a specificity of ≈100%. Diagnosis may also be made retrospectively on serology, which becomes positive approximately 10 days after the onset of illness. Culture (takes 2–10 days) is possible from sputum, tracheal aspirates and blood: laboratories will inoculate appropriate media if requested ☎.

**Complications:** Very rarely, *Legionella pneumophila* can cause renal and cutaneous abscesses, peritonitis, endocarditis and haemodialysis fistula infection.

**Treatment and prevention:** (➢30) Always perform tests for Legionnaire's disease (urinary ELISA recommended) for patients with **severe** pneumonia, immunosuppressed patients (recipients of transplants, cancer chemotherapy or long-term immunosuppression), and anyone presenting with pneumonia during *Legionella* outbreak investigations. Additionally, consider urinary ELISA for patients with pneumonia who have spent one or more days away from home within the 2–10 day incubation period.

## Hospital-acquired pneumonia (HAP)

Pneumonia occurring >48 h after hospital admission has a different aetiology and requires different treatment. Ventilator-associated pneumonia (VAP) may be regarded as a particular subgroup of HAP.

**Risk factors:** Age, co-existing illness, immobility, reduced conscious level, dysphagia, instrumentation of respiratory/GI tract. Debility and use of broad-spectrum antibiotics lead to colonization of the upper respiratory tract by coliforms. Infection also occurs by haematogenous spread in patients with sepsis elsewhere.

**Clinical features:** Fever, purulent respiratory secretions, respiratory symptoms/signs, new CXR signs.

**Organisms:** Depends on duration of hospital stay and presence of risk factors. See Table 3.4. If HAP occurs within 5 days of admission, *Streptococcus pneumoniae*, *Haemophilus influenzae* and *Staphylococcus aureus* are likely. Thereafter, coliforms and pseudomonads become more likely as colonization is established.

**Microbiological investigations:** Blood culture. Sputum and tracheal aspirate cultures are unrepresentative of lower respiratory flora.

**Table 3.3** Treatment of community-acquired pneumonia once microbial aetiology is established

| Organism | Preferred | Alternative |
| --- | --- | --- |
| Streptococcus pneumoniae | Amoxicillin 500 mg – 1 g q8h oral or benzylpenicillin 1.2 g q6h iv | Erythromycin 500 mg q6h oral or clarithromycin 500 mg q12h oral or parenteral cephalosporin |
| Mycoplasma pneumoniae or Chlamydia pneumoniae | Erythromycin 500 mg q6h oral or clarithromycin 500 mg q12h oral (either may be given iv) | Tetracycline 250–500 mg q6h oral or ciprofloxacin 250 mg q12h oral |
| Chlamydia psittaci or Coxiella burnetii | Tetracycline 250–500 mg q6h oral or 500 mg q12h iv | Erythromycin 500 mg q6h oral or clarithromycin 500 mg q12h oral (either may be given iv) |
| Legionella pneumophila | Clarithromycin 500 mg q12h oral or iv, ± rifampicin 600 mg q12h oral or iv | Ciprofloxacin 500–750 mg q12h oral or 400 mg q12h iv |
| Haemophilus influenzae | Non-β-lactamase-producing: Amoxicillin 500 mg q8h oral or Ampicillin 500 mg q6h iv β-lactamase-producing: co-amoxiclav 625 mg q8h oral or 1.2 g q8h iv | Parenteral cephalosporin or ciprofloxacin 500–750 mg q12h oral or 400 mg q12h iv |
| Coliforms | Parenteral cephalosporin | Ciprofloxacin 400 mg q12h iv or imipenem 500 mg q6h iv or meropenem 0.5–1 g q8h iv |
| Pseudomonas aeruginosa | Ceftazidime 2 g q8h iv **plus** gentamicin or tobramycin △ | Ciprofloxacin 400 mg q12h iv or piperacillin 4 g q8h iv **plus** gentamicin or tobramycin △ |
| Staphylococcus aureus | Non-MRSA: flucloxacillin 1–2 g q6h iv ± rifampicin 600 mg q12h oral or iv MRSA: vancomycin 1 g q12h iv △ | Teicoplanin 400 mg q12h iv ± rifampicin 600 mg q12h oral or iv |

From BTS guidelines—Thorax 2001; 56: Suppl. IV.

Bronchoscopy with brushing or lavage are more accurate. Pleural fluid should be aspirated if present.

**Differential diagnosis:** Pulmonary embolism, ARDS, pulmonary oedema, pulmonary haemorrhage.

**Antibiotic management:** see Table 3.4.

&#9136; American Thoracic Society guidelines, Am J Respir Crit Care Med 1996; 153: 1711

**Ventilator-associated pneumonia** (VAP), defined as pneumonia developing in a mechanically ventilated patient later than 48 h after intubation, presents with new or progressive CXR changes, fever, neutrophilia, and purulent tracheobronchial secretions. Differential diagnosis includes non-infectious causes such as ARDS, aspiration, PE and atelectasis; clinical diagnosis is difficult and correlates poorly with the results of quantitative lower airway cultures obtained by bronchoscopy. Many units

Table 3.4 Hospital-acquired pneumonia

| Category | Likely organisms | Recommended antibiotics |
|---|---|---|
| Patients with **no unusual risk factors** who have:<br>**Mild to moderate HAP**<br>or<br>**Severe HAP occurring 'early'** (within 5 days of admission) | 'Core' organisms: *Klebsiella* spp., *Proteus* spp., *Serratia marcescens*, *Enterobacter* spp., *Streptococcus pneumoniae*, *Haemophilus influenzae* and *Staphylococcus aureus*, *Escherichia coli* | Parenteral cephalosporin<br>or<br>co-amoxiclav<br>or<br>levofloxacin |
| **Mild to moderate HAP with unusual risk factors for particular organisms:**<br>Recent thoracoabdominal surgery, dysphagia, witnessed aspiration, dental sepsis | Core organisms plus anaerobes | Use co-amoxiclav *or* clindamycin |
| Coma, diabetes, head trauma, neurosurgery, renal failure | *Staphylococcus aureus* more likely | Consider adding vancomycin if MRSA likely |
| High-dose steroids, *Legionella* endemic in hospital | *Legionella* spp. | Add macrolide ± rifampicin ± fluoroquinolone |
| High-dose steroids, previous antibiotics, prolonged ITU stay, structural lung disease such as bronchiectasis | *Pseudomonas aeruginosa* | Treat as late severe HAP |
| **Severe HAP occurring 'late'** (>5 days after admission), or in patient with unusual risk factors | Core organisms plus *Pseudomonas aeruginosa*, *Staphylococcus aureus* (inc. MRSA) *Acinetobacter* spp. | *Aminoglycoside *or* fluoroquinolone, **plus** piperacillin-tazobactam *or* imipenem **plus** vancomycin |

* BTS recommendation. We would suggest vancomycin **plus *either*** piperacillin-tazobactam *or* imi-/meropenem *or* fluoroquinolone, influenced by local resistance patterns.

HAP, hospital-acquired pneumonia; ITU, intensive therapy unit; MRSA, methicillin-resistant *Staphylococcus aureus*.

use protected specimen bronchial brushings or broncho-alveolar lavage and quantitative culture to direct management. Tracheal aspirates are not useful, because tracheobronchial bacterial colonization is common in critically ill patients.

Selective bowel/gut decontamination (SBD/SGD) with oral non-absorbable and systemic antibiotics (e.g. Selective Parenteral and Enteral Antisepsis Regimen (SPEAR) comprising long-term oral/topical aminoglycoside, polymyxin and nystatin with initial parenteral cefotaxime) has been used in high-risk ICU patients, and aims to reduce aerobic Gram-negative rod colonization while preserving anaerobic mucosal flora. Efficacy at reducing mortality, ventilator-associated pneumonia and septicaemia is not strong and the relevant trials are not of high quality. Many are concerned over encouragement of antimicrobial resistance.

## Pneumonia in children

Acute respiratory tract infections are more common in childhood and may be severe, in particular in children with pre-existing illness such as congenital cardiac disease, bronchopulmonary dysplasia, severe asthma or cystic fibrosis.

Pneumonia is most likely to be viral in aetiol-

**Table 3.5** Causes of pneumonia in children

| Age group | Common organisms |
| --- | --- |
| Birth to 3 weeks | Gp. B β-haemolytic streptococci, coliforms, *Listeria monocytogenes*, *Streptococcus pneumoniae*. Viral infection unusual |
| 3 weeks to 4 months | *Chlamydia trachomatis*, respiratory syncytial virus, parainfluenza, *Staphylococcus aureus*, *Streptococcus pneumoniae*, *Haemophilus influenzae* |
| 4 months to 5 yrs | Respiratory syncytial virus, parainfluenza, adenovirus, influenza A & B, *Haemophilus influenzae*, *Streptococcus pneumoniae*, *Staphylococcus aureus*, *Mycoplasma pneumoniae* (unusual) |
| 5 yrs to 15 yrs | *Mycoplasma pneumoniae*, *Streptococcus pneumoniae*, *Haemophilus influenzae* |

ogy in children (➤23). Other organisms are seen at different ages (see Table 3.5). In small babies, pneumonia is often accompanied by air-trapping, leading to wheeze and hyperinflation (see acute bronchiolitis ➤23). *Chlamydia trachomatis*, acquired at birth, can cause pneumonia in children from 3 weeks to 3 months (➤141).

# Lung abscess

Necrosis of lung parenchyma due to bacterial infection, leading to a cavitated pus-containing lesion.

**Risk factors:** Following aspiration pneumonia or trauma. Secondary to local bronchial obstruction by clots, pus, foreign body or tumour. The following specific bacterial pneumonias tend to cavitate: *Staphylococcus aureus*, *Klebsiella pneumoniae*, *Pseudomonas aeruginosa*. Septic pulmonary emboli, often due to *Staphylococcus aureus*, occur in IVDUs, particularly in the presence of tricuspid valve endocarditis. *Nocardia* spp. and *Aspergillus* spp. in immunocompromised patients.

**Clinical features:** Patients may have risk factors for aspiration pneumonia (➤28). They may present acutely, days after a recognized aspiration event or pneumonia, or onset may be more insidious over weeks. Fever, fatigue, cough, sputum (often copious and offensive). Weight loss, clubbing and anaemia.

**Organisms:** After aspiration: Upper respiratory tract anaerobic organisms (*Peptostreptococcus* spp., *Bacteroides* spp. (not *fragilis* group), *Fusobacterium* spp.), *Streptococcus 'milleri'*, and Gram-negative aerobic bacilli. After pneumonia: *Staphylococcus aureus*, *Klebsiella pneumoniae*, *Pseudomonas aeruginosa*. Rare causes include *Actinomyces israelii*, *Nocardia asteroides* and fungi.

**Microbiological investigations:** Gram stain and culture of sputum. This may be unhelpful in predominantly anaerobic infections. Blood cultures. If there is an associated pleural effusion, thoracocentesis is indicated to exclude empyema. Bronchoscopy is usually indicated to obtain material for culture, assist drainage and to exclude the presence of bronchial obstruction. Percutaneous aspiration (CT guided).

**Other investigations:** Neutrophil leucocytosis is usual, but may wane in chronic cases. Chest X-ray shows a cavitating pulmonary lesion with a fluid level. Multiple peripheral lesions suggest septic pulmonary emboli. CT scan is a sensitive method of diagnosis and may guide fine-needle aspiration for culture and cytology.

**Antibiotic management:** Benzylpenicillin + metronidazole are commonly used, but therapy should be guided by the results of microbiology, and specialist chest referral is recommended. In hospital-acquired cases, *Staphylococcus aureus* and coliforms are more likely and piperacillin/tazobactam is a good first choice. Vancomycin should be included for empirical therapy if local prevalence of MRSA is high. Duration of therapy is controversial—at least 1 month.

**Supportive management:** Bronchoscopy and physiotherapy may be required to assist drainage. Surgical resection may be required rarely for lesions that fail to respond to antibiotics.

**Complications:** Metastatic infection. Empyema. Bronchopleural fistula.

# Empyema

Pus within the pleural cavity.

**Risk factors:** Secondary to bacterial pneumonia, particularly after infection with *Staphylococcus aureus*, anaerobes or Gram-negative aerobic bacilli. Empyema is now unusual after pneumococcal pneumonia, unless treatment is delayed. Pulmonary infections with *Actinomyces israelii* and *Nocardia asteroides* tend to involve the pleura. Secondary to ruptured oesophagus, subphrenic or hepatic abscess. Post thoracic surgery or penetrating chest injury. Pleural tuberculosis may present as empyema.

**Clinical features:** Persistent fever in one of the situations listed above. Weight loss, and dyspnoea if the empyema is large. Purulent sputum if there is a bronchopleural fistula. On examination, clubbing and signs of pleural effusion.

**Organisms:** Dependent on the clinical situation: Upper respiratory tract anaerobic organisms (*Peptostreptococcus* spp., *Bacteroides* spp. (not *fragilis* group), *Fusobacterium* spp.), *Staphylococcus aureus*, *Klebsiella pneumoniae*, *Pseudomonas aeruginosa*, *Streptococcus pneumoniae* and *Streptococcus 'milleri'*. Rarely, *Actinomyces israelii*, *Nocardia asteroides*. *Mycobacterium tuberculosis*.

**Microbiological investigations:** Diagnostic aspiration of fluid through a wide-bore needle. Delivery of pus in a sealed syringe will improve recovery of anaerobes.

**Other investigations:** Neutrophil leucocytosis. Chest X-ray and CT scan will delineate the extent of the infection.

**Management:** Drainage via intercostal tube is nearly always essential, and resolution is more rapid if loculated collections are broken down. Amoxicillin + metronidazole is rational initial therapy and can be guided by the results of culture. Prolonged therapy is rarely required; complete, maintained drainage is essential.

# Chapter 4

# Mycobacteria and mycobacterial infections (Table 4.1)

**Table 4.1** Classification

| Genus | Species | Notes |
|---|---|---|
| Mycobacterium | tuberculosis | Causing tuberculosis (TB➤38) |
| | bovis | Less frequent cause of TB |
| | africanum | Causes some cases of tuberculosis in equatorial Africa |
| | (microti) | The vole tubercle bacillus, now a very rare isolate from human infections |
| | BCG | Used for vaccination against tuberculosis (➤46) |
| | leprae | Causes leprosy |
| | avium-intracellulare, kansasii, marinum, ulcerans, scrofulaceum, xenopi, szulgai, malmoense, haemophilum, chelonei, fortuitum, etc. | 'Atypical' mycobacteria, or 'mycobacteria other than TB' (MOTT). Environmental saprophytes causing a variety of opportunistic infections |
| | (gordonae, terrae, flavescens, smegmatis.) | Also 'atypical' mycobacteria. Environmental saprophytes, very rare pathogens |

Slowly multiplying Gram-positive bacilli and cocco-bacilli. Cell wall is composed of a core of three macromolecules covalently linked (peptidoglycan, arabinogalactan and mycolic acids) and a lipopolysaccharide, lipoarabinomannan. Mycolic acid accounts for >50% of the cell wall by weight; this structure is responsible for the staining characteristics which define the genus. Mycobacteria are resistant to decolorization by acid or alcohol after staining by dyes such as carbol-fuchsin (acid-fast bacilli, AFB; acid- and alcohol-fast bacilli, AAFB). They are sensitive to alcohols and aldehydes, but resistant to many other disinfectants and to drying.

## Microbiological diagnosis of mycobacterial infection

All processing of sputum and specimens for mycobacterial diagnosis performed in containment level 3 laboratory. Different diagnostic laboratories vary in whether mycobacterial investigations are performed routinely or only on request for particular specimens. **Always warn the laboratory if mycobacterial involvement is suspected clinically.** Slow growth makes direct microscopical detection in clinical specimens of prime importance—the most sensitive method is auramine phenol (AP)-stained smears, examined in fluorescence microscope. Ziehl–Nielsen staining (with hot carbol-fuchsin; ZN) now usually not used in primary diagnosis. Microscopical morphology sometimes can suggest involvement of MOTT rather than tubercle bacilli, but this is non-specific.

Most mycobacteria (including *Mycobacterium tuberculosis*) take up to 8 weeks to grow on primary isolation, but often only 2–3 weeks on subculture. Modern liquid culture systems produce positive results in 10–20 days in most cases. So-called 'rapid growers' (*chelonei* and *fortuitum*) take up to 7 days to grow on subculture. *Mycobacterium leprae* has never been cultivated *in vitro*. Most mycobacteria will grow somewhat on a variety of nutritative media, but Lowenstein–Jensen (LJ) medium commonly used, containing eggs, glycerol, salts, malachite green and selective antibiotics.

**Preliminary identification** of mycobacteria in diagnostic laboratories is by optimal growth temperature, speed of growth, colonial and bacterial morphology, and pigment production in light or dark under aerobic conditions; confirmation and sensitivity testing: ✛.

**Positive culture for tubercle bacilli is always clinically significant**, but isolation of MOTT requires careful assessment, because some are frequent contaminants (e.g. *xenopi*, *kansasii* and *gordonae* common in water). Often necessary to demonstrate persistent positivity of smears/cultures before starting treatment. Possibility of significant MOTT infection much higher in immunocompromised patients: ≈10% mycobacterial infection in transplant recipients is non-tuberculous.

Two **rapid molecular methods** (PCR and EMTD) are now widely available for the rapid detection of mycobacteria in clinical specimens. Both of these tests are complementary to microscopy and culture, their main advantage being speed rather than sensitivity. Current PCR assays are positive on >90% of smear-positive sputa, and ≈50% of smear negative, culture-positive sputa. These methods and older methods based on hybridization of species-specific DNA probes can also be used for rapid speciation of positive cultures. PCR is also used for the rapid detection of rifampicin resistance genes (➢39).

# Tuberculosis (TB)

✉ ① Open cases (chest, urine, wound).

**TB infection** may be defined as a state in which the *Mycobacterium tuberculosis* (or *bovis* etc. ➢37) has established itself in the body, without symptoms or evidence of disease, in contrast to **TB disease**, where there are symptoms and signs of damage to one or more organs.

**Epidemiology:** TB remains a major cause of mortality in the developing world, particularly in countries with a high prevalence of HIV infection. WHO reported ≈8.4 million cases in 1999 (8.0 million in 1997). The rise was due largely to a 20% increase in African countries most affected by HIV. WHO estimates 10.2 million cases in 2005.

💻 www.who.int/gtb

In developing countries (and in the UK in the past) most children are infected by TB, but only ≈10% progress to clinical disease. Currently in the UK, TB infection is rare in childhood; most infected persons are middle-aged or elderly, or are immigrants from endemic areas (e.g. 20–30× incidence in immigrants from Indian subcontinent, with higher prevalence of extra-pulmonary TB). Reactivation of pulmonary TB is therefore usually seen in patients from these risk groups; factors predisposing to reactivation include alcoholism, diabetes mellitus, malnutrition, immunosuppression (drugs, HIV, cytotoxic therapy) and malignancy.

Prevalence rising in the UK since 1990, having declined 10% per year for many decades before (Σ ≈ 6800, ≈400 deaths).

💻 www.phls.co.uk/facts/TB/index

**Pathogenesis:** Infection is initially acquired by the respiratory aerosol route. Organisms replicate in the lung and travel to the hilar lymph nodes, from where they are disseminated throughout the body. Further replication is usually halted at this stage by the development of cell-mediated immunity (CMI), but complete eradication of organisms does not take place. Later in life, infection can reactivate, particularly if CMI is impaired by one of the risk factors listed above. Molecular pathogenesis of TB is poorly understood. No recognized toxins or histolytic enzymes, but glycolipid found in more virulent strains ⇒ mitochondrial damage. Research is focused on factors which contribute to **survival within macrophages** by inhibiting phagolysosome formation and the role of cell wall constituents (e.g. mycolic acid) in eliciting **local cell-mediated inflammatory response**, with release of TNF and IL-1, leading to local tissue damage.

**Drug resistance:** During the 1990s, multidrug-resistant TB (**MDRTB**) has emerged as a global threat to TB control. TB may be resistant to one or more drugs; isolated isoniazid resistance is relatively common (≈3% of UK isolates). Isolated rifampicin resistance is very rare, and rifampicin resistance is usually a marker for MDRTB, defined as resistance to isoniazid and rifampicin, with or without resistance to other agents.

Accurate data on the **global prevalence** of MDRTB are difficult to obtain; rates vary widely and are highest in 'second-world' areas where rifampicin has been available, but where poor socio-economic conditions have contributed to poor compliance. Hence, MDRTB has not been linked to HIV in Africa, because rifampicin has only recently been available in many poor African countries. Table 4.2 shows a representative subset of data recently published by WHO.

**Table 4.2** Global prevalence of MDRTB (% of new or previously treated cases)

| | New cases | Previously treated cases |
|---|---|---|
| Estonia | 14 | 38 |
| Latvia | 9 | 24 |
| China (Henan) | 11 | 35 |
| USA | 1.2 | 6 |
| England and Wales | 0.8 | 13 |
| Uganda | 0.5 | 4.4 |
| Sierra Leone | 0.9 | 23 |
| Median (all countries) | 1 | 9 |

↳ Espinal M, N Engl J Med 2001; 344:1294
🖳 www.who.int/gtb

A variety of mutations are responsible for resistance to isoniazid and other drugs, but virtually all rifampicin resistance is caused by point mutations in one 81 base-pair region of the mycobacterial RNA polymerase gene (*rpoB*), the product of which is the cellular target for rifampicin. This region is therefore an ideal target for **molecular assays for the rapid detection of rifampicin (and thus multidrug) resistance**, and there are now several commercial assays available.

## Clinical features
### Pulmonary tuberculosis

**Primary infection** is usually asymptomatic in the healthy, well-nourished individual, manifest only by a conversion from tuberculin-negative to -positive (see below). Some patients, especially children, may complain of fever, cough and dyspnoea. CXR is usually normal or may show areas of infiltration (usually in the middle or lower zones) with unilateral hilar or paratracheal lymphadenopathy ('Ghon complex'). Fifteen per cent of patients with abnormal CXR have bilateral hilar lymphadenopathy. Rare allergic manifestations associated with primary infection include erythema nodosum (➤118), phlyctenular conjunctivitis (➤107) and a sterile polyarthritis (Poncet's disease). Primary infection is usually curtailed by host CMI. Occasionally, particularly in children under 5 yrs, massive dissemination occurs, resulting in miliary TB (see below). Some 10% of young adults with symptomatic primary tuberculosis progress within a few months to cavitary TB. This **progressive primary TB** is similar to reactivated disease (see below)—the presence of lymphadenopathy or a recent conversion from tuberculin negative to positive may suggest progressive primary rather than reactivated disease. Patients are often very unwell with fever, cough and weight loss.

**Miliary TB** (so called because of the millet-seed sized lesions that form in all areas of high blood flow, particularly the viscera, bone marrow and eyes) occurs following dissemination of bacilli, typically in children with acute infection. Miliary TB may also occur during reactivation (**late generalized TB**), particularly in elderly or immunocompromised patients, in which case its onset is more insidious, e.g. as a PUO (➤179), although patients may experience sudden severe deterioration. Symptoms include fever, night sweats and weight loss. Anaemia, leucocytosis or leucopenia, thrombocytopenia and DIC may occur. Miliary lesions may be visible on the CXR as 2–4-mm nodules, but these are absent particularly during the first 10 days of disease. TB meningitis (see below), usually presenting with headache, may occur as a complication.

Reactivated TB presents months to years after primary infection. Symptoms include cough, haemoptysis (≈25%), fever (15–40%), night sweats (60%), fatigue (60%), anorexia and weight loss. Some 20% of patients with radiological evidence of active TB are asymptomatic. CXR usually shows consolidation with cavitation and fibrosis, most commonly in the upper zones. Lymphadenopathy is rare. Fibrosis, calcification and loss of volume may be seen in chronic disease. Disease may progress very rapidly over months, or very insidiously over years.

### Pulmonary complications

TB pleurisy may occur shortly after primary infection or during reactivated disease. Fever, pleuritic chest pain and dry cough are common. AFBs are rarely seen in pleural fluid. Diagnosis is made by culture or, more often, by histology of pleural biopsy. Spontaneous resolution frequently occurs, but there is a high risk of reactivated disease in the following 5 yrs, and treatment is indicated.

Empyema (➤36) results from rupture of tuberculous cavity into the pleural cavity. Bronchiectasis may result from compression of bronchi (usually middle lobe) by enlarged lymph nodes. Haemoptysis is usually mild and recurrent, but severe, life-threatening episodes may occur rarely from erosion of a pulmonary artery by a TB cavity. Aspergilloma (➤365) may develop in a healed TB cavity, causing haemoptysis. Anti-fungal treatment is usually unsuccessful, and resection of the affected lobe may be required.

### Extrapulmonary tuberculosis

TB lymphadenitis ('scrofula') is commonest in Asian and African immigrants. Lymph nodes of the head and neck are almost always affected (≈5% have mediastinal lymphadenitis). Disease is bilateral in 25%, and only ≈20% have constitutional symptoms. Usually presents as a discrete, rubbery, non-tender lymph node ('cold abscess'), which may discharge, giving rise to a chronic sinus.

Genitourinary TB results from reactivation of bacilli disseminated during primary infection. Renal parenchymal disease, with progressive destruction of the kidney, is usually clinically silent. Involvement of the ureter and bladder follow with obstructive uropathy and ulceration, fibrosis and shrinkage of the bladder. Symptoms include dysuria, frequency, haematuria and flank pain. Sterile pyuria is typical, and TB should be considered in all patients with this. Diagnosis is by microscopy and culture of early morning urine (positive in ≈90% if three samples are sent). IVU may show renal calcification, short rigid ureter, thick-walled non-distensible bladder and urethral stricture. Salpingitis, endometritis and epididymo-orchitis also occur. Adrenal involvement usually occurs in association with miliary disease and may cause hypoadrenalism.

Gastrointestinal TB may accompany pulmonary disease from swallowed bacilli, most commonly causing ileitis with anorexia, weight loss, altered bowel habit and abdominal pain. Perforation, obstruction and fistula formation may occur. Peritoneal TB, which usually spreads from an infected mesenteric lymph node, presents insidiously with fever, weight loss, anorexia, abdominal swelling and irregular bowel habit and is not usually associated with pulmonary disease.

Bone and joint involvement most commonly affects the vertebral column (50%), hip (15%), knee (15%) and other large joints. Vertebral disease ('Pott's disease') typically affects the anterior part of the lower thoracic or lumbar vertebral bodies. Back pain, fever and weight loss progressing to kyphosis or paraplegia may be seen. Extension to form paravertebral or psoas abscess may occur. Mycobacteria are typically present in very low numbers in bony lesions and cultures of bone aspirations, and biopsy may be smear and culture negative or slow to become positive.

**CNS involvement** typically causes a basal meningitis with entrapment of cranial nerves and vasculitis affecting cerebral arteries. Onset is usually insidious over several weeks, but may be acute, especially in children. Headache, fever and altered mental state are the commonest presenting symptoms. Cranial nerve lesions (esp. VI, III and IV) and evidence of raised intracranial pressure may occur, followed by progression to coma and fits. Cerebral vasculitis typically affecting the anterior and middle cerebral arteries may result in infarction and hemiplegia. AFBs are seen in smears of CSF in <20% of cases; yield is increased if a large volume (≥10 mL) of CSF is sent for examination. Other CSF changes include low glucose, markedly raised protein and usually lymphocytic pleocytosis (➤97). Rarer neurological complications of TB include cerebral tuberculoma, acute transverse myelitis and radiculitis.

**Pericarditis** may occur with pulmonary TB or as the sole manifestation of infection. It may present with pericardial pain and a friction rub or with massive effusion and tamponade. Steroids speed resolution and should be given in addition to chemotherapy. Constrictive pericarditis may follow acute pericarditis within weeks, or may occur many years later. It typically presents insidiously with dyspnoea, oedema, hepatosplenomegaly, raised venous pressure on inspiration and pericardial calcification on CXR. Surgical pericardectomy is usually required.

**TB and HIV:** HIV infection predisposes to reactivation of TB, which may occur at any time during the course of HIV disease, and often precedes other opportunistic infections. TB at any site, including the lungs, is an AIDS-defining illness (➤146). Extrapulmonary TB and involvement of the lower lung fields are commoner in HIV patients. Patients usually respond well to standard anti-TB drugs (➤42), although the incidence of MDRTB is generally higher in HIV+ persons in UK.

**Organisms:** *Mycobacterium tuberculosis* currently accounts for almost all UK TB. *Mycobacterium bovis*, which is now very rare in UK (Σ ≈ 40), is similar to *M. tuberculosis*, but produces weaker growth on LJ medium. Causes bovine tuberculosis; classically involving infection of the human ileocaecum or cervical lymph nodes (scrofula) from oral ingestion of milk from infected herds. Milk contamination interrupted by pasteurization and testing of herds. Much *M. bovis* infection in developed world is now imported, reactivation, or pulmonary acquired from human cases. Resistant to pyrazinamide; recommended therapy is isoniazid/rifampicin for 9 months, with ethambutol for first 2 months.

**Microbiological investigations:** Diagnosis depends on microscopy and culture of mycobacteria (➤37), molecular diagnostic methods (➤38) and on histological findings. In suspected pulmonary TB, three sputum specimens should be examined. Other relevant specimens include early morning urine (≥150 mL) and gastric washings. Decontamination of sputum to kill non-mycobacteria (e.g. by incubation with sodium hydroxide) is followed by culture. Normally sterile samples (e.g. CSF) are cultured directly after concentration by centrifugation. Buff, dry, heaped colonies. Liquid media (e.g. Kirchner) more sensitive and rapid. Automated culture systems economical in areas of high prevalence. Fibre-optic bronchoscopy, with broncho-alveolar lavage and transbronchial biopsy, has a high yield of positive results. In suspected extrapulmonary TB, relevant tissue samples should be examined, but microscopy is frequently negative, and diagnosis is often made on histology of tissue samples (esp. pleural biopsy, lymph node, liver, bone marrow). Histological features include AFBs and caseating granulomata with epithelioid macrophages and multinucleate (Langhan's) giant cells.

Culture confirmation allowing speciation and sensitivity testing may take up to 8 weeks; rapid liquid culture and molecular methods are now available (➤38).

**Tuberculin testing** is the demonstration of cell-mediated immunity to purified mycobacterial proteins ('tuberculin') by intradermal injection. It may be performed by a number of means. The Heaf test uses a special multi-pronged injector. Reactions are graded 0–4; ≥ grade 2 is regarded as positive. For routine ward use, the Mantoux test is more convenient: 0.1 mL of tuberculin (1 : 10 000 containing one tuberculin unit, TU) is injected intradermally in the upper third of the flexor aspect of the forearm. The injection site is carefully marked and read at 48–96 h. *Palpable* induration >5 mm in diameter constitutes a positive response. If negative, the test should be repeated with 0.1 mL of 1 : 1000 tuberculin (10 TU). Tuberculin testing varies in usefulness depending on the population studied. Previous BCG immunization will cause a positive result. The test may be negative in up to 25% of patients with active TB, particularly in miliary disease. It is most useful in children who have not received BCG and in the surveillance of contacts of cases, in whom a conversion from negative to positive indicates recent infection and a need for prophylactic therapy (see below).

In the US, BCG is not used, so a positive tuberculin test is taken as evidence of TB infection (➤38) and is an indication for a course of pre-emptive isoniazid therapy (➤44).

**Other investigations:** Normochromic normocytic anaemia, hyponatraemia due to inappropriate ADH secretion, mild hypercalcaemia and a raised ESR are common.

## Management of TB
### Principles of anti-TB chemotherapy

Multidrug therapy is required to prevent the emergence of resistant organisms especially in high-inoculum disease and to kill organisms metabolizing at different rates in different cellu-lar environments. Thus, isoniazid is good at killing mycobacteria that are actively dividing, but it is less effective against semi-dormant organisms. Pyrazinamide is particularly active against mycobacteria which are semi-dormant in acid intracellular environments, and rifampicin is considered effective against inter-mittently metabolizing organisms because of its very rapid onset of action.

It is strongly recommended that all TB should be managed by, or in close collaboration with, respiratory physicians with relevant experience and direct access to specialist nursing staff ☏.

## First-line antituberculous drugs

**Rifampicin: Range of activity:** broad, including many mycobacteria, staphylococci, strepto-cocci, neisserias, *Haemophilus* spp., *Brucella* spp., *Legionella* spp., *Chlamydia* spp., *Coxiella burnetii*. One-step mutation to resistance of target RNA polymerase, hence use in combination for all indications except meningococcal and haemophilus prophylaxis. **Administration:** Well absorbed orally (iv available); CSF ✓, urine ✓. Available in combination with other antituberculous drugs to aid compliance. **Adverse effects:** Transiently raised hepatic transaminases common, but significant hepatotoxicity infrequent except in those with pre-existing liver disease. Usually mild rashes and GI disturbance (occasional *Clostridium difficile*-associated diarrhoea); orange-coloured urine, saliva and tears (stains soft contact lenses); induction of liver microsomal enzymes interferes with activity of oral contraceptives and other steroids, phenytoin, sulphonylureas, anticoagulants, ciclosporin. (Give double the dose of any maintenance steroids when starting rifampicin.) Rare thrombocytopenia. Intermittent treatment associated with side effects in up to 30%: influenza-like syndrome, shortness of breath, thrombocytopenia, hypotension, haemolysis, renal failure. **Rifabutin** is similar to rifampicin, and is used for prophylaxis of MAI infection in patients with AIDS (➤168) and for treatment of other mycobacterial infections. It is a less powerful inducer of cytochrome P450 and has less serious interactions with anti-HIV therapy, making it useful in the treatment of TB in patients on HAART.

**Isoniazid: Range of activity:** used for treatment and prophylaxis of *Mycobacterium tuberculosis*; other mycobacteria usually resistant. **Administration:** Oral and parenteral preparations available; CSF ✓, urine ✓. **Adverse effects:** Causes peripheral neuropathy (particularly likely in alcoholics, diabetics, malnourished and patients with chronic renal failure and is preventable by giving pyridoxine 10 mg od). Rare hepatotoxicity, optic neuritis, psychosis, nausea, vomiting, rashes, fever. Potentiates phenytoin, ethosuximide and carbemazepine.

**Ethambutol: Range of activity:** tubercle bacilli and other mycobacteria. **Administration:** Oral only; CSF ✓ with meningitis, urine ✓. **Adverse effects:** Dose-dependent visual disturbance (loss of acuity, visual fields or colour blindness)—rare at 15 mg/kg. Check vision with Snellen chart before treatment and warn patients to stop drug and report any change in vision. Reduce dose in renal failure.

**Pyrazinamide: Range of activity:** *Mycobacterium tuberculosis*, especially intracellular organisms at acid pH, and early in the course of treatment. Inactive against *M. bovis* and MAI. **Administration:** Well absorbed orally; CSF ✓, urine ✓. **Adverse effects:** Common mild arthralgia. Occasional hepatotoxicity, rashes, nausea, gout.

## Recommended treatment regimens
See Tables 4.3, 4.4.

**Table 4.3** British Thoracic Society recommendations for treatment of tuberculosis in adults and children

|  | Initial phase | Months | Continuation phase | Months |
|---|---|---|---|---|
| Pulmonary and extrapulmonary TB | H, R, Z, E* | 2 | H, R | 4 |
| If pyrazinamide is not tolerated | H, R, E | 2 | H, R | 7 |
| Meningitis and other CNS TB | H, R, Z, E | 2 | H, R | 10 |

H, isoniazid; R, rifampicin; Z, pyrazinamide; E, ethambutol.

* **Ethambutol** is added if there is reason to suspect drug-resistant organisms; it may be omitted in previously untreated, indigenous, Caucasian patients in UK, who are known to be HIV– (or have very low likelihood of HIV on risk assessment) and who are not contacts of a known resistant case. Ethambutol can be used in children and unconscious patients because the risk of ocular toxicity is very low at a dose of 15 mg/kg.

**Liver function tests** should be checked before starting therapy. Transient asymptomatic increases in serum transaminases are very common after starting treatment. Discontinuation is **not** indicated unless there are symptoms of hepatitis (anorexia, vomiting, hepatomegaly) or jaundice. It is not necessary to monitor LFTs except in patients known to have pre-existing liver disease. For detailed guidance on management of abnormal LFTs, see BTS guidelines.

**Steroids** are used in life-threatening or widespread TB in an attempt to reduce acute inflammation and allow time for drugs to work. They are usually indicated for pericarditis, extensive pulmonary disease, moderate or severe meningitis, ureteric TB and pleural effusion.

**If there is a positive culture but sensitivity data are delayed**, initial phase should be extended until sensitivity data are available.

**Disseminated TB** should be treated as CNS TB unless CNS infection has been excluded clinically, including lumbar puncture.

Table 4.4 Doses of antituberculous drugs—all are given as a single daily dose

| Drug | Dose | | Frequency |
|------|------|------|-----------|
| | Daily therapy | Intermittent supervised therapy | |
| Isoniazid | 300 mg q24h<br>Child: 5 mg/kg (max. 300 mg) | 15 mg/kg (max. 900 mg) | 3 times weekly |
| Rifampicin | Weight <50 kg: 450 mg q24h<br>≥50 kg: 600 mg q24h<br>Child: 10 mg/kg<br>(max. 600 mg) | 600–900 mg<br>Child: 15 mg/kg (max. 900 mg) | 3 times weekly |
| Pyrazinamide | Weight <50 kg: 1.5 g q24h<br>≥50 kg: 2 g q24h<br>Child: 35 mg/kg | Weight <50 kg: 2 g,<br>≥50 kg: 2.5 g<br>Child: 50 mg/kg | 3 times weekly |
| Ethambutol | 15 mg/kg | 30 mg/kg | 3 times weekly |

↦ BTS guidelines, Thorax 1998; 53:536–48
🖥 www.brit-thoracic.org.uk/

**Intermittent supervised therapy** (see Table 4.3 and 4.4 for regimens) is recommended for patients who may be non-compliant. Directly observed therapy (DOTS) has been widely promoted by WHO as a method of improving cure rate and reducing the incidence of drug resistance.

**Treatment of MDRTB** must always be by specialists with relevant experience, access to isolation facilities and in close collaboration with local microbiologists and reference labs ☎. Detailed guidelines have been published. Treatment should be supervised throughout. Usually five or more drugs to which the organism is known to be sensitive are given until sputum culture is negative, followed by three or more drugs for 9 or more months. HIV status should be checked. Second-line drugs are shown in Table 4.5.

**Management of TB in renal failure:** No dosage adjustment is required for pyrazinamide or rifampicin (HD: <5%). The dose of isoniazid should be reduced to a maximum of 200 mg in patients with severe renal failure (i.e. creatinine >700 μmol/L. HD: >50%, PD: 20–50%. Give usual dose post HD). Streptomycin and ethambutol should be avoided in renal failure. If used, doses should be reduced, and serum levels assayed 🗎.

## Control and prevention of TB

Some 10% of household contacts of sputum smear-positive ('open') TB cases will develop active disease. This figure is ≈2% for smear-negative and extrapulmonary cases. Smear-positive drug sensitive cases are considered non-infectious after 2 weeks' therapy which includes isoniazid and rifampicin.

**Chemoprophylaxis** refers to treatment of people who have TB infection but no TB disease (i.e. they are well, with normal CXR, positive tuberculin test); often started as a consequence of contact tracing. Regimens include isoniazid alone for 6 months or isoniazid + rifampicin for 3 months. Rifampicin alone for 6 months is used in contacts of known isoniazid-resistant cases. Chemoprophylaxis of **MDRTB** is difficult, and not usually given because of the risk of engendering even more resistance. Chemoprophylaxis is recommended in the UK for **HIV+ patients** who have had recent close contact with an infectious case (isoniazid + rifampicin for 3 months). US guidelines continue to recommend chemoprophylaxis in all HIV+ persons with positive tuberculin tests as well as after contact (isoniazid for 9 months **or** rifampicin for 4 months **or** rifampicin + pyrazinamide for 2 months; rifampicin + pyrazinamide prophylaxis has been associated with severe hepatitis

**Table 4.5** Second-line antituberculous drugs. ⟿ Thorax 1998; 53:536–48

| Drug | Dose Child | Adult | Adverse effects and comments |
|------|------------|-------|------------------------------|
| Clofazamine | | 300 mg q24h | Headache, diarrhoea, red skin discoloration |
| Cycloserine | 10 mg/kg q24h | 250–500 mg q24h | Depression, fits, headache, dizziness, psychosis, rash ⌂ |
| Ethionamide | 15–20 mg/kg q24h | <50 kg: 375 mg q12h ≥50 kg: 500 mg q12h | Gastrointestinal, hepatitis. Avoid in pregnancy (possibly teratogenic) |
| Thiocetazone | 4 mg/kg q24h | 150 mg q24h | Gastrointestinal, vertigo, conjunctivitis, rash. Avoid in HIV+ (Stevens–Johnson syndrome) |
| Para-aminosalicylic acid (PAS) | 300 mg/kg q24h | 5 g q12h | Gastrointestinal, hepatitis, fever, rash |
| Streptomycin (➤402) | | 15 mg/kg (max 1 g) q24h | Ototoxicity, nephrotoxicity. Avoid in pregnancy ⌂ |
| Capreomycin | | 15 mg/kg q24h or 1 g q24h | Rash, leucopenia, thrombocytopenia, nephrotoxicity, abnormal LFTs |

and is recommended only for patients who would not be likely to complete one of the other regimens).

Secondary prophylaxis (i.e. continuous prophylaxis after successful treatment of HIV-associated TB) is no longer recommended.

**Examination of contacts** is the responsibility of the local authority (health board in Scotland) and is usually undertaken by a designated chest physician. Notification is essential. Close contacts are defined as those sharing a household with the index case—occasionally a contact at work will also be regarded as close. Close contacts of all cases of TB should be examined. Casual contacts are at low risk, but should be examined if they are unusually susceptible (e.g. children or immunosuppressed adults) or if the index case is thought to be highly infectious. Examination of contacts is aimed at detecting cases of pulmonary TB, offering BCG to those who are tuberculin-negative and chemoprophylaxis to those without evidence of active disease but who may have been infected. Detailed advice is given in BTS guidelines.

**Immigrants** from the Indian subcontinent, Africa and other high-risk areas such as Vietnam should be evaluated for TB infection and disease. If tuberculin-negative, they should be offered BCG. If tuberculin-positive, they should be referred for CXR and clinical assessment. Chemoprophylaxis is recommended for children and adults under 35 yrs with Heaf test grades 3 or 4 (2–4 if there is no history of BCG). BCG should be offered at birth to all children of immigrants from high-risk areas.

## Control of TB in hospital

**Drug-sensitive TB:** Smear-positive patients should be nursed in a single room for the first 2 weeks of treatment. No further precautions (such as gowns or masks) are necessary, but it is reasonable to wear masks during respiratory physiotherapy. Adults with smear-negative and extrapulmonary disease can be nursed on the open ward. Children should be nursed in a single room until the source case has been identified, as it is likely that this person will be among those visiting the child. If a patient in a general ward is found to have TB, then other patients should be followed up as close contacts (see above). Special rules apply for patients who are HIV+ (➤167).

**MDRTB:** The following factors suggest an increased risk of MDRTB: previous TB treatment, HIV+, known contact of MDRTB, failure to respond to conventional anti-TB therapy, prolonged smear positivity (>4 months) or positive sputum culture (>5 months). Detailed guidance on the isolation of patients with or at risk of MDRTB has been published by the UK Departments of Health and the BTS; transfer to units with appropriate facilities is essential. Briefly, patients should be nursed in negative pressure isolation and staff and visitors should wear dust/mist respirator masks (*not* ordinary surgical masks). Isolation continues until successive sputum cultures are negative, the patient has tolerated and responded to therapy, and has stopped coughing ☎.

📖 www.doh.gov.uk/tbguide.htm
↦ Thorax 2000; 55:887–901

## Vaccination

**BCG immunization** uses a live attenuated strain of *Mycobacterium bovis* (**B**acillus **C**almette–**G**uérin). It is contraindicated in patients with immunosuppression (inc. steroids, cytotoxics and HIV), malignancy, hypogammaglobulinaemia, pregnancy, intercurrent febrile illness, tuberculin positivity or generalized septic skin infection. The efficacy of BCG varies with different populations, probably due to patterns of previous exposure to *M. tuberculosis* and atypical mycobacteria, and it should be given before the age of maximum incidence of generalized TB infection in a population. In British children it is estimated to give ≈70% protection. It is currently recommended in the UK for members of the following groups if they are tuberculin-negative and have no history of successful BCG vaccination: children aged 10–13 yrs, students, health-care professionals, veterinary staff dealing with animals known to harbour tuberculosis, contacts of patients with active disease, immigrants from endemic areas (esp. Indian subcontinent, Vietnam, sub-Saharan Africa), travellers to Asia, Africa or Central and S. America who intend to stay for >1 month. Children born to immigrants from India, Africa, Vietnam and other high-risk areas should be offered BCG at birth. BCG also offers some protection against *Mycobacterium leprae*.

## Leprosy ✉ ①

**Epidemiology and transmission:** Leprosy is widespread throughout the world, wherever there is poverty and overcrowding. WHO estimates >12 million cases worldwide, in Africa, Asia and Latin America. Transmission is thought to occur most often by respiratory droplet spread from untreated lepromatous leprosy patients, whose nasal secretions contain large numbers of bacilli. Exposure to *Mycobacterium leprae* is much commoner than clinical disease.

**Pathogenesis:** Manifestations of disease are determined by host immunity. Persons with strong cell-mediated immunity (CMI) against the organism develop tuberculoid leprosy (TT), in which there is a vigorous granulomatous response and very few bacilli are found in lesions. Those with weak or absent CMI against *Mycobacterium leprae* develop lepromatous leprosy (LL) with no granulomatous response and massive infiltration of skin and nerves by mycobacteria. Between these extremes there is a continuum from borderline tuberculoid (BT) through borderline (BB) to borderline lepromatous (BL). Patients with BB or BL tend to downgrade to LL with time. *Mycobacterium leprae* predominantly affects nerves and skin; tissue damage may be caused by infiltration of organisms or by the host granulomatous response.

**Clinical features:** Clinical disease develops insidiously after a prolonged incubation period (≈2–5 yrs for TT, 8–12 yrs for LL). **TT** is characterized by one to three localized asymmetrical hypopigmented macules with sharp, raised edges. Lesions are usually anaesthetic due to damage to nerves within the skin, and there may also be thickening of the peripheral nerve related to the lesion. **LL** has a more insidious onset. Lesions are very numerous, ill-defined, widely distributed and tend to be symmetrical. The skin is thickened, but not usually anaesthetic until late in disease. Thickening of facial skin and loss of the outer third of the eyebrow ('madarosis') cause the typical 'leonine' facies. Widespread thickening of multiple peripheral nerves occurs — those most often affected, and which should be deliberately palpated if leprosy is suspected, include the ulnar, median, radial, common peroneal, posterior tibial and greater auricular nerves. Nasal stuffiness, anosmia and epistaxis are common. Septal perforation and collapse of the bridge of the nose may occur. Bony lesions, glomerulonephritis and amyloidosis also occur. Patients with borderline leprosy present a spectrum of clinical features between these two extremes.

**Deformities** result from a combination of anaesthesia, paralysis and hypohidrosis (due to autonomic neuropathy) leading to misuse, trauma, secondary infection and tissue loss. **Ocular involvement** causes blindness in ≈10% of leprosy patients. Mechanisms include keratitis, iritis, corneal anaesthesia and exposure due to lagophthalmos secondary to facial nerve involvement.

**Reactions** are episodes of acute inflammation of skin, eyes or nerves which affect ≈25% of leprosy patients. **Reversal reactions** (type 1 reaction) occur in patients with borderline leprosy usually after therapy has begun, and cause acute inflammation of nerves and skin lesions, often with sudden loss of nerve function. **Erythema nodosum leprosum** (ENL, type 2 reaction) occurs in LL, causing a characteristic skin lesion, iritis, episcleritis and neuritis. ENL usually starts during the second year of therapy. Both of these reactions should be treated with anti-inflammatory agents (see below), but antimycobacterial treatment should not be discontinued.

**Investigations:** Diagnosis is clinical. In borderline and LL, acid-fast bacilli may be demonstrated in slit-skin smears. Biopsy may also be helpful.

**Organism:** *Mycobacterium leprae.*

**Management:** For 'paucibacillary' disease, (TT or BT, with negative slit-skin smear) rifampicin and dapsone are given for 6 months. For 'multibacillary' disease (positive slit-skin smear, borderline or LL), rifampicin, dapsone and clofazimine are given for at least 2 years. Reactions are treated with clofazimine, thalidomide and steroids. Patients require education to avoid trauma to anaesthetic limbs. Plastic surgery may be required to correct or compensate for deformities. Isolation ① is recommended for smear-positive patients until adequately treated ☎.

## Atypical mycobacteria ('MOTT')
### *Mycobacterium avium-intracellulare*
(Also known as the MAI complex.)

Present in moist environments, and causes tuberculosis in birds and animals. Closely related to a variety of other animal pathogens. Present in ≈50% of HIV+ with advanced immunodeficiency (➤168), also rarely in **organ transplant recipients and others with deficient cell-mediated immunity**. Disseminated and pulmonary infection, lymphadenitis. Seen, and isolated by conventional AFB techniques, in many specimens from such patients: sputum, marrow aspirate, intestinal biopsy, faeces. Granulomata rare; usually only AFB-stuffed macrophages are seen. Frequent chronic bacteraemia detectable by special blood culture techniques (e.g. lysis centrifugation, mycobacterial broths; ☎). Treatment (➤168); *in vitro* sensitivity or resistance not always matched by *in vivo* response. Typing available (➤).

**Local lymph-node infection** ('scrofula', especially unilateral cervical) is also rarely seen in immunologically normal children; usually treatable by excision alone.

### *Mycobacterium kansasii*
Elongated, beaded bacilli, frequently found in piped water supplies (so beware of contamina-

tion of specimens). Causes pulmonary infections in elderly patients with pre-existing lung damage (emphysema, bronchiectasis, pulmonary fibrosis, silicosis etc.) and sometimes pulmonary and other infections in those with deficient CMI, including AIDS; clinically indistinguishable from TB. Effective regimens include rifampicin, isoniazid and ethambutol for 12–24 months; ciprofloxacin and clarithromycin also used.

### Mycobacterium marinum

Elongated, beaded bacilli—the 'fish tubercle bacillus'. Associated with skin granulomas and ulcers after contact of abrasions with water ('swimming-pool granuloma', 'fish fancier's finger'). Rare associated lymphangitis. Diagnosis by microscopy and culture of biopsies of advancing edge of lesions (grows only at low temperature). Usually self-limiting, but responds to co-trimoxazole, tetracycline, ciprofloxacin, or rifampicin plus ethambutol. Modern swimming-pool maintenance eliminates contamination.

### Mycobacterium ulcerans

Very slow growth, at low temperature only. Causes 'Buruli' or 'Bairnsdale' ulcer; chronic, progressive, undermining skin ulceration in tropical countries. Necrosis of underlying dermis. Geographically localized, especially to wetlands, where it is probably present on vegetation. Eventually self-heals (associated with appearance of CMI to the organism), but excision speeds resolution. Possible additional value of antibiotics (e.g. rifampicin plus clofazimine, or co-trimoxazole).

### Mycobacterium scrofulaceum

Is ubiquitous in the environment, and occasionally causes unilateral lymph-node infection in children, treatable by excision. Very rare pulmonary infections (as *Mycobacterium kansasii*). Treatment as for MAI.

### Mycobacterium xenopi, szulgai and malmoense

Rare causes of pulmonary (as *Mycobacterium kansasii*) and lymphatic infection. *Xenopi* commonly contaminates piped water systems, and *malmoense* may require up to 10 weeks' incubation on solid media. Unpredictable response to therapy (☎).

### Mycobacterium haemophilum

Rarely associated with skin nodules in organ transplant recipients. Rifampicin, doxycycline and co-trimoxazole have been used in therapy.

### Mycobacterium chelonei (or chelonae) and fortuitum

'Rapid growers', present in moist environments, that most commonly cause localized, chronic infection of injection abscesses and traumatic wounds. Usually respond to drainage and curettage. Very rare pulmonary and disseminated infections. *Chelonae* is relatively resistant to glutaraldehyde and has contaminated bronchoscope washer-disinfectors, causing diagnostic confusion when bronchial aspirates are stained for AFB. Both resistant to conventional TB chemotherapy, but *fortuitum* usually sensitive to ciprofloxacin, macrolides, co-trimoxazole, or imipenem. *Chelonei* often more resistant, but tobramycin, amikacin, erythromycin and clarithromycin have been used (☎).

# Chapter 5

# Cardiac infections

## Infective endocarditis (IE)

**Definition:** Bacterial, fungal, rickettsial or chlamydial infection of heart valves or mural endocardium. Infection of the vascular endothelium of patent ductus arteriosus, A–V fistulae and coarctation produce a similar clinical pattern. $\Sigma \sim 1000$.

**Risk factors:** IE due to virulent organisms such as *Staphylococcus aureus* (➤249), can occur in the absence of cardiac risk factors and typically present acutely (hours to days). Infection by less virulent organisms such as viridans streptococci (➤259) normally presents less acutely (weeks) and usually requires pre-existing endocardial damage. Platelet thrombi adhere to damaged endocardium and provide a nidus for bacterial adhesion and invasion.

**Predisposing cardiac lesions:** Endocardial damage arises in areas of turbulence, where a high-pressure jet of blood enters a low-pressure chamber, e.g. on the atrial side of the mitral valve (MV) and the wall of the left atrium in mitral regurgitation. Classically, IE affects valves damaged by rheumatic heart disease, but this is becoming less common ($\approx$30% of recent published series). Congenital and degenerative heart disease and MV prolapse predispose to IE; 20–40% of cases have no identifiable lesion.

**Source of bacteraemia:** Viridans streptococci are oral commensals, and some patients have a history of periodontal disease or recent dental work. In hospital patients, intravenous catheters, in particular central lines, are possible sources of infection. Urinary and GI tracts are common sources in the elderly, particularly of enterococci.

**Age:** Incidence increases with age; IE often presents insidiously in the elderly.

**Clinical features:** IE may present acutely over days, with swinging fever, rigors and arthralgia. Commonly, *Staphylococcus aureus* IE presents as fever, collapse and meningism in the elderly, with no localizing clues. May present insidiously over weeks with weakness, anorexia, fatigue, sweats, weight loss and arthralgia. **Fever** is usually remitting and low grade in these subacute presentations. IE is unlikely if fever is absent. **Heart murmur** is present in $\approx$85% of cases; the aortic valve (AV) and MV are most often affected. Tricuspid valve (TV) endocarditis is rare except in IVDUs. **Changing murmurs** are rare — any change is usually due to worsening AV or MV regurgitation in the context of worsening heart failure. A murmur is often absent early (particularly in staphylococcal IE, in which $\approx$30% have no murmur at presentation), in mural endocarditis, in congenital bicuspid AV IE, in the elderly and in isolated TV IE.

**Classical peripheral signs** include splenomegaly ($\approx$30%), petechiae ($\approx$30%) (particularly conjunctival), Osler's nodes (10–25%), Janeway lesions, clubbing ($\approx$10%) and splinter haemorrhages. One or more of these signs is present in $\approx$50% of cases.

**Embolism** to the limbs, kidneys, mesentery, and CNS (leading to stroke, brain abscess, mononeuritis, meningitis, mycotic aneurysm) occurs in $\approx$30–50% of cases.

Standardized criteria for the assessment of possible IE, known as **modified Duke criteria**, have been published (Table 5.1).

↦ Li, Clin Infect Dis 2000; 30:633

**Organisms:** For native valve endocarditis: viridans streptococci ($\approx$40%), enterococci ($\approx$10%), other streptococci ($\approx$20%). GAS are rare. *Staphylococcus aureus* and *Staphylococcus epidermidis* (often nosocomial) account for

**Table 5.1** Modified Duke criteria for assessment of possible infective endocarditis

---

*Major criteria*

Microbiological

Typical IE organism from two separate blood cultures (viridans streptococcus, *Streptococcus bovis*, HACEK group, *Staphylococcus aureus*, community-acquired enterococcal bacteraemia without obvious source)

or

Organism consistent with IE from persistently positive blood cultures

or

Single positive blood culture for *Coxiella burnetii* or *C. burnetii* phase I IgG titre >1 : 800

Evidence of endocardial involvement

New valvular regurgitation

or

Positive echocardiogram

*Minor criteria*

Predisposition to IE (e.g. cardiac abnormality, IVDU)

Fever >38°C

Vascular phenomena not including petechiae or splinter haemorrhages

Immunological phenomena (rheumatoid factor, Osler's nodes, Roth spots, glomerulonephritis)

Microbiological findings (positive blood cultures that do not meet major criteria)

---

Cases are defined as **definite** if they fulfil 2 major criteria, 1 major plus 3 minor or 5 minor criteria, and **possible** if they fulfil 1 major and 1 minor or 3 minor criteria. ⊷ Li, Clin Infect Dis 2000; 30: 633.

≈20%. Miscellaneous others include *Haemophilus* spp. and other HACEK organisms, *Streptococcus pneumoniae*, *Neisseria gonorrhoeae*. Gram-negative aerobic bacilli, including *Pseudomonas aeruginosa*, are rare except in prosthetic valve IE (PVE) or nosocomial IE. Rarely, *Coxiella burnetii*, *Brucella* spp. or fungi (uncommon except in the context of IVDU, severe intercurrent illness or PVE, but incidence rising).

**Microbiological investigations: Blood cultures** are positive in ≈90% of cases but careful assessment of certain isolates, e.g. CNSt, is essential. Bacteraemia is usually continuous, so in unwell patient, three sets may be taken from separate venepunctures in 1 h prior to starting therapy. In less acute cases, three or four sets should be sent over a 48-h period. With viridans streptococci, three blood cultures of adequate volume (15–20 mL) give ≈98% pick-up rate. Failures usually follow antibiotic treatment. If IE is suspected in a patient who has already received antibiotics, daily further cultures should be taken over a 4–5-day period after therapy has been stopped. If blood cultures are negative after 48 h incubation, consider the causes of **culture-negative IE** (*Coxiella burnetii*, *Chlamydia psittaci*, *Brucella* spp., fungi, nutritionally-variant streptococci, *Bartonella* spp., *Legionella* spp. etc. *Abiotropha* spp. (≻255) may be seen in blood cultures, but fail to grow on solid media.) Serology for *Coxiella burnetii*, *Chlamydia* spp., *Brucella*, fungi etc. may be required. Close liaison with the microbiology laboratory is essential. The laboratory may arrange detailed antibiotic sensitivity tests but serum bactericidal levels are no longer recommended.

⊷ Millar B. Rev Medical Microbiol 2000; 11: 59

**Other investigations:** Raised ESR and C-reactive protein. Normochromic, normocytic anaemia. Normal or raised neutrophil count. Thrombocytopenia. Positive rheumatoid factor. Microscopic haematuria. **Echocardiography** may show vegetations, determine the site and extent of cardiac damage and the need for surgical intervention. Sensitivity of transthoracic ECHO is ≈60–80%; vegetations <3 mm may not be seen. Transoesophageal ECHO (TOE) is much more sensitive (≈95%) than transthoracic. A normal TOE does not exclude IE, but makes it very unlikely. Slowly growing organisms (e.g. HACEK, fungi) form the biggest vegetations.

**Complications:** Immune complex mediated effects include **arthritis** and **glomerulonephritis** (GN). GN is usually focal, with haematuria and proteinuria but normal renal function. Rarely, diffuse GN with impairment of renal function develops. **Cardiac** complications include heart failure due to valve damage, conduction defects (due to extension of infection from the valve ring into the conducting system), arrythmias and MI due to coronary embolism. **Peripheral emboli** and metastatic abscesses may occur at presentation or during treatment.

---

**Indications for surgery in IE**

Valve replacement is indicated for progressive severe heart failure, especially with AV rupture or regurgitation, or evidence of other structural damage such as ruptured chordae; persistent bacteraemia despite appropriate antibiotic therapy (which usually implies valve ring abscess or a 'hard' organism such as an enterococcus); relapse after second course of antibiotics; extension of infection into the conducting system with refractory heart block or bundle branch block, or into the pericardium with septic pericarditis. After surgery, at least 2 weeks' antibiotic therapy is given, extended to at least 4 weeks if Gram stain or culture of the resected valve shows bacteria, or if blood cultures are positive at the time of operation.

---

**Response to treatment:** Prolonged administration of bactericidal antibiotics is required for cure and to prevent relapse. Anaemia and splenomegaly may take months to resolve. Recurrent fever may be due to microbiological treatment failure, line infection, drug fever or metastatic abscess. Consider also deep vein thrombosis, urinary tract infection and other complications of hospital admission.

**Antibiotic management:** Early liaison with cardiology and cardiothoracic surgery is essential. Close liaison with the microbiology department is essential in all cases since antibiotic sensitivity *in vitro* determines treatment. If IE is suspected treatment should start as soon as three sets of blood cultures have been drawn. Until results are known, give benzylpenicillin and gentamicin (Table 5.2) unless *Staphylococcus aureus* is strongly suspected, in which case give vancomycin and gentamicin.

**Differential diagnosis:** Most other febrile illnesses, but also atrial myxoma and acute rheumatic fever.

**Bacteraemia without evidence of IE:** Patients with *Staphylococcus aureus* bacteraemia should be assessed for IE and treated for at least 2 weeks. Repeat blood cultures daily for 3–5 days. If there is prolonged bacteraemia or slow clinical response or no obvious source of infection, IE should be strongly suspected and treatment should be extended to 4 weeks. **Sustained** bacteraemia with viridans streptococci or *Staphylococcus epidermidis* should be treated as IE.

## IE in intravenous drug users

Intravenous drug users with IE usually have no history of cardiac disease, and the clinical picture is atypical in several respects:

**Clinical features:** Tricuspid valve IE accounts for more than 50% of cases. Presentation is often with septic pulmonary emboli, causing cough, dyspnoea and pleurisy. Tricuspid murmurs are usually absent. Mortality is lower, and TV IE may respond to short course therapy. If AV or MV is affected, presentation is more typical.

**Organisms:** *Staphylococcus aureus* (60%), streptococci and enterococci (20%). Less often, *Pseudomonas* spp., aerobic Gram-negative rods, *Candida* spp.; 5% of IE in this group is polymicrobial.

**Other investigations:** Chest X-ray may show multiple peripheral lesions with a tendency to cavitate.

**Antibiotic management:** Two weeks therapy with flucloxacillin is often sufficient in TV IE due to *Staphylococcus aureus*. Oral treatment, e.g. with rifampicin and ciprofloxacin may be necessary in patients who cannot comply with iv therapy.

**Table 5.2** Antibiotic treatment of native valve infective endocarditis

| Organism | Antibiotic sensitivity | Treatment | For penicillin allergic patients |
|---|---|---|---|
| Viridans streptococci *Streptococcus bovis* (➢260; investigations for colonic polyp or carcinoma are indicated) | Usually highly sensitive to benzylpenicillin (MIC ≤ 0.1 mg/L) | Benzylpenicillin 7.2 g/day in 6 divided doses by iv bolus **plus** gentamicin 80 mg q12h ☏ for 2 weeks* | Vancomycin 1 g q12h ☏ or teicoplanin 400 mg q12h for 3 doses then 400 mg q24h, **plus** gentamicin 80 mg q12h ☏ for 2 weeks |
| | If MIC > 0.1 mg/L | Benzylpenicillin 7.2 g/day in 6 divided doses by iv bolus plus gentamicin 80 mg q12h ☏ for 4 weeks | |
| Enterococci | Gentamicin-sensitive/ low level resistance (MIC < 100 mg/L) | Ampicillin or amoxicillin 12 g/day in 6 divided doses by iv bolus **plus** gentamicin 80 mg q12h ☏ for 4 weeks | Vancomycin 1 g q12h ☏ or teicoplanin 400 mg q12h for 3 doses then 400 mg q24h, **plus** gentamicin 80 mg q12h ☏ for 4 weeks |
| | Gentamicin high-level resistance (MIC ≥ 2000 mg/L) | Ampicillin or amoxicillin 12 g/day ± streptomycin if sensitive | |
| Staphylococci | Penicillin-sensitive | Benzylpenicillin 7.2 g/day in 6 divided doses by iv bolus for 4 weeks **plus** gentamicin 80–120 mg q8h ☏ for first week | Vancomycin ☏ 1 g q12h for 4 weeks **plus** gentamicin 80–120 mg q8h ☏ for first week |
| | Penicillin-resistant, non-MRSA | Flucloxacillin 12 g/day in 6 divided doses by iv bolus for 4 weeks** **plus** gentamicin 80–120 mg q8h ☏ for first week | |
| | Methicillin-resistant staphylococci (MRSA) | Vancomycin ☏ 1 g q12h for 4 weeks **plus** gentamicin 80–120 mg q8h ☏ for first week | |
| *Streptococcus pneumoniae, Neisseria meningitidis* | Penicillin-sensitive ☎ | Benzylpenicillin 20 MU/ day for 4–6 weeks | Parenteral cephalosporin (high-dose) for 4–6 weeks |
| *Haemophilus* spp. and other fastidious Gram-negative rods (➢296) | Guided by results of culture and sensitivity | Ampicillin or amoxicillin 12 g/day in 6 divided doses by iv bolus **plus** gentamicin 80–120 mg q8h ☏ for 4 weeks | |
| *Pseudomonas* spp. ☎ | Largely a disease of IVDUs and PVE. Right-sided IE, worth trying antibiotics alone. Left-sided IE merits immediate valve replacement followed by 6 weeks of antibiotics | Azlocillin 15 g/day **plus** gentamicin 80–120 mg q8h ☏ for 6 weeks | Ceftazidime 2 g q8h **plus** gentamicin 80–120 mg q8h ☏ for 4–6 weeks |

\* Two weeks' therapy is sufficient if **all** the following criteria are met: MIC ≤ 0.1 mg/L, no evidence of thromboembolic disease, native valve infection, no vegetations > 5 mm on ECHO, clinical response with resolution of fever and symptoms within 7 days, no cardiovascular risk factors such as heart failure, aortic regurgitation or conduction defect. If not, 4 weeks' therapy is given.
\*\* Two weeks' therapy with flucloxacillin alone may be sufficient in staphylococcal tricuspid endocarditis.
☏ Gentamicin levels must be measured at least twice weekly (➢404).
☏ Vancomycin dose adjustment: initially 1 g q12h. Determine level and adjust dose to achieve 1 h post infusion peak of ≈30 mg/L and trough of 5–10 mg/L.

⊶ BSAC guidelines, Heart 1998; 79: 207

⊶ AHA Wilson, JAMA 1995; 274: 1706

🖥 www.americanheart.org/presenter.jhtml?identifier =1231

⊶ Bayer, Circulation 1998; 98: 2936

🖥 circ.ahajournals.org/cgi/content/full/98/25/2936

## Prosthetic valve endocarditis (PVE)

This affects mechanical valves more commonly than bioprosthetic grafts, and affects the AV more than the MV. With mechanical valves, infection consists of ring abscess in tissue behind the valve, with extension into adjacent structures. The valve may leak (commonly presenting as aortic regurgitation) or become obstructed (commoner with MV). Conduction defects also occur. Infection of bioprosthetic valves is often confined to the valve leaflets but ring abscesses may develop.

**Clinical features:** Risk is highest in first 3 months post-operatively. Fever and cardiac findings (e.g. an aortic regurgitant murmur), embolic phenomena and heart failure. In *Candida* spp. IE blood cultures may take 72–96 h to become positive. *Aspergillus* IE is almost always blood culture negative and usually presents as peripheral embolus, the diagnosis being confirmed on histology of the resected embolic material.

**Organisms:** Infection occurring less than 3–4 months after operation is normally acquired perioperatively and is usually caused by *Staphylococcus aureus, Staphylococcus epidermidis*, aerobic Gram-negative rods, coryneforms or fungi. Concomitant sternal wound sepsis is common. Later infections are due to a similar spectrum of organisms as native valve IE and are acquired in the same ways.

**Antibiotic management:** Guided by microbiological results. Empirical treatment should consist of vancomycin + treatment dose gentamicin ⚠ plus parenteral cephalosporin if valve is >12 months old, because of possibility of HACEK infection (➤306). Usually given for at least 6 weeks.

## Prophylaxis against infective endocarditis

Prophylaxis is indicated for patients with a history of rheumatic heart disease, congenital heart disease (except uncomplicated atrial septal defect), other forms of valvular heart disease including a history of native valve repair, mitral valve prolapse (if there is a systolic murmur), surgically constructed systemic–pulmonary shunt, and hypertrophic obstructive cardiomyopathy. Patients with prosthetic valves and previous history of endocarditis are considered to be at particularly high risk. See Table 5.3.

## Viral pericarditis

**Clinical features:** There may be a history of a flu-like illness. Onset is usually acute with substernal pain relieved by sitting forward. There may be a pericardial rub, and in the presence of large amounts of pericardial fluid, signs of cardiac tamponade (hypotension, tachycardia, muffled heart sounds, raised venous pressure which rises further on inspiration).

**Organisms:** Most cases are due to enteroviruses, in particular, coxsackie A and B and echoviruses. Influenza, mumps, varicella zoster and EBV have all been reported as rare causes.

**Microbiological investigations:** Serology for viral causes. If effusion is large and patient is unwell, pericardiocentesis may be required, and fluid obtained should of course be examined for bacteria including mycobacteria.

**Other investigations:** ECG shows widespread concave-upwards ST elevation. Chest X-ray may show cardiomegaly. Echocardiography may show pericardial fluid.

**Differential diagnosis:** Non-infectious causes of pericarditis include uraemia, myocardial infarction, Dressler's syndrome, trauma, connective-tissue diseases, acute rheumatic fever, malignant infiltration.

**Supportive management:** Anti-inflammatory agents such as aspirin or indomethacin may be given. Most cases resolve spontaneously after 2–6 weeks.

**Complications:** 15–20% of cases recur. There may be associated myocarditis.

**Table 5.3** Prophylaxis against infective endocarditis

| Procedure | Recommended regimen | If penicillin allergic or prescribed penicillin more than once in the preceding month |
|---|---|---|
| Dental extractions, scaling or periodontal surgery under **local or no anaesthesia.** (Fillings and other procedures not causing gum trauma do **not** require prophylaxis) | Amoxicillin, 3 g po, under supervision, 1 h prior to procedure. Children <10 yrs: $\frac{1}{2}$ adult dose; <5 yrs: $\frac{1}{4}$ adult dose | Clindamycin 600 mg po, under supervision, 1 h prior to procedure. Children 5–10 yrs: 300 mg; <5 yrs, 150 mg **or** Erythromycin stearate, 1.5 g po, under supervision, 1 h prior to procedure plus 0.5 g 6 h later. Children <10 yrs: $\frac{1}{2}$ adult dose; <5 yrs: $\frac{1}{4}$ adult dose |
| Dental extractions, scaling or periodontal surgery under **general anaesthesia** | Amoxicillin 1 g iv just before induction plus 0.5 g po under supervision, 6 h later. Children < 10 yrs: $\frac{1}{2}$ adult dose **or** Amoxicillin 3 g po under supervision, 4 h before anaesthesia followed by 3 g po as soon as possible after operation. Children <10 yrs: $\frac{1}{2}$ adult dose; <5 yrs: $\frac{1}{4}$ adult dose **or** Amoxicillin 3 g po and probenecid 1 g po under supervision, 4 h before anaesthesia | See below under 'Special-risk patients' |
| **Special-risk patients** who should be referred to hospital: (i) Patients with prosthetic valves who are to have a general anaesthetic; (ii) Patients who are to have a general anaesthetic and who are allergic to penicillin or have had penicillin more than once in the preceding month; (iii) Patients with a previous history of endocarditis **or** *\*Genitourinary surgery or instrumentation* **or** *\*Obstetric, gynaecological and gastrointestinal procedures in patients with prosthetic valves or a history of endocarditis* | Amoxicillin 1 g iv (in water for injection) plus gentamicin 120 mg im just before induction, then amoxicillin 0.5 g po 6 h later. Children under 10: amoxicillin, $\frac{1}{2}$ adult dose plus gentamicin 2 mg/kg | Teicoplanin 400 mg iv plus gentamicin 120 mg iv just before induction or 15 min before surgical procedure. Children under 14: teicoplanin, 6 mg/kg iv plus gentamicin 2 mg/kg iv **or** *Clindamycin 300 mg iv over 10 min just before induction or 15 min before surgical procedure plus 150 mg po or iv 6 h later. Children <10 yrs: $\frac{1}{2}$ adult dose; <5 yrs: $\frac{1}{4}$ adult dose **or** Vancomycin 1 g by slow iv infusion over 60 min followed by gentamicin 120 mg iv Children under 10: vancomycin, 20 mg/kg iv plus gentamicin 2 mg/kg iv |
| **Surgery or instrumentation of upper respiratory tract** | As for dental procedures, but post-operative antibiotics may need to be given parenterally due to difficulty in swallowing | |

\* Clindamycin is not suitable for genitourinary, obstetric, gynaecological and gastrointestinal procedures. If urine is known to be infected, prophylaxis should be extended to include cover against the pathogens involved ☎.

☏ BSAC, Lancet 1990; 335: 89; Lancet 1992; 339: 1292; Lancet 1997; 350: 1100

# Pyogenic pericarditis

**Risk factors:** Bacterial pericarditis nearly always arises in the context of severe intercurrent illness: e.g. after thoracic surgery, by contiguous spread from infection in the pleura, lungs, subphrenic space or endocardium, or by haematogenous spread from septic foci elsewhere.

**Clinical features:** Presentation is usually acute, with fever, tachycardia and signs of cardiac decompensation. Features of viral pericarditis such as pain relieved by sitting forward, rub and typical ECG changes are usually absent.

**Organisms:** *Streptococcus pneumoniae, Staphylococcus aureus.* Gram-negative aerobic bacilli. Less often *Neisseria meningitidis, Neisseria gonorrhoeae, Haemophilus influenzae.* Many other organisms have been reported as very rare causes.

**Microbiological investigations:** Blood culture. Pericardiocentesis may be required for diagnosis, or relief of tamponade.

**Other investigations:** Chest X-ray may show cardiomegaly. Echocardiography will show pericardial fluid.

**Differential diagnosis:** Tuberculous or viral pericarditis. Acute rheumatic fever. Non-infectious causes of pericarditis.

**Antibiotic management:** Prolonged intravenous antibiotics guided by sensitivity testing, similar to regimens listed for IE.

**Supportive management:** Most patients will be extremely unwell and will require intensive investigation and supportive management, often in the intensive-care unit.

# Tuberculous pericarditis ✉

**Risk factors:** Many patients have history of concurrent pulmonary tuberculosis, but pericarditis can be the sole manifestation of TB.

**Clinical features:** Onset is usually insidious, with slow accumulation of pericardial fluid, but rarely TB pericarditis may present as an acute fibrinous pericarditis. Patients may also have fever, weight loss and fatigue.

**Organisms:** *Mycobacterium tuberculosis, Mycobacterium bovis.*

**Microbiological investigations:** Diagnosis may be difficult, since acid-fast bacilli are not usually seen in the pericardial fluid. Pericardial biopsy may show granulomata. Granulomatous pericarditis is due to tuberculosis until proven otherwise.

**Management:** (➤43).

# Myocarditis

Myocarditis is an inflammation of cardiac muscle. Most cases are viral, although myocarditis is also seen as a feature of Lyme disease.

**Clinical features:** Presentation ranges from a symptomless finding to fulminant heart failure. Patients are usually febrile and tachycardic, with dyspnoea and fatigue. On examination, there may be cardiomegaly and murmurs of mitral and tricuspid regurgitation. There may be hypotension and signs of congestive cardiac failure. Arrhythmias and heart block may occur. There may be associated features of pericarditis.

**Organisms:** Coxsackievirus A & B, echovirus. Many other viruses have been reported as rare causes. *Borrelia burgdorferi.* Myocarditis is also a feature of some systemic infections including *Trypanosoma cruzi, Toxoplasma gondii, Neisseria meningitidis, Corynebacterium diphtheriae.*

**Microbiological investigations:** Serology may help to confirm the viral aetiology. Lyme disease (➤323).

**Other investigations:** ECG may show

widespread ST and T wave changes. Most patients recover fully. Myocardial biopsy may be required in those who do not.

**Differential diagnosis:** Pericarditis. Idiopathic congestive cardiomyopathy. Acute rheumatic fever.

# Chapter 6

# Gastrointestinal infections

## Normal bowel flora

A knowledge of the constituents of the normal bowel flora is useful in the understanding of intra-abdominal sepsis (Table 6.1).

## Infectious diarrhoea ②

Patients presenting in the community with recent onset of diarrhoea are usually managed initially as if they have infectious gastroenteritis. Diarrhoea may be defined as three or more loose stools within 24 h. Patients often also have abdominal pain, nausea and vomiting, fever, blood in the stools, faecal urgency and tenesmus. Infectious diarrhoea may helpfully be classified into secretory diarrhoea and invasive enteritis (Tables 6.2, 6.3). Food poisoning (bacterial, viral or toxic) and dysentery are notifiable diseases (Table 6.4). Viral infections are greatly under-reported and are the commonest causes of infectious enteritis in the UK.

**Risk factors:** Usually acquired by ingestion of the infectious agent in food; some are at higher risk (previous gastric surgery, hypochlorhydria, immunodeficiency). Recent antibiotic use predisposes to antibiotic-associated diarrhoea. Microbiological diagnosis may be suggested by the clinical features, other cases in the community and the travel and food history.

**Microbiological investigations:** Stool microscopy for blood and pus cells. Pus cells are absent in viral gastroenteritis. Examination for ova, cysts and parasites is indicated if there is a history of travel. Stool electron microscopy may confirm viral gastroenteritis. Rotavirus genome can be detected by electrophoresis (PAGE). Stool culture for specific pathogens including *Salmonella* spp., *E. coli* O157, *Shigella* spp.

and *Campylobacter jejuni*. ☎ Always inform the laboratory of travel history and if diarrhoea is bloody. Modified Ziehl–Nielsen stain is used to demonstrate *Cryptosporidium parvum* (➤230, Σ ≈5000) which is particularly common in children under 5 yrs and the immunocompromised.

**Other investigations:** All patients should have baseline full blood count and U&Es. If there is blood in the stools, ask for a blood film to be examined to exclude fragmented RBCs (in case the patient has *E. coli* O157 and haemolytic uraemic syndrome). Sigmoidoscopy may reveal changes of pseudomembranous colitis (due to *Clostridium difficile* ➤63), ulceration due to *Entamoeba histolytica*, and allow biopsy to exclude non-infectious causes of diarrhoea such as inflammatory bowel disease (IBD).

**Differential diagnosis:** IBD, diverticulosis, colonic carcinoma, ischaemic colitis, malabsorption.

### Practice point

Up to 30% of patients presenting with diarrhoea, particularly among the elderly, have some other diagnosis—such as bacteraemia due to urinary tract infection or pneumonia.

**Antibiotic management:** Antibiotics are generally **not** indicated for infectious diarrhoea. Antibiotics **are** indicated in the following circumstances:

**For particular pathogens:**
• **Salmonellosis** with bacteraemia or severe illness. Ciprofloxacin is the drug of choice in the UK at present, particularly as clinical trials

**Table 6.1** Normal bowel flora

| Region | Flora |
|---|---|
| Stomach | Usually sterile, unless achlorhydric, when flora resembles that of small intestine |
| Small intestine | Usually contains small numbers of lactobacilli, enterococci and diphtheroids. Diabetes or abnormal anatomy (e.g. following surgery to create a blind loop, or in diverticulosis) may allow bacterial overgrowth with malabsorption and diarrhoea |
| Large intestine | Bacteria account for 30% of the wet weight of faeces. **Strict anaerobes outnumber the aerobic Gram-negative rods ('coliforms') by at least 100 : 1** |

**Table 6.2** Predominantly secretory diarrhoea

| Organism | Incubation period | Typical duration | Clinical features C | V | F | B | Comments |
|---|---|---|---|---|---|---|---|
| *E. coli* (enterotoxigenic (ETEC) and other adherent strains, e.g. EAggEC, DAEC ➤275) | 12–72 h | 2–4 days | + | – | – | – | No routine therapy is indicated, although oral ciprofloxacin shortens the duration of the attack. Typically transmitted by meat, salads, milk, water ✉ |
| Viral diarrhoea | 1–3 days | 3–9 days | + | + | + | – | ➤350 |
| *Bacillus cereus* ✉ (➤266) | 1–6 h | <1 day | + | + + | – | – | Heat-stable toxin preformed in food, typically rice or meat. Incubation period extended and diarrhoea worse if toxin produced by bacterial multiplication in gut |
| *Cryptosporidium parvum* (➤230) | 7–14 days | 10–14 days | + | + | ± | + | Mainly in children. Severe chronic disease in HIV+ patients (➤160) |
| *Clostridium perfringens* (➤314) ✉ | 8–12 h | 1 day | + | ± | + | – | Toxin produced in gut. Usually after ingestion of food, typically meat, kept warm allowing germination of spores and bacterial growth |
| *Staphylococcus aureus* (➤249) ✉ | 2–7 h | <1 day | + | + + | ± | – | Toxin preformed in food. Typically dairy produce, meat products |
| *Vibrio cholerae* (➤285) ✉ | 1–5 days | Variable | – | + | – | – | Severe secretory diarrhoea. Diagnosis suggested by travel to endemic/epidemic area |

C, cramps; V, vomiting; F, fever; B, blood in stools.

**Table 6.3** 'Invasive' enteritis

| Organism | Incubation period | Typical duration (days) | Clinical features | | | | Comments |
|---|---|---|---|---|---|---|---|
| | | | C | V | F | B | |
| Non-typhoidal Salmonella spp. (➤281) | 8–48 h | 4–7 | + | + | + | ± | May rarely cause systemic illness with bacteraemia and metastatic infection |
| Shigellae (➤282) ⊠ Escherichia coli (EIEC ➤277) | 12–96 h | 5–7 | + | + | + | + | Very small infective dose. Faeco-oral spread. Complications include toxic megacolon, reactive arthritis |
| Campylobacter jejuni (➤288) | 1–10 days | 2–20 | + | + | + | + | From meat, esp. poultry, and dairy produce |
| Escherichia coli O157 (VTEC, syn. EHEC ➤276) | 1–5 days | 1–4 | + | + | + | + | Bloody diarrhoea due to verotoxin production. Associated with HUS, especially in children |
| Clostridium difficile (➤319) | 4–9 days after antibiotics | Variable | + | ± | + | + | Antibiotic-associated diarrhoea (➤63) |
| Yersinia enterocolitica (➤284) | 3–7 days | 10–14 | + | + | + | − | Requires special culture techniques. Unusual in UK. Extra-intestinal manifestations are common. Usually from pork or dairy produce |
| Vibrio parahaemolyticus | 24–72 h | 2–10 | + | + | + | + | Usually transmitted by shellfish (➤60, 287) |
| Giardia lamblia (➤218) | 7–21 days | Variable | + | + | ± | − | May cause chronic steatorrhoea and malabsorption |
| Entamoeba histolytica (➤218) ⊠ | Variable; 14–28 days | Variable | + | ± | ± | + | Diagnosis suggested by travel history. Complications include liver abscess, amoeboma, cutaneous ulceration |

C, cramps; V, vomiting; F, fever; B, blood in stools; HUS, haemolytic uraemic syndrome.

suggest that it does not predispose towards the carrier state. In infants under 3 months and in children with underlying illness, parenteral cephalosporin.

• **Shigellosis** due to *Shigella dysenteriae* should be treated with ciprofloxacin (➤282), although milder cases, due to *Shigella sonnei*, usually resolve without antibiotics. Co-trimoxazole is also often recommended.

Nalidixic acid or parenteral cephalosporin are alternatives for use in children.

• *Campylobacter jejuni* infection may respond to erythromycin (➤288). Quinolone resistance is common due to use of similar antibiotics in the poultry industry.

• **Antibiotic-associated diarrhoea** due to *Clostridium difficile* should be treated with oral metronidazole or vancomycin (➤63).

**Table 6.4** Fish and shellfish poisoning

| Disease | Source and toxin | Mechanism | Epidemiology and presentation | Mortality | Confirmation and treatment |
|---|---|---|---|---|---|
| Scombroid fish poisoning | Histamine from bacterial histidine breakdown; tuna, mackerel and other scombroid fish (rarely herring, sardines, anchovies) | Histamine reaction | Worldwide; Minutes–hours → flushing, headache, dizziness and urticarial rash lasting up to 12–24 h | Rare | Histamine levels in suspect fish: antihistamines; iv cimetidine also reported effective |
| Ciguatera fish poisoning | Ciguatoxins; large carnivorous reef fish which have concentrated toxins from dinoflagellate | Blocks $Ca^{2+}$ regulation of $Na^+$ channels | Common in subtropical & tropical waters; 2–30 h → variable blood pressure, nausea, vomiting, diarrhoea, abdominal pain, myalgia, neurological symptoms lasting 24–48 h | <12% | Clinical diagnosis, symptomatic management; iv mannitol may be effective. May lead to 'sensitization', with serious reactions to minor exposure in the future |
| Pufferfish poisoning | Heat-stable tetrodotoxin; pufferfish ('fugu'), shellfish, frogs, newts and salamanders | Blocks axonal transmission ($Na^+$ channels) | Japan, and rarely in eastern USA; usually 10–45 min → paraesthesiae, weakness, salivation, hypotension respiratory paralysis lasting several days | 60% in first 24 h | Airway support, volume expansion, gastric lavage; anticholinesterases may be of value |
| Paralytic shellfish poisoning | Heat-stable saxitoxin; clams, mussels, oysters, scallops, cockles which have concentrated toxic dinoflagellates during 'red tides' | Like tetrodotoxin | Usually cold waters, estimated 1600 cases *per annum* worldwide; 30 min–3 h → paraesthesiae of mouth and extremities, nausea, vomiting, | <10% | Suspect shellfish assayed for mouse toxicity (➔); supportive, gastric lavage |

| | | | | | |
|---|---|---|---|---|---|
| | | | diarrhoea, ataxia, cranial nerve lesions lasting up to 7 days | | Supportive |
| Neurotoxic shellfish poisoning | Brevitoxins; shellfish having ingested toxic dinoflagellates during 'red tides', also aerosolization from surf | Probably like tetrodotoxin | Gulf coasts of Florida and Texas; <3h → paraesthesiae, ataxia, vertigo, nausea, vomiting, diarrhoea, abdominal pain lasting up to 9h. Inhalation leads to cough, wheezing, sneezing, conjunctivitis | Rare | |
| Amnesic shellfish poisoning | Heat-stable domoic acid (neuroexcitatory, like glutamic acid); diatoms ingested by mussels | Hippocampal necrosis | Estuaries of Atlantic, Pacific and Indian Oceans; 15min–36h → nausea, vomiting, GI bleeds, headache; anterograde memory loss lasting up to 2yrs | 3% | – |
| Diarrhoeal shellfish poisoning | Okadaic acid; shellfish having ingested toxic dinoflagellate | Increases gastrointestinal mucosal permeability | Japan, Netherlands, Chile, Italy; 30min–30h → nausea, vomiting, diarrhoea, abdominal cramps lasting up to 2 days | Usually mild | – |
| *Pfiesteria* poisoning | Exposure to water contaminated with dinoflagellate *Pfiesteria piscicida* | Unknown | Rivers of Maryland and North Carolina; memory loss, respiratory distress, headache, nausea, vomiting conjunctivitis | – | – |

- **Giardiasis** (➤218).
- **Amoebiasis** (➤218).
- **Microsporidiosis** (➤231).

**For patients at higher risk of severe illness**, empirical quinolone therapy is often recommended:

- Age > 60 yrs.
- Hypochlorhydria or antacid therapy.
- History of inflammatory bowel disease.
- Prosthetic intravascular device.
- Aortic or ventricular aneurysm.
- Immunosuppressed (inc. steroids).
- Other chronic illness (renal, diabetes, rheumatoid disease/SLE).
- ACE inhibitors, diuretics or β-blockers.
- Dysenteric symptoms (fever, severe abdominal pain, bloody diarrhoea, tenesmus).

The role of antibiotics in *E. coli* O157 infection remains controversial; there is no unequivocal clinical evidence to indicate benefit or harm, although there is *in vitro* evidence that some antibiotics may increase toxin production. At present we do not recommend antibiotic treatment in known or suspected *E. coli* O157 infection.

**Supportive management: Rehydration** is the key to management of diarrhoea from whatever cause. The clinical features of dehydration are due to combined salt and water loss. Table 6.5 summarizes the features of dehydration. These features can be used to assess the need for fluid replacement **when there is no other underlying medical condition**.

Oral rehydration is adequate for the majority of **mild** cases, and is best given as a solution containing both salt and sugar, which are actively taken up together in the small intestine. Commercial rehydration fluids are available (Dioralyte). Home-made recipes are widely

**Table 6.5** Assessment of dehydration

| | Degree of dehydration | | |
| --- | --- | --- | --- |
| | **Mild** | **Moderate** | **Severe** |
| Typical scenarios | 24-h diarrhoea, 24-h vomiting | 48-h diarrhoea, diabetic ketoacidosis, vomiting of pyloric stenosis, salt-losing chronic renal failure | Fulminating diarrhoea (>10 stools/day), >48 h toxin-mediated explosive diarrhoea |
| Average water loss | 1–2 L | 2–4.5 L | 4.5–8.5 L |
| Average sodium loss | 2.5–5 mmol/kg | 5–10 mmol/kg | 10–20 mmol/kg |
| Common symptoms | Lassitude, anorexia, nausea, light-headedness, postural hypotension | Apathy, tiredness, giddiness, nausea, headache, muscle cramps | Profound apathy, weakness, confusion, coma |
| Common signs | Nil of note | Pinched face, dry tongue, sunken eyes, reduced skin turgor, postural hypotension (systolic BP >90 mmHg), tachycardia, oliguria | Shock, tachycardia, marked peripheral vasoconstriction, systolic BP < 90 mmHg, uraemia, oliguria |
| Other features | | Hyponatraemia if water has been taken as fluid replacement | |

➥ Farthing *et al.*, J Infection 1996; 33: 143

used in developing countries: for example, four tablespoons of sugar, $^3/_4$ teaspoon of salt, one teaspoon of sodium bicarbonate mixed in 250 mL of orange juice and made up to 1 L with water.

For patients with **moderate and severe** dehydration, estimate current deficit, add daily requirement and additional ongoing losses and replace this iv over first 24 h. Daily requirement for an adult of average size is $\approx 2$ L of water in 24 h, and $\approx 70$–100 mmol of sodium. A suitable allowance for the daily requirement would therefore be 1.5 L of 5% dextrose plus 0.5 L of normal saline. The deficit and ongoing losses should all be replaced as normal saline. Vomit should be replaced as 0.5 N saline (i.e. half as normal saline, half as 5% dextrose). Give K+ as indicated by U&E result.

In patients with **severe** dehydration, 20% of replacement fluid should be given as isotonic (1.26%) sodium bicarbonate.

Antispasmodic agents such as loperamide may be used for mild diarrhoea without blood, but they should not be used if there are features to suggest dysentery.

↦ BIS guidelines for management of gastroenteritis: Farthing *et al.*, J Infection 1996; 33: 143

# Control of gastrointestinal infections

National PHLS guidelines are published, but local rules, which may be less stringent, often exist. Responsibility for investigation and control of GI infections in the community rests with the Consultant in Communicable Disease Control (CCDC) (Consultant in Public Health Medicine, CPHM, in Scotland), to whom all cases of suspected food poisoning or dysentery should be notified.

In general, patients should not return to work/school until they have been free of diarrhoea for 48 h. More stringent rules apply for particular organisms (e.g. *S. typhi*, *E. coli* O157) in particular groups (e.g. young children, food handlers) ☎.

↦ Comm Dis Report 1995, Suppl. 11
💻 www.phls.co.uk/advice/schools/summary.htm

**Antibiotic-associated diarrhoea (AAD)** ②
Certain agents, notably clindamycin, amp/ amoxicillin, co-amoxiclav and parenteral cephalosporins are particularly likely to cause diarrhoea, although almost all antibiotics have been implicated. Most cases are due to infection by toxin-producing *Clostridium difficile*, growth of which is promoted by alteration in other bowel flora. *Clostridium difficile* produces a colitis, which in its most severe form causes colonic ulceration with pseudomembrane formation ('pseudomembranous colitis'). AAD is an important and expensive cause of nosocomial morbidity and mortality.

**Risk factors:** Age and antibiotic use, particularly those listed above. Rarely reported in the absence of antibiotic use (e.g. in association with anti-cancer chemotherapy). *Clostridium difficile* can be recovered easily from surfaces within the rooms of patients with AAD, especially if they are incontinent, and from the hands of their medical attendants. The carriage rate in hospital patients on admission is $\approx$1% and the organism is usually acquired nosocomially. CDAD is rising in incidence ($\Sigma$ 15 000 toxin reports in 2000).

**Clinical features:** Asymptomatic carriage is common. Diarrhoea may be mild or very severe. Abdominal cramps, fever and leucocytosis occur. Sigmoidoscopy may show ulceration and pseudomembranes in severe cases, although disease can be restricted to ascending colon. Toxic megacolon and perforation occur rarely. Relapse after apparently successful treatment is common ($\approx$25%), and persistent diarrhoea leading to hypoalbuminaemia can occur.

**Microbiological investigations:** Assay for *Clostridium difficile* toxin in stool (➤319). Culture is also possible, but is slower and not specific for the disease. Avoid sending multiple repeat faecal samples from patients with symptomatic relapse, or to assess 'clearance' because continued presence of toxin or organism is common ($\approx$25%) and not predictive of response or relapse.

**Antibiotic management:** Stop the precipitating antibiotic whenever possible. Metronidazole
*(Continued...)*

400 mg 8-hly, **po**, or vancomycin 125 mg 6-hly, **po** Vancomycin is much more expensive and might encourage colonization by vancomycin-resistant enterococci, but may be slightly more effective. IV metronidazole (not vancomycin) may be effective in patients unable to take oral therapy. Either agent should be given for 10 days, and if there no response the other may be substituted. Relapse should be treated with a further course. Various strategies have been suggested for preventing relapse, but none has been subjected to clinical trial. These include tapering doses of vancomycin over several weeks, very low-dose vancomycin therapy for 3 weeks post-treatment, cholestyramine and even enemas containing normal bowel organisms. About 50% of relapses are in fact due to reinfection, and infection control measures are important.

**Prevention:** Isolation during diarrhoea and for 3 days thereafter. The use of gloves for routine handling of all body fluids has been shown to reduce the transmission of *Clostridium difficile* and the incidence of AAD. Bedpan washers may not kill the spores of *Clostridium difficile*, and bedpans used by infected patients should be autoclaved. Control of antibiotic prescribing. Cleaning of rooms after discharge or transfer of patients.

**Antibiotic-associated diarrhoea without** *Clostridium difficile:* Some patients with antibiotic-associated diarrhoea have negative tests for *Clostridium difficile* toxin. These patients tend to be less ill, with few constitutional symptoms. Other putative causes of AAD include *Clostridium perfringens, Staphylococcus aureus, Bacteroides fragilis* and *Candida* spp.

**Whipple's disease (➢272)**
Extremely rare multi-system disorder due to systemic infection by *Tropheryma whipplei*. Most prominently affects the small intestine and its lymphatics, but organisms can be demonstrated in all body tissues, including CNS. Presents with recurrent attacks of arthritis, weakness, weight loss, cough, fever and persistent diarrhoea. Ascites, oedema, splenomegaly and encephalopathy occur. Uniformly fatal prior to introduction of antibiotics.
*(Continued...)*

Diagnosis is usually made on the basis of characteristic histological and ultrastructural changes seen on small bowel biopsy.

Consider Whipple's disease as part of the differential diagnosis of the following conditions when more common causes have been excluded: unexplained malabsorption with systemic disease; sarcoid-like systemic granulomatous disease; neurological disease with myoclonus, dementia and supranuclear ophthalmoplegia; culture-negative endocarditis; unexplained uveitis.

**Traveller's diarrhoea**
International travellers frequently develop diarrhoea. A wide range of organisms may be responsible, including ETEC, shigellae, salmonellae, *Campylobacter* spp., *Giardia lamblia*, and rarely *Entamoeba histolytica*. Travellers who may have difficulty obtaining medical attention should carry standby medication (➢195).

## *Helicobacter pylori* infection

Associated with gastritis and gastric/duodenal ulceration (➢289).

## Cholecystitis

The biliary tract is normally sterile; infection becomes established (bactibilia) secondary to stones or anatomical abnormality, such as malignant or inflammatory strictures. Bacteria may reach the bile via the ampulla of Vater, or from the portal or systemic circulations.

**Risk factors:** Cholecystitis is associated with calculi in ≈95% of cases. Acalculous cholecystitis typically occurs in elderly debilitated patients with severe intercurrent illness. Cholecystitis is a post-operative complication which may follow any operation, due to biliary stasis associated with recumbency and dehydration.

**Clinical features:** Fever, rigors, nausea and vomiting, right upper quadrant pain. On examination, tender right upper quadrant and possibly a tender, palpable, enlarged gallbladder. There may be evidence of associated bacteraemia with hypotension and confusion. Emphysematous cholecystitis is a rare condition due to infection by *Clostridium perfringens*, sometimes in mixed culture with Gram-negative aerobes. There is gas formation within the gallbladder and risk of gangrene and perforation.

**Organisms:** Bowel flora, usually in mixed culture: coliforms, enterococci and anaerobes, including *Bacteroides fragilis* and *Clostridium perfringens*.

**Microbiological investigations:** Blood culture. Culture of bile if available (e.g. after ERCP or surgical intervention).

**Other investigations:** Ultrasound demonstrates bile duct obstruction, detects 95% of stones and allows assessment of the gallbladder wall, which is usually thickened.

**Antibiotic management:** In mildly ill patients, give co-amoxiclav. In more severe cases, use benzylpenicillin + gentamicin + metronidazole **or** parenteral cephalosporin + metronidazole. No antibiotic regimen will reliably sterilize an obstructed biliary tree. Antibiotics which usually penetrate well into bile do not do so in this situation.

**Supportive management:** Initial management of acute cholecystitis is with antibiotics, analgesia, fluid therapy and nasogastric suction if the patient is vomiting. The timing of cholecystectomy after cholecystitis is a matter of controversy and requires experienced surgical judgement.

**Complications:** Septicaemia, ascending cholangitis, pancreatitis, liver abscess, perforation and peritonitis. Complications are more frequent in the elderly.

## Ascending cholangitis

Ascending cholangitis is usually associated with partial or complete biliary obstruction due to stones or strictures (malignant or inflammatory). The classic features are fever with rigors, abdominal pain and jaundice ('Charcot's triad'). There may be associated evidence of bacteraemia and sepsis syndrome with shock and confusion. Liver abscess, frequently multiple, may develop. This severe infection requires combined surgical and medical treatment. Antibiotic therapy should be as above. Surgical decompression of the gallbladder is usually urgently required, and may often be achieved endoscopically.

## Peritonitis

Localized or generalized inflammation of the peritoneal cavity, due to micro-organisms or irritant chemicals (e.g. bile, stomach contents).

**Risk factors:** Ruptured viscus (e.g. appendix, diverticulum, peptic ulcer, perforated bowel as a complication of enteric fever), ischaemic bowel (e.g. vascular insufficiency, strangulated hernia), trauma, post-operative infection or leakage, pelvic inflammatory disease (including perihepatitis in Fitz-Hugh–Curtis syndrome), ruptured abscess. Unusual causes include spontaneous bacterial peritonitis, peritoneal dialysis peritonitis and tuberculous peritonitis.

**Clinical features:** There may be features of the underlying illness. Fever, vomiting, abdominal pain with tenderness, guarding and evidence of paralytic ileus (absent bowel sounds). Hypotension and tachycardia are initially due to hypovolaemia due to loss of intravascular fluid into the peritoneal cavity. If bacteraemia and sepsis syndrome develop they also contribute to hypotension and confusion.

**Organisms:** Mixed infection with bowel flora: coliforms, anaerobes, *Enterococcus* spp., *Streptococcus* 'milleri'.

**Microbiological investigations:** Culture of blood and peritoneal fluid.

**Other investigations:** Leucocytosis, abnormal liver function tests and raised amylase are common. Chest and abdomen X-ray may show subdiaphragmatic gas if there has been perforation of a viscus.

**Differential diagnosis:** The differential diagnosis of the 'acute abdomen' includes appendicitis, perforated peptic ulcer, cholecystitis, pancreatitis, renal and biliary colic, inflammatory bowel disease, gynaecological causes including ruptured ectopic pregnancy and ovarian torsion, retroperitoneal haemorrhage and leaking aortic aneurysm. Non-surgical causes include basal pneumonia; others, such as familial Mediterranean fever and porphyria, are very rare.

**Antibiotic management:** Benzylpenicillin + gentamicin + metronidazole **or** parenteral cephalosporin + metronidazole **or** co-amoxiclav. Vancomycin + gentamicin + metronidazole may be needed in the penicillin- and cephalosporin-allergic patient.

**Supportive management:** Antibiotics are used to speed recovery and prevent bacteraemia — definitive treatment requires surgery for the underlying cause. Instillation of topical antibiotics at operation has not been shown to be of benefit.

# Peritoneal dialysis (CAPD) peritonitis

Patients on chronic ambulatory peritoneal dialysis (CAPD) have a permanent indwelling catheter in the peritoneal cavity. Fluid is instilled and withdrawn three or four times daily, and there is therefore a risk of peritoneal infection. Scrupulous attention to aseptic technique is essential when handling CAPD catheters, and has been shown to reduce the incidence of peritonitis to well below one episode per patient-year.

**Clinical features:** Abdominal pain and cloudiness of the peritoneal fluid.

**Organisms:** A vast range, of which the commonest are *Staphylococcus epidermidis*, *Staphylococcus aureus*, coliforms, *Streptococcus* spp.

**Microbiological investigations:** Microscopy showing >100 cells/μL suggests infection. Gram stain is positive in 50% of cases, more commonly with Gram-positive infection.

**Antibiotic management:** All renal units will have a local protocol for the management of CAPD peritonitis. If this is not available, the following regimen, which gives up to three intraperitoneal (ip) doses of vancomycin 7 days apart, may be used:
- Send whole bag of peritoneal fluid to laboratory for culture.
- Into the first bag of dialysis fluid, give vancomycin 2 g (adjusted for body weight as below) + heparin 1000 IU ip. Fluid should be instilled over at least 30 min and remain in peritoneal cavity for ≥6 h. Also give ciprofloxacin 1 g po stat.
- Start ciprofloxacin 500 mg po 12 hly thereafter.
- Continue heparin whilst bags remain cloudy.
- Dose of ip vancomycin: 20–40 kg, 1 g; 40–70 kg, 1.5 g; ≥70 kg, 2 g. Subsequent doses of vancomycin are given at 7-day intervals (i.e. days 7 and 14). Levels should be measured between days 1 and 7. These are likely to be higher than usually encountered, but doses should only be reduced if levels exceed 60 mg/L.
- If Gram-positive organism is isolated, discontinue ciprofloxacin and continue vancomycin for 14 days (i.e. three doses). If Gram-negative organism isolated, stop vancomycin and continue ciprofloxacin for 14 days (or modify according to results of culture). If there is no growth after 4 days and there have been no previous episodes of Gram-negative peritonitis, stop ciprofloxacin and continue vancomycin for 14 days.

# Spontaneous bacterial peritonitis

**Risk factors:** Cirrhosis, nephrotic syndrome, girls under 10 yrs with no previous history of ill health.

**Clinical features:** As for peritonitis above, although presentation in the cirrhotic patient may be clinically silent.

**Organisms:** Cirrhosis: coliforms, *Streptococcus pneumoniae*, other *Streptococcus* spp.; Nephrotic patients and young girls: *Streptococcus pneumoniae*, β-haemolytic streptococci.

**Microbiological investigations:** Culture of blood and peritoneal fluid. Peritoneal aspiration should always be carried out in cirrhotic and nephrotic patients who are non-specifically unwell. WBC >250 cells/μL suggests infection.

**Antibiotic management:** Initially parenteral cephalosporin **or** benzylpenicillin + gentamicin, then guided by the results of culture.

## Intra-abdominal abscess

**Risk factors:** Appendicitis, diverticulitis, pancreatitis, genitourinary tract disease, biliary disease. Less commonly tumour, trauma, perforated peptic ulcer.

**Clinical features:** Fever, abdominal pain and sometimes localizing signs such as a palpable mass, depending on the underlying pathology.

**Organisms:** Coliforms, anaerobes, streptococci including *Streptococcus 'milleri'*, *Enterococcus* spp. Actinomycosis may develop in longstanding abscesses (➤321).

**Investigations:** Blood culture. Aspiration of pus if possible. Ultrasound, CT and radiolabelled white cell scans are used to establish the size and site of the abscess.

**Antibiotic management:** In the absence of material for microbiology, benzylpenicillin + gentamicin + metronidazole **or** parenteral cephalosporin + metronidazole **or** co-amoxiclav. Vancomycin + gentamicin + metronidazole may be needed in the penicillin- and cephalosporin-allergic patient.

**Supportive management:** Drainage is almost always required; in some cases, this can be achieved by percutaneous drainage under radiological guidance. For a well-localized appendix abscess, when there is no evidence of generalized peritonitis, patients are frequently treated with antibiotics and observed. Two-thirds will settle and can then have interval appendicectomy. If the clinical state deteriorates, urgent surgery is required.

Management of abscesses at particular sites, such as in the pancreas, spleen or liver is discussed separately below.

## Diverticulitis

Diverticula are small herniations of the colonic mucosa. Diverticulosis is common and increasing in incidence in the developed world. Infection of a diverticulum leads to diverticulitis, which results from pericolic inflammation and microabscess formation. Generalized peritonitis or abscess may also develop.

**Clinical features:** Abdominal pain and tenderness, frequently left lower quadrant ('left-sided appendicitis'), fever, nausea and vomiting. There may be a palpable mass.

**Organisms:** As for intra-abdominal abscess.

**Microbiological investigations:** Blood cultures if systemically affected.

**Other investigations:** Usually none acutely. After acute symptoms have settled, sigmoidoscopy and barium enema may be needed to exclude other pathology.

**Differential diagnosis:** Carcinoma of the colon, inflammatory bowel disease, mesenteric ischaemia and pelvic inflammatory disease.

**Antibiotic management:** Intravenous antibiotics as for intra-abdominal abscess.

**Supportive management:** Nasogastric aspiration. Intravenous fluids.

## Pyogenic liver abscess

A collection of pus within the liver parenchyma, usually secondary to infection elsewhere in the abdomen.

**Risk factors:** Cholangitis, haematogenous spread from the gut via the portal vein ('portal pyaemia'), most often secondary to appendicitis, direct extension from contiguous infection, post-traumatic, secondary infection of liver tumour; 20% of cases are of unknown cause. Compared with amoebic abscess, patients are older and lack a recent travel history, and pyogenic abscesses are often multiple/multilocular.

**Clinical features:** Fever, nausea and vomiting, weight loss. Right upper quadrant tenderness, hepatomegaly, jaundice, raised right hemidiaphragm and pleural effusion.

**Organisms:** Frequently mixed: coliforms, anaerobes, streptococci (in particular *Streptococcus 'milleri'*, *Enterococcus* spp.), *Staphylococcus aureus*, *Pseudomonas* spp.

> **Practice point**
>
> Suspect amoebic liver abscess (➤219) in a patient with high fever and rigors and a travel history. Early USS liver scan is required.

**Microbiological investigations:** Culture of abscess contents is essential. Blood culture.

**Other investigations:** Leucocytosis, raised alkaline phosphatase, milder elevations of transaminases and bilirubin. Reduced albumin. Ultrasound or CT will be required to establish the size and site, and guide aspiration.

**Differential diagnosis:** Cholangitis, amoebic liver abscess, subphrenic abscess, tumour.

**Antibiotic management:** Guided by the results of microbiology: initial therapy as for intra-abdominal abscess above. Prolonged therapy is required to prevent relapse: at least 1 month, increasing to 4 months in the case of multiple abscesses.

**Supportive management:** Drainage is the most important component of therapy. Percutaneous drain insertion under USS or CT control may be possible.

## Pancreatic abscess

Acute pancreatitis is a sterile process, and antibiotics do not accelerate recovery, except in the presence of intercurrent biliary disease.

Pancreatic abscess refers to a collection of infected pus in the pancreas or due to an infected pseudocyst. Abscess complicates ≈5% of cases of acute pancreatitis, and is commoner when pancreatitis is secondary to biliary disease. Prophylactic antibiotics do not reduce this incidence.

**Clinical features:** Fever, abdominal pain and tenderness, ileus, persisting for greater than 10 days in a patient presenting with acute pancreatitis.

**Organisms:** Coliforms, enterococci, occasionally *Staphylococcus aureus*. Anaerobic infection is unusual, but superinfection with yeasts (particularly *Candida albicans*) is common.

**Microbiological investigations:** Blood culture and culture of aspirated pus if possible.

**Other investigations:** Leucocytosis and raised serum amylase are common, but do not distinguish from acute non-infective pancreatitis. Air bubbles in the pancreas on plain X-ray are pathognomonic. Ultrasound, CT and radio-labelled white cell scan will demonstrate the collection. CT scanning is the modality of choice, and may also allow guided aspiration and drainage.

**Antibiotic management:** Antibiotics are given to prevent bacteraemia and aid healing. Benzylpenicillin + gentamicin **or** parenteral cephalosporin. Metronidazole is added if clinical response is poor, or if investigation of aspirated material suggests anaerobic infection. Antifungal treatment may also be required ☏ (➤371).

**Supportive management:** Drainage, either at laparotomy or percutaneously under radiological control, is required.

**Complications:** Probably as a result of activated pancreatic enzymes, pancreatic abscesses have a tendency to spread, unlike other intra-abdominal collections. Extension may occur along the retroperitoneum in any direction, and pancreatic abscesses may extend and discharge at distant sites, e.g. the scrotum or the neck.

# Splenic abscess

**Risk factors:** Splenic abscesses arise in three situations:
• Metastatic seeding during bacteraemia. This accounts for the majority of cases and is particularly common in IVDUs and may accompany IE (➤51).
• Secondary to infection associated with infarction from blunt trauma or haemoglobinopathy.
• By direct extension from contiguous infection in the abdomen.

**Clinical features:** Fever, left upper quadrant pain. Left-sided chest signs, e.g. pleural effusion. Splenomegaly is present in 50%. Splenic rub is rare. Multilocular splenic abscesses are much more likely to be clinically silent and carry a higher mortality.

**Organisms:** Depending on the clinical situation: *Staphylococcus aureus* ($\approx$25%, particularly likely in IVDUs), coliforms ($\approx$25%), enterococci ($\approx$10%), *Salmonella* spp. (particularly in patients with AIDS, who may also develop splenic abscess due to MAI ➤168). Fungi (*Candida* spp., *Aspergillus* spp.) are increasing in frequency and are hospital-acquired. Anaerobes ($\approx$20%). Mixed infections are common.

**Microbiological investigations:** Culture of blood and aspirated material if available. Resected spleen should be submitted for culture.

**Other investigations:** Ultrasound, radionuclear white cell scan and CT scan; CT is superior for multilocular abscesses. IE should be suspected and excluded (➤49).

**Antibiotic management:** As for intra-abdominal abscess, then guided by microbiology results. Blood culture is positive in $\approx$50% of cases.

**Supportive management:** Splenectomy is almost always required.

# Retroperitoneal abscess

**Risk factors:** Direct extension of pyelonephritis, spinal osteomyelitis, other intra-abdominal sepsis, traumatic haemorrhage, bacteraemia.

**Clinical features:** Fever, abdominal pain, flank and lumbar pain. A palpable mass may be present. If extension into the psoas sheath has occurred, there may be pain on hip flexion.

**Organisms:** *Staphylococcus aureus*, often with a history of cutaneous infection. Coliforms, particularly if secondary to pyelonephritis. Less often mixed infections including anaerobes. See also vertebral osteomyelitis (➤124). Rarely *Mycobacterium tuberculosis*.

**Microbiological investigations:** Culture of blood and aspirated material if available.

**Other investigations:** Plain X-ray, CT and radionuclear white cell scan.

**Antibiotic management:** Benzylpenicillin + gentamicin + metronidazole **or** parenteral cephalosporin + metronidazole, depending on risk factors and guided by microbiology.

**Supportive management:** Surgical drainage is required.

# Chapter 7

# Hepatitis

The clinical features of acute viral hepatitis are similar for all hepatitis viruses, although they differ considerably in severity, tempo and likelihood of progression to chronic infection. Many other viruses cause hepatitis as part of systemic infection, including EBV, CMV and yellow fever virus. Hepatitis also occurs with bacterial infections, either as part of a specific syndrome, such as leptospirosis, or as a non-specific feature of severe sepsis. Acute hepatitis is also caused by drugs, e.g. alcohol, chlorpromazine, antituberculous drugs and halothane.

**Clinical features:** Anorexia, nausea and vomiting. Fever, chills, headache, fatigue and myalgia. Right upper quadrant pain and tenderness. Jaundice develops in a proportion of patients, initially with pale stools and dark urine. The speed of onset and clinical course varies depending on the virus involved. Patients usually feel better with the onset of jaundice.

**Fulminant hepatitis** describes the development of liver failure during viral hepatitis. **Cholestatic hepatitis** is characterized by prolonged severe jaundice with pruritis persisting for several months after the acute attack.

## Hepatitis A (HAV) ✉ ② (➤348)

**Transmission:** Faeco-oral, either by contaminated water/food or person-to-person. Infection is widespread in the developing world, affecting mainly children. In the UK, infection is commoner with low socio-economic status. Outbreaks occur in institutions, particularly primary schools.

**Incubation period:** 2–6 weeks.

**Clinical features:** Usually asymptomatic under

2 yrs of age; 70% of adults become jaundiced. Onset occurs over days.

**Progression to chronic liver disease:** Does not occur.

**Complications:** Fulminant hepatitis is rare (<0.2%). Cholestatic hepatitis (very rare). Relapsing hepatitis occurs, but is very rare.

**Serodiagnosis:** Total Ig or IgG indicate previous exposure. Anti-HAV IgM indicates recent infection and is required for diagnosis of current hepatitis.

**Immunization:** ➤192.

**Treatment of contacts:** Close personal contacts should receive pooled human immunoglobulin. They should also receive active immunization with an accelerated schedule (➤192). Immunization may also be required to terminate outbreaks in institutions.

**Isolation policy:** If patients require hospitalization, ②. Virus is present in stools for 1–2 weeks before the onset of jaundice and for 1 week after.

## Hepatitis B (HBV) ✉③ (➤344)

A full account of the replication cycle of HBV is beyond our scope. HBV replication involves reverse transcription of RNA to DNA. This step is the target for lamivudine therapy.

**Transmission:** Parenteral. Transmission occurs through percutaneous exposure (needle-stick, needle-sharing, blood transfusion), sexual contact and vertically by maternal–neonatal infection. Maternofetal transmission occurs, but accounts for only 5% of vertical transmission.

**Epidemiology:** Very common worldwide—up to 20% of the population of SE Asia and sub-Saharan Africa have evidence of previous infection, and there are >170 million chronically infected persons. Vertical transmission is common in endemic areas. Affected children are usually infected at birth and become carriers. Immunization of neonates (active immunization plus immunoglobulin, ➤73) reduces vertical transmission by ≈90%. Infection is rarer in the developed world. Groups at particular risk include IVDUs, homosexual men, prostitutes, health-care workers, haemodialysis patients (now regularly screened). Σ ≈1000 notifications p.a.

**Incubation period:** 2–6 months.

**Clinical features:** Usually asymptomatic in infants; 25% of adults have jaundice. Onset usually insidious. Occasionally associated with 'serum sickness'-like illness attributed to immune complex deposition with symmetrical distal polyarthritis, angio-oedema, urticaria and rarely glomerulonephritis.

**Complications:** Fulminant hepatitis is rare (≈1%). Cholestatic hepatitis (very rare).

**Progression to chronic liver disease:** 95% of acute cases recover completely. Chronic infection with development of chronic active hepatitis develops in ≈5%. In these patients, there is an estimated annual incidence of cirrhosis of ≈2.5% (≈15% at 5 yrs). Hepatocellular carcinoma (HCC) occurs mainly in patients with cirrhosis, but can occur in context of chronic active hepatitis.

**Serodiagnosis:** There are several serological markers of HBV infection:

**HBV surface antigen (HBsAg)** is the key marker of HBV infection, present in serum during acute and chronic infection. HBsAg appears in serum 1–10 weeks after exposure, before the onset of symptoms or raised ALT. In patients who recover, HBsAg becomes un-detectable after 4–6 months. Persistence of HBsAg for more than 6 months implies chronic infection. Clearance of HBsAg is followed by development of **anti-HBs**. Rarely, anti-HBs may not appear until several weeks after HBsAg is lost. During this 'window period', diagnosis is by the detection of IgM anti-HBc. Some HbsAg+ patients also have anti-HBs. They should be regarded as carriers.

**HBV core antigen (HBcAg)** is an intracellular protein, which is not found in serum. Anti-HBc IgM is detected during acute infection and may be the only indicator of HBV if there is a window period (see above). IgM may remain detectable up to years after the acute infection, and may reappear during exacerbations of chronic hepatitis B. **IgG anti-HBc** persists life-long, with anti-HBs in patients who recover, and with HBsAg in chronic infection. Isolated anti-HBc with neither HBsAg nor anti-HBs sometimes occurs and indicates either (i) the window period of acute hepatitis B (mostly IgM); (ii) many years after recovery from acute hepatitis B when anti-HBs has fallen to un-detectable levels; or (iii) after many years of chronic HBV infection when the HBsAg has been cleared (which occurs in ≈1% of carriers). Individuals with isolated anti-HBc may be infectious, and will not be detected if HBsAg is used as the only screening test for infectivity.

**Hepatitis B e antigen (HBeAg)** is a marker of viral replication and high infectivity; usually associated with the presence of HBV DNA in serum. Loss of HBeAg and development of **anti-HBe** occurs early during acute infection, before HBsAg to anti-HBs seroconversion. In chronic infection, HBeAg may persist and is associated with high infectivity ('supercarriers') and active liver disease. Loss of HBeAg and development of anti-HBe is usually associated with the loss of HBV DNA from serum and remission of hepatitis. Some patients continue to have active liver disease and detectable HBV DNA after HBeAg seroconversion. In some cases, this is due to the presence of a mutation that prevents the production of HBeAg (so-called 'precore mutants').

**HBV DNA** can be detected in serum by a variety of methods; PCR is most widely used, and current assays have a sensitivity of 50 copies/mL. After apparent recovery from acute HBV, DNA may remain detectable by PCR in serum for many years, suggesting that virus persists after 'recovery' but is contained by the immune system. HBV DNA levels may be used to determine the likelihood of response to therapy, to assess response to therapy and to determine infectivity in health-care workers.

**Serodiagnosis in practice:**

•   **Diagnosis of cause of jaundice:** HBsAg is present in serum from 1 to 7 weeks before the onset of jaundice and for up to 6 weeks thereafter in uncomplicated cases. Approximately 15% of cases will be HBsAg-negative by the time they present. They will have IgM anti-HBC antibodies. IgG anti-HBC indicates previous exposure but does not establish the cause of recent disease.

•   **Assessment of infectivity and risk of progression:** HBsAg indicates that the patient is potentially infectious and is at risk of progression to chronic hepatitis. Ninety-nine per cent of patients developing chronic hepatitis are HBsAg-positive. HBeAg implies very high infectivity and increased risk of progression.

•   **Clinical staff doing 'exposure-prone' procedures (EPP):** Current UK Department of Health guidelines stipulate that all such staff must be immunized against HBV infection. Staff who are HBeAg-positive must not carry out such procedures. Staff with evidence of HBV infection but who are HBeAg-negative are tested for HBV DNA; if >1000 copies/mL, then they are considered infectious and must not perform EPP.

🖳 tap.ccta.gov.uk/doh/coin4.nsf/page/HSC-
2000-020

**Management:** The management of cirrhosis, and the role of transplantation are beyond the scope of this manual.

Specific antiviral therapy is now available for chronic HBV; this rapidly-evolving area is a specialist subject ☏. **Interferon alpha** (IFN) is recommended for patients with positive HBeAg, positive HBV DNA, raised ALT and chronic hepatitis on liver biopsy. Treatment is associated with a transient rise in ALT and is

effective in ≈35% of patients; benefit is usually sustained in those who respond initially. Factors predicting a good response to therapy include high ALT, low DNA, active histology, female sex, adult-acquired HBV and absence of coinfection with HCV and HIV. Duration of therapy is usually 3–6 months (longer in some groups, e.g. those with precore mutants). Long-term efficacy in terms of prevention of cirrhosis and HCC remains to be seen, but early studies suggest that progression is rare in responders. Pegylated IFN probably gives a better response rate. **Lamivudine**, originally developed as an anti-HIV drug (➤150), is also active against HBV. It is well tolerated and treatment for 12 months is associated with normalization of the serum ALT in ≈50–70% of patients, HBeAg loss in ≈30% and HBeAg seroconversion in ≈15–20%. Lamivudine-resistant mutants arise in 15–30% at the end of year of treatment, and in 60% after 3 yrs. Lamivudine appears to be effective in patients with precore mutants. Other antiviral agents with activity against HBV include tenofovir (➤150) and famciclovir (➤361). Monotherapy with a single antiviral agent or interferon is unlikely to be sufficient for the eradication of HBV infection in the majority of patients who are chronically infected. The role of combination therapy for hepatitis B is currently being defined. Up-to-date guidelines can be found at:

🖳

www.aasld.org/pdffiles/chronichepatolendorse.pdf

**Immunization:** Effective vaccine containing recombinant HBV surface antigen is available and is recommended in the UK for high-risk groups including:

•   IVDUs.

•   Individuals who change sexual partners frequently (including homosexuals).

•   Close family contacts of a case or carrier.

•   Haemophiliacs and others receiving regular blood products, and their carers.

•   Patients with chronic renal failure (including haemodialysis).

•   Health-care personnel and other occupational risk groups such as morticians and embalmers.

•   Staff and patients of day-care or residential

accommodation for those with severe learning difficulties.

• Inmates of custodial institutions.

• Those travelling to areas of high prevalence who are at increased risk or who plan to remain there for lengthy periods (➤194).

• Families adopting children from countries with a high prevalence of hepatitis B.

Vaccine should also be given to infants born to mothers who *either* have had hepatitis B during pregnancy, *or* are positive for both hepatitis B surface antigen and hepatitis B e antigen *or* are surface antigen-positive without e markers (or where they have not been determined); active immunization of the infant is started immediately after delivery, and hepatitis B immunoglobulin is given at the same time as the vaccine. Infants born to mothers who are positive for hepatitis B surface antigen and for e antigen antibody should receive the vaccine but not the immunoglobulin.

Vaccine is usually given at months 0, 1 and 6, and takes up to 6 months to confer adequate protection; the duration of immunity is not known precisely, but a single booster 5 yrs after the primary course may be sufficient to maintain immunity for those who continue to be at risk. Immunized health-care workers usually have the level of anti-HBsAg antibodies estimated to determine the need for further doses of vaccine. It is currently believed that once an individual has achieved a protective level (>100 miU/mL), no further boosters are required.

Specific hepatitis B immunoglobulin (HBIG) is available for use with the vaccine in infants and in post-exposure prophylaxis.

Action to be taken after accidental exposure to possible HBV depends on the HBV status of the source patient (positive, negative or unknown) and the vaccination status of the injured person. If the injured person is not known to be immune, and the source is not known to be HBsAg-negative, then an accelerated course of vaccine should be given (months 0, 1 and 2). If the source is known or strongly suspected to be HBsAg-positive, then HBIG should also be given. Health-care workers who are known to be vaccine non-responders should receive HBIG. For PEP against HIV ➤155.

A combined hepatitis A and hepatitis B vaccine is also available (➤192).

In many countries with high HBV seroprevalence, universal immunization against HBV is carried out, and there are moves to introduce this in the UK.

**Isolation policy:** ③ At home, transmission may occur by sharing of razors, toothbrushes etc., and patients should be aware of this. Vaccination is recommended for sexual partners and close household contacts.

## Hepatitis D (HDV, Delta virus) ✉

**Virus:** An RNA virus which is defective in the sense that it requires HBV for its replication.

**Transmission:** As for HBV.

**Incubation period:** Days to weeks.

**Clinical features:** Acute hepatitis, often in a patient previously known to be HBsAg positive. Infection with HBV and HDV may be simultaneous, in which case the illness is indistinguishable from HBV infection alone, although there may be higher incidence of fulminant liver failure.

**Progression to chronic liver disease:** The risk of progression to CAH and cirrhosis, and the incidence of HCC are increased by HDV superinfection in a patient already infected with HBV.

**Serodiagnosis:** Anti-HDV IgG and IgM, and HDV antigen and RNA can be demonstrated in serum.

**Immunization:** Not available.

## Hepatitis C (HCV) ✉ (➤354)

**Transmission:** Parenteral. HCV accounts for 90% of transfusion-associated hepatitis; blood is now screened for HCV and post-transfusion hepatitis is now rare. Seroprevalence in UK IVDUs is typically 60–80%. Transmission to health-care workers by needle-stick has been reported; estimated overall risk ≈3% per event (➤155). Sexual transmission occurs but appears to be infrequent; prevalence in monogamous partners of HCV+ patients is ≈5%. Vertical transmission occurs; risk is ≈5%, ≈10% if mother is HIV+.

**Incubation period:** 2–26 weeks, mean 8 weeks.

**Clinical features:** Frequently asymptomatic. Less than 25% of adults are jaundiced, and fulminant hepatitis is extremely rare. Several extrahepatic disorders are associated with chronic viraemic HCV, including cryoglobulinaemia, lymphoma, cutaneous vasculitis, Raynaud's disease, porphyria cutanea tarda, arthralgia, neuropathy, sicca syndrome, glomerulonephritis and autoimmune thyroid disease.

**Progression to chronic liver disease:** Chronic infection develops in ≥80% of patients, most of whom will have persistently abnormal LFTs, detectable HCV RNA by PCR and abnormal liver histology. Progression to cirrhosis is typically slow (median 30 yrs in one meta-analysis ⌐ Poynard, Lancet 1997; 349: 825) thus, the true lifetime incidence of cirrhosis and hepatocellular carcinoma (HCC) has been difficult to define. Currently estimated that ≈50% of infected persons will develop cirrhosis, and ≈10% will have clinically significant liver disease. The 10-yr survival after diagnosis of compensated cirrhosis is ≈80%; 5-yr survival after decompensated cirrhosis is ≈50%. High level of viraemia, genotype 1 (esp. 1b), high degree of viral genetic diversity, male sex, age >40 yrs, alcohol intake >50 g/day, acquisition by blood transfusion and coinfection with HIV or HBV all predict more rapid progression.

**Diagnosis:** Early antibody tests lacked sensitivity and specificity, but modern ELISA is sensitive and specific and becomes positive a mean of 10 weeks after infection. PCR for HCV RNA is routinely available. Twenty per cent of patients with antibodies will have persistently negative PCR; these have a good prognosis and are almost certainly not infectious. Positive PCR indicates chronic infection and is usually associated with histological abnormalities on liver biopsy. PCR can also be used to diagnose infection before the development of positive antibody tests, e.g. after known exposure, or in patient coinfected with HIV who may not mount an antibody response. Quantitative PCR is available. High level viraemia (>2 × $10^6$ copies/mL) is associated with worse prognosis and implies need for extended duration of therapy. Similar molecular techniques are used to determine genotype. Genotypes 1–3 are common; 1, and esp. 1b, are associated with worse prognosis and reduced response to therapy. ALT is often elevated in chronic infection, but does not correlate well with histology.

**Immunization:** Not available.

**Management:** Subcutaneous interferon alpha (IFN-α) results in normalization of ALT, loss of viraemia and improvements in histology in some patients. Several trials have demonstrated improvements in response rates with combination of IFN-α and ribavarin (RBV). RBV alone is not effective. Host factors (female sex, low alcohol intake, youth) and viral factors (nongenotype 1) predict better response to therapy. Pegylated interferon is IFN-α covalently attached to polyethylene glycol, resulting in a preparation which can be injected once weekly, achieves sustained IFN-α levels and improves response rate. Response rates vary from ≈5% for IFN-α monotherapy with genotype 1, to ≈80% with pegIFN-α/RBV in patients with genotype 2 or 3. Side effects of therapy include myelosuppression, depression and haemolysis. Current UK guidelines recommend 6 months of IFN-α/RBV for patients whose liver biopsies show moderate fibrosis or inflammation, extended to 12 months if genotype 1 and HCV RNA >2 × $10^6$ copies/mL. US guidelines are broadly similar, but suggest that patients with normal ALT should not undergo biopsy and should be treated expectantly. This is a rapidly evolving field, and therapy should only be undertaken in specialist centres ☎.

🖥 odp.od.nih.gov/consensus/cons/
105/105_statement.htm

🖥 www.bsg.org.uk/pdf_word_docs/
clinguidehepc.pdf

**Table 7.1** Causes of granulomatous hepatitis

| Category | Conditions |
| --- | --- |
| **Infections** | |
| Mycobacteria | ***Mycobacterium tuberculosis*** (the commonest cause worldwide ➤38), *Mycobacterium leprae* (➤46), atypical mycobacteria (➤47) |
| Bacteria | *Brucella* spp.(➤303), *Francisella tularensis* (➤284), *Yersinia enterocolitica* (➤293), *Burkholderia pseudomallei* (➤307) |
| Spirochaetes | *Treponema pallidum* (➤89) |
| Fungi | Blastomycosis (➤370), histoplasmosis (➤369), coccidioidomycosis (➤369), cryptococcosis (➤368). |
| Protozoa | *Leishmania major* (➤222), ***Toxoplasma gondii*** (➤137) |
| Helminths | ***Schistosoma* spp.**(➤226), *Toxocara canis* (➤236), *Ascaris lumbricoides* (➤233) |
| Rickettsia | *Coxiella burnetti* (➤332), *Rickettsia conori* (➤329) |
| Viruses | EBV (➤133), CMV (➤339) |
| **Non-infectious causes** | |
| Chemicals | Beryllium, copper, drugs |
| Others | **Sarcoidosis**, Crohn's disease, ulcerative colitis, primary biliary cirrhosis, hypogammaglobulinaemia, systemic lupus erythematosus, **Hodgkin's lymphoma** |

Commoner causes in **bold** type.

# Hepatitis E (HEV) ✉

**Virus:** A newly recognized RNA virus, with similarities to caliciviruses (➤350).

**Transmission:** Faeco-oral, as for HAV. Typically waterborne. Prevalent in the developing world, esp. Asia, Africa, Middle East, and Central America, where it is a common cause of hepatitis in adults. Person-to-person spread is unusual.

**Incubation period:** 15–60 days.

**Clinical features:** Usually more severe than HAV, with a much higher incidence of fulminant hepatic failure. The mortality is particularly high during pregnancy, up to 25%. Vertical infection occurs and neonatal infection can be severe or fatal.

**Progression to chronic liver disease:** Does not occur.

**Serodiagnosis:** Antibody testing is now widely available, but antigen testing is only available via research laboratories.

# Hepatitis G

Two flaviviruses, hepatitis G virus (HGV) and hepatitis GB virus type C (HGBV-C), have recently been described and subsequently been shown to be virtually identical isolates of the same virus. HGV is distributed worldwide, and can be transmitted by blood transfusion. Prevalence in blood donors is ≈1.7% (USA), but is higher in groups with risk factors for other blood-borne viruses, e.g. 11% in Japanese HCV patients, ≈20% in some studies of dialysis patients. The exact role, if any, of HGV in producing disease in humans remains unclear, and there is no clear evidence that it causes hepatitis. Follow-up of IVDUs over a 6.5-yr period in one US centre found evidence of HGV infection (either RNA or antibody) in 110 of 116 patients followed. Seventy had anti-HGV antibodies but were never positive for HGV RNA, 40 had HGV RNA but no antibody. All eight patients who cleared HGV RNA were antibody-positive, and there were no new infections in 61 antibody-positive subjects. Thus, anti-HGV antibodies appear to be highly associated with viral clearance and protection from reinfection. Evidence is accumulating for a protective effect of chronic HGV infection on patients coinfected with HIV.

## Granulomatous hepatitis

The discovery of granulomata at liver biopsy is not unusual. Often the diagnosis is obvious in the context of the patient's other signs. In many cases this is not so, and the diagnosis may be found among the conditions listed in Table 7.1. In most series, ≈10% remain undiagnosed.

# Chapter 8

# Urinary tract infection (UTI)

UTI covers a spectrum of illness from asymptomatic bacteriuria to acute pyelonephritis (APN) with septic shock. **Cystitis** describes a superficial mucosal infection confined to the lower urinary tract (UT). **APN** is due to infection and inflammation of the renal parenchyma. **Chronic pyelonephritis** is a histological pattern of diffuse interstitial inflammation which may be due to many causes, some of them infective. It may follow acute pyelonephritis in childhood, particularly in association with vesicoureteral reflux (VUR).

UTI may be usefully classified into uncomplicated (acute cystitis in females) and complicated (UTI with APN in females, all UTIs in males). Special cases include children, UTI during pregnancy and catheter-associated infections.

Community-acquired UTI usually occurs by ascending infection following colonization of the vagina, periurethral area and anterior urethra by uropathogenic bacteria.

**Risk factors:** Vary with age:
• Neonates–1 yr: Functional or anatomical abnormalities (e.g. congenital stenosis, urethral valves).
• 1–15 yrs: Infection more common in girls, particularly associated with VUR. Infection during first 5 yrs is associated with VUR or congenital abnormalities and may give rise to renal scarring and subsequent risk of chronic pyelonephritis.
• 16–35 yrs: Risk of infection increases in females, associated with sexual intercourse. Diaphragm and spermicide use convey higher risk.
• After 35 yrs the sex incidence starts to equalize—risk factors include gynaecological surgery and bladder prolapse in women, prostatic hypertrophy and chronic prostatitis in men and stones, tumours and catheter use in both sexes.
• Prolonged recumbency, catheter use, dehydration and antibiotic use, which promote introital colonization and cross-infection by uropathogenic strains, increase the risk of UTI for hospital in-patients.

UTI is normally prevented by mucosal defences (e.g. secreted proteins which prevent bacterial adhesion), the composition of the urine (low pH, high urea, high osmolarity) and mechanical factors (e.g. regular complete emptying of the bladder).

**Clinical features: Adults**: Dysuria, urgency, frequency, low-grade fever, suprapubic discomfort and cloudy, bloodstained urine. Flank pain and tenderness with rigors and vomiting suggest APN, but lack of these clinical features does not reliably exclude it. **Young children** present more non-specifically with fever, abdominal pain, vomiting and poor feeding. **Infection in neonates** presents as failure to thrive, vomiting, fever and jaundice and is frequently associated with bacteraemia. **UTI in the elderly** is common and may present non-specifically with nocturia, incontinence and confusion.

**Organisms:** *Escherichia coli* (80%)—a limited range of *E. coli* serogroups which have surface molecules that allow them to adhere to UT epithelium ('adhesins') are 'uropathogenic', accounting for most UTIs (➤278). Other coliforms such as *Klebsiella* spp., *Proteus* spp., *Enterobacter* spp. are isolated less often, but are more likely to be antibiotic-resistant. *Staphylococcus saprophyticus* is a relatively common cause of uncomplicated UTI in young women. Hospital infections (particularly catheter-associated or in patients on antibiotics) are associated with a wider range of organisms, including *Pseudomonas aeruginosa, Staphylococcus epidermidis,* yeasts and *Enterococcus* spp. *Staphylococcus aureus* bacteriuria may follow haematogenous seeding of the kidney from infection elsewhere. Adenovirus infection is a rare cause of epidemic haemorrhagic cystitis in children.

**Microbiological investigations:** It is good practice to send a mid-stream urine (MSU) for microscopy and culture in all patients before starting therapy. Some question the cost-effectiveness of this in uncomplicated UTI, but it allows monitoring of antibiotic resistance rates. Dipstix have a high false-negative rate and are not cost- or clinically effective. **Interpreting the results of MSU:** Epithelial cells suggest contamination of the specimen by skin organisms. Pus cells are usually present in UTI. Their absence favours contamination. Pyuria without bacterial growth may be due to previous antibiotics, tumour, stones, urethritis or tuberculosis. A bacterial count of $>10^5$ organisms/mL is considered to indicate UTI, but many patients with clinical evidence of infection have lower counts. Some authorities consider counts over $10^2$ organisms/mL significant if they represent a pure growth of a known urinary pathogen, but few laboratories culture to detect this low level. Suprapubic puncture is rarely used, but is useful if an aseptically taken specimen is essential. Blood cultures should be taken if systemic infection is a possibility. Chlamydial infection may need to be excluded (➤87).

**Other investigations:** Urological assessment (ultrasound scan, in the first instance, followed by IVP) for **stones, tumours and anatomical abnormalities** should be carried out in recurrent uncomplicated UTI, all complicated UTIs and in all males, children and infants. Rectal examination is required in men.

**Differential diagnosis:** Urethritis is suggested by pyuria without bacteriuria. Historical clues include a change in sexual partner, gradual onset of relatively mild dysuria, urethral or vaginal discharge and associated cervicitis (➤87). Candidal or bacterial vaginitis and genital herpes often cause burning 'external'

dysuria. Genitourinary tuberculosis should be considered, especially in the elderly and in immigrants.

**Antibiotic management:** All symptomatic UTIs should be treated. For **uncomplicated UTI**, a large range of oral antibiotics is available: trimethoprim, co-amoxiclav, oral cephalosporin (e.g. cephalexin) norfloxacin or ciprofloxacin. Amoxicillin is less suitable due to ≈50% resistance rates. Single-dose oral therapy (SDT) with co-amoxiclav (500/125 mg), norfloxacin (400 mg) or trimethoprim (400 mg) is slightly less effective than treatment for 7 days, but has a lower incidence of side effects. Three-day treatment regimens are as effective as 7-day schedules, with no more side effects than SDT, and are recommended for uncomplicated UTI when there is no suggestion of upper tract involvement, or complication such as pregnancy. Short-course therapy is not suitable for children. For **complicated UTI**, 7–14 days' treatment is recommended (APN: 14 days). In **severe illness**, intravenous therapy is required initially. Amoxicillin + gentamicin **or** co-amoxiclav **or** cefotaxime **or** ciprofloxacin are all suitable whilst awaiting the results of urine and blood cultures. All empirical regimens should be based on local contemporary resistance data.

**Supportive management:** Patients should drink as much fluid as possible. Intravenous rehydration may be necessary particularly if vomiting is a prominent symptom. Urinary obstruction is the most common cause of treatment failure and will require surgery or nephrostomy. In hyperglycaemic diabetics, fermentation of glucose by coliforms can produce gas in the renal parenchyma (emphysematous pyelonephritis). Less severe cases may be managed medically, but surgery, including nephrectomy, may be required.

**Complications:** Renal abscess, bacteraemia with sepsis syndrome.

## Asymptomatic bacteriuria

The prevalence of asymptomatic bacteriuria is 1% in children and rises to 4% in adult women and 10–20% in elderly women. The significance of this finding varies with the clinical context. Pregnant women should be screened for bacteriuria at booking and treated (10–14 days normally recommended) if two MSUs are positive. UTI is common during pregnancy, often develops into APN (≈30%) and may result in prematurity and fetal loss. Amoxicillin, cefalexin and nitrofurantoin are safe. **Avoid** tetracyclines (dental discoloration), fluoro-quinolones (possible fetal arthropathy) and trimethoprim (risk of teratogenicity) during pregnancy, and sulphonamides (risk of neo-natal jaundice) during the last trimester. Monthly MSUs should then be performed until delivery. There is little evidence that treating adults, including the elderly, with asympto-matic bacteriuria is beneficial except in patients with neutropenia or immunosuppression. Children should be treated with antibiotics, and investigated for UT abnormality.

## Catheter-associated UTI

The risk of bacteriuria with an indwelling catheter is proportional to duration since inser-tion, and is reduced by careful asepsis during insertion and maintenance of a closed system of drainage. Infection is often asymptomatic, but is the commonest cause of hospital-acquired Gram-negative bacteraemia. Scrupulous aseptic technique at insertion may delay infection. Many recommend a single-dose of intravenous gentamicin at catheterization. Asymptomatic catheter UTI should not be treated. If infection is symptomatic, it is unlikely to be eradicated by antibiotics whilst the catheter remains *in situ*. Try to remove the catheter, begin treatment and then recatheterize if necessary. Antiseptic or antibiotic irrigation is of no benefit.

## Acute urethral syndrome (AUS)

This describes acute dysuria and frequency in women whose MSU is sterile or contains only low bacterial counts. Vaginitis and sexually transmitted causes of urethritis should be excluded. Most women with this syndrome have acute bacterial urethrocystitis, and should be treated with antibiotics as above.

## Recurrent UTI

Many women have occasional attacks of cystitis, but some have frequent recurrences (e.g. more than twice/yr). Patients with recurrent UTI require urological evaluation for UT abnormal-ity, but in the majority none will be found. Risk factors such as diaphragm and spermicide use should be avoided, and patients should void after sexual intercourse. Antibiotic pro-phylaxis may be needed. Successful regimens include continuous low-dose therapy (e.g. co-amoxiclav 375 mg q24h, trimethoprim 100 mg q24h, cephalexin 250 mg q24h or norfloxacin 400 mg q24h), self-administered single-dose or short course therapy or postcoital single-dose prophylaxis.

## Acute bacterial prostatitis

**Risk factors:** Usually none; may follow urethral instrumentation or surgery.

**Clinical features:** Fever, perineal pain, symp-toms of UTI. Rectal examination reveals a swollen, tender prostate. Patients are often very unwell with bacteraemia.

**Organisms:** Coliforms including *Escherichia coli* (25%), less often *Pseudomonas aeruginosa*, *Enterococcus* spp.

**Microbiological investigations:** MSU: Pyuria and bacteriuria are usually present. Blood cul-tures if unwell. Results of urine culture should guide antibiotic therapy; prostatic massage is **not** required.

**Antibiotic management:** Ciprofloxacin. Par-enteral cephalosporin if bacteraemic. Anti-biotics should be given for 4 weeks to prevent relapse.

**Complications:** Prostatic abscess may develop. This may rupture spontaneously into the urethra, or more rarely the rectum, or it may require cystoscopic drainage. Urological advice should be sought ☎ and antibiotic cover extended to cover anaerobes.

# Chronic prostatitis

This is a difficult diagnosis to make; urological opinion should be sought. In some men, the prostate may serve as a reservoir of infection, resulting in recurrent UTI. **Prostatic localization studies** involve collecting urine samples before and after prostatic massage. Expressed prostatic secretions are also collected and quantitative bacterial culture is used to determine the likelihood of persistent bacterial prostatitis. There is rarely a history of acute prostatitis. Some patients complain of perineal or low back pain and may have difficulty voiding. The prostate is sometimes tender on palpation. Chronic prostatitis may follow chlamydial urethritis (➤87) and treatment with doxycycline for 4 weeks helps some patients.

# Epididymitis

Inflammation of the epididymis is acquired via ascending infection from the urethra, particularly if the urethra is instrumented in the presence of bacteriuria. Pain, fever and swelling of the epididymis are present and symptoms of concurrent UTI or urethritis may also be present. In sexually active men, infection may follow urethritis due to chlamydiae or *Neisseria gonorrhoea*, which should be treated appropriately (➤87). Non-sexually transmitted epididymitis is caused by coliforms, *Enterococcus* spp. and occasionally *Staphylococcus* spp. or *Streptococcus* spp. Other causes include *Mycoplasma* spp. and viruses. Non-sexually acquired infection should be treated with trimethoprim or a fluoroquinolone for 2 weeks. TB should be considered in appropriate risk groups.

# Orchitis

Orchitis is usually viral, associated in particular with mumps (➤128). Pyogenic orchitis usually arises as a complication of epididymitis, due to the same organisms. Parenteral antibiotics are required and urgent urological advice should be sought, in particular to exclude testicular torsion.

# Intrarenal and perinephric abscess

**Risk factors: Renal cortical abscesses:** haematogenous spread of *Staphylococcus aureus* (most commonly) usually from a skin infection. IVDU, diabetes mellitus and haemodialysis predispose. **Corticomedullary abscesses:** ascending infection usually secondary to UT abnormality, especially calculi and obstruction in adults and vesicoureteric reflux in children.

**Clinical features:** Onset is characteristically insidious. Fever, rigors and flank pain. There may be renal angle tenderness with a flank bulge or kyphosis. Corticomedullary abscess is usually associated with nausea and vomiting and urinary symptoms, but these are usually absent in cortical abscess, which rarely communicates with the lower UT.

**Organisms:** *Staphylococcus aureus* (cortical abscess); coliforms, in particular *Escherichia coli* and *Proteus* spp. (corticomedullary abscess).

**Microbiological investigations:** MSU (often normal in cortical abscess). Blood culture. Culture of aspirated pus.

**Other investigations:** Ultrasound and/or CT scan are required to localize the abscess, and may be used to guide aspiration or percutaneous drain insertion.

**Differential diagnosis:** Renal carcinoma.

**Antibiotic management:** For staphylococcal cortical abscess, high-dose flucloxacillin (2 g 6hly, iv) for 2 weeks (± iv gentamicin or oral fucidin) followed by 2 weeks of oral flucloxacillin. For corticomedullary abscess, gentamicin plus either ampicillin or ciprofloxacin initially, guided thereafter by the results of cultures.

**Supportive management:** Smaller abscesses are treated with antibiotics alone, but large abscesses or those that fail to respond after 2–4 days' therapy with appropriate antibiotics will require drainage (often percutaneous). Obstruction should be relieved if present.

**Complications:** Rupture through the renal capsule leads to **perinephric abscess**. Onset is often insidious, with symptoms as above; extension towards the diaphragm causes pleuritic pain and raised fixed hemidiaphragm with pleural effusion. There may be signs of psoas irritation with scoliosis and pain on hip flexion. Drainage is always required.

Prolonged severe infection, particularly with *Proteus* spp. and obstruction may lead to **xan-thogranulomatous pyelonephritis**. The renal pelvis is dilated, often with a staghorn calculus. There may be an abscess cavity, and the surrounding tissue is replaced by a yellow zone, histology of which shows macrophages laden with cholesterol and lipid material. Nephrectomy is usually required.

**Practice point**

Urine culture positive for *Staphylococcus aureus* in patients who have not been catheterized should suggest previous staphylococcal bacteraemia and possible secondary renal abscess.

# Chapter 9

# Gynaecological and obstetric infections

**Normal flora of the vagina and cervix** include non-sporing anaerobes (not *Bacteroides fragilis* group), lactobacilli, *Staphylococcus epidermidis*, diphtheroids and less commonly coliforms, *Enterococcus* spp., *Candida* spp., group B β-haemolytic streptococci and *Staphylococcus aureus*. The composition of this flora changes before and after puberty and the menopause, and during the menstrual cycle. Use of antibiotics favours an increase in coliforms and *Candida* spp., and a decrease in lactobacilli.

## Vulvovaginal candidiasis

**Risk factors:** Pregnancy, diabetes mellitus, oral contraceptive pill, antibiotics, immunosuppression (e.g. therapeutic or HIV-related (➤160)).

**Clinical features:** Pruritis, 'external' dysuria and dyspareunia, vaginal discharge. On examination, vulval erythema and excoriation and vaginal discharge.

**Organisms:** *Candida albicans* (➤367), less often other *Candida* spp.

**Microbiological investigations:** Gram stain and culture of high vaginal swab (HVS). As *Candida albicans* is a frequent commensal (20% of asymptomatic women), diagnosis depends on the association of positive culture result with appropriate history and clinical findings.

**Differential diagnosis:** Trichomoniasis (➤92), bacterial vaginosis.

**Antibiotic management:** Clotrimazole, econazole and miconazole are all available in a variety of topical preparations, including single-dose pessaries. Nystatin is an alternative. In severe cases or in the immunocompromised, oral fluconazole may be required.

**Comments: Chronic recurrent candidiasis** is probably due to failure of eradication of infection during treatment of acute attacks. Recurrences should be treated for longer than usual or with a course of oral fluconazole, which will abolish gut colonization, which may act as a reservoir. Reinfection from a partner is possible—20% of male partners have penile colonization, and topical therapy is recommended. Prolonged suppressive therapy with fluconazole (100 mg weekly) may rarely be necessary. Some refractory cases are due to antifungal resistance, so identification and susceptibility testing may be useful ☎.

It has also been suggested that some women with recurrent candidiasis have immune hypersensitivity to low numbers of *Candida*.

> **Practice point**
>
> Some topical vaginal preparations may damage condoms and diaphragms. Up-to-date information is available in datasheets or the BNF.

## Bacterial vaginosis

*Gardnerella vaginalis* (➤302) is a vaginal commensal organism. Under certain circumstances, it acts in synergy with other commensal anaerobes to multiply and inhibit the growth of lactobacilli and other vaginal flora. Σ 62 000.

**Clinical features:** Many patients are asymptomatic. Mild vaginal discharge with a fishy odour and pruritis may occur. On examination, there is little or no vaginal inflammation. Discharge is thin, grey and homogenous. When potassium hydroxide is added, a fishy odour is liberated ('whiff test').

**Organisms:** *Gardnerella vaginalis* is a vaginal commensal organism, so isolation by culture is not significant. Quantification and culture for anaerobes is not routinely practicable.

**Microbiological investigations:** Microscopy of wet preparation characteristically shows 'clue cells'—squamous epithelial cells studded with *Gardnerella*. Diagnosis depends on the presence of three out of four of the following: positive whiff test, clue cells, characteristic vaginal discharge and vaginal pH > 5.0.

**Differential diagnosis:** Candidiasis (➤82), trichomoniasis (➤92), gonorrhoea (➤86), non-specific cervicitis (➤87).

**Antibiotic management:** Metronidazole (400 mg q8h for one week) or topical clindamycin (2% cream, 5 g q24h for 1 week). Metronidazole is relatively contraindicated during pregnancy. Ampicillin is effective in some cases and has been used during pregnancy. Asymptomatic cases should not be treated; yeast superinfection reported in up to 20% after oral metronidazole.

**Complications:** Bacterial vaginosis is associated with increased risk of premature labour, chorioamnionitis, and puerperal sepsis, but the value of screening and treating asymptomatic pregnant women remains to be established.

## Puerperal infection

Endometrial infection following delivery; causes ~30% of puerperal fevers.

**Risk factors:** Caesarian section is associated with a greatly increased risk (20–55% incidence without prophylaxis vs. 2–5% for vaginal delivery). Other factors include prolonged labour, retained products of conception and prolonged rupture of membranes.

**Clinical features:** Fever, uterine tenderness, foul lochia, leucocytosis. Malaise, abdominal pain and rigors.

**Organisms:** Mixed aerobic and anaerobic genital flora including coliforms, *Streptococcus 'milleri'*, *Enterococcus* spp., group B β-haemolytic streptococci, anaerobic streptococci, *Bacteroides* spp., *Gardnerella vaginalis*, genital *Mycoplasma* spp., *Clostridium* spp.

**Microbiological investigations:** Culture of lochia and blood.

**Differential diagnosis:** Pyelonephritis or UTI (40% of puerperal fevers), wound infection (~7% of puerperal fevers).

**Antibiotic management:** Parenteral cephalosporin + metronidazole **or** clindamycin + gentamicin.

**Complications:** Pelvic abscess formation. Sepsis syndrome (➤185). **Septic pelvic thrombophlebitis** is an uncommon but important complication. It is due to mixed aerobic and anaerobic flora, but in particular, *Bacteroides* spp. It presents in two ways. **Ovarian vein thrombosis** presents with acute onset of severe abdominal pain and signs of peritonism. 50% of cases have a palpable abdominal mass. In other patients onset is gradual, with spiking fevers that are unresponsive to antibiotics. Septic pulmonary embolism (➤35) may follow. Venography and CT scanning are required. Treatment consists of antibiotic therapy as above, with heparinization and consideration of surgical intervention ☎.

## Infected abortion

Infection is associated with illegal and occasionally therapeutic abortion. The history of illegal or attempted abortion may not be obtained, and the diagnosis should be considered in any febrile woman with vaginal bleeding during the first half of pregnancy.

**Risk factors:** Incomplete removal of the products of conception. Uterine perforation. Pre-existing untreated infection with *Neisseria gonorrhoeae* or *Chlamydia trachomatis*.

**Clinical features:** Fever, rigors, abdominal pain, pelvic tenderness, history of passage of products of conception. Uterine perforation may follow with evidence of pelvic abscess or peritonitis. On examination, there may be a tender, enlarged uterus, foul cervical discharge and open os with evidence of passage of products of conception or instrumentation.

**Organisms:** As for puerperal infection, plus *Neisseria gonorrhoeae* and *Chlamydia trachomatis*. Clostridial infection ('uterine gas gangrene') may sometimes cause full-blown clostridial septicaemia with haemolysis, jaundice, shock, renal failure and disseminated intravascular coagulation (➤115, 314).

**Microbiological investigations:** Gram stain and culture of discharge. Blood cultures.

**Other investigations:** Imaging, usually ultrasound, to define pelvic abscess.

**Antibiotic management:** As for puerperal sepsis, plus doxycycline if chlamydia involved.

**Supportive management:** Removal of remaining products of conception and exclusion of uterine perforation.

**Complications:** See puerperal sepsis (➤83).

## Intra-amniotic infection

Amniotic fluid infection usually follows rupture of the membranes, although it may occur as a complication of instrumentation, e.g. amniocentesis.

**Clinical features:** Fever, maternal and foetal tachycardia, uterine tenderness, malodorous amniotic fluid.

**Organisms:** As for puerperal infection.

**Microbiological investigations:** Culture of amniotic fluid and blood.

**Antibiotic management:** Parenteral cephalosporin + metronidazole.

**Supportive management:** Prompt delivery is required. Antibiotics should be given intrapartum rather than waiting until post-delivery.

Prophylactic ampicillin and erythromycin are recommended by some experts for mothers with preterm premature rupture of membranes without evidence of intra-amniotic infection, to prolong pregnancy.

> **Practice point**
>
> Certain vaginal infections are suspected of causing premature rupture of membranes (e.g. bacterial vaginosis ➤82, heavy colonization with group B β-haemolytic streptococci ➤140); appropriate treatment may prevent this complication.

## Bartholinitis

Infection of Bartholin's glands may present as a localized abscess or as cellulitis of the surrounding skin. Infection is usually due to mixed genital flora (➤82); *Neisseria gonorrhoeae* is a rarer cause which must be excluded by Gram stain and culture (including endocervical, rectal and throat swabs). For localized abscess, surgical incision and drainage is required. For cellulitis, co-amoxiclav **or** amoxicillin + metronidazole may be given. For severe infection, give parenteral cephalosporin + metronidazole **or** clindamycin + gentamicin.

## Toxic shock syndrome (TSS)

**Risk factors:** Most cases are associated with tampon use in menstruating women, but it can complicate any focal staphylococcal infection. Menstrual cases have been reported in women who have not used tampons; non-menstrual cases have occurred secondary to surgical wound infection, nasal packing, postpartum, due to infection of intrauterine contraceptive devices and in association with post-influenzal staphylococcal pneumonia (➤28). The incidence of menstrual cases has fallen dramatically since the withdrawal of high absorbency tampons. $\Sigma \approx 18$.

**Pathogenesis:** A number of staphylococcal superantigen toxins have been associated with TSS, including toxic shock syndrome toxin (TSST-1, >90% of menstrual cases, ≈50% of non-menstrual cases), enterotoxin B (≈40% of non-menstrual, TSST-1 negative cases), less frequently enterotoxins A–D (➤249).

**Clinical features:** Median onset in menstrual cases is 2 days after onset of menses. Diagnosis is clinical, since *Staphylococcus aureus* may not always be isolated. **Diagnostic criteria** have been established to allow recognition and surveillance. Patients should have **all** of the following: fever (≥38.9°C); diffuse macular rash, which should desquamate 1–2 weeks after the onset of illness; hypotension (SBP ≤90 mmHg); **plus** at least **three** of the following categories of multi-organ involvement: (1) vomiting or diarrhoea; (2) severe myalgia with elevated creatine phosphokinase (≥2 × normal); (3) mucous hyperaemia affecting vagina, oropharynx or conjunctiva; (4) renal failure (creatinine ≥2 × normal) or pyuria in the absence of UTI; (5) abnormal liver function tests; (6) thrombocytopenia (≤100 × 10$^9$/L); (7) disorientation or altered conscious level without focal neurological signs. These criteria were established for epidemiological surveillance and should not be used to preclude treatment if the suspicion of TSS is high.

**Organisms:** *Staphylococcus aureus*. A similar illness may rarely be caused by exotoxin producing β-haemolytic streptococci.

**Microbiological investigations:** Culture of blood, vagina, nares, urine and, if there is doubt about the diagnosis, CSF may be required, in particular to exclude other infections such as meningococcaemia (➤185). Isolated organisms can be tested for toxin production *in vitro*; convalescent serology is also useful ☎.

**Differential diagnosis:** Meningococcaemia (➤185), scarlet fever (➤135), Gram-negative bacteraemia (➤185).

**Antibiotic management:** Antibiotics prevent relapse, but have not been shown to modify the course of the illness, which is toxin-mediated. However, *in vitro* studies suggest that antibiotics that inhibit protein synthesis may reduce toxin production and therefore we recommend clindamycin **plus** flucloxacillin. Flucloxacillin (1 g 6 hly) should be given iv for a week, then orally for another week to ensure eradication. If meningococcaemia cannot be excluded, then give parenteral cephalosporin initially instead of the flucloxacillin. IV immunoglobulin has been advocated, but has not been demonstrated to be effective. High-dose steroids (methylprednisolone 10–30 mg/kg/day) have also been advocated. Retrospective studies suggest benefit, but there has been no definitive controlled trial.

**Supportive management:** Supportive management is most important. Fluid replacement and monitoring, pressor agents and other intensive care therapies may be required (➤187).

# Chapter 10

# Sexually transmitted diseases (STDs)

(For HIV infection ➤143).

Sexual contact is critical to the transmission of all the conditions described in this section, although it is not necessarily the only route of acquisition. There are certain important concepts unique to the management of STDs.

• STDs are diseases of lifestyle. The risk of transmission is related primarily to the number of partners, and the same risk factors apply for most STDs. These include frequency of partner change, lower socio-economic status and non-barrier contraception.

• Patients with one STD are therefore likely to have others. All patients should be evaluated for other STDs, including urethritis and syphilis. It may also be appropriate to discuss the need for serological testing for HIV infection.

• Contact tracing is very important. Since many STDs are asymptomatic and/or difficult to exclude clinically, it is often appropriate to treat asymptomatic contacts presumptively. **Referral to a genitourinary medicine (GUM) clinic is essential for all the conditions described in this chapter.**

• Patients attending STD clinics are drawn predominantly from less advantaged socio-economic groups, and frequently reattend with newly acquired infections. Clinic attendance is an opportunity for discussion and education about risk reduction, contraception and other matters of sexual health, and allows provision of services such as cervical smear testing to groups who are otherwise unlikely to have contact with health services.

• The UK incidence of all STDs has increased between 1995 and 2000, particularly in teenage females and homosexual men, a trend attributed to increasing practise of unsafe sexual behaviours in these groups.

Detailed and up-to-date UK guidance on management of all STDs is available at:

🖥 www.mssvd.org.uk/CEG/ceguidelines.htm

Guidelines for managing outbreaks of sexually transmitted infections are at:

🖥 www.phls.co.uk/topics_az/hiv_and_sti/
guidelines/sti_outbreakplan.pdf.

## Gonorrhoea

**Epidemiology:** Common worldwide. Risk factors as for other STDs. $\Sigma$: ≈20 000 in 2000, vs. ≈10 000 in 1995. Disproportionately more common among gay men and ethnic minorities. In 2000, 9% of UK isolates were penicillin-resistant, 4% resistant to ciprofloxacin and 40% resistant to tetracycline.

🖥 www.phls.co.uk/facts/sti/files/grasp_report.pdf

**Clinical features:** *Neisseria gonorrhoeae* causes mucosal infection of the urethra, cervix, rectum, conjunctiva and pharynx. Asymptomatic infection is common at all sites. Symptomatic infection in males causes urethritis with copious purulent urethral discharge and dysuria, after an incubation period of 2–5 days. Local complications include epididymitis (➤80) and rarely periurethral abscess. Infection in women is usually a cervicitis, which can be asymptomatic or cause discharge, dysuria and itching. Concurrent urethritis and proctitis is usual. Infection of Bartholin and Skene glands may occur (➤84). Infection of the vaginal epithelium occurs in prepubertal girls. Anorectal infection occurs in homosexual men, but is unusual in heterosexual males. It is usually asymptomatic, but if not there is discharge, pain and tenesmus. Ophthalmia neonatorum (➤107, ②) and disseminated infection both occur in neonates.

**Organisms:** *Neisseria gonorrhoeae* (➤300)

**Microbiological investigations:** Gram stain and culture of material from urethra, endocervix, rectum or pharynx. Gram-negative intracellular diplococci may be seen. Antibiotic sensitivity should always be performed. Screening for other STDs, in particular syphilis, is essential (➤86).

**Differential diagnosis:** Chlamydia and other causes of non-specific urethritis (NSU). Vaginal candidiasis, trichomoniasis and bacterial vaginosis.

**Antibiotic management:** For infections acquired in UK: ciprofloxacin 500 mg single dose **or** ofloxacin 400 mg single dose **or** ampicillin 3.5 g *plus* probenecid 1 g (if local penicillin resistance rate <5%). For known resistance, or in cases acquired outside UK before sensitivity known, consider cefotaxime (500 mg) **or** ceftriaxone (250 mg) **or** spectinomycin (2 g), all im single dose. For pharyngeal gonorrhoea, ciprofloxacin or ceftriaxone should be given. Many physicians treat all patients with gonorrhoea for possible concomitant chlamydial infection (e.g. ceftriaxone, single dose, plus doxycycline for 1 week). Screening/treatment of sexual partners is essential; referral to GUM clinic is highly recommended.

**Complications:** Pelvic inflammatory disease (➤92). **Disseminated gonococcal infection (DGI)** occurs in 1–2% of untreated cases, causing bacteraemia with a pustular rash and asymmetrical polyarthritis affecting mainly hands, wrists, ankles and knees (➤120). Endocarditis and meningitis occur very rarely.

## Chlamydia infections

**Epidemiology:** Very common worldwide. Risk factor as other STDs (➤86). UK incidence continues to increase steadily. Σ ≈60000 reported cases in 2000 (doubled since 1995).

**Clinical features:** Infection is very commonly asymptomatic, particularly in women (≤70%). Untreated infection can persist for many years.

Symptomatic infection in men causes urethritis with dysuria and mucopurulent discharge, usually less copious than in gonorrhoea. Epididymitis may occur. In women, mucopurulent cervicitis with discharge and associated urethritis. Proctitis and pharyngitis occur in either sex. Chlamydial urethritis can be prolonged or present as apparent treatment failure after confirmed gonorrhoea ('postgonococcal urethritis'). Conjunctivitis (➤107, ②) and pneumonia (➤142) occur in infants born to infected mothers.

**Organisms:** *Chlamydia trachomatis*, trachoma biovar, serovars D–K (➤329).

**Microbiological investigations:** Culture is no longer routinely performed. Antigen detection (e.g. ELISA) has been available since 1984, but has relatively poor sensitivity. Tests for chlamydia DNA (PCR or ligase chain reaction—LCR) are now widely available, with high sensitivity and specificity, and can be performed on endocervical swabs, urine and vulvovaginal swabs. These tests are now the first-line investigation for all specimen types. Best sensitivity is obtained with urine (males) and endocervical swabs (female).

**Differential diagnosis:** Gonococcal urethritis (➤86). Non-specific urethritis may also be caused by *Ureaplasma urealyticum* (➤330). Genital herpes simplex (➤88) may cause urethritis, with severe dysuria but little discharge. *Trichomonas vaginalis* (➤92) infection in men may cause urethritis, but is usually asymptomatic.

**Antibiotic management:** Azithromycin 1 g single dose or doxycycline 100 mg q12h for 7 days or erythromycin 500 mg q6h for 7 days or ofloxacin 400 mg q24h for 7 days. Referral to GUM clinic is highly recommended.

**Complications:** Pelvic inflammatory disease (➤92). Reiter's disease (➤122). Perihepatitis (Fitz-Hugh–Curtis syndrome). Conjunctivitis (➤106).

**Comments: Recurrent disease** is usually due to reinfection, often because of inadequate treatment of sexual partners. Since infection in women is usually asymptomatic, female partners of men with NSU should be treated whether or not there is clinical evidence of infection. The availability of sensitive non-invasive tests for chlamydia introduces the possibility of screening. Criteria for screening programmes vary, but UK Dept of Health has suggested opportunistic screening of women having their first cervical smear.

🖥 www.doh.gov.uk/nshs/

# Genital herpes

Primary herpes simplex virus (HSV) infection is followed by latent infection of sacral ganglia, and subsequent reactivation, which may be subclinical or symptomatic.

**Epidemiology:** Infection is common worldwide. The incidence has increased in recent decades in the UK, as a result of changes in sexual behaviour, and a reduction in childhood infection by HSV-1, but no significant increase since 1995. Σ ≈18000. Severity of HSV-2 infection is reduced by prior exposure to HSV-1 and vice versa.

**Clinical features:** The incubation period is 3–7 days, (range 1– >14 days) although ≥60% of primary infections are asymptomatic. New diagnoses of genital herpes are equally likely to be caused by HSV-1 or HSV-2, but the recurrence rate is much higher for HSV-2 than HSV-1. Subclinical reactivation and viral shedding occur more frequently than overt recurrent disease. The **first clinical attack of genital herpes** may therefore be due to primary infection, or may represent a first reactivation episode ('initial non-primary herpes'). First attacks, whether primary or initial non-primary, are more severe than recurrences. Local burning and tenderness are followed by a vesicular eruption, usually bilateral. In moist areas, the vesicles rupture, leaving shallow, very tender ulcers. In drier areas, vesicles may remain intact to develop into pustules and scabs. New lesions continue to appear for about 1 week. In men, the glans penis, prepuce and shaft of the penis are usually involved. Lesions occur less frequently on the scrotum and thighs. In

women, lesions form initially on the external genitalia and vulva, but the cervix is usually subsequently involved and there is usually a watery vaginal discharge. Urethritis and dysuria occur in both sexes. Constitutional symptoms and local lymphadenopathy are usual. Resolution occurs over 1–3 weeks. Herpetic proctitis, with rectal discharge, pain, tenesmus and sometimes urinary retention, may occur in either sex.

One or more **recurrent attacks** are experienced by 60–80% of patients during the first year after the first episode. Recurrences are less severe and of shorter duration, and constitutional symptoms, lymphadenopathy and urethritis are unusual. Frequent and severe recurrent infection occur in immunocompromised patients (➤174). HIV+ patients may develop chronic anal ulceration (➤159). **Asymptomatic viral shedding** occurs most commonly in patients with genital HSV-2 infection, in the first year after infection and in individuals with frequent symptomatic recurrences.

**Organisms:** Herpes simplex virus types 2 and 1 (➤334).

**Microbiological investigations:** Culture of virus from lesions. Serology is often unhelpful, as it does not reliably distinguish between types 1 and 2. Rapid diagnostic methods for demonstration of viral antigens are available, using type-specific antibodies. PCR is now widely available and is more sensitive than culture, particularly in lesions more than a few days old.

**Differential diagnosis:** Other causes of genital ulceration, in particular syphilis (➤89) and in the tropics, chancroid, lymphogranuloma venereum and granuloma inguinale (➤94). Dark ground examination of material from lesions may be indicated. Less common causes of genital ulceration include Behçet's disease, herpes zoster, candidiasis and impetigo.

**Specific management:** Aciclovir (ACV), valaciclovir, and famciclovir all reduce the severity and duration of episodes, but do not alter the natural history of the disease. Intravenous therapy is only indicated when the patient cannot swallow or tolerate oral medication because of vomiting. Treatment should commence as soon as possible for maximum benefit. Systemic antivirals are of less benefit in recurrent attacks, which tend to be short and self-limiting. Topical ACV is of marginal benefit only. ACV (400 mg q12h) is effective prophylaxis for patients with frequent recurrences (e.g. >four attacks per year). Intravenous ACV is indicated for severe, disseminated or neonatal infection (➢362).

**Complications:** Neonatal infection (➢129). Bacterial and candidal superinfection occur rarely. Herpetic whitlow (➢338). Viral meningitis may complicate first attacks of genital herpes (➢100). Severe disseminated infection occurs rarely in the immunocompetent (➢338). If catheterization is required, suprapubic catheterization is preferred to prevent theoretical risk of ascending infection, to reduce the pain associated with the procedure and to allow normal micturition to be restored without multiple removals and recatheterizations.

# Syphilis②

**Risk factors:** As for other STDs (➢86).

**Epidemiology:** Common worldwide. $\Sigma \approx 500$ in 2000, up from $\approx 170$ in 1995. Concurrent HIV infection alters the course of infection, with more frequent and rapid onset of neurological disease, and treatment failures with standard antibiotic regimens.

**Transmission:** By sexual contact and vertically. Very rarely by blood transfusion. *Treponema pallidum* cannot penetrate intact skin, but infection may occur through macroscopically invisible cuts and abrasions.

**Clinical features: Primary syphilis:** 14–20 days (range 10–90) after inoculation, a red painless **papule** develops and ulcerates to form a **chancre**, usually 0.5–2 cm in diameter, painless with a clean base and an indurated edge. Moderate bilateral local lymphadenopathy is usual. Chancres are usually located on penis, fourchette or cervix, but may be anywhere, e.g.

mouth, hands, anus and rectum. Multiple chancres are sometimes seen. Spontaneous resolution occurs after 3–8 weeks.

**Secondary syphilis** follows systemic dissemination of organisms from the chancre; 4–10 weeks after the development of the chancre, a generalized symmetrical scaly papular rash develops, involving trunk and extremities including palms and soles. The papules may be smooth, pustular or itchy. Mucosal ulcers are common. Condylomata lata are raised grey-white lesions found in warm moist areas. Unlike the rash, they are highly contagious. Malaise, fever, sore throat, lymphadenopathy and myalgia are common, sometimes with subclinical hepatitis and periostitis. Neurological disease may rarely present during the secondary stage ('early neurosyphilis') with meningitis, headache, cranial nerve lesions, intranuclear ophthalmoplegia, cerebrovascular accident or signs of spinal cord involvement. Early neurosyphilis is more common in patients coinfected with HIV. Iritis, arthritis and glomerulonephritis occur infrequently. Spontaneous resolution occurs after 3–12 weeks, after which patients are said to have entered **latency**. Without treatment, 25% have recrudescence of secondary disease during the first year of latency.

After a variable latent period (2–20 yrs), **tertiary syphilis** (late benign syphilis, visceral syphilis, cardiovascular syphilis or neurosyphilis) develops in a minority of patients. **Late benign syphilis** describes the development of large granulomatous lesions ('gumma'), in skin and soft tissues, particularly on the head, neck and arms. Gummata may be indurated, nodular or ulcerated. **Visceral syphilis** describes the development of gummata in the viscera and bones. Lesions affecting the palate, pharynx, nasal septum or tongue can be locally destructive. Bony lesions are particularly painful. Other organs that can be involved include liver, testis, eye, stomach and rarely lungs. **Cardiovascular syphilis** affects the aorta and is due to endarteritis of the vasa vasorum. Aortic regurgitation occurs more commonly than aneurysm and presents with angina and dyspnoea secondary to left ventricular failure. Aneurysm typically affects the ascending aorta, and may involve the ostia of the coronary arteries. The arch and descending aorta are less frequently affected. VDRL (Venereal Disease Reference Laboratory) may be negative, suggesting that development of aneurysm is due to ongoing mechanical damage in a previously inflamed aorta. **Neurosyphilis** includes asymptomatic latent syphilis in which the CSF is found to be abnormal, meningovascular syphilis, general paresis of the insane (GPI) and tabes dorsalis. *Meningovascular syphilis* presents approximately 5 yrs after primary infection, either as a cerebral pachymeningitis with headaches, fits and limb paralysis, or more commonly as a chronic diffuse basal meningitis, causing headaches and isolated cranial nerve palsies. There may be mental changes, with memory impairment and poor concentration. In severe cases, there are multiple cranial nerve palsies and severe mental deterioration leading to stupor. Cerebral artery thrombosis can occur, leading to stroke. Meningovascular syphilis may also affect the spinal cord causing cervical myelopathy or hemiplegia. *GPI* describes severe cerebral atrophy developing 10–20 yrs after primary infection, with gradual onset of confusion, hallucinations, delusions, fits and severe cognitive deficit. On examination, there are coarse tremor of the lips and tongue, brisk tendon reflexes and extensor plantars. *Tabes dorsalis* develops 15–35 yrs after primary infection. There is atrophy of the dorsal columns of the spinal cord below the cervical region, with autonomic neuropathy and cranial nerve lesions. Patients present with ataxia, sensory loss, lightning pains and sphincter disturbance. Classical signs on examination include sensory loss, areflexia and Argyll Robertson pupils (irregular pupils that may constrict to accommodation but do not react to light).

The risk of **congenital syphilis** is highest during early syphilis (1° or 2°). Treatment of the mother before 16 weeks' gestation will prevent congenital disease. Neonates may present with fulminant disease; hepatitis, pulmonary haemorrhage and intercurrent bacterial infection are common and mortality is high. In less severe early congenital syphilis, signs develop over the first 2–10 weeks of life, including vesicular or bullous rash involving the sole and palms, rhinitis (snuffles) and evidence of widespread visceral involvement. Features of late congenital syphilis develop throughout childhood and include interstitial keratitis, Clutton's joints, Hutchinson's teeth, meningoencephalitis and skeletal changes. Diagnosis is by serology or dark-ground examination of material from mucosal lesions.

**Organisms:** *Treponema pallidum* (➤322).

**Microbiological investigations:** Diagnosis of primary syphilis is confirmed by **dark-ground microscope examination** of material from the base of the chancre for spirochaetes. An alternative method of identifying *T. pallidum* from lesions is direct fluorescent antibody testing (DFA-TP). This technique has the advantage of permitting the identification of the organism when smears cannot be examined immediately and is specific for *T. pallidum* antigens. PCR (➤) is sometimes used to confirm diagnosis, particularly in oral lesions which can be contaminated by oral communal spirochaetes.

Two types of **serological tests** are used (Table 10.1). *Non-specific tests* include VDRL and RPR (Rapid Plasma Reagin). These tests are based on the original Wassermann reaction (WR) and detect antibodies against cardiolipin, which is found in mammalian cell membranes, and is incorporated by the spirochaete into its outer membrane. False positives in non-specific tests are seen in a large number of conditions, including acute viral infections, connective tissue diseases, pregnancy and leprosy. The value of non-specific tests is that titres fall after successful treatment of syphilis. A reappearance or fourfold rise in titre of VDRL is regarded as evidence of relapse or reinfection. *Specific tests*, including fluorescent *Treponema* antigen tests (FTA and FTA-ABS), *Treponema pallidum* haemagglutination test (TPHA) and treponemal enzyme immunoassay (EIA) use *Treponema pallidum* antigens as targets. They are specific for syphilis, but remain positive for life and are not useful for assessing success of treatment. Their value lies in confirming the diagnosis of primary syphilis, as they become positive before VDRL in this situation, and excluding

**Table 10.1** Serological diagnosis of syphilis

| Clinical situation | Non-specific serology (e.g. VDRL) | Specific serology (e.g. TPHA) |
|---|---|---|
| Primary syphilis* | Positive in ≈75% | Positive in ≈90% |
| Secondary syphilis | Positive at high titre in ≈100% | Positive in ≈100% |
| Latent infection | May remain positive. Titre falls with time and after treatment. Rise in titre suggests reinfection | Remains positive |
| Late benign syphilis | Usually strongly positive | Remains positive |
| Syphilitic aortitis | Positive in only 60% of cases | Remains positive |
| Late neurosyphilis† | May be negative or weakly positive | Remains positive |

* Definitive disgnosis by dark-ground examination of chancre.
† CSF may show pleocytosis with raised protein and positive VDRL.

syphilis in suspected secondary and tertiary disease. False-positive reactions occur in Lyme disease (➤323) and other spirochaetal infections (➤322). Patients with syphilis and late-stage HIV infection may lose all antibody responses (➤165).

**Antibiotic management:** Referral to GUM clinic is essential. Published guidelines all stipulate benzathine penicillin as first line, but this is no longer available in the UK. Most now use (and BNF recommends) doxycycline or tetracycline or erythromycin. Early syphilis is treated for 14 days; late latent syphilis is treated with doxycycline for 28 days.

**Isolation:** Body fluid precautions should be observed for the first 24 h of treatment of patients with primary and secondary disease.

**Complications: Jarisch–Herxheimer reaction** is a hypersensitivity reaction precipitated by lysis of organisms. It occurs 1–6 h after initiating treatment in many patients and consists of fever, rash, lymphadenopathy and hypotension.

## Genital warts

**Clinical features:** After an incubation period of about 4–6 weeks, warts ('condylomata acumi-

nata') develop as small irregular papules around the external genitalia, in the perianal region and less often in the vagina, urethra and on the cervix. Subclinical infection of surrounding epithelium is the rule. On the cervix, the presence of infected epithelium may be demonstrated by the application of acetic acid, which turns infected areas white. Biopsy of aceto-white areas is indicated to confirm infection and exclude intraepithelial neoplasia.

**Organisms:** Human papillomavirus. Some types are associated with warts, whereas others are associated with cervical cancer (➤342).

**Microbiological investigations:** Viral culture is not possible. DNA hybridization methods and PCR are available for determining which HPV type is present. These techniques have hitherto been used mainly in epidemiological studies; their value in the management of individual patients is currently being studied.

**Differential diagnosis:** Moles and skin tags. Syphilis (condylomata lata) (➤89), molluscum contagiosum (➤119).

**Management:** Specific antiviral therapy is not available; therapy is directed towards removal of warts and relief of symptoms. Caustic agents such as podophyllin or trichloracetic acid are effective in ≈50% of cases, but have a high rate of recurrence. Podophyllin is very irritant, and excess topical application can lead to systemic toxicity with nausea, vomiting, lethargy and neuropathy. It is anti-mitotic and contraindicated in pregnancy and infancy. 5-Fluorouracil has a higher success rate, but can be extremely irritating. Systemic and intralesional interferon is effective, but is not yet in widespread use, not least due to its cost. Recurrence is common when treatment is discontinued. Imiquimod is a recently developed immune response modifier, which acts by local cytokine induction. It is applied topically as a 5% cream and has shown significant effect in clearing warts with few recurrences in limited clinical experience. Cryotherapy is widely used. Laser therapy is particularly useful for cervical lesions. If external warts are very numerous, surgical removal may be necessary.

**Complications: Juvenile-onset respiratory papillomata** are due to infection with HPVs causing mucosal warts, probably acquired intrapartum from the maternal genital tract.

## Trichomoniasis

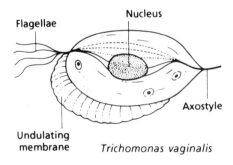

Trichomonas vaginalis

Transmission occurs by sexual contact. Although *Trichomonas vaginalis* can survive in urine on towels or clothing for several hours, non-sexual transmission is believed to be very rare. Symptoms are more likely to occur during pregnancy or menstruation when the vaginal pH is highest, as this favours parasite replication. Σ >6000, but rare outside GUM clinics.

**Clinical features:** Infection in men is usually asymptomatic; there may be mild dysuria. Up to 50% of infected women are asymptomatic. Symptoms may develop after an incubation period of 1–4 weeks with yellow vaginal discharge, frequently copious, frothy and offensive. Dysuria, dyspareunia, lower abdominal pain and vulval itching also occur. On examination, there may be erythema of the vaginal walls and cervix, which may be friable with punctate haemorrhages ('strawberry cervix').

**Organisms:** *Trichomonas vaginalis.*

**Microbiological investigations:** Microscopy (phase-contrast or dark-ground best) of wet preparation of vaginal discharge usually shows motile flagellated protozoa. Culture is also possible in liquid medium (Feinberg's). Organisms may also be seen on fixed cervical smears examined cytologically.

**Antibiotic management:** Metronidazole (2 g single dose). Sexual partners should be treated. Asymptomatic patients should be treated, except during pregnancy, when metronidazole is relatively contraindicated. It may be given after the first trimester if symptoms are severe.

**Differential diagnosis:** Candidiasis (➤82), bacterial vaginosis (➤82), gonorrhoea (➤86), non-specific cervicitis (➤87).

## Pelvic inflammatory disease (PID) (syn. salpingitis)

PID complicates 10–15% of cases of gonococcal and chlamydial cervicitis. Damage caused by these organisms also facilitates entry of aerobic and anaerobic vaginal flora (➤82) into the Fallopian tube, so that many infections are polymicrobial.

**Risk factors:** Commonest in teenage girls with multiple sexual partners and non-barrier methods of contraception, especially intra-uterine device (IUD). Previous PID predisposes to further episodes.

**Clinical features:** Fever, pelvic pain, abdominal tenderness, adnexal and cervical tenderness, vaginal discharge. Symptoms do not correlate well with the presence of infection and the likelihood of subsequent complications. Right upper quadrant pain occurs due to peri-hepatitis in $\approx$10% (Fitz-Hugh–Curtis syndrome ➤87).

**Organisms:** *Neisseria gonorrhoeae, Chlamydia trachomatis.* Infection is often polymicrobial with mixed aerobic and anaerobic genital flora, including *Bacteroides* spp., *Escherichia coli, Gardnerella vaginalis. Mycoplasma hominis* and *Ureaplasma urealyticum* have also been implicated in PID.

**Microbiological investigations:** Microscopy and culture of endocervical swab should be done but, with the exception of *Neisseria gonorrhoeae*, does not accurately reflect contents of Fallopian tube. Material from peritoneal cavity and tube obtained by laparoscopy may be available.

**Other investigations:** In view of difficulty of diagnosis, leucocytosis and raised ESR may be helpful indicators of ongoing infection. Laparoscopy is frequently done to confirm diagnosis. Ultrasound may be used to examine for tubo-ovarian abscess, but appearances do not otherwise correlate well with clinical symptoms or microbiological results.

**Differential diagnosis:** Ectopic pregnancy, appendicitis, ruptured or haemorrhagic ovarian cyst, endometriosis.

**Antibiotic management:** Admission for intravenous therapy will often be required. Cover for aerobic and anaerobic organisms is recommended. Suitable regimens include:
- a single dose of parenteral cephalosporin, then doxycycline *plus* metronidazole
- or clindamycin *plus* gentamicin followed by either oral clindamycin or doxycycline *plus* metronidazole
- or ofloxacin *plus* metronidazole.

IUD should be removed after antibiotic therapy has commenced.

**Complications:** Infertility, chronic pelvic pain. **Tubo-ovarian abscess** (TOA) presents with similar symptoms to uncomplicated PID, and should be excluded by ultrasound (or CT) scan if patient is unwell or if symptoms fail to settle. Early gynaecological referral is essential as a ruptured TOA requires immediate surgery. Intravenous antibiotics should be given. Surgery may be required if there is no response after 72 h or if clinical features suggest rupture. An adnexal mass >8 cm in diameter is unlikely to respond to antibiotic therapy alone. Percutaneous and laparoscopic drainage is sometimes employed as an alternative to laparotomy.

# Tropical genital ulceration

The prevalence of genital ulceration in patients presenting with STDs is much higher in the developing world than in the UK. This has recently acquired greater significance, as it is now believed that genital ulceration is an important factor in the heterosexual transmission of HIV in Africa and Asia.

## Chancroid (syn. Soft sore)

Common throughout the tropics and subtropics, but very rarely imported into the UK. Previously the commonest cause of tropical genital ulceration, but recent studies suggest incidence is falling, possibly due to changing patterns of HIV and HSV infection.

**Clinical features:** Incubation period is $\approx$1 week. Painful papules develop on external genitalia of both sexes and rapidly ulcerate. Ulcer is typically sloughy, irregular, painful, non-indurated and haemorrhagic. 'Kissing' lesions develop on adjacent skin surfaces such as scrotum or thigh. Cervical and vaginal wall ulcers are rare. Suppurative local lymphadenopathy is common, progressing to bubo and sinus formation. Local complications include phimosis and urethral stricture.

**Organisms:** *Haemophilus ducreyi* (➤298).

**Microbiological investigations:** Gram stain ('shoal of fish' appearance) and culture of material obtained from ulcer or aspirated from lymph nodes. Concurrent syphilis and gonor-rhoea should be excluded. PCR possible, but is not widely available.

**Antibiotic management:** Erythromycin for 1 week, **or** azithromycin **or** ciprofloxacin **or** parenteral cephalosporin, all as a single dose. Patients with HIV may respond less well.

**Supportive management:** Aspiration of bubo may be required.

## Lymphogranuloma venereum (LGV)②

LGV causes inconspicuous genital ulceration, followed by severe local sequelae. Clinical infection is much commoner in men than women. Asymptomatic infection in women may serve as a reservoir. LGV occurs throughout the tropics, but is very rarely imported into the UK.

**Clinical features:** Incubation period is 3–30 days. Primary lesion is an inconspicuous, transient, painless genital ulcer which heals without scarring and is recalled by ≈20% of cases. Extremely tender local lymphadenopathy then develops, with fever, headache, weight loss and sometimes meningoencephalitis, pneumonia, arthritis and erythema nodosum. Lymphadenopathy may be very marked, with cleavage of the inflammatory mass by the inguinal ligament (the 'groove' sign). Multiple abscesses with sinus formation may follow, with fibrosis of the sacral and iliac lymphatics leading to lymphoedema of the perineum. Haemorrhagic proctitis with perirectal abscess, rectal stricture and fistula formation may occur.

**Organisms:** *Chlamydia trachomatis* serovars L1, L2 and L3.

**Microbiological investigations:** Diagnosis is based on clinical features. Serology for anti-chlamydial antibodies is also helpful. Immuno-fluorescent and ELISA antigen capture assays for chlamydial antigens are available but are not specific for LGV serovars. Culture is possible but not widely available in the countries where LGV occurs.

**Antibiotic management:** Doxycycline **or** erythromycin for 3 weeks.

**Supportive management:** Aspiration of lymph nodes may be required to avert sinus formation, but surgical debridement should be avoided.

## Granuloma inguinale
(syn. donovaniasis)

Endemic in South India, Papua New Guinea and certain Caribbean islands. Non-sexual transmission also occurs; infection is common in children in endemic areas.

**Clinical features:** Painless, non-purulent, 'beefy-red' ulcer progressively enlarging over months to 5 cm or more in diameter, commonly on the prepuce or labia. Local extension, healing and fibrosis may all occur simultaneously. Secondary infection may cause increased purulence and necrosis. Other cutaneous sites may be involved, often in patients who also have genital disease. Metastatic haematogenous spread to bones, joints and liver has been reported very rarely. Regional lymphadenopathy is rare.

**Organisms:** *Calymmatobacterium granulomatis* has recently been officially redesignated *Klebsiella granulomatis* (➤297).

**Microbiological investigations:** Microscopy of Giemsa-stained material from ulcers shows bipolar intracellular bacteria, visible as 'Donovan bodies' with characteristic safety pin appearance. Culture and serology are not available.

**Antibiotic management:** Azithromycin (1 g weekly) **or** erythromycin **or** co-trimoxazole **or** doxycycline for 3 weeks.

## Pubic lice

**Clinical features:** Severe pruritis. 1–2 mm grey-brown lice and 0.5 mm ovoid nits attached to hairshafts may be seen. Tiny red dots on affected skin are louse excreta. Pubic, axillary, chest and abdominal hair may be infested. Eyelashes may also be involved (➤104).

**Organisms:** *Pthirus pubis.*

**Management:** Preparations containing permethrin, phenothrin and malathion are effective. All hairy parts of the body should be treated. Retreatment after 1 week is recommended.

## Scabies

Scabies may be acquired by any close contact, including household contact as well as sexually. ①

**Risk factors:** Poor hygiene. Crowded housing. Sexual contact. Prolonged contact (>20 min) needed for transmission.

**Clinical features:** Incubation period is approximately 4 weeks. Severe pruritus. Infestation is usually confined to the interdigital areas and the flexor surfaces of the wrists, where papulovesicular lesions and scaly plaques may be seen. Classical linear burrows are often very difficult to see. Excoriation is usual. Other areas, including the genitalia, buttocks, thighs, breasts, belt line, umbilicus, feet, ankles, elbows and axillae are often infested.

**Organisms:** *Sarcoptes scabiei.*

**Microbiological investigations:** Diagnosis is clinical, and may be confirmed by microscopical demonstration of mites or eggs in skin scrapings.

**Management:** Malathion or permethrin preparations may be used. The whole body below the chin must be treated, paying particular attention to the finger webs and under the edges of the finger nails. Ivermectin (single dose 200 μg/kg) has been used in combination with topical agents in the treatment of Norwegian scabies that does not respond to topical treatment alone.

**Complications:** In immunosuppressed patients, **Norwegian scabies** may develop. This is characterized by very heavy infestation with little or no itching. There is widespread keratosis and erythema, and these patients are highly infectious. Patients with HIV infection develop papulosquamous lesions along lines of skin cleavage (➤159).

# Chapter 11

# CNS infections

## Bacterial meningitis ✉①

Infection and inflammation of the arachnoid and pia mater and the cerebrospinal fluid (CSF). Detailed UK guidelines for management of meningitis in adults have been published by the BIS (↪ Begg, J Infection 1999; 39:1).

**Risk factors and organisms:** Most cases are caused by *Neisseria meningitidis* Σ ≈2800 and *Streptococcus pneumoniae* Σ ≈250. *Haemophilus influenzae* type b has become very rare since the introduction of vaccination. Likely organisms vary depending on the age of the patient and a large number of risk factors.

Commonest organisms by **age group: <1 month:** Gram-negative bacilli, group B β-haemolytic streptococci, *Listeria monocytogenes*. **1 month–5 yrs:** *Streptococcus pneumoniae, Neisseria meningitidis, Haemophilus influenzae* type b. **6–59 yrs:** *Streptococcus pneumoniae, Neisseria meningitidis.* **>59 yrs:** *Streptococcus pneumoniae,* Gram-negative bacilli, *Listeria monocytogenes.*

Other **specific risk factors** include: **Open cranial trauma:** coliforms, *Staphylococcus aureus,* pseudomonads. **Closed trauma** (e.g. with fracture into sinuses): *Streptococcus pneumoniae, Haemophilus influenzae* type b, polymicrobial meningitis, with coliforms and non-sporing anaerobes. **Meningitis following neurosurgery** may involve typical surgical pathogens such as *Staphylococcus aureus, Staphylococcus epidermidis* and coryneforms, (often in association with shunts and prosthetic material), wet-source environmental organisms such as coliforms and pseudomonads, or nasopharyngeal flora such as staphylococci, streptococci, *Neisseria meningitidis* and coliforms (often after fracture or transmucosal pharyngeal operative approaches). **Otitis media and sinusitis:** *Streptococcus pneumoniae, Haemophilus influenzae* type b, coliforms, non-sporing anaerobes, other streptococci. **Complement deficiency:** Recurrent infection with *Haemophilus influenzae* type b, *Streptococcus pneumoniae, Neisseria meningitidis.* **Immunosuppressed patients:** Fungal meningitis (➤101) and *Listeria monocytogenes* (➤267), as well as all bacteria listed. **Neonatal ICU** may have outbreaks of meningitis due to *Citrobacter koseri, Campylobacter jejuni, Klebsiella* spp. and *Serratia* spp.

Very rare causes include *Leptospira interrogans, Nocardia asteroides, Treponema pallidum, Borrelia burgdorferi, Brucella* spp., *Francisella tularensis.* 1% are polymicrobial, usually associated with CSF leak or invasive tumour.

***Salmonella* spp.** are common in neonates worldwide. In China and Hong Kong, the commonest cause of meningitis is *Streptococcus suis* (Gp R) acquired from pigs (also recognized as an industrial disease of butchers). **Eosinophilic meningitis** in tropical areas may be caused by a number of helminths including *Gnathostoma* spp. and *Angiostrongylus* spp. (➤237).

**Exposure history** is particularly relevant to *Neisseria meningitidis*, which may cause epidemics in institutions such as colleges, barracks and schools. Asymptomatic nasal carriage rate is typically 25% for UK adults. Meningococcal meningitis is endemic in the developing world; in sub-Saharan Africa, periodic epidemics occur in the 'meningitis belt' (➤193).

**Clinical features:** Onset may be rapid (<1 day) or subacute (1–3 days), frequently with symptoms of URTI. Classical features of meningism are **headache, fever, photophobia** and **neck stiffness,** but these are not all always present (e.g. neck stiffness absent in 18% in one series).

**Table 11.1** Interpretation of CSF findings

| Infection | Cells/μL | Cell type | Appearance | Protein | Glucose |
|---|---|---|---|---|---|
| Meningitis | | | | | |
|   Bacterial | 500–10 000 | PMN | Turbid | ↑ or ↑↑ | ↓ or ↓↓ |
|   Viral | 50–1 000 | Monocytes | Clear | N or ↑ | N |
|   TB | 50–1 000 | Monocytes | Opalescent | ↑ or ↑↑ | ↓ or ↓↓ |
| Brain abscess | 5–100 | PMN, monocytes | Clear | ↑ or ↑↑ | N |
| Viral encephalitis | 5–100 | Monocytes | Clear | N or ↑ | N |
| Parameningeal abscess | 5–100 | PMN, monocytes | Clear | ↑ or ↑↑ | N |

↑ Raised, ↓ low, N normal, PMN, neutrophils. CSF glucose should be > 0.5 × blood glucose. Normal protein concentration is ≤ 0.4 g/L. CSF lactate and LDH levels are not specific enough to be useful in routine clinical practice. Always collect CSF in three bottles and number them. This allows differentiation between uniformly bloody CSF of subarachnoid haemorrhage, and sequentially falling RBC count of traumatic tap. Cell counts are at best approximate guides to the most likely organisms. Retain CSF for PCR testing for viruses and meningococci.

Conscious level ranges from fully alert, confused (≈45%) to unconscious (≈25%). To demonstrate **Kernig's sign**, flex the hip and the knee, and then attempt to extend the knee. Muscle spasm in the hamstrings prevents knee extension if there is meningeal irritation. Brudzinski's sign is used in children; when the neck is flexed, the knees and hips also flex. Focal neurological signs (10–20%), fits (15–30%). Meningococcal septicaemia is associated with a characteristic **petechial rash** (present in ≈50%); similar rashes occur rarely in other septicaemias (e.g. *Staphylococcus aureus*). **Raised intracranial pressure** (ICP) may lead to coma, hypertension and bradycardia. **Presentation in infants is non-specific**, with fever, vomiting, behavioural change. Neck stiffness is not usually present. Bulging fontanelle may be present late in disease.

**Microbiological investigations: Lumbar puncture** (LP) should be performed as soon as possible. Contraindications to LP include suspected raised ICP or intracranial space-occupying lesion, focal neurological signs, coagulopathy, severe cutaneous sepsis in the lumbar region, severe respiratory distress, or haemodynamic instability. Many experts would defer LP in patients with petechial rash or other evidence of meningococcaemia, particularly in children. **Give empirical treatment before sending the patient to CT scanning.** Interpretation of CSF findings is summarized in Table 11.1.

**CSF Gram stain** may be diagnostic, allowing definitive narrow-spectrum antibiotic therapy. In immunosuppressed patients, request India ink staining for fungi, and send serum and CSF for cryptococcal antigen (➤369). Fungal and viral culture should be requested if appropriate. Mycobacterial stain and culture requires larger volume of CSF (≥10 mL). CSF should be sent for cytology if malignancy is considered possible.

**Raised opening pressure:** Normal <18 cmH₂O. If pressure is greater than 45 cmH₂O, remove only the CSF in the manometer and give iv 20% mannitol (1 g/kg by rapid infusion) and dexamethasone (4 mg 6hly). Be prepared to repeat the mannitol. Intubation and hyperventilation may be required if signs of cerebral herniation develop.

**Equivocal CSF results:** Rarely, CSF is normal in early bacterial meningitis. In early viral meningitis, low/moderate cell counts with PMN and monocytes may be seen. Prior treatment with antibiotics inadequate to treat meningitis may cause low cell count, lymphocyte predominance, negative CSF and blood culture and abnormal Gram stain appearances. In these situations, it may be appropriate to observe, repeat the LP after a few hours, or commence treatment. If in doubt, treat. CSF is often normal in meningococcaemia.

**Table 11.2** Empirical therapy in suspected bacterial meningitis

| Clinical situation | Antibiotic regimen |
|---|---|
| **Adults—community-acquired meningitis or closed head trauma** | |
| Meningitis with typical meningococcal rash | Benzylpenicillin 2.4 g q4 h *or* ampicillin 2 g q4 h (BIS recommendation—we prefer high-dose parenteral cephalosporin, e.g. ceftriaxone 2 g q12 h) |
| Adults without typical meningococcal rash | |
| Aged 18–50 | High-dose parenteral cephalosporin, e.g. ceftriaxone 2 g q12 h. |
| | If LP delayed *or* patient from area of high prevalence of penicillin-resistant pneumococcus (e.g. Spain, Eastern Europe), add vancomycin 1 g q12 h *or* rifampicin 600 mg q12 h iv. |
| Aged over 50 | As above, plus ampicillin 2 g q4 h (to cover *Listeria*) |
| Patients with definite history of anaphylaxis to β-lactams | |
| Aged 18–50 | Chloramphenicol 25 mg/kg q6 h **plus** vancomycin 1 g q12 h. |
| Aged over 50 | As above, **plus** co-trimoxazole (to cover *Listeria*) |
| **Open head trauma, post-neurosurgical patient** | Parenteral cephalosporin + gentamicin ± metronidazole initially then guided by microbiology |
| **Child with community-acquired meningitis** | Cefotaxime, **or** chloramphenicol + vancomycin |
| **Neonate < 1 month old** | Ampicillin + gentamicin, **or** cefotaxime + gentamicin |

↪ **Begg**, J Infection 1999; 39: 1

**Blood cultures** are often positive in untreated meningitis and more often negative than CSF culture in partially treated cases. Culture of *Neisseria meningitidis* by some laboratories may require special medium ('meningitis bottle' ➤ 11). If **rash** is present, it can be scarified gently with a needle, swabbed and an impression smear made. Gram stain may reveal *Neisseria meningitidis* or *Staphylococcus aureus*. Nose and throat swabs are usually sent.

**Serology and PCR** (blood and CSF) are now routinely available, but are generally only useful in retrospect. Serum is usually sent on days 0, 4 and 14. A high proportion of diagnoses is now made by non-culture techniques because of increasing early antibiotic therapy.

**Other investigations:** If diagnosis is not clear cut, chest X-ray and CT head scan may be needed. Peripheral blood leucocytosis occurs in both viral and bacterial meningitis.

**Differential diagnosis:** Bacteraemia due to *Staphylococcus aureus* or coliforms. Meningism commonly accompanies community-acquired *Staphylococcus aureus* endocarditis. Viral and fungal meningitis. Subarachnoid haemorrhage. Meningism may rarely occur in Behçet's disease and familial Mediterranean fever.

**Antibiotic management:** Antibiotics should be given intravenously in high dose without delay. Early treatment improves prognosis in all cases. Once an organism is isolated or identified on Gram stain, therapy can be targeted appropriately. See Tables 11.2–11.4. Patients with *Neisseria meningitidis* treated with penicillin require subsequent subsequent rifampicin, ciprofloxacin or ceftriaxone to eradicate throat carriage (➤ 100).

**Table 11.3**  Treatment of bacterial meningitis once CSF microscopy findings are available

| | |
|---|---|
| Gram-negative diplococci visible | Benzylpenicillin 2.4 g q4 h or ampicillin 2 g q4 h (BIS recommendation—we prefer high-dose parenteral cephalosporin, e.g. ceftriaxone 2 g q12 h) |
| Gram-positive diplococci | High-dose parenteral cephalosporin, e.g. ceftriaxone 2 g q12 h. If condition deteriorates or patient from area of high prevalence of penicillin-resistant pneumococcus (e.g. Spain, E. Europe), add vancomycin 1 g q12 h or rifampicin 600 mg q12 h iv |
| Gram-positive coccobacilli suggestive of *Listeria* | Ampicillin 2 g q4 h **plus** gentamicin 5 mg/kg q24 h |

**Table 11.4**  Treatment of meningitis once pathogens have been cultured

| | Treatment | Duration (days) |
|---|---|---|
| *Neisseria meningitidis* | Benzylpenicillin 2.4 g q4h or ampicillin 2 g q4h (BIS recommendation—we prefer high-dose parenteral cephalosporin, e.g. ceftriaxone 2 g q12h). If there is a definite history of anaphylaxis to β-lactams, chloramphenicol 25 mg/kg q6h | 7–10 |
| *Streptococcus pneumoniae* | High-dose parenteral cephalosporin, e.g. ceftriaxone 2 g q12h. If condition deteriorates or patient from area of high prevalence of penicillin-resistant pneumococcus (e.g. Spain, E. Europe), add vancomycin 1 g q12h or rifampicin 600 mg q12h iv, pending sensitivity results | 10–14 |
| Penicillin and cephalosporin resistant *Streptococcus pneumoniae* | High-dose parenteral cephalosporin, e.g. ceftriaxone 2 g q12h, **plus** vancomycin 1 g q12h or rifampicin 600 mg q12h iv | 10–14 |
| *Listeria monocytogenes* | Ampicillin 2 g q4h **plus** gentamicin 5 mg/kg q24h | 21–28 |
| *Haemophilus influenzae* | Parenteral cephalosporin | 7–10 |
| *Staphylococcus aureus* | Flucloxacillin **or** parenteral cephalosporin **plus** either rifampicin or fusidic acid | 28 |
| Coliforms | Parenteral cephalosporin **or** meropenem, possibly with gentamicin guided closely by microbiology | |

**Supportive management:** Steroids have been shown to reduce the incidence of neurological sequelae in children and should now be routinely used. Dexamethasone 0.4 mg/kg 12hly for 2 days, starting with the first dose of antibiotic. Their use in adults remains controversial, and there are no good published trials. BIS guidelines support the use of steroids (single dose of dexamethasone, before or with first dose of antibiotics) in adults with signs of raised ICP, raised opening pressure or cerebral oedema on CT scan. US guidelines do not support their use. We do not recommend the use of steroids and consider that other agents to reduce ICP (e.g. mannitol) should only be used in neurosurgical intensive care units or similar, where there is the facility to monitor ICP. Patients should be kept euvolaemic; fluid restriction has not been shown to reduce cerebral oedema. Patients with sepsis syndrome require full supportive therapy (➤187). Very ill patients may require intubation and ventilation.

**Complications:** Cranial nerve palsy (III, VI, VIII). Fits and focal neurological deficit (e.g. hemiparesis). Shock and sepsis syndrome (➤185). 10% of patients with *Neisseria meningitidis* develop serum sickness-like illness at 4–10 days, with arthritis, fever and pericarditis, which must be distinguished from persisting metastatic infection.

**Comments:** *Haemophilus influenzae* meningitis is very rare in adults — cranial trauma with CSF leak, otitis media, sinusitis and underlying immunodeficiency should be excluded. The same factors should be excluded in **recurrent meningitis.** Mollaret's meningitis describes a rare condition of recurrent brief episodes of meningitis alternating with asymptomatic intervals. CSF shows pleocytosis and characteristic epithelial cells. No infectious cause is found and the prognosis is good.

**Prophylaxis:** To be effective, household contacts should receive prophylaxis quickly; this usually involves liaison between hospital clinicians, GPs, public health doctors and microbiologists. ***Neisseria meningitidis:*** Household and intimate contacts should receive rifampicin 600 mg 12hly for 2 days. (Children: >1 month old, 10 mg/kg up to 600 mg 12hly; <1 month old, 5 mg/kg 12hly.) Alternatives include ciprofloxacin and ceftriaxone ☎. Prophylaxis should be given as soon as possible; taking nose swabs from contacts is not helpful, as 25% of normal population are carriers. **Patients** should also receive rifampicin as treatment regimens may not eradicate nasal carriage. **Hospital** staff only need prophylaxis if they have performed mouth-to-mouth resuscitation or had other mucosal contamination, otherwise the risk of side effects outweighs the risk of infection. **Meningococcal vaccines** against group C, and groups A and C are available (➤193), and are sometimes used in outbreaks within closed communities such as boarding schools. Vaccination is also recommended for travellers to the 'meningitis belt' of sub-Saharan Africa, and for pilgrims to Mecca (➤193). ***Haemophilus influenzae* type b:** Prophylaxis is given to **all** household contacts of cases if there is a sibling under 4 years considered to be at risk. Recommended treatment is rifampicin 600 mg 24hly for 4 days (children's doses as above).

## Viral meningitis

'Aseptic' meningitis indicates no bacterial cause can be found. The majority are viral. A large number of viruses have been implicated, and depending on the agent, incubation periods, modes of transmission and associated clinical features vary. Viral meningitis is commonest in children and adolescents, and is a common cause of hospital admission in the UK. It is essential to exclude bacterial meningitis.

**Clinical features:** Headache, fever, neck stiffness, photophobia, irritability. There may also be signs of underlying associated virus infection such as parotitis (mumps), pharyngitis, GI disturbance or rash.

**Organisms:** Enteroviruses (Coxsackie A & B, echoviruses, polioviruses ➤347), herpesviruses (HSV-1 and HSV-2, EBV, VZV ➤334), mumps (➤128), measles (➤126), arenaviruses (lymphocytic choriomeningitis ➤356), adenoviruses (➤334).

**Microbiological investigations:** CSF changes are discussed above. Attempt virus culture from CSF, throat swab or stools. Many patients have a peripheral blood leucocytosis.

**Differential diagnosis:** Essential to consider and exclude bacterial, mycobacterial and fungal meningitis. Other very rare causes of aseptic meningitis include syphilis (➤89), leptospirosis (➤327), Lyme disease (➤323) and eosinophilic meningitis (➤237).

## Fungal meningitis

Fungal meningitis is usually associated with immunodeficiency such as HIV infection, and is usually due to *Cryptococcus neoformans* (➤164). Diagnosis is made by India ink staining of CSF and antigen detection in CSF and serum. Other fungal meningitides are rare in the UK; fungal infections that cause invasive disease in the immunocompetent host such as *Histoplasma capsulatum*, *Blastomyces dermatitidis* and *Coccidioides immitis* are geographically restricted in their distribution (➤369). They should be considered if there is an appropriate travel history. *Candida* spp. (➤367) are associated with meningitis in neonates and in patients with CSF shunts.

## CSF shunt infections

CSF shunt infections occur in up to 50% depending on the patient group studied, the duration of follow-up and the device used. The majority present within 2 months of surgery and are due to skin flora, suggesting contamination at the time of operation. *Staphylococcus epidermidis, Staphylococcus aureus,* coryne-

forms and coliforms are most often isolated, but a very large range of other organisms have been reported. Signs of infection can be subtle and non-specific: fever, erythema over the course of the catheter or malfunctioning of the shunt. A minority of patients have symptoms of meningitis. An infected ventriculoperitoneal shunt may present with abdominal symptoms. Treatment usually comprises removal of all or part of the shunt, culture of blood and CSF and prolonged administration of antibiotics, often including intrathecal injection of antibiotics via the externalized shunt.

## Chronic meningitis

Symptoms and signs of meningeal irritation lasting longer than 4 weeks with CSF pleocytosis. Tuberculosis is the commonest infectious cause and must be vigorously pursued (➤41). Other infectious causes include syphilis (➤89), Lyme disease (➤323), listeriosis (➤267) fungal meningitis (➤101), brucellosis (➤303), and helminth infections such as schistosomiasis, cysticercosis and hydatid disease (➤206, 233). Non-infectious causes include carcinomatous meningitis and lymphoma and very rarely connective-tissue diseases such as systemic lupus erythematosus and sarcoid.

## Herpes simplex encephalitis ✉

Encephalitis implies infection of the brain parenchyma. The commonest, and treatable, cause of viral encephalitis in the UK is herpes simplex virus (HSV).

**Risk factors:** HSE occurs in otherwise healthy individuals, but the incidence is higher in the immunocompromised, such as HIV-infected patients. Most episodes are believed to result from reactivation of latent virus rather than primary infection.

**Clinical features:** Onset may be abrupt or insidious. There is often a brief prodrome with headache, fever, lethargy, behavioural change and somnolence, followed by rapid progression to severe CNS dysfunction often with focal

**Table 11.5** Viruses associated with encephalitis ☒

| Disease | Geographical distribution | Vector | Months of greatest risk | Usual incubation (days) |
|---|---|---|---|---|
| **Herpes viruses (➤334)** | | | | |
| Herpes simplex | Worldwide | — | Any | |
| **Togaviruses (➤352)** | | | | |
| Western equine encephalitis | Western North America, S. America | M | JJAS | 5–15 |
| Eastern equine encephalitis | Eastern USA | M | JJA | 5–15 |
| Venezuelan equine encephalitis | South America | M | Rainy months | 2–6 |
| **Flaviviruses (➤352)** | | | | |
| St Louis encephalitis | USA | M | JJA | 5–15 |
| Japanese B encephalitis | SE Asia | M | MJJAS | 5–15 |
| Murray Valley encephalitis | South Australia | M | JFMAM | 5–15 |
| West Nile encephalitis | N. Africa, SE Asia | M | JJAS | 3–12 |
| Tick-borne encephalitis | Central Europe, Asia | T | JJA | 7–14 |
| Powassan encephalitis | Northern USA, southern Canada | T | JJAS | 7–14 |
| Rocio | Brazil | M | FMAMJJ | 5–15 |
| **Bunyaviruses (➤354)** | | | | |
| California encephalitis | Western USA | M | JJASO | 5–15 |
| La Crosse | Mid-Western USA | M | JJAS | 5–15 |

M, mosquito; T, tick.

(usually temporal lobe) signs, seizures and coma. Patients do not usually have concurrent cold sores or genital herpes. Mortality is 60–80% untreated.

**Organisms:** HSV-1 (encephalitis in adults), HSV-2 (meningitis in adults, encephalitis in neonates).

**Microbiological investigations:** LP to exclude bacterial, fungal and mycobacterial meningitis (➤97). PCR for HSV in CSF is sensitive and specific and is now routinely available. Serum/CSF serological titres against HSV rise during infection, but in general this occurs too late, and the results are insufficiently sensitive, for them to be clinically useful except in retrospect. Brain biopsy for histology and viral culture is required for definitive diagnosis; need for early biopsy in all cases remains controversial. Most physicians would treat on the basis of

CT, EEG and clinical signs and observe response to aciclovir.

**Other investigations:** CT scan shows low-density lesions with ring enhancement, particularly in the temporal lobe. EEG may show focal temporal lobe abnormality. Both CT and EEG may be normal early in the illness, and if the diagnosis is strongly suspected, they should be repeated after 48 h. MRI is more sensitive.

**Differential diagnosis:** Meningitis, brain abscess, cerebrovascular accident and tumour. Other viral encephalitides include rabies and the arthropod-borne flaviviruses, togaviruses and bunyaviruses. These are geographically restricted and should be considered if there is an appropriate travel history (see Table 11.5). Enteroviruses and mumps, which more often produce meningitis, may cause a mild self-limiting encephalitis. West Nile virus is a mosquito-borne avian zoonosis causing an illness similar to dengue. Previously restricted to Africa, Eastern Europe and Asia, cases were reported in New York in 1999 and Israel in 2000. Some 1% of cases were complicated by encephalitis (➤354).

**Antibiotic management:** Aciclovir 10 mg/kg iv 8hly for 10 days. Treatment reduces the mortality to ≈25%.

**Supportive management:** Anticonvulsants, intubation and ventilation may all be required. There may be long-term neurological sequelae in survivors.

> **Practice point**
>
> Start antiviral treatment whenever the diagnosis of HSE is suspected, even in the absence of typical CT appearances.

# Cerebral abscess

Localized collection of pus within the brain parenchyma.

**Risk factors:** Up to 80% have an identifiable predisposing cause including recent neurosurgery, contiguous parameningeal infection (sinusitis, otitis, mastoiditis, dental abscess), distant infection with metastatic spread (lung abscess, empyema, endocarditis), cranial trauma. Congenital heart disease with right-to-left shunt greatly increases risk.

**Clinical features:** Symptoms and signs of intracranial mass with focal signs and evidence of raised ICP. Headache, fever, changes in mental status, nausea and vomiting, fits. Onset usually occurs over 1–4 weeks, but may be slower. There may signs of primary infection elsewhere.

**Organisms:** 50% are mixed infections. *Staphylococcus aureus, Streptococcus pneumoniae, Streptococcus 'milleri',* coliforms, *Haemophilus influenzae* and other fastidious Gram-negative rods, *Pseudomonas aeruginosa,* non-sporing anaerobes. Aspirated material is sterile in up to 15% of cases, usually after antibiotic therapy.

**Microbiological investigations:** If cerebral abscess is suspected, LP is **contraindicated** even in the absence of papilloedema, due to the risk of neurological deterioration and the fact that CSF findings are rarely helpful (➤97). If signs suggest possible cerebral abscess or meningitis, treatment for the latter should be started whilst a CT scan is obtained. Blood cultures and culture of any other infected sites such as empyema, sinus aspirate.

**Other investigations:** Leucocytosis is common. CT head scan shows ring-enhancing lesion with surrounding oedema. In early disease CT may be normal or show low-density lesion only.

**Differential diagnosis:** Meningitis (including mycobacterial and fungal). Cerebrovascular accident, tumour, viral encephalitis. Tuberculoma, cryptococcoma or toxoplasma encephalitis in the immunocompromised patient. Rarely cysticercosis, hydatid disease.

**Antibiotic management:** Parenteral cephalosporin + metronidazole may be used initially, guided thereafter by the results of aspiration, microscopy and culture of abscess contents. The clinical setting and risk factors present may suggest likely pathogens.

**Supportive management:** The optimum timing of aspiration and/or open drainage are matters for expert neurosurgical opinion ☎. Small abscesses in otherwise healthy people have been treated with antibiotic therapy alone. Anticonvulsants, careful attention to fluid balance and nutrition, intubation and ventilation may all be required. Dexamethasone and mannitol may be used to control cerebral oedema, but steroids should not be given routinely as animal studies suggest they delay resolution.

**Complications:** Rupture into CSF, recurrence, residual neurological deficit, epilepsy.

# Chapter 12

# Eye infections

## Topical antibiotics for ophthalmic use

Chloramphenicol is widely used, although agranulocytosis after ophthalmic use has been reported very rarely. Fusidic acid preparations are useful for staphylococcal infection, and contain such high concentrations of antibiotic that they are effective against most Gram-positive infections. Gentamicin, neomycin, ciprofloxacin and ofloxacin are also available. Fusidic acid and the quinolones penetrate the cornea to achieve therapeutic concentrations in the anterior chamber. Tetracycline drops are available for *Chlamydia trachomatis* infection, but systemic treatment is also required in this situation. Severe ophthalmic infections are treated by combinations of antibiotics given topically, subconjunctivally, intravitreally and/or systemically; ophthalmological and microbiological opinion should be sought ☎.

## Stye ('hordeolum') and chalazion

Acute bacterial infection of one of the glands of Zeiss, adjacent to the eyelash follicles. Infection of the Meibomian glands may present acutely as an 'internal stye' or as a chronic painless cyst, known as a chalazion.

**Clinical features:** Painful, red, localized swelling at the lid margin, with surrounding erythema. The Meibomian glands are located deeper in the tarsal plate, and infection there tends to produce more pain and swelling, usually visible on the conjunctival surface of the lid. Infection may spread from an internal stye to cause preseptal cellulitis (➤109).

**Organisms:** Usually *Staphylococcus aureus* or culture-negative.

**Microbiological investigations:** Not usually indicated. Gram stain and culture of expressed material may be helpful.

**Antibiotic management:** Local antibiotic ointment/drops.

**Supportive management:** Warm compresses may give symptomatic relief. Incision and drainage may be required, particularly for chalazia.

## Blepharitis

Diffuse inflammation of the eyelids or their margins.

**Risk factors:** Blepharitis is usually associated with seborrhoeic dermatitis, which causes scalp irritation and dandruff. It may also be associated with acne rosacea, or with pubic lice, which may infest the scalp, axillae and eyelashes of sexually active adults, and children, who may acquire the infection by non-venereal contact.

**Clinical features:** Chronic bilateral irritation and hyperaemia of the lid margins, with scaling of the skin, flakes of epithelium clinging to the lashes and destruction of lash follicles. There may be superficial ulceration of the lid margins. The roots of the lashes should be examined carefully to exclude the presence of lice and their eggs (nits).

**Organisms:** *Staphylococcus aureus* is often isolated, and is believed to play a role in pathogenesis, although asymptomatic carriage of *Staphylococcus aureus* is also common.

**Antibiotic management:** Long-term treatment with topical antibiotic ointment/drops. If associated with acne rosacea, oral tetracycline for 2–4 weeks is effective. Lice should be treated by topical application of carbaryl, malathion or permethrin preparations to scalp, axillae and pubic areas (➤95). Eyelid infestation may be treated by coating with vaseline for 3–4 days, although cutting back of the lashes to remove nits may be required.

**Supportive management:** Regular careful cleaning of the eyelids and removal of scaling with plain water and cotton wool buds. Treatment of seborrhoeic dermatitis (➤117) with topical miconazole/hydrocortisone ointment and ketoconazole shampoo.

## Conjunctivitis

Conjunctivitis may be bacterial, chlamydial, viral or allergic. Some chlamydial and viral agents, such as *Chlamydia trachomatis*, cause specific and characteristic syndromes; other causes of bacterial and viral conjunctivitis are not distinguishable clinically. Conjunctivitis is also seen as a minor part of systemic infections such as influenza, leptospirosis, rubella or measles. The major clinical features of conjunctivitis are itching and burning of the eyes, with a serous or purulent discharge. Pain is mild, photophobia and lacrimation are usually absent and there is no impairment of vision, unless infection progresses to keratitis and corneal ulceration, which are discussed separately below. There is erythema of both tarsal and bulbar conjunctivae; in viral infection, this is 'follicular', with tiny translucent follicles of lymphoid hyperplasia over the conjunctival surface.

**Differential diagnosis of acute conjunctivitis:** A number of clinical features help to differentiate acute conjunctivitis, which may usually be treated by the non-specialist, from other causes of acute red eye which require urgent ophthalmic referral. Conjunctivitis is rarely painful. Grittiness and irritation are common, but significant pain suggests corneal involvement or intraocular disease. Visual acuity is normal; sometimes vision is impaired by a film of mucopus over the cornea, but this can be removed by blinking. Vasodilation and redness is spread all over the conjunctivae, or is most obvious nearest the fornices. Conjunctival vasodilation found only around the limbus strongly suggests corneal or intraocular disease. The cornea should be clear and give a sharp, bright reflection. Keratitis causes dulling of the corneal reflection.

> **Practice point**
>
> Conjunctivitis is a clinical diagnosis of exclusion, made in a patient with a red eye and discharge and only if the vision is normal and there is no evidence of keratitis, iritis, or angle closure glaucoma.

### Bacterial conjunctivitis

Much less common than viral conjunctivitis.

**Clinical features:** Infection is usually unilateral initially, spreading to the other eye within a few days. The discharge is usually thick and purulent.

**Organisms:** *Staphylococcus aureus, Streptococcus pneumoniae, Haemophilus influenzae. Staphylococcus aureus* and coliforms may occasionally cause chronic low-grade conjunctivitis. Rarely, *Neisseria gonorrhoeae, Neisseria meningitidis, Moraxella lacunata, Corynebacterium diphtheriae.*

**Microbiological investigations:** Gram stain and culture of discharge. Fluorescence microscopy for chlamydial inclusion bodies. Viral culture.

**Other investigations:** Fluorescent staining to rule out corneal ulcer and abrasion should always be performed.

**Differential diagnosis:** Keratitis. Subconjunctival haematoma. Allergic, viral or chlamydial conjunctivitis.

**Antibiotic management:** Local antibiotic ointment/drops.

**Supportive management:** Topical steroids should not be given because of the possibility of herpetic dendritic ulcer (➢107). Do not apply an eye-patch.

**Complications:** More virulent organisms such as *Neisseria gonorrhoeae*, *Pseudomonas aeruginosa*, *Moraxella lacunata* and *Streptococcus pneumoniae* may cause corneal ulceration. Infection by these organisms and *Neisseria meningitidis* and GAS may necessitate admission for systemic antibiotic therapy.

## Viral conjunctivitis

Many viruses cause conjunctivitis as part of systemic or upper respiratory infection. Certain specific agents cause more severe disease—see below.

**Clinical features:** As for bacterial conjunctivitis. The discharge is thinner and watery, and the conjunctivitis is follicular and less florid. There is often local lymphadenopathy. Purulent discharge suggests bacterial superinfection.

**Microbiological investigations, differential diagnosis:** As for bacterial conjunctivitis.

**Antibiotic management:** Local antibiotic ointment/drops may be given to prevent bacterial superinfection, as well as specific antiviral medication if appropriate (see below).

## Specific forms of conjunctivitis
### Adenovirus conjunctivitis

**Risk factors:** Exposure to other infected children, hence 'swimming-pool conjunctivitis'.

**Clinical features:** Severe conjunctivitis with fever, sore throat and preauricular lymphadenopathy. There may be punctate keratitis, progressing to corneal ulceration, which may persist for months.

**Organisms:** Adenovirus, particularly types 8, 10 and 19.

> **Practice point**
>
> Adenovirus infection is highly contagious, and careful handwashing by patient and physician and disinfection of medical equipment is required to avoid spread.

## Acute haemorrhagic conjunctivitis

**Risk factors:** Crowding and poor hygiene, particularly in the developing world.

**Clinical features:** Severe eyelid oedema and irritation, conjunctivitis and subconjunctival haemorrhage, typically lasting a week to 10 days. Punctate keratitis may develop and there may be signs of systemic viral infection.

**Organisms:** Enterovirus type 70, coxsackievirus A24, adenovirus 11.

## Herpes simplex conjunctivitis

Primary infection by HSV is a rare cause of conjunctivitis. Herpetic vesicles may be seen on the eyelids. The majority of patients with HSV conjunctivitis go on to develop corneal lesions, usually after 7–10 days. Recurrent HSV usually causes HSV keratoconjunctivitis (see below).

## Chlamydia trachomatis infections

*Chlamydia trachomatis* (➢329) causes two distinct ocular syndromes—**adult inclusion conjunctivitis** (IC), which is a sexually transmitted infection due to serotypes D–K, and **trachoma**, a chronic follicular keratoconjunctivitis caused by serotypes A, B and C, which leads over years to corneal scarring and opacity. Trachoma is a major cause of blindness in the developing world. *Chlamydia trachomatis* is also an important cause of ophthalmia neonatorum (➢107).

**Risk factors:** IC predominantly affects sexually active young adults. Trachoma is a disease of poverty, related to frequent reinfection spread by flies, fomites and person to person.

**Clinical features:** IC presents as follicular conjunctivitis, which may persist for months untreated. The lower lid is preferentially affected. In trachoma, follicular conjunctivitis is followed by keratitis, corneal vascularization, scarring and scar retraction. Much of the corneal damage is secondary to distortion of the eyelids by scarring and secondary bacterial keratitis.

**Microbiological investigations:** Diagnosis is confirmed by demonstrating basophilic cytoplasmic inclusion bodies on Giemsa stain or immunofluorescence microscopy of conjunctival scrapings.

**Differential diagnosis:** Viral conjunctivitis, herpes simplex keratitis.

**Antibiotic management:** Oral erythromycin **or** tetracycline, for 3 weeks in IC and for 3–6 weeks in trachoma. In trachoma-endemic areas, re-infection is common and treatment of infected individuals may be secondary to public health measures aimed at reducing transmission rates.

**Complications:** If untreated, IC may fail to recover and may develop the features of trachoma.

### Ophthalmia neonatorum ✉ ②

Infectious conjunctivitis in the neonatal period. Infection is acquired during passage through the birth canal, and may be due to *Neisseria gonorrhoeae, Chlamydia trachomatis, Staphylococcus aureus, Streptococcus pneumoniae* and rarely HSV. Treatment depends on the infecting organism. *Neisseria gonorrhoeae* infection merits systemic treatment with benzylpenicillin, unless penicillinase-producing organisms are isolated or locally prevalent. Chlamydial conjunctivitis requires topical tetracycline and systemic erythromycin to prevent respiratory infection. Other bacterial causes may be treated topically. HSV requires topical aciclovir.

### Phlyctenular conjunctivitis

A localized hypersensitivity reaction, usually secondary to pulmonary tuberculosis (➤37). A raised pinkish nodule (the 'phlycten') appears on the bulbar conjunctiva, usually close to the limbus. It subsequently ulcerates and heals with minimal or no scarring. This process takes about 2 weeks. Symptoms are few, unless the phlycten encroaches on the cornea, where it may cause pain, photophobia and visual loss associated with scarring. Topical steroids accelerate healing and minimize scarring. Patients must be fully assessed for intercurrent pulmonary TB.

### Molluscum contagiosum (➤119)

Infection with the poxvirus that causes molluscum contagiosum may involve the eyelid margins and cause follicular conjunctivitis. Careful examination is required to exclude the presence of the characteristic umbilicated papules, which may hide close to the eyelash roots. Treatment is by mechanical removal of the lesions by excision, cryotherapy or curettage.

## Keratitis

Infectious inflammation of the cornea. Keratitis merits urgent referral to an ophthalmologist, since visual impairment may develop rapidly. ☎

**Risk factors:** Bacterial keratitis usually follows trauma (which may be minor). Soft contact lenses are a particular risk factor for *Pseudomonas aeruginosa* and *Acanthamoeba* infection, because of contamination of lens solutions.

**Clinical features:** Unilateral red eye with moderate to severe pain, photophobia, lacrimation and **impaired vision**. There is usually no exudate. Fluoroscein staining will help to reveal defects in the corneal epithelium. Herpes simplex virus (HSV) causes a characteristic dendritic ulcer. Herpes zoster (➤132) affecting the ophthalmic division of the trigeminal nerve may cause keratitis in 75% of cases. Vesicles on the tip of the nose imply involvement of the nasociliary nerve, and this increases the likelihood of corneal involvement.

**Organisms:** HSV. Varicella zoster virus. *Staphylococcus aureus, Staphylococcus epidermidis, Bacillus cereus*, group A β-haemolytic streptococci (GAS), *Streptococcus pneumoniae, Moraxella lacunata*, pseudomonads. Rarely fungi (commoner in the tropics, esp. *Fusarium* spp.) and *Acanthamoeba* spp. (➤231).

**Microbiological investigations:** Bacterial fungal and viral culture of conjunctival scrapings. Fluorescent antibody stains and special culture techniques are needed to demonstrate *Acanthamoeba* ➤. Corneal biopsy may be required to diagnose fungal keratitis.

**Antibiotic management:** Ophthalmological referral and specialist management are essential. Debridement is often performed. For HSV and zoster, topical and systemic aciclovir should be given. Topical steroids may be required, but should only be given under experienced ophthalmological supervision. Bacterial keratitis is treated with very frequent instillation of antibiotic drops, plus parenteral antibiotics in severe cases. Fungal keratitis has been treated with topical amphotericin, miconazole and econazole. *Acanthamoeba* keratitis is treated with topical dibromopropamidine, chlorhexidine, hexamidine diisothionate and polyhexamethylene biguanide, usually in combination ☎. Neomycin is no longer considered appropriate therapy, because it is not active against cysts and resistance is common.

**Comments:** If keratitis is related to contact lens use, it is essential to ensure adequate and ongoing disinfection of lenses and equipment to avoid recurrence.

## Uveitis

The uveal tract consists of the iris, ciliary body and choroid.

### Anterior uveitis (syn. iridocyclitis)
Inflammation of iris and ciliary body.

**Clinical features:** Unilateral red eye, deep ocular pain with a tender eyeball, irregular or constricted pupil, photophobia and tearing.

**Organisms:** Anterior uveitis is a minor feature of a number of infections, including mumps (➤128), rubella (➤127), measles (➤126), HSV (➤334), herpes zoster (➤132) and secondary syphilis (➤89), and more rarely, *Neisseria gonorrhoeae* (➤86), leptospirosis (➤327), brucellosis (➤303) and Lyme disease (➤323). It is also a feature of Reiter's syndrome (➤122), but it is more commonly seen as a complication of non-infectious diseases, including connective-tissue diseases, inflammatory bowel disease, Behçet's disease and sarcoidosis.

**Differential diagnosis:** Acute glaucoma usually causes a cloudy cornea and a dilated pupil. Conjunctivitis (➤105).

### Posterior uveitis (syn. chorioretinitis)
Indicates inflammation of the choroid, usually with extension to the adjacent retina.

**Clinical features:** Gradual onset of painless visual loss. Ophthalmoscopy reveals retinal scarring.

**Organisms:** *Toxoplasma gondii* (➤137), *Toxocara* spp. (➤236), *Mycobacterium tuberculosis*, usually associated with miliary TB (➤39), very rarely *Histoplasma capsulatum*, if there is an appropriate travel history (➤369). HSV (➤334) and CMV (➤339). VZV may cause chorioretinitis, particularly after an attack of herpes zoster (➤132). In the immunocompromised, *Cryptococcus neoformans* (➤368), CMV (➤166), *Pneumocystis carinii*, e.g. in HIV patients treated with aerosolized pentamidine as prophylaxis against pulmonary pneumocystis.

**Microbiological investigations:** Depending on the clinical situation, appropriate tests to look for extraocular infection by pathogens mentioned, including staining, culture and antigen detection in aspirated material. Serological testing may be helpful. The ophthalmoscopic appearances may be sufficiently characteristic to allow an informed guess.

**Comments:** Urgent ophthalmological referral is required for both forms of uveitis. Aspiration of aqueous or vitreous humour may allow identification of the causative organism.

# Endophthalmitis

Suppurative infection of the vitreous with abscess formation.

**Risk factors:** Exogenous infection secondary to trauma, surgery (risk after phacoemulsification and intraocular lens implantation ≈0.1%), penetrating corneal ulcer. Endogenous metastatic infection during bacteraemia or fungaemia (risk factors include immunocompromise, immunosuppressive drugs, prolonged iv access, IVDU).

**Clinical features:** Pain, photophobia, headache and reduced visual acuity. Conjunctival injection, eyelid swelling, hypopyon and reduced red reflex.

**Organisms: Following surgery:** *Staphylococcus epidermidis* (≈70%), coryneforms, *Staphylococcus aureus*. **Following trauma:** *Staphylococcus aureus*, *Bacillus cereus*, GAS, coliforms, pseudomonads, anaerobes. **Bacteraemic infection:** *Candida* spp., *Staphylococcus aureus*, *Streptococcus pneumoniae*, GAS, coryneforms. Many other possible causes.

**Microbiological investigations:** Gram stain and culture of aspirated material. Blood cultures.

**Antibiotic management:** Systemic, topical and intravitreal antibiotics, guided by the results of microscopy and culture. Specialist referral is obviously very urgent; vitrectomy may be a vital component of therapy ☎.

    ☞ Callegan M, Clin Micro Rev 2002; 15: 111

# Orbital infections

Infection confined to the eyelid and superficial tissues anterior to the orbital septum is referred to as **preseptal cellulitis**. Deeper infection is referred to as **periorbital** or **orbital cellulitis**.

## Preseptal cellulitis

**Risk factors:** Usually secondary to laceration or minor trauma. Occasionally secondary to facial cellulitis or an infected Meibomian cyst (➤104).

**Clinical features:** Pain, swelling and erythema of the eyelid. Low-grade fever. Proptosis and impairment of ocular mobility are **not** seen; if present, they suggest orbital cellulitis.

**Organisms:** *Staphylococcus aureus*, GAS, *Haemophilus influenzae* (particularly in children prior to introduction of Hib vaccination). Anaerobic infection may follow trauma, especially bite injuries, and is suggested by foul-smelling discharge and tissue necrosis.

**Microbiological investigations:** Gram stain and culture of pus. Blood cultures.

**Other investigations:** CT/MRI may be required to exclude orbital spread.

**Antibiotic management:** Flucloxacillin. If *Haemophilus influenzae* is suspected, then give parenteral cephalosporin **or** co-amoxiclav. See also bites (➤114).

## Orbital cellulitis

Infection within the tissues of the orbit.

**Risk factors:** Usually by direct spread from ethmoid or frontal sinusitis (➤17). Less often following surgery or trauma, otitis media, dental infection or facial cellulitis.

**Clinical features:** Fever, headache, toxaemia, eyelid oedema, rhinorrhoea, pain and tenderness over the eye. Limited, painful eye movement. As infection progresses there may be displacement of the globe by subperiosteal collection of pus extending directly from the infected adjacent sinus, ophthalmoplegia and severely reduced visual acuity.

    **Cavernous sinus thrombosis** may occur with headache, eye pain, neck stiffness, swelling over the forehead and eyelids. Ophthalmoplegia and papilloedema may occur. The patient is extremely unwell, with altered level of consciousness.

**Organisms:** *Streptococcus pneumoniae*, *Staphylococcus aureus* (especially post surgery or trauma), GAS, *Streptococcus* '*milleri*', *Haemophilus influenzae* and other fastidious

Gram-negative rods, anaerobes. In elderly diabetics or immunocompromised patients, fungal sinusitis due to zygomycetes and other filamentous fungi may involve the orbit (➤369).

**Microbiological investigations:** Gram stain and culture of aspirated material. Blood culture. LP may be indicated if there is meningism. Biopsy may be needed to establish the diagnosis of fungal infection.

**Other investigations:** Sinus X-rays, CT/MRI scanning to examine sinuses and delineate extent of infection.

**Differential diagnosis:** Preseptal cellulitis—in this condition, limitation of eye movement and impaired visual acuity do not occur.

**Antibiotic management:** Initially cefotaxime + metronidazole, guided thereafter by microbiology results. Urgent surgery plus high-dose lipid preparation of amphotericin in zygomycosis (➤369).

**Supportive management:** Surgical intervention to drain collections may be required.

**Complications:** Meningitis.

# Dacryocystitis

Infection of the lacrimal sac, usually secondary to obstruction of the nasolacrimal duct.

**Clinical features:** Pain, swelling and tenderness in the nasal corner of the eye below the mediocanthal ligament.

**Organisms:** *Staphylococcus aureus*, *Streptococcus pneumoniae*, GAS; *Actinomyces israelii*.

**Microbiological investigations:** Gram stain and culture of pus.

**Antibiotic management:** Local antibiotic ointment/drops **and** systemic flucloxacillin are required. *Actinomyces israelii* infection responds to local debridement.

**Supportive management:** Ophthalmological referral for duct irrigation or drainage is usually required ☎.

# Chapter 13

# Skin infections

Features of normal skin that prevent infection include the physical integrity, dryness and regular shedding of the stratum corneum, free fatty acids and low pH of sebum, and normal cellular and humoral immune function. The normal cutaneous flora (Table 13.1) consists of a restricted range of organisms, most of which may be opportunist pathogens in certain circumstances.

## Impetigo ①

Superficial infection of the stratum corneum, usually confined to the face.

**Risk factors:** Minor trauma, underlying dermatitis (e.g. atopic eczema). Nasal carriage of *Staphylococcus aureus*. Commonest in children.

**Clinical features:** Vesicles and pustules on an erythematous base, which burst leaving yellow-brown scabs. It is non-scarring. Persistence of flaccid blisters ('bullous impetigo') suggests staphylococcal infection (usually due to phage type 71). **Ecthyma** is a variant of impetigo which is common in debilitated, malnourished or alcoholic patients. Infection by the *Staphylococcus aureus* or group A β-haemolytic streptococci (GAS) causes scarring ulceration on the legs.

**Organisms:** *Staphylococcus aureus* or GAS, often mixed.

**Microbiological investigations:** Usually unnecessary.

**Antibiotic management:** Topical mupirocin **or** oral flucloxacillin.

## Folliculitis

Inflammation of the hair follicles.

**Risk factors:** Commonest in children. Moist, warm conditions and tight clothing predispose.

**Clinical features:** Erythematous papules and pustules around hairs, usually occurring in crops.

**Organisms:** *Staphylococcus aureus. Pseudomonas aeruginosa* causes 'hot-tub folliculitis', associated with use of contaminated jacuzzis and hot tubs.

**Antibiotic management:** Flucloxacillin may be used in extensive or prolonged folliculitis. Hot-tub folliculitis is usually self-limited.

## Cutaneous abscesses (boils, furuncles and carbuncles)

Localized pyogenic skin infection, usually arising in an infected hair follicle.

**Risk factors:** Boils and carbuncles are common infections in normal hosts. Recurrent infection may indicate diabetes mellitus, poor hygiene or nasal carriage of virulent *Staphylococcus aureus* strains.

**Clinical features:** A tender nodule, usually surmounted by a pustule through which a hair emerges. A **furuncle** is an isolated cutaneous abscess or boil. Systemic features of infection are unusual. When several adjacent furuncles coalesce and drain through multiple orifices, this is termed a **carbuncle**, and fever and toxaemia are more likely.

**Table 13.1** Normal cutaneous flora

| Organism | | Location | Disease associations |
|---|---|---|---|
| *Staphylococcus aureus* | ➤249 | Anterior nares, skin folds | See text |
| *Staphylococcus epidermidis* | ➤253 | All skin | Prosthetic materials and line infections |
| *Micrococcus* spp. | ➤250 | | |
| *Corynebacterium* spp. 'diphtheroids' | ➤269 | Moist areas | Erythrasma (➤117), prosthetic materials and line infections |
| *Bacillus* spp. | ➤263 | | |
| *Brevibacterium* spp. | ➤264 | | |
| Gram-negative bacilli, commonly *Acinetobacter* spp. | | Moist skin | UTI (➤77), prosthetic materials and line infections |
| *Propionibacterium acnes* | ➤270 | Sebaceous glands | Acne vulgaris (➤116) |
| *Pityrosporum orbiculare* | ➤117 | Back and chest | Pityriasis versicolor, seborrhoeic dermatitis (➤117) |
| *Candida albicans* | ➤367 | Mucous membranes and moist skin | Candidiasis |

**Organisms:** *Staphylococcus aureus*, but often culture-negative. Mixed infection by coliforms, anaerobes and other Gram-positive cocci is more likely in perineal abscesses.

**Microbiological investigations:** Gram stain and culture of pus. Blood cultures in severe infection.

**Antibiotic management:** Flucloxacillin if there is significant surrounding cellulitis (➤113), or failure to resolve. Co-amoxiclav is suitable for initial treatment of perineal abscesses, until results of microbiology are available.

**Supportive management:** Incision and drainage is usually required. Patients at risk of endocarditis should receive antibiotic prophylaxis for this procedure. For patients with prosthetic valves, flucloxacillin 1 g iv before and 6 h after, **plus** gentamicin 120 mg with first dose. For non-prosthetic valves, flucloxacillin, 500 mg po at the same timings.

**Complications:** Systemic infection with metastatic abscess.

## Special forms of cutaneous abscess
### Boils on the upper lip and nose

Boils in the 'dangerous triangle' carry the special risk of cavernous sinus thrombosis. They should not be incised or manipulated. Warm soaks may encourage pointing. Flucloxacillin should be given.

### Perianal abscess

If infected with gut flora, often associated with fistula-in-ano.

### Hydradenitis suppurativa

A chronic suppurative disease of apocrine glands in genital, axillary and perianal areas. Plugging of glands leads to proximal dilatation, rupture and infection with local normal flora. Sinus track formation and scarring follow.

**Organisms:** Mixed flora, including non-sporing anaerobes, *Streptococcus* 'milleri', staphylococci, diphtheroids and coliforms.

**Management:** Incision and drainage of abscesses, antibiotics if inflamed and systemically unwell: flucloxacillin **plus** metronidazole, or co-amoxiclav.

### Breast abscess

May occur during lactation. *Staphylococcus aureus*, β-haemolytic streptococci and normal skin flora are usually involved. Incision and drainage may be required. Flucloxacillin or co-amoxiclav may be given. Recurrent abscesses, often associated with diabetes mellitus or nipple inversion, may involve mixed anaerobic flora and may require excision of nipple ducts.

# Cellulitis

Acute spreading infection of the subcutaneous tissues.

**Risk factors:** Minor trauma, dermatitis. Peripheral vascular disease. Impaired lymphatic drainage, often following previous attacks of cellulitis. Site of saphenous vein harvest for coronary artery bypass surgery.

**Clinical features:** Erythema, tenderness, swelling and warmth. Bullae and desquamation may occur. Fever, rigors. Lymphadenitis.

**Organisms:** GAS, *Staphylococcus aureus*. See also wound infections (➤113). Rarely *Pasteurella multocida* (bite wounds ➤114).

**Microbiological investigations:** Local cultures may occasionally be helpful but are usually negative. Swab any visible lesions (e.g. cracked skin between toes). Blood cultures.

**Differential diagnosis:** Venous thrombosis.

**Antibiotic management:** In mild cases, oral flucloxacillin; in severe infections or if oral therapy fails, give iv flucloxacillin and benzylpenicillin. Alternatives include clindamycin or parenteral cephalosporin. In children with facial cellulitis, initial therapy should include cover for *Haemophilus influenzae*: co-amoxiclav or parenteral cephalosporin.

**Complications:** Permanent scarring, lymphatic damage and lymphoedema, recurrence.

## Particular forms of cellulitis
### Erysipelas ①

A clinically distinct form of cellulitis with a sharply demarcated raised edge, which may advance rapidly and tends to occur on the face and limbs. It is usually due to GAS.

### Erysipeloid

A rare infection due to *Erysipelothrix rhusiopathiae* (➤271). It presents as a tender, purple, well-demarcated cellulitis of the fingers or hand in those who handle raw fish and poultry. Give benzylpenicillin (erythromycin if penicillin allergic).

### *Haemophilus influenzae* facial cellulitis

Typically causes a purple cellulitis with indistinct margins over the face and arms. Previously predominantly in children, but very rare since the advent of Hib vaccination.

### Blistering distal dactylitis

Due to GAS with or without *Staphylococcus aureus*. It presents as a painful superficial bulla over the finger pulp in children. Incision and drainage and systemic flucloxacillin are required.

# Wound infection

**Risk factors:** Damage to the physical integrity of the skin is the most important risk factor for infection. Wound infection may follow traumatic or surgical wounds. Predisposing factors include chronic illness and debility, diabetes, cirrhosis and alcoholism, trauma to mucosae allowing inoculation of normal flora, foreign body, *Staphylococcus aureus* nasal carriage. Less common risk factors are shown in Table 13.2.

**Clinical features:** Erythema, warmth, tenderness, swelling and a purulent exudate. Postoperative fever. Failure to heal and dehiscence

**Table 13.2** Special forms of wound infection

| Risk factors | Organisms | Management | Comments |
|---|---|---|---|
| Freshwater contamination | *Aeromonas hydrophila* (➤286) | Parenteral cephalosporin | |
| Seawater contamination | *Vibrio vulnificus* (➤286) and other vibrios | Parenteral cephalosporin **or** doxycycline **plus** gentamicin | May range from mild cellulitis to severe bacterial myositis |
| Animal bites (monkey bites carry a special risk of monkey herpes B infection ☎) | *Pasteurella multocida* (➤303), *Capnocytophaga canimorsus* (DF-2) (➤302), non-sporing anaerobes, oral streptococci, staphylococci | Thorough cleansing. Give prophylactic antibiotics. Co-amoxiclav, **or** co-trimoxazole **plus** metronidazole | Establish need for tetanus treatment (➤315). Consider rabies if appropriate travel history (➤358) |
| Human bites | Non-sporing anaerobes, oral streptococci, staphylococci, *Eikenella corrodens* (➤306) | Thorough cleansing. Give prophylactic antibiotics. Co-amoxiclav, **or** erythromycin **plus** metronidazole | |
| Swimming pool granuloma (fish-tank granuloma) | *Mycobacterium marinum* | Rifampicin and ethambutol | (➤48) |

are important sequelae of surgical wound infection.

**Organisms:** *Staphylococcus aureus,* GAS. Contaminated accidental wounds and abdominal surgical wounds may be infected by normal local mucosal flora including coliforms, *Clostridium* spp. and non-sporing anaerobes, and *Streptococcus* 'milleri'.

**Microbiological investigations:** Gram stain and culture of pus. Blood cultures if unwell.

**Antibiotic management:** Topical antibiotics are **not** indicated. Initial treatment depends on clinical situation and results of microbiology. Flucloxacillin may be given initially, unless the wound is heavily contaminated or is an abdominal or mucosal surgical wound, in which case cover should be extended to coliforms and anaerobes, e.g. benzylpenicillin + gentamicin + metronidazole, **or** parenteral cephalosporin + metronidazole.

**Supportive management:** Drain pus, debride devitalized tissue and remove foreign bodies — this is more important than choice of antibiotic therapy. Establish tetanus vaccination status (➤315).

# Severe tissue infections

These may be classified by microbial aetiology, e.g. due to a single species such as GAS or *Clostridium perfringens,* or polymicrobial, often due to a mixture of Gram-negative aerobes and anaerobes. They may also be classified by anatomical site of infection, e.g. myositis, fasciitis. Certain clinical syndromes such as clostridial myonecrosis, or necrotizing fasciitis due to GAS are well-defined, but very similar clinical features may result from polymicrobial infections, in which case the results of Gram stain and culture may identify only a subset of the organisms responsible. **Early surgical referral** is essential, as prompt debridement is necessary to avoid a fatal outcome in most severe tissue infections. **High-dose parenteral antibiotics**, including cover for Gram-negative aerobes and anaerobes, clostridia and GAS should be used in all cases initially (e.g. penicillin + gentamicin + metronidazole).

## Gas gangrene (clostridial myonecrosis)

Necrotizing gas-forming infection of muscle with systemic toxaemia. The presence of gas in the tissues is not pathognomic of clostridial infection—it may also occur in infection by coliforms or non-sporing anaerobes.

**Risk factors:** This rare condition usually follows traumatic injury with wound contamination. Anaerobic devitalized tissue provides the environment for clostridial growth. Also occurs rarely following intestinal or biliary surgery and very rarely spontaneously, either by contiguous or metastatic spread from a colonic carcinoma or diverticular abscess, or in neutropenic patients.

**Clinical features:** Severe necrotizing cellulitis and myositis with tissue gas and severe systemic toxaemia. Usually occurs 1–4 days after trauma (range 8 h–3 weeks). Pain, fever, hypotension, oedema of affected skin with haemorrhagic bullae and unpleasant odour. At operation, muscles have a characteristic appearance, initially pale and oedematous, with tissue gas and a serous discharge, progressing to frank gangrene. Intravascular haemolysis, DIC and renal failure are also seen. Frequently fatal, even with optimum management.

**Organisms:** *Clostridium perfringens* (80%), *Clostridium novyi* (*oedematiens*), *Clostridium septicum*.

**Microbiological investigations:** Microscopy of tissue samples shows brick-shaped Gram-positive rods and scanty pus cells. Culture may be positive, but **the diagnosis is clinical** because of the urgent need for surgical debridement.

**Other investigations:** USS and CT may help to localize and delineate infection.

**Differential diagnosis:** Necrotizing fasciitis (see below).

**Antibiotic management:** Benzylpenicillin + gentamicin + metronidazole should be given to cover the possibility of mixed or secondary infection with coliforms and non-sporing anaerobes.

**Supportive management:** Resection of all dead tissue is essential. Hyperbaric oxygen therapy is believed to help, although there has been no controlled clinical trial.

**Comments:** See also puerperal uterine infection by *Clostridium perfringens* (➤84).

> **Practice point**
>
> Fatal *Clostridium novyi* infection has recently been associated with subcutaneous injection of contaminated heroin.

## Necrotizing fasciitis

(Including synergistic gangrene, streptococcal gangrene, 'hospital gangrene'.)

Acute necrotizing cellulitis involving the dermis, subcutaneous fat and superficial fascia.

**Risk factors:** Usually postsurgical, with exposure to bowel flora. May be spontaneous, following e.g. urinary tract infection, urethral diverticula or perianal suppuration. Predisposing factors include diabetes, age, gross obesity and intercurrent illness. May complicate minor skin wounds, particularly if due to GAS. Necrotizing fasciitis due to GAS has been referred to in the past as 'hospital gangrene'.

**Clinical features:** Rapidly spreading painful cellulitis, often with tissue gas and foul odour. Physical signs such as erythema and induration may be less than expected given the degree of tissue destruction subsequently found at operation. Diagnosis is often suggested by a failure to improve on antibiotics, very rapid progression, systemic toxicity or development of cutaneous anaesthesia and gangrene. At surgical exploration, there is disintegration of the superficial fascial plane with extensive undermining.

**Fournier's gangrene** is a particular form of necrotizing fasciitis affecting the male genitalia. Patients are usually >50 yrs and are often diabetic. Infection may follow surgery, minor trauma, local sepsis or UTI. Onset may be rapid with systemic toxicity, genital swelling and gangrene, which may extend up the abdominal wall and down the thighs. The penile and scrotal skin may slough.

**Organisms:** Mixed infection with coliforms and anaerobes, or GAS ($\approx 30\%$).

**Microbiological investigations:** Gram stain and culture of exudate, biopsy material or tissue fluid aspirated from the advancing edge. Blood cultures.

**Other investigations:** X-rays, CT, MRI and USS may demonstrate tissue gas and help to delineate infection.

**Differential diagnosis:** Streptococcal cellulitis (➤113). Clostridial myonecrosis (➤115).

**Surgical management:** Early surgical intervention to deroof undermined areas and remove all necrotic tissue. **Radical debridement is essential.**

**Antibiotic management:** High-dose penicillin + gentamicin + metronidazole initially, guided thereafter by the results of microbiology. Clindamycin may be especially effective for severe GAS infection, perhaps by inhibiting protein toxin synthesis.

### Meleney's synergistic gangrene

A rare, slowly progressive synergistic wound infection that occurs following surgery and is usually caused by *Streptococcus 'milleri'* and *Staphylococcus aureus* and may involve non-sporing anaerobes. It is not associated with systemic toxicity. Surgical debridement, flucloxacillin + metronidazole are indicated.

## Bacterial myositis (pyomyositis)

Bacterial infection of muscle. Rare in the developed world, commoner in the tropics ('tropical pyomyositis').

**Risk factors:** 25% have antecedent trauma. Other cases occur in apparently healthy individuals and are presumed secondary to bacteraemia.

**Clinical features:** Induration and tenderness of muscles, usually quadriceps, progressing to fluctuance and abscess formation. 40% have multiple abscesses.

**Organisms:** *Staphylococcus aureus,* GAS, *Aeromonas* spp., as well as many other less common organisms.

**Microbiological investigations:** Gram stain and culture of aspirated material. Blood cultures.

**Other investigations:** Leucocytosis. Creatine kinase is usually normal. USS, CT and MRI will delineate abscesses and guide aspiration for diagnosis and treatment.

**Differential diagnosis:** Cysticercosis (➤238), trichinosis (➤241).

**Surgical management:** Aspiration or incision and drainage.

**Antibiotic management:** Flucloxacillin initially, guided thereafter by microbiology.

## Acne vulgaris

Inflammation of the seborrhoeic follicles. Acne is multifactorial in origin, due to increased, androgen-driven sebum production, hyperkeratosis of the follicular epithelium with plug formation and growth within the follicle of *Propionibacterium acnes*. Treatment should be started early to avoid scarring.

**Management: Mild cases:** Regular thorough cleansing followed by application of benzoyl peroxide or azelaic acid. **Moderate cases:** Long-term topical or oral tetracycline (250 mg 12hly po) or erythromycin (250 mg 12hly po). Topical clindamycin is also very effective. **Severe cases**

merit dermatological referral for consideration of topical retinoin or systemic isotretinoin. Because of the real risk of teratogenicity, the latter is only available for use under consultant dermatologist supervision.

## Seborrhoeic dermatitis

Scaling and greasiness of the scalp, forehead, interscapular, sternal and intertriginous regions, caused by hypersensitivity to, and overgrowth of, commensal skin fungi, in particular *Pityrosporum orbiculare*. Ketoconazole shampoo and topical miconazole/hydrocortisone cream are effective. Topical hydrocortisone alone is often sufficient.

## Cutaneous fungal infections ('dermatophytoses')

Ringworm (tinea) is particularly common in children, and in adults with poor personal hygiene or occupational exposure to animals.

**Clinical features:** Vary depending on the site of infection. **Tinea capitis** (scalp ringworm) presents as an area of erythema and scaling on the scalp with hair loss. Pustules may develop. **Kerion** describes a large, boggy, inflammatory mass on the scalp, with multiple pustules and overlying hair loss. Infection is acquired by person-to-person spread or via fomites such as infected hairbrushes or bedding. **Tinea barbae** affects the beard area, usually in men with rural occupations or animal contact. **Tinea corporis** presents as a pruritic scaly erythematous papule with a raised edge and central healing. **Tinea cruris** describes infection of the groin. It is common in men and humidity and tight-fitting clothing are predisposing factors. **Majocchi's granuloma** occurs on the legs and arms, particularly in women after shaving. It presents as multiple red pustules that coalesce to form an inflamed plaque. **Tinea pedis** (athlete's foot) causes itching, soreness and maceration between the toes. Warmth, humidity and occlusion predispose. Fungal infection of the **nails** causes subungual hyperkeratosis, with lifting of the free edge of the nail.

**Organisms:** *Microsporum* spp., *Trichophyton* spp. (recently rising incidence in the UK), *Epidermophyton* spp.

**Microbiological investigations:** Microscopy of KOH preparation of scrapings or hair. Culture.

**Differential diagnosis:** Seborrhoeic dermatitis, psoriasis, eczema.

**Antibiotic management:** Topical miconazole, ketoconazole **or** clotrimazole. Systemic treatment with terbinafine or itraconazole if topical treatment fails, or if infection is extensive, multicentric or difficult to treat. Fungal nail infections require terbinafine treatment for 6–12 weeks.

**Supportive management:** Attention to risk factors, such as close-fitting clothes or shoes.

**Pityriasis versicolor** ('tinea versicolor') is a common superficial infection caused by the commensal skin fungus *Pityrosporum orbiculare* (also known as *Malassezia furfur*, *Pityrosporum ovale*, or *Malassezia ovalis*). Hypopigmented, light brown, or salmon-coloured, often scaly, macules, most commonly on the upper trunk and extremities, and less often on the face and intertriginous areas. Commonest in tropics. Diagnosis is confirmed by microscopy of skin scrapings. Topical antifungals are usually effective (treat for 2 weeks, although skin may take months to regain normal appearance). Oral itraconazole or fluconazole is also effective (esp. for extensive disease), but terbinafine is *not* effective.

## Erythrasma

Superficial cutaneous infection by *Corynebacterium minutissimum*, commonest in tropical climates.

**Clinical features:** Maceration, scaling and erythema in toe webs. Red-brown well-demarcated irregular patches over dry skin. Skin fluoresces red/pink in UV light (Wood's lamp).

**Management:** Topical miconazole. Vigorous washing. Whitfield's ointment.

**Table 13.3** Causes of erythema nodosum

| | |
|---|---|
| Streptococcal infection | (➤254) |
| Sulphonamides | (➤405) |
| Sarcoidosis | |
| Tuberculosis | (➤37) |
| Lymphogranuloma venereum | (➤94) |
| Cat scratch disease | (➤309) |
| Psittacosis | (➤329) |
| Infectious mononucleosis | (➤133) |
| Tularaemia | (➤307) |
| Histoplasmosis | (➤369) |
| *Yersinia* spp. | (➤294) |
| Leprosy | (➤46) |
| Blastomycosis | (➤370) |
| Coccidioidomycosis | (➤369) |
| Ulcerative colitis | |
| Crohn's disease | |
| Leukaemia | |
| Lymphoma | |
| Pregnancy | |
| Oral contraceptive pill | |

## Erythema nodosum (EN)

Tender red swellings on the front of the shins, and sometimes also on the thighs and forearms. Pathologically there is small-vessel vasculitis in the deep dermis and subcutaneous tissue. A number of infectious and non-infectious diseases are associated with EN (Table 13.3).

## Herpes simplex skin infections

Herpes simplex virus (HSV) does not usually infect intact skin; primary cutaneous infection is associated with trauma or pre-existing skin disease. Primary infections may be asymptomatic. Both primary and recurrent disease are associated with the development of painful vesicles that progress to pustules and then scabs, healing without scarring.

### Primary cutaneous HSV infection

**Clinical features:** Traumatic herpes ('herpes gladiatorum', 'scrumpox') results from contamination of broken skin by infectious saliva or vesicle fluid. There is a localized vesicular rash with lymphadenopathy, fever and constitutional symptoms. Recurrences are common. There may be a prodrome of itching, pain or paraesthesia, and lymphadenopathy is common. HSV infection may be severe if it occurs in patients with eczema or other skin disease (e.g. pemphigus or burns) which allow extensive viral replication and easy spread. Severe infection in patients with atopic eczema (**Kaposi's varicelliform eruption** syn. **eczema herpeticum**) may cause widespread vesicular rash and severe constitutional symptoms and may follow primary or recurrent infection. In young children, the infection may be fatal due to disseminated visceral involvement. HSV may cause **paronychia** ('whitlow'), particularly in health professionals exposed to HSV-1 infected saliva, in children with herpes stomatitis (➤129), and in adults with genital herpes. Two to 7 days after exposure, itching, pain and erythema of the terminal phalanx develop, followed by a vesicular eruption which resolves after ≈10 days. Pain may be severe; recurrence and local lymphadenopathy are common.

**Organisms:** Most cutaneous HSV infections are due to HSV-1.

**Microbiological investigations:** Examination of vesicle fluid (culture, immunofluorescence or PCR). Serology.

### Recurrent cutaneous HSV infection

Recurrent infection occurs after the unusual cutaneous primary infections described above, but the most common manifestation is **herpes labialis** ('cold sores') which are due to reactivation of HSV-1 infection in the trigeminal ganglion. Genital herpes due to reactivation, usually of HSV-2, in the sacral ganglia, is discussed elsewhere (➤88).

**Clinical features:** After a prodrome of pain and itching lasting from 6 to 48 h, a small cluster of erythematous papules develops on the lip, usually at the vermilion border, and most commonly on the outer third of the lower lip. The papules rapidly develop into vesicles, which crust over and heal within 2–3 days. Herpes labialis is frequently precipitated by external stimuli, such as bright sunlight, or by intercurrent illness or fever. Classically, the sores appear during the course of bacterial pneumonia (hence 'fever sores').

**Management:** Oral aciclovir may shorten the duration of the primary attack, but it is less effective for recurrent attacks. Topical aciclovir is not very effective and is not recommended. **Kaposi's varicelliform eruption** is an indication for urgent systemic (usually iv) aciclovir.

## Molluscum contagiosum

A wart-like skin condition caused by poxvirus infection.

**Risk factors:** Infection occurs worldwide. It is commonest in young adults. Transmission occurs by direct contact, including sexual contact.

**Clinical features:** Firm raised umbilicated flesh coloured nodules develop on the skin anywhere on the body except the palms and soles. Typically occur on the face and genitalia. Lesions may persist for months or years.

**Organisms:** Family *Poxviridae*, genus *Molluscipoxvirus* (➤341).

**Microbiological investigations:** Diagnosis is clinical. Routine culture of virus is not possible.

**Supportive management:** There is no specific antiviral therapy. Treatment depends on ablation of lesions by curettage, cryotherapy or topical agents such as trichloracetic acid.

**Comments:** In immunocompromised patients, particularly those with AIDS, molluscum contagiosum causes bigger and more numerous lesions, which may be very disfiguring. Regular cryotherapy may be required.

## Orf (syn. contagious pustular dermatosis)

This occupational disease of those who work with sheep is caused by a parapoxvirus (➤341) and is acquired by direct contact with infected animals. It produces a raised fleshy purple plaque 1–2 cm in diameter on the hands or fingers of infected farmers and veterinary surgeons. A central vesicle develops, often with haemorrhage into the base. Spontaneous resolution occurs over a few weeks. Recovery may be complicated by the development of a widespread itchy vesicular eruption, which has been described as a form of erythema multiforme and which is thought to be a manifestation of hypersensitivity.

# Chapter 14

# Bone and joint infections

## Septic arthritis

Bacterial joint infection.

**Risk factors:** Usually secondary to haematogenous seeding of the highly vascular synovial membrane during bacteraemia; occasionally due to direct spread from bone or adjacent tissues. Pre-existing joint disease (e.g. rheumatoid arthritis (RA), crystal synovitis, severe osteoarthritis, haemarthrosis) and chronic systemic disease (e.g. malignancy) or IVDU predispose. Direct intra-articular inoculation, iatrogenic or traumatic, is a rare cause of infection, except in the case of prosthetic joint infection. Risks estimated at 0.007% for intra-articular injection, 0.04–0.4% for arthroscopy. In young adults, consider disseminated gonococcal infection (➤86).

**Clinical features:** Rapid onset, over hours or days, of monoarthritis affecting (in descending order of frequency) knee, hip, ankle, wrist, shoulder, elbow or other synovial joint. 15–20% have more than one affected joint (especially in *Neisseria* infection and Lyme disease). Joint is swollen, tender, red, warm and has very limited range of movement due to pain. Fever and leucocytosis are common, but may be absent. Signs may be minimal with infected prosthetic joint or at certain locations, e.g. sacroiliac joints. There may evidence of a source of bacteraemia.

Gonococcal arthritis is a feature of disseminated gonococcal infection (➤86). It is three times commoner in women. Only 25%, mostly men, report concurrent symptoms of genital gonorrhoea. The incubation time ranges from 1 day to 2 months after sexual exposure. Usual presentation is migratory polyarthralgia followed by synovitis and tenosynovitis at more than one site (knees, wrists, ankles, hand and foot tendon sheaths). Most have skin lesions (macules, papules and pustules) although these may be scanty. Septic arthritis also occurs during **meningococcaemia** (➤185) although *Neisseria meningitidis* infection is more often associated with a sterile immune-mediated oligoarthritis.

**Organisms:** Adults: *Staphylococcus aureus* (90% of cases complicating RA), streptococci, coliforms (particularly with malignancy, immunosuppression or IVDU), rarely *Streptococcus pneumoniae*. *Neisseria gonorrhoeae* and *meningitidis*. In children under 2 yrs: *Haemophilus influenzae*, *Staphylococcus aureus*. In neonates, *Staphylococcus aureus*, coliforms and Gp B β-haemolytic streptococci. Arthritis is also associated with *Brucella* spp. (➤303), and *Salmonella* spp. (➤280), particularly in developing world. *Mycobacterium tuberculosis* (➤40).

**Microbiological investigations:** Immediate joint aspiration is mandatory. Fluid may be inoculated direct into blood culture bottles, but these are optimized for culture when they contain blood, so also send some in a sterile universal for Gram stain and conventional culture. Neutrophil counts on synovial fluid are usually high (50 000–150 000 WBC/μL), but do not differentiate from non-infectious causes. Fluid should always be examined for crystals, but their presence does not exclude sepsis, particularly as crystal arthropathy predisposes to septic arthritis. Sensitivity of Gram stain 11–80%, depending on causative organism (Gram-positives are more readily visualized). Synovial fluid culture is positive in >90% of cases due to *Staphylococcus aureus*, and blood cultures are positive in ≈50%. Mycobacterial and fungal cultures should be requested in more chronic cases in groups at risk. USS, CT and MRI may be used to assess the presence of, and assist drainage of, effusions from joints otherwise difficult to aspirate, such as hip and sacroiliacs. Synovial biopsy may be necessary to diagnose TB. In gonococcal arthritis, blood cultures are positive in <10% and synovial fluid culture in ≈25%; genital cultures (➤87) are positive in the majority. PCR assays are showing promise.

**Other investigations:** X-rays may be normal early in disease. Earliest finding is joint effusion with displacement of the fat pads, followed by periarticular osteoporosis, joint space narrowing and erosions. Bone scan can be helpful in localizing infection, and differentiating between septic arthritis and overlying cellulitis.

**Differential diagnosis:** RA, crystal synovitis, seronegative spondarthritides, Reiter's syndrome (➤122), viral arthritis (e.g. due to rubella (➤127), rubella vaccination, parvovirus (➤341) or hepatitis B (➤70)), reactive arthritis (➤122), Lyme disease (➤323).

**Antibiotic management:** Depends on clinical situation and results of initial Gram stain and culture. **Gram-positive cocci seen:** flucloxacillin (≥2 g q6h), unless there is reason to suspect MRSA (➤251) when vancomycin should be used. **Gram-negative cocci seen:** parenteral cephalosporin. If *Neisseria gonorrhoeae* subsequently grown and shown to be penicillin-sensitive, change to benzylpenicillin. **Gram-negative bacilli seen:** parenteral cephalosporin + gentamicin. **Negative Gram stain:** Adult with risk factors listed above: flucloxacillin + gentamicin. Children and healthy young adults: parenteral cephalosporin. Therapy can be modified when culture results are available. Disseminated gonococcal infection characteristically responds rapidly (within 1–3 days) to appropriate antibiotics. Duration of therapy: 21 days for *Neisseria gonorrhoeae*. Other organisms 3–4 weeks, depending on response.

**Supportive management:** Joint drainage is required and may be achieved by needle aspiration of peripheral joints. Axial joints usually need open surgical drainage. Rheumatological and/or orthopaedic referral is strongly recommended ☎.

**Complications:** During recovery, a sterile 'post-infectious' arthritis may affect the joint. Differentiation from relapse depends on Gram stain and culture of synovial fluid. Some 50% have residual sequelae after successful antimicrobial therapy (chronic pain, restriction of movement) commoner in elderly, in pre-existing joint disease, in shoulder and hip infection and with treatment delay >1 week.

> **Practice point**
>
> Acute monoarthritis is septic until proven otherwise, and should be aspirated.

## Prosthetic joint infection

Approximately 1% of joint prostheses will become infected. The majority are acquired during the original operation; occasionally infected later by bacteraemia. This almost always occurs secondary to an established septic focus elsewhere in the body; transient bacteraemia from e.g. dental extractions or endoscopy has never been proven to result in prosthetic joint infection.

**Clinical features:** Loosening of the prosthesis is more common and does not necessarily indicate infection, but may predispose towards it. Fever and local signs may be absent. Progressive pain made worse by activity is characteristic, although a good range of passive movement may be preserved.

**Organisms:** *Staphylococcus aureus* and *epidermidis*, coliforms, enterococci; many other species reported less often.

**Investigations:** ESR and CRP are usually raised and this may be useful evidence of infection. Indium white cell scan may also be helpful. Aspiration around the prosthesis may yield the causative organism.

**Management:** Often entails removal and revision of the prosthesis.

# Reiter's syndrome (RS)

Immune-mediated arthritis, conjunctivitis and mucocutaneous lesions associated with urethritis due to *Chlamydia trachomatis* ($\blacktriangleright$87), or bacillary dysentery.

**Risk factors:** Strongly associated with possession of HLA B27; 80% of cases are B27 positive. Commoner in males.

**Clinical features:** Onset occurs between a few days and 4 weeks after infectious illness. Acute-onset asymmetrical oligoarthritis affecting, in decreasing order of frequency, ankles, knees, metatarsophalangeal joints, proximal interphalangeal toe joints, wrists. Sternocostal and sacroiliac joints may also be affected. Most patients have two or more affected joints. Inflammation occurs at the points of insertion of tendons ('enthesopathy'), causing Achilles tendinitis and 'sausage' swelling of digits. Conjunctivitis is usually bilateral and mild. Rarely anterior uveitis develops. Urethritis presents as mucopurulent urethral discharge with dysuria. The meatus may be swollen and red. In post-dysenteric RS, sterile urethritis may develop 1–2 weeks after diarrhoea. Skin lesions include superficial painless ulceration of the glans penis, which may be localized or may encircle the glans (circinate balanitis), and crusted scaling papules usually on the soles, palms, trunk and genitals (keratoderma blenorrhagica). Oral ulceration also occurs. Eye and skin involvement is unusual after dysentery. Arthritis resolves slowly over months, and does not usually cause permanent joint damage, although this may occur. Recurrences occur, and may be triggered by sexual exposure. Heart block and aortic regurgitation occur rarely in patients with severe longstanding disease.

**Organisms:** *Chlamydia trachomatis* ($\blacktriangleright$329), *Salmonella* spp. ($\blacktriangleright$281), *Shigella* spp. ($\blacktriangleright$282), *Yersinia enterocolitica* ($\blacktriangleright$284).

**Microbiological investigations:** Urethral smear and culture for *Chlamydia trachomatis* and *Neisseria gonorrhoeae* ($\blacktriangleright$87). Aspiration and culture of synovial fluid to exclude septic arthritis ($\blacktriangleright$120). Synovial fluid usually contains 5000–20 000 WBC/$\mu$L (usually >50 000 WBC/$\mu$L in septic arthritis) and culture is negative. Stool culture. *Yersinia* serology ($\blacktriangleright$284).

**Other investigations:** Leucocytosis and raised ESR are common.

**Differential diagnosis:** Gonococcal arthritis ($\blacktriangleright$86). Rheumatoid arthritis, psoriatic arthritis, ankylosing spondylitis, inflammatory bowel disease.

**Antibiotic management:** Doxycycline should be given for chlamydial urethritis. Prolonged doxycycline treatment for 3 months speeds resolution of arthritis in post venereal but not dysenteric cases.

**Supportive management:** Non-steroidal anti-inflammatory drugs. Intra-articular steroid injections and immunosuppression in severe cases. Rheumatological referral is recommended.

**Comments:** The term **reactive arthritis** is used to describe post-dysentery arthritis without the eye or cutaneous features of Reiter's disease.

# Viral arthritis

A symmetrical peripheral arthritis, superficially resembling rheumatoid arthritis, may complicate a number of infections, particularly parvovirus ($\blacktriangleright$341), rubella and rubella immunization ($\blacktriangleright$127) and hepatitis B ($\blacktriangleright$70), but also mumps ($\blacktriangleright$128), enteroviruses ($\blacktriangleright$347), herpesviruses ($\blacktriangleright$334) and adenoviruses ($\blacktriangleright$334). Joint symptoms are usually mild, of sudden onset and brief duration, and often occur early in the illness at the same time as skin rash. Joint damage can be more severe and persistent, particularly after parvovirus and rubella infections. Serological confirmation of infection should be sought, as a firm diagnosis helps to differentiate from rheumatoid arthritis. Arthritis is a prominent feature of some-arthropod-borne alphavirus infections such as chikungunya, o'nyong-nyong, Ross River virus and Sindbis (➤352).

# Osteomyelitis

Infection of bone, including periosteum, cortical bone and medullary cavity, leading to progressive destruction of bone and deposition of new bone. May be acute (over weeks) or chronic (months to years). **Sequestrum** is dead bone that is devoid of blood supply. It acts as a foreign body and must be removed before antibiotics will be effective. Periosteal new bone formation is referred to as **involucrum**. Osteomyelitis arises by two main mechanisms: **haematogenous** spread during bacteraemia and by spread from a **contiguous focus** of infection.

**Risk factors:** Bacteraemia. Contiguous soft-tissue infection, such as frontal sinusitis, leading to local osteomyelitis with oedema of the forehead ('Pott's puffy tumour'). Local pre-disposing factors include previous major trauma, particularly open fractures, foreign bodies, including prosthetic implants, vascular insufficiency. Cranial radiotherapy may cause osteoradionecrosis, which predisposes to sub-sequent osteomyelitis. Sickle-cell disease, diabetes mellitus, IVDU are also risk factors.

**Clinical features:** Fever, rigors, bone pain, local swelling, tenderness and erythema. These classic features are seen in acute haematogenous osteomyelitis, and are often mild or absent in disease due to contiguous infection. **Haematogenous** infection classically affects the metaphyses of long bones (esp. tibia and femur) in children and the vertebrae of adults. **Contiguous** osteomyelitis is commonly secondary to open fractures, hip replacements and in the sacrum secondary to decubitus ulcers. **Brodie's tumour** (primary subacute pyogenic osteomyelitis) presents subacutely with pain and low-grade fever. It affects the lower limb in patients under 20 yrs. **Chronic osteomyelitis** usually presents with sinus formation and discharge. Systemic features are uncommon, and local signs tend to be less prevalent. It is difficult to eradicate without extensive surgical debridement.

**Organisms:** *Staphylococcus aureus* causes 42–95% overall. **Neonates:** *Staphylococcus aureus*, group B β-haemolytic streptococci, coliforms (especially *Salmonella* spp. worldwide). **Children <6 yrs:** *Staphylococcus aureus*, *Staphylococcus epidermidis*, streptococci, *Haemophilus influenzae*. **Adults:** *Staphylococcus aureus*. **Elderly/immunocompromised patients:** *Staphylococcus aureus*, coliforms, pseudomonads. **Children with sickle-cell disease:** *Salmonella* spp. Mixed infection is common in disease due to vascular insufficiency. Anaerobic infection occurs particularly in the diabetic foot (➤125), dental sepsis, in lower limb fractures, in osteomyelitis underlying venous ulceration and in deep human bite wounds. Brodie's tumour is always due to *Staphylococcus aureus*.

**Microbiological investigations:** Accurate microbiological diagnosis is very important. Send blood cultures if systemically unwell. Culture of sinus pus should be performed, but may not accurately reflect organisms present in bone, unless *Staphylococcus aureus* is isolated. Needle aspiration under radiological guidance should be performed early. Open biopsy is more sensitive and has been found to alter management in ≈50% of cases of osteomyelitis associated with open wounds.

**Other investigations:** Leucocytosis and raised ESR are likely. **Plain X-rays are usually normal early in disease.** Soft-tissue swelling and periosteal elevation are seen after 1–2 weeks and lytic changes and sclerosis even later. Technetium bone scan is sensitive and is usually positive at presentation. It may be difficult to interpret if there is contiguous soft-tissue infection. CT and MRI scanning are particularly helpful for vertebral disease. Alkaline phosphatase is usually normal.

**Differential diagnosis:** Includes sickle-cell crisis, primary and metastatic tumour, tuberculous osteomyelitis (➤40).

**Antibiotic management:** Antibiotics penetrate bone poorly, so prolonged treatment is required, initially parenteral. Antibiotic-impregnated beads and other inserts are commonly used (gentamicin, vancomycin, clindamycin etc.). **Empirical therapy** before organism is isolated: **Neonates:** Flucloxacillin + gentamicin. **Children <6 yrs:** Flucloxacillin + ampicillin **or** co-amoxiclav **or** parenteral cephalosporin. **Adults:** Flucloxacillin (+gentamicin if elderly or immunocompromised). Clindamycin is an alternative in penicillin allergics. **Treatment of particular organisms:** *Staphylococcus aureus*: flucloxacillin (+oral fucidin if severe). MRSA: vancomycin. Streptococci: benzylpenicillin. *Haemophilus influenzae*: ampicillin if sensitive, **or** parenteral cephalosporin. Coliforms: parenteral cephalosporin **or** ciprofloxacin. *Pseudomonas aeruginosa*: azlocillin or ceftazidime ± gentamicin. Treat for at least 4 weeks, although good results have been reported with 3 weeks' therapy of acute, uncomplicated, haematogenous osteomyelitis. Long-term parenteral therapy is used in the USA but evidence of superiority over iv to oral switch therapy is lacking and the latter is often preferred in Europe. **Suppression of chronic osteomyelitis:** flucloxacillin (for Gram-positives); ciprofloxacin (for Gram-negatives). Oral treatment of Gram-negative osteomyelitis possible with ciprofloxacin, but only where the organism has been isolated and shown to be sensitive and compliance guaranteed.

**Supportive management:** Drainage is indicated if there is a poor response to appropriate antibiotic therapy. Surgery may be required for diagnosis or for debridement and removal of sequestra. Osteomyelitis of the femoral head is usually drained to prevent the development of septic arthritis. Early orthopaedic consultation and close liaison with microbiology are essential.

**Complications:** Recurrence. Chronic osteomyelitis may lead to amyloidosis. Rarely, carcinoma may occur in the sinus tract.

**Comments:** Septic arthritis is an unusual complication in adults, because the epiphyseal plate provides a physical barrier to spread of infection. It is much more likely in infants, in whom the plate has yet to develop.

# Vertebral osteomyelitis

Osteomyelitis of the vertebral body is usually haematogenous in origin; retrograde venous spread from the genitourinary tract occurs rarely.

**Risk factors:** Patients are usually elderly. IVDU also predisposes.

**Clinical features:** Usually presents subacutely. Clinical signs may be minimal, and diagnosis is frequently delayed. Back pain, spinal tenderness and raised ESR in an elderly patient should alert. Neurological complications such as root pain, paraplegia, or meningitis are rare. May present as psoas abscess.

**Organisms:** *Staphylococcus aureus* (55%), *Salmonella* spp., coliforms (22%), *Pseudomonas aeruginosa* (esp. IVDU), streptococci, fastidious Gram-negative bacteria (➤296). *Mycobacterium tuberculosis*.

**Microbiological investigations:** Blood cultures. Biopsy is essential. Open biopsy is much more sensitive than needle aspiration.

**Other investigations:** Raised ESR. Plain X-rays may be normal in early disease. Radiological involvement of the disc favours infection (pyogenic or TB) rather than tumour. Isotope bone scan is positive early in disease. MRI is the most sensitive mode of imaging.

**Differential diagnosis:** Tuberculous osteomyelitis. Metastatic carcinoma.

**Antibiotic management:** As above for osteomyelitis. Treat for 8 weeks for *Staphylococ-*

*cus aureus.* Duration for other organisms is uncertain, but 4–8 weeks generally used.

# Diabetic foot infections

A common cause of hospital admission and amputation. Diabetics are prone both to cellulitis, due to group A β-haemolytic streptococci, and to deep necrotic mixed infections.

**Risk factors:** Ischaemia due to peripheral vascular disease, neuropathy and defective immune function, particularly phagocytosis, contribute to pathogenesis. Apart from poor diabetic control, smoking, hypertension and hyperlipidaemia.

**Clinical features:** Commoner in elderly type 2 diabetics. Many patients have longstanding ulceration. Warmth, redness, swelling and exudate suggest infection, but tenderness is usually absent due to neuropathy. There may be crepitus and foul odour. Concomitant evidence of peripheral vascular disease (absent pulses, bruits, atrophic skin) and neuropathy. Unexplained poor diabetic control may indicate infection. Fever is unusual.

**Organisms:** Polymicrobial infection is usual. *Staphylococcus aureus,* non-sporing anaerobes, *Staphylococcus epidermidis,* streptococci including β-haemolytic groups A and B and *Streptococcus 'milleri',* enterococci, pseudomonads, coliforms, anaerobes and coryneforms.

**Microbiological investigations:** Local sinus cultures may be misleading, unless *Staphylococcus aureus* is isolated. Isolation of coliforms and pseudomonads from ulcers and sinuses is particularly likely to represent superficial colonization. Curettings from ulcer base, or material removed at surgical debridement, are more likely to represent organisms responsible. Blood culture if systemically unwell.

**Other investigations:** Plain X-ray to look for osteomyelitis and gas in tissues. Bone scan may be difficult to interpret because of overlying soft-tissue infection. CRP, ESR and WBC are often unhelpful in diagnosis or for monitoring response to therapy.

**Antibiotic management:** For mild cases, co-amoxiclav **or** flucloxacillin + metronidazole **or** clindamycin. In severe infection, clindamycin **or** flucloxacillin + gentamicin + metronidazole **or** parenteral cephalosporin + metronidazole **or** flucloxacillin + ciprofloxacin + metronidazole.

**Supportive management:** Control hyperglycaemia. A full discussion of the indications for and timing of reconstructive surgery and amputation is beyond the scope of this manual. Early orthopaedic consultation is advised.

**Comments:** Prevention of diabetic foot ulcers depends on good glycaemic control, careful foot care with regular chiropody, correctly fitting shoes and patient education, and attention to other risk factors such as smoking.

# Chapter 15

# Paediatric infections

## Common viral infections of childhood

**Measles** ✉ ① (syn. rubeola, morbilli)
**Organism:** Family Paramyxovirus, genus *Morbillivirus* (➤346).

**Epidemiology:** Prior to immunization, infection was widespread in all communities (>90% infected by age 20). Much less common since immunization, usually occurring in unimmunized adolescents. Measles-related deaths now extremely rare in the UK. In developing countries, infection occurs in epidemics and is an important cause of death.

**Reservoir:** Man.

**Transmission:** Highly contagious. Droplet spread via respiratory route.

**Incubation period:** 7–18 days. Mean 10 days to prodrome, 14 days to rash.

**Infectious period:** Just before onset of symptoms to 4 days after appearance of rash.

**Clinical features:** 2–4 days **prodrome** with malaise, fever, coryza, conjunctivitis and cough. Fever peaks after the onset of rash and resolves over the next 3 days. Fever persisting beyond the third day of rash suggests secondary bacterial infection. **Koplik's spots** are pathognomonic. They are 1–2 mm white spots on an erythematous base on the buccal mucosa, appearing first opposite the lower molar teeth, 2 days before the rash. **Rash** appears 2–4 days after onset — a blanching erythematous maculopapular eruption starting behind the ears, rapidly involving the forehead and then spreading caudally so that the face, trunk, buttocks and legs are involved by the third day. May be confluent. As it fades, it leaves non-blanching 'staining' due to capillary haemorrhage. Rash lasts 1 week, and ends with fine desquamation. Soles and palms are spared and do not desquamate (in contrast to scarlet fever ➤135).

The majority have **pulmonary involvement**, which although usually mild, accounts for 90% of deaths due to measles. Direct viral involvement causes bronchiolitis and giant-cell pneumonia, giving bilateral hyperinflation and diffuse fluffy infiltrates on CXR. It may be difficult to distinguish from secondary bacterial pneumonia, usually due to *Staphylococcus aureus*, *Haemophilus influenzae*, or group A β-haemolytic streptococci. Severe infection is particularly likely in immunocompromised patients and in malnourished children.

Diarrhoea, vomiting, abdominal pain, severe pharyngitis and cervical lymphadenopathy may occur. In severe cases, generalized lymphadenopathy and splenomegaly may be seen. Myocarditis, pericarditis and hepatitis occur rarely. Encephalitis, which may be severe and leave permanent neurological sequelae, occurs in ≈1 in 1000 cases.

**Modified measles** describes a less severe form, often with a prolonged incubation period, seen in those with partial immunity (infants with maternal antibodies, recipients of immunoglobulin, previously immunized patients).

**Atypical measles** is a rare form occurring in previously immunized individuals. Early symptoms include high fever and headache. The rash appears peripherally and may be maculopapular, urticarial or vesicular. Pulmonary involvement with dyspnoea and nodular changes on CXR are common. Patients are often very unwell, and the illness may last 2 weeks or more. Diagnosis is confirmed by demonstrating a large rise in specific antibodies.

**Investigations:** Diagnosis is clinical, but can be confirmed by serology.

**Specific management:** None.

**Supportive management:** Symptomatic relief. Treatment of complications, including antibiotics for secondary bacterial infection.

**Complications:** Bacterial otitis media (➢17) and pneumonia (➢25). **Subacute sclerosing panencephalitis (SSPE)** is a very rare (≈1 in 100 000 cases) complication due to persistent measles infection. Onset is insidious and occurs 6–8 yrs after measles, with behavioural and intellectual changes progressing to myoclonic spasms, focal neurological deficits, coma and death, usually within 3 years.

**Immunization:** Single-dose live vaccine (as component of MMR) gives 90–95% protection (➢417). Measles vaccine is also effective as postexposure prophylaxis if given within 72 h of exposure. **Human normal immunoglobulin** (HNIG) is effective if given within 72 h after exposure, and may be useful if given up to 6 days after exposure. May be given to prevent or attenuate attacks in contacts who are pregnant, immunocompromised or under 12 months of age ☎.

**Comments:** Infection in pregnancy may cause abortion or stillbirth, but does not cause congenital malformation. Infants born to immune mothers are protected by maternal antibody for 6–9 months. These antibodies interfere with immunization, which is therefore not recommended in the UK before age 12 months. In developing countries, where death due to measles is common before that age, it may need to be given earlier, and repeated.

## Rubella ✉ ① (syn. German measles)
**Organism:** Family Togaviridae, genus *Rubivirus*. (➢352).

**Epidemiology:** A worldwide disease of childhood. Its significance lies entirely in the ability of maternal infection during pregnancy to cause congenital malformation (➢128).

**Reservoir:** Man.

**Transmission:** Droplet spread by the respiratory route.

**Incubation period:** 16–18 days (range 14–23).

**Infectious period:** One week before and 4 days after the onset of rash. Infants with congenital rubella syndrome (CRS) may continue to excrete virus in pharyngeal secretions and urine for many months after birth.

**Clinical features:** Frequently asymptomatic, especially in children. Adults may have 1–5 day prodrome with headache, fever and upper respiratory symptoms. Onset of disease in children occurs with rash; this consists of discrete maculopapular patches of erythema, starting on the face and spreading to the rest of the body. There may be generalized and particularly postauricular lymphadenopathy, splenomegaly and conjunctivitis. Arthralgia occurs in the majority of adults. Some patients develop a symmetrical peripheral arthritis (➢122). This usually lasts 5–10 days and resolves, but it may be severe or persistent, resembling rheumatoid arthritis. Thrombocytopenia, Guillain–Barré syndrome and encephalitis (one in 5000 cases) occur rarely.

**Investigations:** Clinical diagnosis is unreliable, and serological confirmation must be sought whenever pregnancy is a possibility. Acute infection is diagnosed by demonstrating specific IgM or a greater than fourfold rise in IgG titres between acute and convalescent sera. Serum taken earlier than 1 week or later than 3 weeks after onset of rash can give a false negative IgM.

**Exposure to rubella in pregnancy:** Any pregnant woman with suspected rubella or exposure to rubella requires serological screening, irrespective of a history of immunization, clinical rubella or a previous positive rubella antibody test. Serum should be taken as soon as possible ☎. Close liaison with the virology service is required, as further serum samples will be needed. If current rubella infection is confirmed, parents need counselling on the risk of CRS and termination (➤141).

**Immunization:** Immunization with measles/mumps/rubella (MMR) vaccine is currently recommended for all children between 12 and 15 months old. 10–14-yr-old females should be given single-antigen rubella vaccine unless there is documented evidence that they have received MMR. Non-pregnant seronegative women of childbearing age should be vaccinated and advised not to risk pregnancy for 1 month after vaccination. All women should be screened in every pregnancy for rubella antibodies, irrespective of a previous positive antibody report. Immunization of seronegatives should not be performed during pregnancy, although there is no evidence that this would be harmful. Immunization must be given after delivery (➤417).

**Specific management:** None. Human immunoglobulin may be given to pregnant women exposed to rubella who would not consider a termination under any circumstances, although its benefits are controversial.

### Congenital rubella syndrome (CRS)

The risks of CRS following maternal rubella depend on the stage of pregnancy at which infection occurs: <10 weeks, risk ≈90%; 11–12 weeks, ≈30%; 13–20 weeks, <10%; >20 weeks, risk very low.

**Clinical features:** 50% of neonates with CRS appear normal at birth. Affected children usually have low birth weight. Clinical features may be considered in three categories: transient, permanent and developmental. **Transient** features include hepatitis, hepatosplenomegaly and jaundice, thrombocytopenia, chronic rubelliform rash, haemolytic anaemia, hypogammaglobulinaemia, lymphadenopathy, encephalitis and diarrhoea. These features may be severe, but usually resolve over the first few weeks of life. **Permanent** features include the classical triad of patent ductus arteriosus,

cataracts and nerve deafness. Deafness is the commonest manifestation of CRS, affecting ≈80% of cases. It is usually bilateral and reflects central or peripheral neurological damage. Other common defects include pulmonary artery stenosis and pulmonary valvular stenosis, retinopathy, cloudy cornea and glaucoma, microcephaly, mental retardation and spastic diplegia. **Developmental** defects are those which present later in life. Children with CRS have a greatly increased risk of developing insulin-dependent diabetes mellitus (20% by age 35) and hypo- or hyperthyroidism. Hearing loss and ocular defects may also be progressive.

**Diagnosis:** The assessment of a child with congenital defects consistent with intrauterine infection includes consideration of other potential causes (TORCH screening ➤141). Congenital rubella infection is confirmed by identifying anti-rubella IgM in the neonate, isolating rubella virus or demonstrating the persistence of specific IgG after 12 months, when maternally-derived IgG levels should have waned.

## Mumps ✉ ① (syn. infectious parotitis)

**Organism:** Family Paramyxovirus, genus *Paramyxovirus* (➤346).

**Epidemiology:** In the absence of immunization, infection is widespread and frequently asymptomatic.

**Reservoir:** Man.

**Transmission:** Droplet spread by the respiratory route.

**Incubation period:** 12–25 days.

**Infectious period:** 1 week before parotitis and up to 10 days thereafter.

**Clinical features:** There is a 2–3 day prodrome with malaise, headache, fever and anorexia. Progressive pain and swelling develop in one or both parotid glands, peaking at 2–3 days and resolving over the following week. There is often associated swelling of sublingual and submandibular glands. Meningoencephalitis is commoner in postpubertal patients (➤100). It is rarely complicated by permanent nerve deafness (one in 20 000 cases of mumps) or facial palsy. Other rare neurological complications include acute cerebellar ataxia and transverse myelitis. Orchitis occurs in ≈20% of postpubertal males. It is usually unilateral, so sterility is rare. Oophoritis also occurs, causing pelvic pain and tenderness. Orchitis and meningitis can occur before or without parotitis. Pancreatitis occurs in <10% of cases and usually presents with abdominal pain and tenderness, nausea and vomiting days to weeks after parotitis. Resolution usually occurs in 7–10 days. Thyroiditis, myocarditis and arthritis are very rare.

**Investigations:** Diagnosis can be confirmed by specific serology.

**Differential diagnosis:** Bacterial parotitis. Viral and bacterial meningitis (➤96). Bacterial epididymo-orchitis (➤80).

**Immunization:** Immunization is recommended at age 12–15 months as part of the MMR vaccine (➤417). Vaccine may also be given to susceptible adults, but antibody responses develop too slowly for this to be useful as protection after exposure to mumps.

---

**Practice point**

Serum amylase is raised in uncomplicated mumps parotitis, even in the absence of pancreatitis.

---

## Primary herpes simplex virus (HSV) infection (herpetic stomatitis)

**Organism:** Family Herpesviridae, genus herpes simplex virus type 1 and 2 (➤334).

**Epidemiology:** >80% of primary HSV infections are asymptomatic. In children >6 months and <5 yrs old, acute gingivostomatitis may occur. May also occur in adults, in whom it is usually less severe.

**Reservoir:** Man.

**Transmission:** Usually from an adult with herpes labialis, or from another infected child.

**Incubation period:** 3–6 days (range 2–14 days).

**Infectious period:** Virus may be secreted in saliva for many weeks following acute infection. Periods of asymptomatic viral shedding also occur. Isolation ① is recommended for children with disseminated infection.

**Clinical features:** Abrupt onset of fever, anorexia, listlessness and sore mouth, followed by severe ulcerative gingivostomatitis with local lymphadenopathy. Vesicles (1–3 mm) form on buccal mucosa, rupture and coalesce leaving painful ulceration. Salivation and drooling are prominent. Herpetic vesicles may develop in areas contaminated by highly infectious saliva, including perioral skin, eye (➤106), fingers and vulva.

**Investigations:** Diagnosis is confirmed by culture of HSV from saliva, and by a rise in specific antibody titres.

**Differential diagnosis:** *Candida albicans* (➤367). *Capnocytophaga ochracea* (➤302), Vincent's angina (➤18). Other viral causes of oropharyngeal ulceration include coxsackieviruses (hand, foot and mouth disease or herpangina ➤135), and echoviruses (➤349).

**Specific management:** Topical aciclovir is of **no** benefit. Systemic or intravenous aciclovir may speed healing and is particularly useful in the immunocompromised host.

**Supportive management:** Maintenance of adequate fluid input may require parenteral therapy.

**Neonatal HSV infection** is acquired peripartum. Forty per cent of HSV-infected mothers have no history of current infection or genital lesions. Fifty per cent of babies delivered via an actively infected birth canal will become infected, and nearly all of these will manifest disease. Infection may be localized to the eye or

CNS, but usually becomes disseminated with a vesicular rash, hepatomegaly and jaundice, pneumonitis and encephalitis. Treatment with aciclovir is essential.

## Varicella ①
(syn. chickenpox) ⊠ (Scotland only)

**Organism:** Family Herpesviridae, genus varicella zoster virus (VZV, syn. herpes zoster) (➤339).

**Epidemiology:** VZV infection occurs worldwide. Seroprevalence at age 20 is typically ≈95%. Primary infection with VZV causes chickenpox, which is primarily a disease of childhood, although it may occur at any age and is more severe in adults, with a higher incidence of serious complications such as pneumonitis. Reactivation of latent VZV in sensory ganglia causes herpes zoster (syn. shingles). The absolute incidence of zoster is higher in adults, but not if corrected for prior exposure to VZV.

**Reservoir:** Man.

**Transmission:** Person-to-person, by direct contact or droplet spread from cases of chickenpox or herpes zoster.

**Incubation period:** 13–21 days.

**Infectious period:** From 2 days before the onset of rash until the lesions are crusted. Scabs are non-infectious.

**Clinical features:** There is a mild prodrome of malaise, fever, headache and rhinitis. The rash develops as crops of vesicles, each appearing on an erythematous base ('dewdrop on a rose petal'). Vesicles rapidly progress to umbilicated papules, pustules and scabs. Distribution is typically central on head, trunk and arms, and also the palate or gums. New crops continue to appear for up to 7 days. Fever remains elevated for 4–5 days after onset of rash. Bacterial superinfection of the rash is common (esp. GAS). Many patients have mild hepatitis. Mucositis may cause dysuria.

Varicella **pneumonitis** is commoner in immunocompromised patients and adults who smoke or are pregnant. It may progress rapidly, with hypoxia and tachypnoea. CXR shows widespread patchy shadowing. Intubation and ventilation may be required, and there is significant mortality. Residual pulmonary fibrosis and CXR calcifications may occur in survivors. Pulmonary disease during varicella is often due to secondary bacterial pneumonia, usually with *Streptococcus pneumoniae*, *Haemophilus influenzae* or *Staphylococcus aureus*. Staphylococcal septicaemia may occur. **Encephalitis** presenting with cerebellar ataxia occurs very rarely. It may be fatal, but usually resolves in the immunocompetent host. **Thrombocytopenia** and **disseminated intravascular coagulopathy** occur very rarely and may cause haemorrhagic varicella, with bleeding into vesicles. All complications are commoner in the immunocompromised.

**Investigations:** Light microscopy of vesicle contents reveals multinucleate giant cells (Tzanck preparation); electron microscopy shows large numbers of herpesvirus particles. Methods are available for the rapid detection of VZV antigens in vesicle fluid. Retrospectively diagnosis can be confirmed by serology.

**Differential diagnosis:** In atypical cases, vesicular impetigo due to *Staphylococcus aureus* or GAS can be confused (➤111). Other infectious vesicular rashes include herpes simplex infection (➤118), hand, foot and mouth disease (➤135) and disseminated gonococcal infection (➤86). Non-infectious causes include Stevens–Johnson syndrome, pemphigus and pemphigoid.

**Specific management:** Aciclovir shortens and reduces the severity of illness but must be given early (ideally <24 h) to have a significant effect. Detailed UK guidelines have been published. (↪UK guidelines, J Infection 1998; 36: Suppl. 1). Aciclovir is not recommended for routine use in immunocompetent children. Intravenous aciclovir is indicated in the following circumstances: immunocompromised patients (including those with AIDS), neonates and if there is evidence of severe or disseminated disease, in particular, ophthalmic disease, pneumonitis or encephalitis (10 mg/kg q8h for 7–10 days). Dose may need to be reduced in renal failure and a good throughput of fluid should be maintained to avoid crystalluria. Antibiotics may be needed for secondary bacterial infection of rash or lower respiratory tract. Some physicians would give prophylactic parenteral flucloxacillin to all adult cases because of the small risk of staphylococcal septicaemia.

Oral aciclovir may be given to immunocompetent adults with varicella (including during pregnancy, see below) in whom disease is often more severe. Guidelines recommend treating patients who present early (<24 h); those who present later but in whom there is clinical deterioration, evidence of complications or persistent fever/cropping should be admitted for iv therapy ± antibiotics.

**Infection in pregnancy:** Pregnant women with varicella have an increased risk of severe pneumonitis and other severe complications, although the exact rate is uncertain. Pneumonitis is more likely in the last trimester, and in women who smoke, have COPD, are taking steroids or have extensive cutaneous varicella. Aciclovir is not licensed for use in pregnancy, but there is extensive experience suggesting it is safe. Current UK guidelines suggest:

• **If there are signs or symptoms to suggest pneumonitis**, do CXR (with abdominal screening) and check oxygenation. If CXR abnormal or $Po_2$ <10.6 kPa, start iv aciclovir ± antibiotics. If both are normal, observe in hospital for ≥24 h; start oral aciclovir if >20 weeks gestation and rash present ≤24 h. If chest deteriorates, convert to iv aciclovir.

• **If there are no symptoms or signs of pneumonitis and rash present ≥24 h**, withhold aciclovir and review at 24–48 h. Advise patient to report any deterioration.

• **If there are no symptoms or signs of pneumonitis and rash present ≤24 h**, start oral aciclovir and review at 24–48 h. If <20 weeks gestation, this decision is best discussed with a specialist.

**Fetal infection:** If infection occurs at less than 26 weeks gestation, there is a small risk of fetal malformation (microcephaly, hydro-cephalus, limb hypoplasia, cutaneous scarring and ophthalmic defects). The risk is highest during the first trimester (≈3%). Infection just before or shortly after delivery may be followed by neonatal infection, which can be severe.

**Infection in neonates:** Neonates of mothers who develop varicella <5 days before or shortly after delivery will not be protected by maternal IgG and may develop severe disseminated infection. They should receive VZIG (see below) and be monitored for 14–16 days for signs of infection, which should be treated promptly with aciclovir. Some recommend prophylactic aciclovir for these neonates. Herpes zoster during pregnancy poses no threat to mother or child, since by definition, the mother will have anti-VZV IgG, and this will protect the neonate.

💻 www.rcog.org.uk/guidelines/guideline/13.html

**Reye syndrome** was in the past most often associated with varicella and aspirin use in children. Now that the use of aspirin in childhood is discouraged, Reye syndrome has become much less common.

**Immunization:** A live attenuated vaccine is used in some countries (e.g. Japan) but is not licensed in the UK. It is available on a named patient basis for immunocompromised individuals such as children with leukaemia.

**Varicella zoster immune globulin (VZIG)** is prepared from donors with high titre antibodies against VZV and is only available in small quantities. It does not prevent infection, but modifies its severity. It should be given within 72 h, but confers some benefit up to 10 days post exposure. VZIG is indicated for patients who are:

• VZV-seronegative. Many labs offer a rapid service for VZV serostatus, but administration should not be delayed beyond 7 days whilst result is awaited. Antibody testing is recommended in all immunocompromised patients, irrespective of a history of varicella. In pregnancy, only those with no history of varicella need testing;

**and**

• Have a contact history. Significant exposure is defined as household, face-to-face for 5 min, or indoors contact for >15 min with case

of chickenpox, disseminated or exposed (e.g. ophthalmic) zoster, or immunocompromised person with localized zoster (in whom viral shedding may be greater), between 48 h before onset (day of onset for zoster) until cropping has ceased and all lesions crusted;
**and**
• Are at increased risk of complications of VZV infection:
   • Organ transplant recipients on immuno-suppressive drugs.
   • Bone-marrow transplant, radiotherapy or chemotherapy within past 6 months.
   • Steroid therapy (risk defined as children on ≥2 mg/kg/day of prednisolone for >1 week or 1 mg/kg/day of prednisolone for >1 month, within 3 months of exposure, adults on ≥40 mg prednisolone for >1 week or 1 mg/kg/day of prednisolone for >1 month, within 3 months of exposure, or lower doses of steroid in combination with other immunosuppressants.
   • Inherited or acquired defects of cell-mediated immunity (including symptomatic HIV and haematological malignancy).
   • Infants less than 4 weeks old whose mothers develop chickenpox 1 week before to 4 weeks after delivery, or who are exposed to VZV from another source and whose mothers have no history of chickenpox or are seronegative.
   • Infants less than 4 weeks old in contact with VZV who are born at less than 30 weeks' gestation or with birth weight less than 1 kg. These may not have maternal antibody despite a positive maternal history. (This is an American recommendation that is not part of current UK guidelines.)

**Dose of VZIG (always given im)**

| Age (yrs) | Dose (mg) | Vials |
|-----------|-----------|-------|
| 0–5       | 250       | 1     |
| 6–10      | 500       | 2     |
| 11–14     | 750       | 3     |
| ≥15       | 1000      | 4     |

↵ Immunisation against Infectious Disease. London: HMSO, 1996

• Pregnant women (especially <20 weeks' gestation or <5 days pre-term).

## Herpes zoster ① (syn. shingles)

Reactivation of VZV in sensory nerve ganglia causes herpes zoster.

**Epidemiology:** Occurs at any age but is commoner <5 yrs and in the elderly. Commoner in the immunocompromised, in whom disseminated disease is more likely. Second and third attacks occur, but are unusual.

**Clinical features:** Pain, often severe or burning, localized to a single dermatome, followed after 1–4 days by a vesicular eruption which progresses through the same stages as varicella (papules, vesicles, pustules and scabs) and is confined to the same dermatome, with sharp demarcation in the midline. Commonly involved areas are the thoracic dermatomes and the ophthalmic division of the trigeminal nerve (➢107). Healing occurs with scarring after 1–4 weeks.

Patients may be systemically unwell with fever, headache, mild confusion. Rarely viral meningitis or encephalitis may ensue. Acute retinal necrosis occurs rarely, often preceded by ophthalmic zoster. A few disseminated lesions outside the dermatome are commonly seen in normal hosts. In the immunocompromised, widespread progressive dissemination may occur. Very severe zoster can be accompanied by weakness of the muscles supplied by the same spinal root. Involvement of particular nerve roots causes a number of specific syndromes (Table 15.1).

**Management:** Detailed guidelines have been published (↵ UK guidelines, J Infection 1995; 30: 193). Oral aciclovir recommended for >60 yrs, severe pain or shingles outside the thoracic dermatomes. IV aciclovir for immunocompromised (including symptomatic HIV and haematological malignancy). In ophthalmic shingles, red eye or reduced visual acuity merits prompt ophthalmic opinion.

**Postherpetic neuralgia** persisting beyond 1 month after healing is an infrequent occurrence. It is more likely in elderly female patients,

**Table 15.1** Specific syndromes associated with zoster in different dermatomes

| Syndrome | Root | Clinical features |
|---|---|---|
| Ophthalmic (➤107) | VI. Rarely associated with ipsilateral III, IV and VI palsies | Pain in scalp. Corneal lesions and iridocyclitis. Rash over forehead, eyelid and nose. Rash on tip of nose indicates involvement of nasociliary nerve and suggests eye involvement. Rarely complicated by acute retinal necrosis |
| Geniculate (Ramsay–Hunt) | VII Variable involvement of V, IX and X | Pain in ear canal, pinna and scalp. Facial nerve palsy. Tinnitus, vertigo, deafness, dysphagia. Vesicles on external auditory meatus, scalp, pinna and hemitongue |
| Vagal and glossopharyngeal | X, XI | Mucous membrane involvement only—soft palate and posterior pharynx. Pain in throat, dysphagia |
| Sacral | S1–4 | Disturbance of micturition, haematuria |

may be severe, and usually resolves over 6–24 months. Therapeutic modalities include analgesia, tricyclics, protecting the sensitive area (e.g. with an occlusive dressing or cling film) and counter-irritants (capsaicin ointment). **Gabapentin** is often effective and is relatively free of adverse effects. Dose titration up to 600 mg q8h is usually required. Carbemazepine is ineffective.

### Infectious mononucleosis

(IM; syn. glandular fever)

**Organism:** Family Herpesviridae, genus Epstein–Barr virus (EBV) (➤339).

**Epidemiology:** Common in all populations. In developed countries, adult seroprevalence is >90%. Infection under 5 yrs is common (seroprevalence ≈50%) but usually asymptomatic. Further peak of seroconversion occurs during adolescence; 50% of these cases result in IM, the rest being asymptomatic.

**Reservoir:** Man.

**Transmission:** Person-to-person via saliva.

**Incubation period:** 30–45 days.

**Infectious period:** EBV can be recovered from oral secretions for up to 18 months after infection; ≈25% of asymptomatic seropositives shed virus in saliva. Transmission by blood transfusion has occurred.

**Clinical features:** Onset may be sudden or insidious. In young children, fever, sore throat and lymphadenopathy are common. Malaise and anorexia may occur. In adolescents and adults, non-specific features may predominate and tonsillitis is often absent. Physical findings include generalized, particularly cervical, lymphadenopathy (95%), tonsillitis with tonsillar enlargement and exudate (85%), splenomegaly (50–75%), hepatomegaly (10–50%), petechial palatal haemorrhages (10%) and periorbital oedema (30%). Widespread maculopapular rash develops in a few patients; administration of ampicillin induces a florid pruritic rash in nearly all patients with IM. Most attacks resolve fully within 2–3 weeks.

**Investigations:** Peripheral WCC is increased to $10–50 \times 10^9/L$, with an absolute ($>4 \times 10^9/L$) and relative (>50% of total WBC) increase in mononuclear cells, of which ≤20% are atypical lymphocytes. These are activated T lymphocytes, produced in response to virus-induced proliferation of B cells, and have a characteristic morphology with large nuclei, fine reticular chromatin pattern and abundant basophilic, often vacuoloated, cytoplasm. Mild thrombocytopenia is common. Patients usually have mildly abnormal liver function and, occasionally, jaundice.

**Heterophile antibodies:** Patients with IM produce IgM antibodies that bind erythrocytes from other species (sheep and horses) but not guinea-pig kidney. Heterophile antibodies are also found in normal sera, and in some patients with lymphoma, but these usually bind to guinea-pig kidney cells. Several tests are available: the Paul–Bunnell test measures agglutination of sheep RBCs by patient's serum. In the Paul–Bunnell–Davidsohn test, the serum is first pre-absorbed with guinea-pig kidney cells. In the monospot test, formalinized horse RBCs are agglutinated after pre-absorption of serum on guinea-pig kidney cells. These tests are positive in 40% of patients during the first week of illness, 60% by week 2 and 80% by week 3. They are usually negative in children under 5 yrs. A positive test usually persists for 3–6 months after IM, and occasionally up to 1 yr. Patients also make **specific antibodies** against viral antigens, including viral capsid antigen (VCA) and nuclear antigens (EBNA). Anti-VCA IgM is a sensitive and specific indicator of recent infection.

**Differential diagnosis:** Bacterial pharyngitis due to GAS (➤19) and *Arcanobacterium haemolyticum* (➤270). Other causes of mononucleosis, including CMV (➤339) and *Toxoplasma gondii* (➤137) are rare. In these conditions, heterophile antibodies do not occur. Diphtheria (➤268).

**Specific management:** None. Aciclovir is **not** indicated. Steroids may be used for thrombocytopenia, haemolytic anaemia, neurological complications and myocarditis. If tonsillar enlargement threatens to cause airway obstruction prednisolone should be given (60 mg/day for 5–10 days). Tracheotomy may be required.

**Complications:** Tonsillar enlargement may be so severe as to threaten airway obstruction. Splenic rupture occurs in ≈0.2% of patients. Abdominal pain is rare in IM and if it occurs splenic rupture should be excluded. Rarely, profound thrombocytopenia with purpura and haemorrhage occurs. Autoimmune haemolytic anaemia also occurs rarely. Neurological complications include encephalitis presenting with cerebellar ataxia, viral meningitis, Guillain–Barré syndrome, Bell's palsy and transverse myelitis. These affect less than 1% of patients and usually resolve completely, but they account for most of the mortality and long-term morbidity associated with IM. Very rare complications include myocarditis, pericarditis and pneumonitis.

Boys who carry the very rare X-linked immunoproliferative syndrome (XLP) gene have a specific defect of the immune system that renders them susceptible to fatal acute IM, which occurs in >75% of XLP gene carriers. Features include massive hepatic necrosis, pancytopenia and lymphoma. The mean reported age of presentation is 6.5 yrs.

**Comments:** Postinfectious fatigue has been said to be a particular feature of IM, but in practice this is rare. There is no firm evidence to implicate EBV in the aetiology of the chronic fatigue syndrome (CFS ➤339), and EBV serology has no part in the work-up of patients with CFS. Genuinely persistent active EBV infection has been reported very rarely. Patients have very high titre-specific anti-EBV antibodies and a variety of clinical features, including pancytopenia, lymphadenopathy, hepatosplenomegaly, interstitial pneumonitis and hepatitis. They may respond to aciclovir.

EBV is associated with the development of African Burkitt's lymphoma and nasopharyngeal carcinoma, and polyclonal B-cell lymphomas in immunosuppressed patients, particularly those with AIDS (➤169). It is also responsible for oral hairy leukoplakia in HIV infection (➤160).

## Human herpesvirus type 6

Family Herpesviridae, genus human herpesvirus type 6 (HHV6) (➤341)

**Epidemiology:** Infection is worldwide and very common in children >4 months and <3 yrs old. Transmission by saliva.

**Reservoir:** Man.

**Incubation period:** 10 days (range 5–15 days).

**Infectious period:** As with other herpesviruses, asymptomatic carriers may continue to excrete virus for many months.

**Clinical features:** Primary HHV-6 infection in childhood causes **exanthem subitum** (syn. roseola infantum, sixth disease) ①. Abrupt onset of fever lasting 3–5 days, followed by a rash which develops on the back and neck and spreads to the chest and limbs. The feet and face are spared, and the rash typically lasts 2 days. Mild malaise, vomiting, diarrhoea, cough, coryza, pharyngitis and lymphadenopathy may occur. Can be complicated by febrile convulsions, meningitis and encephalitis.

Also associated with a mononucleosis-like syndrome in adults and infection in the immunocompromised (➤341). A link to multiple sclerosis has been suggested but remains theoretical.

**Specific management:** None for exanthem subitum. Infection in the immunocompromised may require treatment (➤341).

### Parvovirus B19—erythema infectiosum ('slapped cheek' disease, fifth disease) ①

Primary infection with parvovirus B19 (➤341) in childhood causes **erythema infectiosum** (syn. fifth disease, slapped cheek disease). After a short prodrome of myalgia, arthralgia, malaise and fever, the typical rash develops on the face. It is sharply demarcated, occasionally with a raised edge ('slapped cheek' appearance). 1–2 days later, a maculopapular rash develops on the trunk, legs, arms and buttocks. After a few days, areas of clearing develop giving the rash a characteristic lacy or reticulate appearance. The rash may fade and reappear over the following 3 weeks. Children are infectious from before the onset of rash, but not thereafter.

Parvovirus is also associated with transient aplastic crisis in patients with pre-existing haemolytic anaemia, arthritis, usually in adults, congenital infection causing hydrops fetalis and chronic infection with anaemia in the immunocompromised (➤342).

### Enteroviral infections

Enteroviral infections account for the majority of childhood febrile exanthemata, but only two—hand foot and mouth disease and herpangina—produce a significantly characteristic clinical picture to allow easy identification. Transmission is typically by orofaecal or respiratory route, and incubation times are short (3–5 days). Viral excretion may persist in stool for several weeks.

### Hand, foot and mouth disease

(syn. enteroviral vesicular stomatitis with exanthem)

**Organism:** Coxsackievirus A16 (plus other serotypes) (➤347).

**Clinical features:** Pharyngitis with vesicles that burst, leaving 5–10 painful oral ulcers. Simultaneous vesicular rash on hands and feet. Resolves within 7–10 days. A very rare severe relapsing form is described.

### Herpangina

(syn. enteroviral vesicular pharyngitis)

**Organism:** Coxsackie A viruses (A1–10, A22) (➤347).

**Clinical features:** Vesicles and ulcers confined to the posterior pharynx, i.e. on the tonsillar pillars, soft palate and uvula. Constitutional symptoms include fever, headache, vomiting and myalgia.

## Specific infections frequently occurring in childhood

### Scarlet fever ①

(syn. scarlatina) ⊠

Scarlet fever is caused by infection with streptococci that produce erythrogenic toxin. It usually accompanies streptococcal pharyngitis (➤19), but may also result from cutaneous infection. Streptococcal erythrogenic toxin is similar to the toxic shock syndrome toxin of *Staphylococcus aureus* (➤249).

**Organism:** Group A β-haemolytic streptococci (≻254)

**Epidemiology:** Scarlet fever was common and frequently fatal in the 19th century, but its severity and frequency have waned since the 1920s. It is now rarely considered serious.

**Clinical features:** 1–2 days after onset of sore throat, rash appears on face, sparing the area around the lips ('circumoral pallor'), and spreading to the neck, chest, back, trunk and limbs. Rash is a diffuse blanching erythema with punctate elevations around hair follicles that give it a characteristic 'sandpaper' feel to the touch. It is accentuated in skin folds by capillary haemorrhage (Pastia's lines). Palms and soles are usually spared. Rash is followed by desquamation, which starts on the hands. The tongue is red with prominent papillae ('strawberry tongue').

**Investigations:** Throat swab. ASOT (≻255).

**Differential diagnosis:** Measles (≻126) and other viral exanthemata. Kawasaki's disease (≻180). *Arcanobacterium haemolyticum* causes rash and pharyngitis (≻270).

**Specific management:** Oral penicillin V or parenteral benzylpenicillin should be given.

**Complications:** Rheumatic fever (≻257), post-streptococcal glomerulonephritis (≻256), erythema nodosum (≻118).

## Toxic epidermal necrolysis

(syn. scalded skin syndrome, Ritter's disease, staphylococcal scarlet fever)
*Staphylococcus aureus* may produce an exotoxin that causes exfoliation of the upper layers of the epidermis (≻249). The initial site of staphylococcal infection may be minor and localized, but general skin colonization may occur rapidly.

**Organism:** *Staphylococcus aureus* (≻249).

**Clinical features:** Abrupt onset of generalized skin erythema, followed after 1–2 days by wrinkling and separation of upper layers with even slight trauma, such as light stroking (Nikolsky's sign). Large sheets of skin may peel off leaving a raw, tender surface. The rash fades over the next few days. There may be associated conjunctivitis, stomatitis and urethritis.

**Investigations:** *Staphylococcus aureus* can usually be cultured from the skin.

**Specific management:** Flucloxacillin is the drug of choice. For penicillin-allergic patients, erythromycin or parenteral cephalosporin is given. Careful fluid balance and replacement of protein loss required for this potentially fatal disorder.

## Pertussis ✉ ①

(syn. whooping cough)

**Organism:** *Bordetella pertussis* (≻301). *Bordetella parapertussis* and *Bordetella bronchiseptica* are unusual causes of a milder illness.

**Epidemiology:** Infection is worldwide, but is unusual in the UK since the advent of vaccination. Fears about vaccine side effects led to a temporary decline in vaccine uptake in the mid-1970s, and a rise in reported cases and deaths. Vaccine uptake in UK now ≈90%. Case fatality rate ≈1:200 under 2 months of age, ≈1:15000 in 1–4-yrs age group. Σ 1140 notified cases, 330 bacteriologically confirmed in 1999, compared with 11000 notifications in 1989. 10% of cases occur in adults (probably underdiagnosed).
   Worldwide pertussis remains a major cause of death with estimated $51 \times 10^6$ cases and $6 \times 10^5$ deaths p.a.

**Reservoir:** *Bordetella pertussis* and *Bordetella parapertussis* have no animal reservoir, but *Bordetella bronchiseptica* causes illness in a wide range of mammals, including farm animals.

**Transmission:** Highly contagious. Person-to-person via the respiratory droplet route.

**Incubation period:** 7 days (range 6–20).

**Infectious period:** From the onset of illness to 2–3 weeks into the paroxysmal stage.

**Clinical features:** Clinical course is considered in three stages: **Catarrhal stage:** Illness commences with symptoms of mild URTI, such as non-paroxysmal cough, coryza, conjunctivitis and sneezing. After 7–10 days, the cough becomes more frequent and intense. Fever is low grade or absent. **Paroxysmal stage:** The cough becomes very severe and frequent. Paroxysms, precipitated by many stimuli including eating, drinking, emotion or exercise, are characterized by repeated staccato coughing during a single prolonged expiration, followed by forceful inspiration giving rise to the 'whoop'. Whoop is often absent in infants and older patients. Paroxysms are associated with vomiting and exhaustion, and may cause facial/eyelid oedema, subconjunctival haemorrhage and erosion of the lingual frenulum. The paroxysmal stage lasts from 2 to 4 weeks. **Convalescent stage:** this lasts 2 weeks to 2 months, during which paroxysms become less severe and less frequent, although still triggered by intercurrent viral respiratory infections. Morbidity and mortality in pertussis occur in infants and are associated with the paroxysms of coughing, which may cause feeding difficulties, choking, anoxia and apnoea.

**Investigations:** During the catarrhal stage, there is a lymphocytosis. CXR may be normal or show dense markings radiating from the heart borders ('shaggy heart sign') due to peribronchial thickening. Culture of the organisms requires special media. Clinical disease very variable, therefore bacteriological confirmation essential. Pernasal swab is the sample of choice. Serology will confirm the diagnosis in retrospect.

**Differential diagnosis:** Other causes of respiratory tract infection (➤23). Inhaled foreign body.

**Specific management:** Erythromycin, given during the first 5 days of illness, shortens the duration of the paroxysmal stage. It should still be given after this time, but in this situation the main benefit is to render the patient non-infectious to others. Treatment should be given for 14 days. Strict isolation is necessary until 5 days' treatment have been completed. Cotrimoxazole is an alternative for patients allergic to erythromycin. Close contacts may also be given a 14-day course of erythromycin.

**Complications:** Atelectasis, particularly of the right upper lobe, is common during the paroxysmal stage. Other pulmonary complications include secondary bacterial infection (due to *Haemophilus influenzae*, *Streptococcus pneumoniae*, GAS, *Staphylococcus aureus*), suggested by fever and CXR changes. Pneumothorax, mediastinal and subcutaneous surgical emphysema and diaphragmatic rupture have been reported. There is no evidence of long-term pulmonary damage in survivors.

Neurological damage, including encephalopathy progressing to coma, and focal deficits including hemiplegia, account for significant morbidity and mortality and are probably caused by anoxia during paroxysms or cerebral haemorrhage.

**Immunization:** Recommended for all babies at 2 months as part of DTP vaccination (➤417). There is no transfer of protective maternal antibodies even in infants of mothers with documented history of pertussis or pertussis vaccination.

## Toxoplasmosis

**Epidemiology and transmission:** Worldwide. Seroprevalence varies with age and between countries (UK: ≈35%, France: ≈85%). Σ ≈800.

**Life cycle:** *Toxoplasma gondii* is an intracellular parasite of macrophages infecting a wide range of birds and mammals. Cats are the definitive hosts for the sexual phase of the life cycle. Infected cats excrete oocysts in faeces, which become infectious 2–3 days after they are passed and may remain infectious for many months in warm moist soil. Ingestion of oocysts by other cats completes the cycle. Ingestion by non-felines (including man) causes acute infection, followed by formation of tissue cysts in many tissues. Cysts contain slowly replicating

**Table 15.2** Interpretation of toxoplasma serology

| Situation | Comments |
| --- | --- |
| Suspected acute toxoplasmosis in immunocompetent patient | Negative serology excludes toxoplasmosis. Seroconversion, a fourfold rise in titre at 3-week interval, or positive IgM supports diagnosis. IgM may persist for several years |
| Ocular disease | Seropositivity is common in most populations. Titres do not correlate with active chorioretinitis, and serology is therefore not usually helpful |
| Suspected toxoplasmosis in immunodeficient patients | Titres do not usually rise during reactivation, and serology is therefore not usually helpful. Only ≈3% of AIDS patients with toxoplasma encephalitis are seronegative for *Toxoplasma gondii* |
| Infection during pregnancy | Documented seroconversion confirms infection. The interpretation of positive serology discovered during pregnancy requires consultation with reference laboratory. Fetal blood sampling may be used to confirm fetal infection |
| Congenital infection | Confirmed by rising titres or +IgM |

parasites ('bradyzoites') and are asymptomatic, but may reactivate during immunodeficiency, to cause clinical disease, particularly in the CNS.

Human infection is acquired by ingestion of infectious oocysts in cat faeces, by eating poorly cooked meat containing tissue cysts, transplacentally, or rarely via blood transfusion.

### Clinical features

**Incubation time:** 5–20 days for acute infectious mononucleosis-like syndrome.

**Symptoms and signs:** Infection is rarely symptomatic in the normal population. *Toxoplasma gondii* causes disease in four situations:

**Acute infectious mononucleosis-like** illness, due to acute primary infection in immunocompetent individuals. Generalized lymphadenopathy, fever, headache, malaise, sore throat, myalgia, hepatosplenomegaly and abnormal liver function tests. Reactive lymphocytosis may occur (➤133).

**Chorioretinitis** (➤108) presents in older children and adults and is usually due to reactivation of congenital infection. Only ≈1% of acquired infections result in eye disease. Chorioretinitis occurs in AIDS patients, usually in association with CNS disease (➤163). It presents with visual loss. On fundoscopy, acute lesions are yellowish patches with surrounding

hyperaemia. Older lesions are atrophic white plaques with distinct borders and choroidal pigmentation.

**Reactivation during immunodeficiency,** particularly AIDS (➤163), typically causing encephalitis.

**Congenital infection** (➤141).

**Investigations:** In acute infection, **lymph-node histology** is characteristic, with follicular hyperplasia and collections of enlarged epithelioid cells with abundant pale cytoplasm, vesicular nuclei and prominent nucleoli. Organisms are rarely seen on histology. Isolation of *Toxoplasma gondii* is complex and expensive and is rarely performed. Diagnosis is usually confirmed by **serology**. A large number of test are available for detecting IgG and IgM antibodies including the Sabin–Feldman dye test, the indirect fluorescent antibody test and complement fixation and agglutination tests (Table 15.2). Since infection is common, interpretation of tests can be difficult; liaison with local and reference labs is essential ☎.

**Management:** Immunocompetent, nonpregnant patients generally do not require treatment unless symptoms are severe or prolonged beyond a few weeks. Treatment is usually given for 2–4 weeks. Treatment is

**Table 15.3** Management of toxoplasmosis

| Situation | Comments |
| --- | --- |
| Acute toxoplasmosis in immunocompetent patient | No therapy required usually |
| Ocular disease | Pyrimethamine, folinic acid and sulphadiazine for 1 month. Steroids and laser may also be used to limit lesion size ☎ |
| Toxoplasmosis in immunodeficient patients | Pyrimethamine, folinic acid and sulphadiazine or clindamycin for 6 weeks, followed by indefinite prophylaxis |
| Infection during pregnancy | Treatment reduces fetal infection rate. Pyrimethamine is contraindicated in first trimester. Ideal treatment regimens not established. Spiramycin or sulphadiazine alone are commonly used for first trimester, followed by pyrimethamine/sulphadiazine continuously or alternating with spiramycin. Consultation with reference lab essential ☎ |
| Congenital infection | Pyrimethamine, folinic acid, and sulphadiazine, alternating with spiramycin, plus steroids. Consultation with reference lab essential ☎ |

required in immunodeficient persons (Table 15.3).

## Bacterial infection in childhood

Children are susceptible to most of the bacterial infections described in the system-based chapters of this manual, but in many cases, the expected range of infecting organisms varies with age.

See:
- Pneumonia in children (➤34).
- Bacterial meningitis (➤96).
- Infectious diarrhoea (➤57).

*Streptococcus pneumoniae, Haemophilus influenzae* and other bacteria are sometimes isolated from blood cultures taken from febrile children who are not severely ill and lack obvious foci of infection ('**occult bacteraemia**'). Antibiotic therapy should be assessed on clinical grounds and careful follow-up instituted.

## Neonatal infections

Infection in the neonate is common and requires a high level of awareness, since neonates rarely manifest classical symptoms of infection seen in older patients. Neonatal sepsis presenting early, within 5 days of birth, is usually due to infection acquired before or during birth (early neonatal infection, ENI). After 7 days or more after birth, it is due to infection acquired after birth (late neonatal infection—LNI). Group B β-haemolytic streptococci (GBS) account for many cases; see Table 15.4.

**Clinical features:** Presenting signs are similar for both categories. Signs of infection are often subtle, and up to 10% of babies with positive blood cultures may appear asymptomatic. Even with proven meningitis neonates rarely have neck stiffness or bulging fontanelle. Fever (50%) or hypothermia (15%), dyspnoea (20%), apnoea (20%), cyanosis (25%), tachycardia or hypotension (25%), anorexia (30%), vomiting (20%), abdominal distension (20%) and diarrhoea (10%), hepatomegaly (30%) and jaundice (30%), bleeding diathesis (2–10%), lethargy (35%), irritability (15%) or fits (15%). Rarely, disseminated enteroviral infection may produce a clinical illness similar to bacterial sepsis.

**Microbiological investigations:** Culture of blood, urine and CSF. CXR. Leucocytosis is common, and immature WBC forms are often seen in normal neonates; the normal ranges for infants differ with age:

**Table 15.4** Comparison of early (ENI) and late neonatal infection (LNI)

|  | ENI | LNI |
|---|---|---|
| Acquisition | Usually from mother | Often by cross-infection (via staff hands) from other babies. Occasional outbreaks from contaminated equipment (e.g. breast pumps) |
| Risk factors | Maternal perinatal infection, including infections causing disseminated intrauterine infection and congenital abnormalities (➤141) genital infections (e.g. HSV ➤129, or *Chlamydia trachomatis* ➤87) and infections acquired close to birth such as intra-amniotic infection (➤84). Prolonged rupture of membranes. Prolonged/difficult labour. Prematurity/low birth weight. Low APGAR score/need for resuscitation. Scalp electrodes | Congenital abnormalities. Prolonged admission to special-care baby unit. Procedures and medical interventions, especially iv lines and umbilical artery catheters Less strongly associated with risk factors for ENI |
| Organisms | Group B β-haemolytic streptococci (GBS ➤258), *Escherichia coli (K1)* (➤279), *Listeria monocytogenes.* Less often *Streptococcus pneumoniae* (associated with severe endometritis ➤84), other coliforms. Rarely anaerobes (particularly with PRM and intra-amniotic infection ➤83), GAS | GBS (➤258), *Listeria monocytogenes*, *Staphylococcus aureus*, *Staphylococcus epidermidis*, *Serratia* spp., *Citrobacter* spp. and other coliforms, *Salmonella* spp. (tropics), *Candida albicans*, *Malassezia furfur* |
| Clinical features | Overwhelming generalized sepsis; ≈30% have meningitis, and mortality is high (≈50%) | Meningitis ± bacteraemia. Skin sepsis. Usually lower mortality but coliform meningitis commonly associated with cerebral abscess |

| Age | Total neutrophils |
|---|---|
| Birth | 1.8–6.0 |
| 12 h | 7.8–14.5 |
| 1 day | 7.2–12.6 |
| 2 days | 3.6–8.1 |
| ≥5 days | 1.8–5.4 |

**Antibiotic management:** Early presumptive treatment with benzylpenicillin and gentamicin should be commenced after cultures have been obtained. If GBS infection is confirmed, benzylpenicillin (+ initial gentamicin) is the agent of choice. Parenteral cephalosporin (± gentamicin) recommended for Gram-negative meningitis and septicaemia.

**Supportive management:** A detailed discussion of the management of severely ill neonates is beyond the scope of this manual. Urgent referral to neonatology/paediatric intensive care is required ☎.

**Prevention of neonatal GBS infection:** Current guidelines for the prevention of neonatal GBS infection, published in the UK and USA, are based on limited evidence. Intrapartum antibiotics reduce the risk of neonatal GBS infection, but need to be targeted to those mothers most at risk of infecting their babies. Approaches based on screening for GBS carriage during pregnancy, or on assessment of maternal risk factors for neonatal infection, have both been recommended in the USA and have been associated with falling rates of GBS sepsis. In the UK, rates of GBS infection are lower, and PHLS have produced interim 'good practice' guidelines pending the results of further studies. These suggest that there is insufficient evidence to recommend screening for vaginal GBS carriage during pregnancy. Intrapartum antibiotic prophylaxis (benzylpenicillin or clindamycin) should be given to mothers who have:

- Had GBS infection in a previous baby.
- Been found incidentally to have GBS in urine or vagina.
- Chorioamnionitis.
- Pre-term delivery.
- Prolonged rupture of membranes.
- Fever in labour.

Neonates should receive antibiotics if they are unwell, if another baby from the same multiple birth has GBS infection, if mother should have had antibiotic prophylaxis but did not, if maternal antibiotics were given less than 4 h prior to delivery or if they are pre-term.

💻 www.phls.org.uk/topics_az/
strepto/goodpracticeStrepto.pdf
💻www.aap.org/policy/re9712.html

## Congenital infection—'TORCH' screening

Disseminated intrauterine infection by a number of organisms causes fetal abnormalities. The acronym TORCH (**T**oxoplasma, **O**ther, **R**ubella, **C**MV, **H**SV) has been used to describe these infections which have the following in common: (1) mild or inapparent infection in the mother; (2) wide range of severity in the infant; (3) similarity of presentation, with growth retardation and congenital defects; (4) diagnosis by serology; (5) long-term sequelae, with progressive disease in childhood and adolescence if untreated.

*Toxoplasma gondii* (➤137)

Rubella (➤127)

CMV (➤339)

Syphilis (➤89)

Parvovirus (➤342)

VZV (➤131)

Other agents that may be transmitted vertically include HIV (➤143), hepatitis B (➤70), EBV (➤133), leptospirosis (➤327), enteroviruses (➤347), *Ureaplasma urealyticum* (➤330) and *Mycoplasma hominis* (➤330).

**HSV** causes neonatal infection (➤129).

## Specific neonatal infections
### Ophthalmia neonatorum ✉②

Conjunctivitis affecting the newborn (➤107).

**Organisms:** *Chlamydia trachomatis*, *Neisseria gonorrhoeae*, *Staphylococcus aureus*.

## Otitis media

Not rare in the neonatal period (➤17).

**Organisms:** Coliforms, *Staphylococcus aureus*, *Haemophilus influenzae*, streptococci.

**Microbiological investigations:** Tympanocentesis may be indicated, particularly if otitis fails to respond promptly to antibiotics, as progression to meningitis or generalized sepsis may occur.

**Antibiotic management:** Ampicillin + gentamicin initially.

## Pneumonia

**Risk factors:** Intrapartum aspiration of maternal cervicovaginal flora, or infected amniotic fluid. Congenital infections.

**Clinical features:** Physical signs of pneumonia are usually absent. Signs of generalized sepsis (➤139), respiratory distress and CXR changes are more often seen.

Organisms: Group B β-haemolytic strepto-cocci, *Staphylococcus aureus*, coliforms, viral infections including RSV (➤23), influenza (➤23).

*Chlamydia trachomatis* causes lower respi-ratory tract infection that develops between 4 and 12 weeks. 50% have a history of conjunc-tivitis. Signs include gradual onset of cough and inspiratory crepitations. CXR shows patchy infiltrates. Many affected children have eosinophilia.

## Necrotizing enterocolitis

A severe condition of unknown cause: the commonest gastrointestinal emergency in the neonate. Pathogenesis may be related to tem-porary anoxia or other trauma to the bowel, allowing invasion of the epithelium by gut organisms.

Risk factors: Occurs sporadically and as nursery epidemics. Associated with prematurity, enteral feeding and umbilical artery catheter use. Usually occurs during the first 3 weeks, peaking at 3–10 days.

Clinical features: Fever, apnoea, lethargy. Abdominal distension, vomiting, blood in stools. In severe cases, there may be signs of peritonitis, crepitus and cellulitis of the anterior abdominal wall. Perforation may occur and healing may be complicated by stricture.

Organisms: The role of bacteria in the aetiology of necrotizing enterocolitis is uncertain and no single causative pathogen has been identified, but coliform predominance in gut flora in NEC is usual. Blood cultures may be positive with intestinal flora.

Investigations: AXR shows ileus, bowel dis-tension, pneumatosis intestinalis (intramural hydrogen bubbles), portal vein gas or free peri-toneal gas.

Antibiotic management: Benzylpenicillin + gentamicin + metronidazole are often used.

Supportive management: It is necessary to stop oral feeding and institute parenteral nutrition. Full paediatric intensive care is required; mortality 9–28%.

## Urinary tract infection

Risk factors: Structural abnormality of the urinary tract.

Clinical features: Non-specific features of infec-tion with fever and vomiting.

Organisms: *Escherichia coli*, *Klebsiella* spp., enterococci.

Microbiological investigations: Clean catch urine or suprapubic aspirate.

Other investigations: Imaging of urinary tract should be performed in all cases to exclude structural abnormality.

## Neonatal skin infections

These include cellulitis, Ritter's disease (toxic epidermal necrolysis or 'scalded skin' syndrome) (➤136), and oomphalitis (infec-tion of the umbilical stump) Oomphalitis may cause ascending phlebitis resulting in peri-tonitis or generalized sepsis. It is usually due to *Staphylococcus aureus*, streptococci and coliforms. Careful local toilet is required. If severe, flucloxacillin and gentamicin may be required.

# Chapter 16

# Human immune deficiency virus (HIV) infection and acquired immune deficiency syndrome (AIDS)

Since the first edition of this book was written in 1994, HIV medicine has progressed at an astounding pace, and has now effectively become a specialty in its own right. Major changes include a new understanding of the dynamics of viral replication, the routine availability of viral load and resistance testing, and the availability of highly active antiretroviral therapy (HAART). This chapter serves as a primer on HIV for the non-specialist, a source of some specific data for the specialist and a source of practical advice on the management of HIV patients presenting away from their usual units, but it cannot be a full text on the use of HAART.

## Epidemiology

AIDS was first described in 1981, and HIV was isolated in 1983. Since then, HIV infection has been reported from almost all countries. At the end of 2000, WHO estimated that there had been ≈58 million infected people worldwide, of whom 22 million have died, including over 4 million children. Sub-Saharan Africa has been most severely affected, accounting for ≈70% of cases, with over 4 million new cases in 2000 and an adult seroprevalence rate of 8.8%, of whom 55% are women. The demographic and social effects of this catastrophe are beyond the scope of this chapter. In the UK, there have been ≈14 000 AIDS cases to 2000, and ≈45 000 reported HIV infections.

Patterns of transmission vary between countries. In the UK, USA and Europe, infection has hitherto largely been associated with homosexual men and intravenous drug users. Heterosexual transmission in the UK has increased in significance, and exceeded the number of cases transmitted by sex between men in 1999 for the first time. In the developing world, heterosexual

transmission has always been more important, and this accounts in part for the greater prevalence of HIV infection there.

**HIV-2** is found mainly in W Africa. It shares only 45% sequence identity with HIV-1 and differs from HIV-1 in the following ways:
- Transmission rates appear to be lower.
- It appears to be less pathogenic *in vitro*.
- It is believed that the time to development of AIDS is longer with HIV-2 than HIV-1.

In the following sections, no further distinction will be made between HIV-1 and HIV-2.

🖥 www.phls.co.uk/
🖥 www.unaids.org/

## Transmission

Well-defined transmission routes exist:
- By **sexual contact**, both homo- and heterosexual, male to female and vice versa. Risk of transmission is highest with rectal intercourse, very early or advanced HIV infection, concomitant genital ulcer disease and other STDs.
- **Blood-borne**, in particular IVDU, but also by transfusion of blood/blood products. In the developed world, blood for transfusion is now screened for anti-HIV antibodies, and high-risk blood and tissue donors are excluded by questionnaire. Blood products are heat-treated.
- **Vertical transmission** (➤156).

Casual and household contact is not associated with transmission.

## Virology

**Key biological features:** HIV-1 and HIV-2 are members of the lentivirus family of human retroviruses (➤351). Virus attaches to host cells via specific binding of the viral envelope glycoprotein gp120 to the host membrane protein CD4 present on helper T lymphocytes,

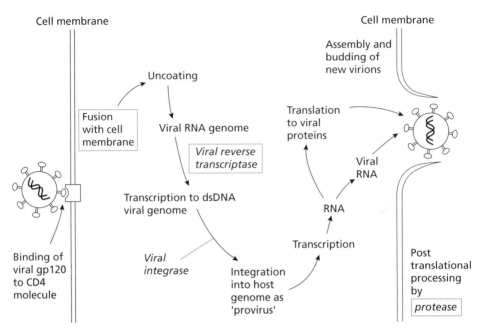

**Figure 16.1** A simplified diagram of the HIV replication cycle. Currently available drugs target viral reverse transcriptase, protease and fusion of the virus with the host cell membrane.

macrophages and other antigen-presenting cells. Chemokine receptors CXCR4 and CCR5 act as co-receptors, and individuals with inherited mutations in these proteins have relative resistance to infection. Fusion of the viral envelope with the cell membrane is mediated by envelope gp41. The viral RNA genome is transcribed into DNA by the viral enzyme reverse transcriptase (RT), and then integrated into the host genome by the viral enzyme integrase (Fig. 16.1).

It has now been established that throughout the course of HIV infection, including during clinical latency, viral replication proceeds at a high level. At least $10^9$ viral particles are produced daily, with destruction of a similar number of CD4+ lymphocytes. It is now possible to quantify virions in plasma ('viral load'); most are the product of continuous rounds of new infection in actively replicating short-lived T lymphocytes, with a very small contribution from long-lived chronically infected cells (mainly macrophages). This rapid high volume turnover of virus, combined with the high error rate of viral reverse transcriptase ($\approx 1$ per 1000 bases transcribed) provides the mechanism for the generation of viral diversity, which is clinically significant for the development of resistance to HAART (➤152), and the development of more virulent viral strains as disease progresses.

➥ Perelson AS, Science 1996; 271: 1582

**Viral load** may be estimated by a number of methods. Quantitative PCR is most widely used. Current routine assays have a lower detection limit of the order of 50 virions/mL and an upper limit of 750 000 virions/mL. High viral loads are expected during seroconversion and in late disease. Within 4–6 months of seroconversion, partial immunological control of viral replication leads to a fall in viral load to a plateau level that varies between individuals ('set point'). Set point correlates with the rate of progression. Thus, an individual with a viral load (off HAART) of 100 000 copies/mL is likely to progress to AIDS more rapidly than average, whereas long-term survivors tend to have untreated viral loads of 5000 copies/mL or below. Viral load increases during intercurrent infections (e.g. *Pneumocystis carinii* pneumonia or PCP), and the set point rises gradually as disease progresses in the untreated patient.

↵ Mellors JW, Ann Intern Med 1995; 122: 573

## Clinical features of HIV infection

A very large number of **immunological defects** have been described in HIV infection, affecting all the components of the immune system. The most important abnormalities are:
• A severe decline in the number of CD4+ helper T lymphocytes, associated clinically with impaired cell-mediated immunity and the development of opportunist infections and malignancies.
• Hypergammaglobulinaemia, which is associated clinically with the development of a wide range of autoantibodies, idiopathic thrombocytopenia and a high incidence of severe drug allergies.

## Stages of HIV infection

**Incubation:** Following infection, there is an asymptomatic period of 2–4 weeks during which all tests for HIV antibodies and antigens are negative.

**Seroconversion** is accompanied by a febrile illness in ≈50% of cases, although it may not be recognized as such. Clinical features are variable, but include fever, malaise, headache, pharyngitis, generalized lymphadenopathy and a maculopapular rash. Features suggesting primary HIV infection rather than any other flu-like illness include the skin rash, mucocutaneous ulceration (mouth, oesophagus, anogenital area), neurological involvement (meningoencephalitis, peripheral neuropathy, retro-orbital pain and photophobia) and oral candidiasis. Initial lymphopenia followed by an atypical lymphocytosis may occur. Mild thrombocytopenia and abnormal liver function tests are common. Specific antibody tests for HIV become positive between 2 and 6 weeks after the onset of the seroconversion illness, but viral load is positive from the onset of symptoms. Differential diagnosis includes rubella (➤127), infectious mononucleosis (➤133), secondary syphilis (➤89) and disseminated gonococcal infection (➤87). Resolution occurs over 2–4 weeks.

**Latency:** Following infection, patients remain free from serious illness for a variable number of years, although viral replication continues at a high level throughout. After an initial asymptomatic period, they may develop constitutional symptoms (e.g. fever, malaise and weight loss), manifestations of mild immunodeficiency (e.g. oral candidiasis, cutaneous herpes zoster or herpes simplex, or bacterial infections) or manifestations of immunodysregulation (e.g. immune thrombocytopenia, multiple drug allergies or seborrhoeic dermatitis). This phase of HIV-related illness was previously referred to as AIDS-related complex (ARC). There may be persistent generalized lymphadenopathy, but this is not a prognostic indicator for progression to AIDS.

**Progression to AIDS** is defined in the UK by development of one of the AIDS-defining illnesses listed in Table 16.1. Prior to the introduction of prophylaxis against PCP, patients often presented with this infection, usually after the CD4 count had fallen below 200 cells/μL. In the USA, a CD4 count below 200 cells/μL is considered diagnostic of AIDS. Although this definition of AIDS has not been formally adopted in the UK, the US surveillance definition provides a useful framework for describing stages of infection (Table 16.2).

**In the absence of HAART,** the median time from infection to the onset of AIDS in the developed world is about 10 years, although some patients progress rapidly within 2 years of infection, and ≈10% will become 'long-term survivors' who have yet to develop clinical illness. Survival following the diagnosis of AIDS also varies widely depending on the nature of the AIDS-defining event, but is about 1–2 yrs in the developed world.

**AIDS in children:** The average age of onset of immunodeficiency in perinatally infected

**Table 16.1** AIDS indicator diseases (UK definition)

| AIDS indicator disease | Comments and qualifications |
| --- | --- |
| Bacterial infections, recurrent or multiple | In a child less than 13 yrs |
| Candidiasis | Affecting oesophagus, trachea, bronchus or lungs |
| Cervical carcinoma | Invasive |
| Coccidioidomycosis | Disseminated or extrapulmonary |
| Cryptococcosis | Extrapulmonary |
| Cryptosporidiosis | With diarrhoea for greater than 1 month |
| Cytomegalovirus disease | Onset after age 1 month, not confined to liver, spleen and lymph nodes |
| Cytomegalovirus retinitis | |
| Encephalopathy (dementia) due to HIV | HIV infection and disabling cognitive and/or motor dysfunction, or milestone loss in a child, with no other causes by CSF examination, brain imaging or postmortem |
| Herpes simplex | Ulcers for greater than 1 month or bronchitis, pneumonitis or oesophagitis |
| Histoplasmosis | Disseminated or extrapulmonary |
| Isosporiasis | With diarrhoea for greater than 1 month |
| Kaposi's sarcoma | |
| Lymphoid interstitial pneumonia and/or pulmonary lymphoid hyperplasia | In a child less than 13 yrs |
| Lymphoma | Burkitt's or immunoblastic or primary in brain |
| Mycobacteriosis, atypical | Disseminated or extrapulmonary |
| Mycobacteriosis (*Mycobacterium tuberculosis*) | Pulmonary tuberculosis |
| *Pneumocystis carinii* pneumonia | |
| Progressive multifocal leukoencephalopathy | |
| Recurrent non-typhoidal salmonella bacteraemia | |
| Recurrent pneumonia | Two episodes within 12 months |
| Toxoplasmosis of brain | Onset after age 1 month |
| Wasting syndrome due to HIV | Weight loss (over 10% of baseline) with no other cause, and 30 days or more of either diarrhoea or weakness with fever |

children in the US is 5–10 months. Few infected infants remain well beyond 3 yrs of age, and their median survival after diagnosis of AIDS is ≈9 months. Children with AIDS present in a number of ways, including failure to thrive and developmental delay, hepatosplenomegaly and lymphadenopathy, recurrent bacterial infection, or with the opportunistic infections

**Table 16.2** US AIDS classification

| CD4 cell categories | Clinical categories | | |
| --- | --- | --- | --- |
| | A<br>Asymptomatic, or PGL<br>or acute HIV infection | B<br>Symptomatic<br>(not A or C) | C<br>AIDS indicator condition<br>(Table 16.1) |
| (1) >500/mm³ (≥29%) | A1 | B1 | C1 |
| (2) 200 to 499/mm³<br>(14–28%) | A2 | B2 | C2 |
| (3) <200/mm³ (<14%) | A3 | B3 | C3 |

All patients in categories A3, B3 and C1–3 defined as having AIDS, based on the presence of an AIDS indicator condition (Table 16.1) and/or a CD4 cell count <200/mm³.

Category B is defined by symptomatic conditions that are not included in Category C and that are (a) attributed to HIV infection or indicative of a defect in cell-mediated immunity, or (b) considered to have a clinical course or management that is complicated by HIV infection. Examples of B conditions include but are not limited to bacillary angiomatosis; thrush; vulvovaginal candidiasis which is persistent, frequent or poorly responsive to therapy; cervical dysplasia (moderate or severe); cervical carcinoma *in situ*; constitutional symptoms such as fever (38.5°C) or diarrhoea >1 month; oral hairy leukoplakia; herpes zoster involving two episodes or >1 dermatome; idiopathic thrombocytopenic purpura (ITP); listeriosis; pelvic inflammatory disease (PID) (especially if complicated by a tubo-ovarian abscess); and peripheral neuropathy.

common in adults, particularly candidiasis and PCP. Some manifestations of AIDS are unique to children, such as salivary gland enlargement and lymphocytic interstitial pneumonia (LIP). Forty per cent of children develop LIP, with nodular peribronchial infiltrates and hilar lymphadenopathy. LIP causes clubbing and progressive shortness of breath, which may respond to steroids; acute deterioration of ventilation is usually due to intercurrent infection. Neurological disease, in particular encephalopathy, is common and often severe.

## Tests for HIV infection

Anti-HIV antibodies are always detectable within 3 months of acquiring infection, and present in almost all patients within 6 weeks. Infection can also be demonstrated by viral culture, antigen detection or PCR for viral RNA. During seroconversion, antibody tests are often negative for the first week of illness. All HIV testing requires experienced pre- and post-test counselling.

## CD4 counts

T lymphocytes may be divided on the basis of surface protein expression into two main categories: CD4+ (helper) T cells and CD8+ (cytotoxic/suppressor) T cells. HIV specifically infects and depletes the CD4+ subset, and the CD4 count falls as immunodeficiency develops. CD4 counts are subject to wide diurnal variation and the counting procedure itself is inaccurate, so at least two counts should be performed before management decisions are made. Some patients with very low counts may remain relatively well. Nevertheless, the CD4 count is the only widely used marker of immunological status and does allow approximate staging of infection.

Normal ranges for CD4 count are: absolute count >500 cells/µL, or 40–70% of total lymphocytes. The CD4/CD8 ratio should be >0.5. There is a small transient decrease in CD4 count during the seroconversion illness. During the latent period, there is a gradual decline in CD4 count. Opportunist infections are unusual before the count falls below 200 cells/μL. Below 100 cells/μL, infections, particularly PCP and disseminated *Mycobacterium aviumintracellulare* (MAI), are usual. Patients with end-stage disease typically have counts <50 cells/μL.

## Management

### General care

**Initial assessment** includes estimation of the likely duration and route of infection, and careful history and examination to exclude ongoing opportunistic infection and malignancy. Previous illnesses, especially STDs, should be reviewed. Baseline investigations should include: CD4 count, viral load, FBC, serology for CMV, toxoplasmosis, hepatitis C, hepatitis B and syphilis. A cervical smear or culposcopy should be performed and repeated at least annually in all HIV+ women. Information, education, social and psychological support are very important, and an integrated approach involving doctors, nurses, health advisors and other professionals is essential.

**Follow-up visits** should include examination for conditions that present insidiously, including skin (seborrhoeic dermatitis, infections, Kaposi's sarcoma or KS), mouth (candidiasis, oral hairy leukoplakia), lymph nodes (*localized* enlargement suggests infection or malignancy), fundi (chorioretinitis) and neurological system (AIDS dementia complex, peripheral neuropathy). CD4 count and viral load are usually monitored every 3 months in patients stabilized on HAART.

## Highly active antiretroviral therapy

The availability of HAART has transformed the outlook of HIV+ patients in the developed world.

**Brief history:** An understanding of the history and chronology of HAART is useful, as many patients received inadequate therapy under previous regimens which influences their current prognosis. Zidovudine (AZT) was available from ≈1987. Early studies of AZT monotherapy showed marginal benefit to patients with advanced disease, with mean increases in survival measured in months. Early treatment of asymptomatic persons with AZT monotherapy did not improve overall prognosis. Two-drug combination therapy was then shown to be superior to monotherapy.

↦ Concorde, Lancet 1994; 343: 871
↦ Delta, Lancet 1996; 348: 283

Triple combination therapy was first shown to be useful in 1995 and was generally in widespread and exclusive use by 1997. The benefits of HAART are so obvious that prolonged controlled trials versus dual therapy have not been possible. The evidence base for current practice is reviewed extensively in current US and UK guidelines, which are constantly updated.

🖳 www.bhiva.org/guidelines.html
🖳 www.hivatis.org/trtgdlns.html

**Principles of therapy:** The principle of HAART is to maintain complete and continuous suppression of viral replication to a point where mutation cannot occur, thus preventing the emergence of viral resistance. In practice, suppression of plasma viral load below 50 copies/mL is associated with prolonged efficacy of treatment, sustained increases in CD4 count and concomitant reversal of immunodeficiency. This is usually achieved by giving three antivirals to which the patient's virus is sensitive. Because viral replication will resume as soon as drug levels fall below the concentration necessary for viral inhibition **adherence** (syn. compliance) is essential. Poor adherence to therapy predicts premature failure of the antiviral regimen. Adherence is influenced by lifestyle factors (e.g. ongoing IVDU), other medical conditions (e.g. dementia), social and personal factors (including significant relationships and support from health-care workers), pill count, dosage schedule and adverse effects of medication.

A major point of controversy remains the correct **timing of the start of therapy**. Most experts agree that treatment should be started before the CD4 count falls below 200, at which point clinically significant immunodeficiency becomes likely. Starting therapy later is associated with slower and less complete immune reconstitution. Some experts would recommend therapy for all HIV+ individuals, but most would wait until the CD4 count was between 200 and 500. A high viral load (e.g. >100 000 copies/mL) predicts rapid progression and suggests an earlier start to therapy. Once started, therapy is intended to continue lifelong. Structured interruption of therapy is currently being investigated. There are theoretical advantages to this, but there is no current experimental evidence to suggest any benefit, and this is **not** currently recommended.

**Commonly used triple regimens** usually include two NRTIs (➤149) with either an NNRTI or a PI. Triple NRTI regimens are used, but doubts exist over their efficacy in patients with high viral loads. Regimens have to be designed with the patient's lifestyle and individual needs in mind. If the first regimen fails (i.e. viral load becomes detectable and starts to rise), further regimens are designed on the basis of previous therapies and resistance testing (➤152).

**Efficacy of therapy** is closely related to adherence and resistance, but in compliant patients who are treatment-naïve, most will achieve an undetectable viral load and a rise in CD4 count to the point where serious opportunistic infections do not occur.

## Specific drugs

Three classes of antiretroviral drug are in widespread use. For doses in renal failure of these specialist medications, please see the manufacturer's data sheet.

🖥 emc.vhn.net

## Nucleoside reverse transcriptase inhibitors (NRTI)

Nucleoside analogues that are preferentially incorporated into the nascent viral DNA chain by viral RT and act as chain terminators.

**Class-specific side effects:** Peripheral neuropathy, pancreatitis.

### ZIDOVUDINE (AZT, RETROVIR)
**Normal dose:** 250 mg q12h.

**Common adverse effects:** Transitory headache and muscle aching with start of treatment. Anaemia, myositis.

**Comments:** Available in combination preparations. Not usually co-administered with D4T, because of intracellular pharmacodynamic antagonism.

### DIDANOSINE (ddI, VIDEX)
**Normal dose:** 400 mg q24h (or 200 mg q12h), reduced to 250 mg q24h if weight <60 kg. New enteric-coated preparation has replaced previous buffered tablets/powders, but ddI must still be taken on an empty stomach. Manufacturer currently recommends taking at least 2 h after food.

**Common adverse effects:** Pancreatitis, peripheral neuropathy, GI upset with older preparations.

**Comments:** Can also be given as a liquid made up in antacid mixture.

### ZALCITABINE (ddC, HIVID)
**Normal dose:** 1.125 mg q12h.

**Common adverse effects:** Peripheral neuropathy, pancreatitis.

**Comments:** Less frequently used now because of the high incidence of peripheral neuropathy.

### STAVUDINE (d4T, ZERIT)

**Normal dose:** 40 mg q12h (30 mg q24h if <60 kg).

**Common adverse effects:** Peripheral neuropathy, pancreatitis.

**Comments:** Not usually co-administered with AZT because of intracellular pharmacodynamic antagonism.

## LAMIVUDINE (3TC, EPIVIR)
**Normal dose:** 150 mg q12h.

**Common adverse effects:** Generally free of adverse effects.

**Comments:** Available in combination preparations. Resistance develops more easily than with other drugs in class, but 3TC-resistant mutants may be more susceptible to AZT and NNRTIs, and have reduced replicative fitness. Studies are in progress to determine the usefulness of continuing 3TC in combination with other agents, even after the development of 3TC-resistant virus. Also has activity against hepatitis B virus (➤72).

## ABACAVIR (ZIAGEN)

**Normal dose:** 300 mg q12h.

**Common adverse effects:** Generally well tolerated, but ≈3% develop a hypersensitivity reaction, which can be severe and even fatal. The reaction develops most often during the first 6 weeks of treatment (peak 10 days) and may involve rash, fever, GI disturbance and constitutional disturbance. Patients are ill and get worse day by day. The reaction resolves when abacavir is stopped, but **rechallenge is absolutely contraindicated**, because this can result in a rapidly fatal reaction. Patients must be given written instructions when they start abacavir, warning of this possibility. Patients with suspected abacavir hypersensitivity should not discontinue medication without consultation with their prescriber, since restarting may not be possible once the opportunity to observe the adverse reaction is lost.

**Comments:** Available in combination preparations.

## TENOFOVIR (VIREAD)
**Normal dose:** 245 mg q24h with food.

**Common adverse effects:** GI upset, headache.

**Comments:** Approved in late 2001 for second-line use only. A nucleotide analogue which is active against HIV with multiple-NRTI resistance (➤152). 3TC-resistant mutants may be hypersensitive to tenofovir. An earlier nucleotide analogue, adefovir, was abandoned, primarily because of nephrotoxicity.

### NEW NRTIS IN DEVELOPMENT
**Emtricitabine (FTC)** is closely related to 3TC, but can be given q24h.

### NUCLEOSIDE COMBINATION PRODUCTS
**Combivir** is zidovudine 300 mg and lamivudine 150 mg.

**Trizivir** is zidovudine 300 mg, lamivudine 150 mg, abacavir 300 mg.

## Non-nucleoside reverse transcriptase inhibitors (NNRTI)

These drugs competitively inhibit RT by binding in the active groove of the enzyme, but they are not incorporated into DNA. Easy to take, with low pill count and few severe side effects. Resistance develops more easily than with protease inhibitors (➤152).

**Class-specific side effects:** Rashes (potentially severe). Nevirapine and efavirenz are enzyme inducers (➤152) and can precipitate opiate withdrawal in methadone users.

### NEVIRAPINE (VIRAMUNE)
**Normal dose:** 200 mg q12h (200 mg q24h for first 2 weeks of treatment).

**Common adverse effects:** Rash, potentially severe. If the rash is blistering or severe, or if there are constitutional symptoms, drug must be stopped. Rechallenge is contraindicated. The incidence of rash is reduced by giving reduced dose for first 2 weeks. If rash develops whilst on 200 mg q24h, the dose must not be increased—this is potentially very dangerous. Hepatitis, potentially severe.

**Table 16.3** Protease inhibitor combination doses

| Drug | Schedule | Daily pill count |
|---|---|---|
| **Ritonavir** (100 mg cap) | 600 mg b.d. | 12 |
| **Indinavir** (400 mg cap) | 800 mg t.d.s. (food restrictions) | 6 |
| Indinavir/ritonavir | 800 mg/100 mg b.d. | 6 |
| **Saquinavir** (200 mg soft gel capsule — Fortovase) | 1200 mg t.d.s | 18 |
| | 1600 mg b.d. | 16 |
| Saquinavir (200 mg hard capsule — Invirase)/ | 1000 mg/100 mg b.d. | 12 |
| ritonavir | 1600 mg/100 mg o.d. | 9 |
| Saquinavir/nelfinavir | 1200 mg/1250 mg b.d. | 22 |
| **Nelfinavir** (250 mg cap) | 750 mg t.d.s. | 9 |
| | 1250 mg b.d. | 10 |
| **Lopinavir/r** | 3 caps b.d. | 6 |
| **Amprenavir** (150 mg cap) | 1200 mg b.d. | 16 |
| Amprenavir/ritonavir | 600 mg/100 mg b.d. | 10 |

### EFAVIRENZ (SUSTIVA)
**Normal dose:** 600 mg q24h.

**Common adverse effects:** Rash, dizziness and ataxia, nightmares, hallucinations. CNS side effects usually wear off after a few doses.

**Comments:** Often given at night to reduce impact of CNS side effects.

### DELAVIRDINE (RESCRIPTOR)
**Normal dose:** 600 mg q12h. Unlicensed in UK.

**Common adverse effects:** Rash.

### NEW NNRTIS IN DEVELOPMENT
At the time of writing (early 2002), no new NNRTIs have progressed beyond phase I or II clinical trial.

## Protease inhibitors (PI)

Drugs that inhibit the viral protease (an enzyme involved in processing viral proteins in the nascent virion). Powerful drugs with less capacity for development of resistance than NNRTIs, but usefulness is reduced by the high frequency of side effects, especially gastrointestinal, and by their potential for drug interactions. Because ritonavir is the most potent known inhibitor of cytochrome P450, it boosts levels of other PIs, and combinations of one PI with a small dose of ritonavir (e.g. 100 mg o.d. or b.d.) are often used to reduce costs and pill count. This is referred to as 'low-dose ritonavir', 'pharmacodynamic boosting', etc. Lopinavir has low-dose ritonavir included in the capsule. Thus, there are many different PI dosing schedules, see Table 16.3.

**Class-specific side effects:** GI upset. Drug-interactions. Hyperlipidaemia, hyperglycaemia. Circumoral paraethesia.

### INDINAVIR (CRIXIVAN)
**Common adverse effects:** GI, hyperbilirubinaemia, crystalluria and renal stones.

**Comments:** To avoid crystalluria, patients must keep well hydrated — >3 L fluid q24h. Patients may take low-fat food only for 2 h before and 1 h after each dose if IDV is given without ritonavir.

### RITONAVIR (NORVIR)
**Common adverse effects:** Circumoral paraesthesia, GI upset if given as single PI in full dose. Many serious drug interactions (➤152).

**Comments:** Mainly used to boost levels of other PIs. Rarely used as a single PI because of adverse effects; these are minimized by starting at lower dose and increasing ('dose titration')▤.

### SAQUINAVIR SOFT GEL CAPSULE (FORTOVASE)
**Common adverse effects:** GI upset, not usually severe.

**Comments:** Original hard-gel formulation (Invirase) was very poorly absorbed and is no longer used except in combination with ritonavir.

### NELFINAVIR (VIRACEPT)
**Common adverse effects:** GI upset.

**Comments:** Taken with food to maximize absorption.

### AMPRENAVIR (AGENERASE)
**Common adverse effects:** GI upset.

**Comments:** Licensed only as a second-line PI, for use when other PIs have failed. Probably less potent than other PIs, but has unique resistance profile (➤152), which may make it useful in this context.

### LOPINAVIR/R (KALETRA)
**Dose and administration:** Three capsules (lopinavir 400 mg, ritonavir 100 mg) q12h. Increased to four caps q12h if given with nevirapine or efavirenz in a patient in whom partial lopinavir resistance is possible.

**Common adverse effects:** GI upset.

**Comments:** Well tolerated. Ritonavir is included to boost lopinavir levels; dose is inadequate for any useful antiviral activity *per se*.

### NEW PIS IN DEVELOPMENT
**Tipranavir, mozenavir** and **atazanavir** are all in phase II/III study and show benefits in dosing schedules and resistance profile. **GW433 908** ('**908**') is a pro-drug of amprenavir with a favourable pharmacodynamic profile.

## Novel antiviral strategies

At the time of writing, drugs that inhibit fusion of the viral envelope with the host cell membrane are in trial. These agents, **T20** (**pentafuside**) and **T1249**, are injected subcutaneously. Other strategies under investigation include agents that inhibit interaction with CD4 or chemokine receptors and integrase inhibitors.

## Drug interactions

PIs and NNRTIs are often inhibitors or inducers of cytochrome P450 (CYP450) in the liver, so drug interactions are important in patients in HAART. Ritonavir is the most potent CYP450 inhibitor known, and is used to boost levels of other PIs (Table 16.3). Potential interactions between HAART agents are shown in Table 16.4; dosage modification is frequently required, depending on the combination used. Other medications contraindicated are shown in Table 16.5. Any prescription in a patient taking ritonavir should be examined for potential interactions. An invaluable source of up-to-date information on this subject is maintained by the University of Liverpool:

💻 www.hiv-druginteractions.org/

## Therapeutic drug monitoring

Plasma levels of HAART agents, particularly PIs, vary widely between individuals and are affected by other drugs, diet, liver disease and compliance. Measuring plasma levels of PIs is often a useful adjunct to ensuring adequate dosing.

## Resistance testing

HIV has enormous capacity for mutation because of high turnover and error-prone transcription (➤144). In the presence of sub-inhibitory levels of HAART agents, resistant virus will arise. Particular mutations in RT and protease are associated with resistance to different agents (Table 16.6). Resistance testing is currently usually performed when patients fail one antiviral regimen. Using viral resistance testing to inform HAART choices has been shown to improve prognosis. Two methods are available:

• **Genotypic resistance testing** uses PCR to

**Table 16.4** Interactions between antivirals. Only clinically significant interactions are shown

| Acting drug | Affected drug | | | | |
| --- | --- | --- | --- | --- | --- |
| | Indinavir | Ritonavir | Saquinavir | Nelfinavir | Amprenavir |
| Indinavir | – | – | AUC↑ ×5 | 84% AUC↑ | 64% AUC↑ |
| Ritonavir | AUC↑ ×5 | | AUC↑ ×20 | AUC↑ ×2.5 | AUC↑ |
| Saquinavir | | | – | | |
| Nelfinavir | 50% AUC↑ | | AUC↑ ×5 | – | |
| Amprenavir | | | | | – |
| Nevirapine | 28% ↓AUC | | 28% ↓AUC | 28% ↓AUC | |
| Delavirdine | | 70% AUC↑ | AUC↑ ×5 | | |
| Efavirenz | | | AUC↓* | | |

AUC, area under curve. Shaded boxes are those that result in dose modifications (➤152).
*Efavirenz and saquinavir should not be given together without ritonavir, because saquinavir levels will be too low.

**Table 16.5** Drugs contraindicated in patients taking protease inhibitors. This is a list of some potentially significant interactions—it is wise to check *any* presciption in a patient receiving highly active antiretroviral therapy (HAART). 📄 🖥 www.hiv-druginteractions.org/

| | | |
| --- | --- | --- |
| *Ritonavir* | *Indinavir* | *Amprenavir* |
| Dextropropoxyphene | Bepridil | Bepridil |
| Pethidine | Rifampicin | Rifampicin |
| Piroxicam | Astemizole | Astemizole |
| Amiodarone | Dihydroergotamine | Dihydroergotamine |
| Bepridil | Ergotamine | Ergotamine |
| Flecainide | Alprazolam | Midazolam |
| Propafenone | Midazolam | Triazolam |
| Quinidine | Triazolam | |
| Rifabutin | | *Delavirdine* |
| Rifampicin | *Saquinavir* | Rifabutin |
| Bupropion | Bepridil | Rifampicin |
| Astemizole | Rifabutin | Astemizole |
| Dihydroergotamine | Rifampicin | Midazolam |
| Ergotamine | Astemizole | Triazolam |
| Clozapine | | |
| Pimozide | *Nelfinavir* | *Efavirenz* |
| Clorazepate | Bepridil | Astemizole |
| Diazepam | Amiodarone | Dihydroergotamine |
| Estazolam | Quinidine | Ergotamine |
| Flurazepam | Rifampicin | Midazolam |
| Midazolam | Astemizole | Triazolam |
| Triazolam | Dihydroergotamine | |
| Zolpidem | Ergotamine | *Nevirapine* |
| | Midazolam | Ketoconazole |
| | Triazolam | |

**Table 16.6** Some examples of HIV mutations contributing to resistance to commonly used antiretrovirals

| Drug | Key resistance mutations | Comments |
| --- | --- | --- |
| **NRTIs** | | |
| AZT | K70R, T215Y/F | |
| 3TC | M184V | Partially reverses T215Y mediated AZT resistance |
| ddI | L74V | Causes increased sensitivity to AZT |
| 'Multi-NRTI' | Q151M | Confers high-level resistance to most NRTIs |
| **NNRTIs** | K103N, Y181C/I | Shared across class |
| **PIs** | | |
| RTV/IDV | I84V, L90M | |
| SQV | I84V, L90M | |
| NFV | D30N, L90M | |
| APV | I50V, I84V | |

NNRTIs, non-nucleoside reverse transcriptase inhibitors; NRTIs, nucleoside reverse transcriptase inhibitors; PIs, protease inhibitors.

First letter represents amino acid present in wild type, last letter represents amino acid present in mutant. Number indicates codon affected, either in RT or protease. These data are shown to illustrate the type of data available and how it is usually presented. Resistance depends not only on the presence of given mutations, but also on interaction between mutations. New data accrue continuously—for a full discussion, see ⌨ hivdb.stanford.edu/hiv/. ⌨ www.tibotecvirco.com.

detect the presence of particular mutations. It requires the patient to be on treatment and to have a detectable viral load (>2000 copies/mL at present). Because it amplifies the virus which is currently circulating in the patient's blood, it only detects resistance to drugs which the patient is currently taking, and it does not detect the presence of small amounts of resistant virus present as a result of previous regimens ('archived resistance'). Genotypic testing is now in routine clinical use in the UK, US and Europe.

• **Phenotypic resistance testing** is performed by culturing virus in the presence of antiviral drugs. It is more complicated and expensive and not widely used routinely at present.

As the transmission of drug-resistant virus increases, it will become more appropriate to perform resistance testing in HAART-naïve patients.

⌨ hivdb.stanford.edu/hiv

## Adverse effects associated with long-term use of HAART

### Metabolic abnormalities

Protease inhibitors are associated with hyperlipidaemia and hyperglycaemia. NRTIs and NNRTIs can cause lactic acidosis, which may present as GI upset, Kussmall respiration, cramps, myalgia and paraesthesiae, and ascending muscular weakness, which resembles Guillain–Barré syndrome.

### Lipodystrophy

Patients on long-term HAART may develop redistribution of body fat, with loss of fat from face and limbs and central obesity. This can be disabling, and also gives rise to a characteristic facial appearance which some patient groups may find stigmatizing. This adverse effect had been thought to be due to PIs, but it may be more common in patients taking D4T. It may improve if treatment is discontinued, but this is not usually possible.

**Table 16.7** Prophylaxis against opportunist infection in HIV

| Organism | Indications for prophylaxis | Regimen | Comments |
|---|---|---|---|
| *Pneumocystis carinii* (➤156) | CD4 count <200 cells/μL or AIDS—may be discontinued if CD4 persistently >200 (➤147) | Co-trimoxazole 480 mg q24h **or** inhaled pentamidine* (300 mg monthly) **or** dapsone 100 mg q24h **or** dapsone 200 mg/week plus pyrimethamine 75 mg/week **or** atovaquone 1500 mg q24h | Breakthrough infection is commoner with inhaled pentamidine, particularly affecting the upper lobes or extrapulmonary sites |
| Herpes simplex virus (➤159) | Recurrent cutaneous herpes | Aciclovir 400 mg q12h | Breakthrough infections may be treated with increased dose |
| Toxoplasmosis (➤163) | Previous toxoplasma encephalitis—may be discontinued if CD4 persistently >200 | Pyrimethamine 25 mg q24h, folinic acid 15 mg q24h and either sulphadiazine 500 mg q6h or clindamycin 300 mg q6h | Co-trimoxazole prophylaxis against PCP reduces the incidence of toxoplasmosis; toxoplasma- seropositive patients with CD4 <100 who are not taking co-trimoxazole should be offered primary prophylaxis with pyrimethamine 100 mg weekly |

PCP, *Pneumocystis carinii* pneumonia.

* A small-particle nebulizer is required. The conventional nebulizer commonly used to administer bronchodilators is not suitable.

## Peripheral neuropathy

NRTIs are associated with painful distal symmetrical peripheral neuropathy, predominantly sensory. This is particularly seen when ddI and D4T are used together (≈10% of patients). Amitriptyline and gabapentin can relieve symptoms, but a change in therapy is often required.

## Prophylaxis against OI

Prophylaxis against OI remains important, esp. in patients who have failed HAART. See Table 16.7. The value of prophylactic treatment for TB is debated. In the US, where BCG is not used, a positive Mantoux (➤42) is taken as evidence of previous TB infection and is an indication for isoniazid prophylaxis (usually given for 9 months). Prophylaxis against atypical mycobacteria (➤168) reduces subsequent infection in patients with low CD4 counts, but organisms are more frequently resistant when infection does occur. UK national guidelines for prophylaxis have not been published. For US guidelines, see:

💻 www.hivatis.org/guidelines

## Postexposure prophylaxis (PEP) against HIV

The following body fluids are considered potentially infectious for HIV: blood, amniotic fluid, CSF, breast milk, pericardial, peritoneal and pleural fluid, saliva in association with dentistry (likely to be contaminated with blood, even when not visibly so), synovial fluid, unfixed human tissues and organs, any other body fluid if visibly bloodstained, exudative or other tissue fluid from burns or skin lesions. Three types of exposure are associated with significant risk:

- **Percutaneous injury** (from needles, instruments, bone fragments, significant bites which break the skin, etc.).
- Exposure of **broken skin** (abrasions, cuts, eczema, etc.).
- Exposure of **mucous membranes**, including the eye.

The risk of acquiring HIV infection following occupational exposure to HIV-infected blood is low. Epidemiological studies have indicated that the average risk for HIV transmission after percutaneous exposure to HIV-infected blood in health-care settings is about three per 1000 injuries. After a mucocutaneous exposure, the average risk is estimated at less than one in 1000. It has been considered that there is no risk of HIV transmission where intact skin is exposed to HIV-infected blood, although PEP might be considered where exposure has been particularly heavy or prolonged.

Factors associated with increased risk of occupationally-acquired HIV infection include:
- Deep injury.
- Visible blood on the device which caused the injury.
- Injury with a needle which had been placed in a source patient's artery or vein.
- Terminal HIV-related illness in the source patient.

Retrospective case–control studies and animal experiments suggest that prompt administration of HAART, ideally within 2 h of exposure, reduces risk of transmission. Despite lack of direct evidence, this has been accepted as policy in Europe, the UK and US. All hospitals should have protocols for administration of PEP, and counselling/testing of staff and source patients. **Familiarize yourself with local policy and seek specialist advice immediately after any potential high-risk exposure.** The use of PEP for non-occupational exposures, including sexual exposure, is controversial.

 www.doh.gov.uk/eaga/index.htm
 www.cdc.gov/mmwr/preview/
mmwrhtml/rr5011a1.htm

## Preventing vertical HIV transmission

The risk of vertical transmission is ≈25% overall, with infection occurring at birth or through breast feeding. Transmission rates vary with maternal viral load, and antiviral therapy during late pregnancy, labour and to the neonate has been shown to reduce infection rates. Risk of transmission is probably <1% if maternal viral load is <50 copies/mL. Current UK strategy for the prevention of vertical transmission depends on:
- Identification of HIV+ mothers through antenatal screening (now offered universally in the UK).
- Use of HAART during pregnancy.
- Neonatal AZT monotherapy.
- Bottle feeding.
- Careful obstetric management, usually including caesarean section.

Early involvement of obstetricians and paediatricians with specialist interest is essential ☎.

# Specific clinical syndromes in HIV-infected patients

## Pulmonary infections in HIV-infected patients

### *Pneumocystis carinii* pneumonia

Exposure to *Pneumocystis carinii* is common in the developed world, and most children have specific antibodies by age 2. Clinical disease occurs only in the context of severe immunodeficiency, such as advanced HIV infection, after transplantation or severe malnutrition. *Pneumocystis carinii* multiplies within the alveolus, damaging the alveolar epithelial cells and causing increased permeability of the alveolar/capillary membrane. This results in low-pressure pulmonary oedema, intrapulmonary shunting, decreased lung compliance and impaired gas exchange. Σ 78 in 1990, 19 in 1999, probably under-reported.

**Risk factors:** PCP is unusual in patients with CD4 counts > 200 cells/μL. It is uncommon in Africa, for reasons that remain unclear. Incidence is reduced by prophylactic treatment (Table 16.7).

**Clinical features:** Insidious onset over weeks or months with fever, fatigue, weight loss and then cough and progressive dyspnoea. Onset may be particularly subtle in patients on prophylaxis.

There may be tachycardia, cyanosis, tachypnoea and confusion. Auscultation may be normal or reveal crepitations. Extrapulmonary pneumocystosis (skin, pleura, viscera, eye and lymph nodes) has been reported rarely.

**Organisms:** *Pneumocystis carinii.* Classified as a fungus on the basis of DNA homology and membrane sterol content (➤364). Recently officially renamed *P. jiroveci* although this name is not in widespread use.

**Microbiological investigations:** Culture is not possible, and diagnosis depends on identification of the organism by microscopy, with special stains or immunofluorescent techniques. Suitable materials include induced sputum (produced by inhaling nebulized 3% saline) or broncho-alveolar lavage. If the diagnosis is strongly suspected clinically, treatment is commenced presumptively, and diagnostic tests arranged as soon as possible thereafter.

**Other investigations:** Patients are usually hypoxic; $Po_2$ may be normal at rest but fall rapidly on exercise. CXR may be normal or may show widespread, diffuse, interstitial shadowing. Focal consolidation suggests bacterial pneumonia, but does not rule out PCP. Cystic changes and pneumatocoeles are common, but lymphadenopathy and pleural effusions are rare.

**Differential diagnosis:** Bacterial pneumonia (➤158), pulmonary Kaposi's sarcoma (➤168).

**Antibiotic management:** Co-trimoxazole, 120 mg/kg/day in divided doses orally or iv. (i.e. 20 mg/kg/day trimethoprim and 100 mg/kg/day sulfamethoxazole). Adverse effects (Table 16.8) are common, particularly hypersensitivity reactions with severe rash and fever (desensitization ➤158). Alternatively, pentamidine, 4 mg/kg/day in 250 mL 5% dextrose iv over 1 h. Adverse effects (Table 16.8) occur, but therapy may usually be continued. The usual

**Table 16.8** Adverse effects and drug interactions in HIV management

| Drug | Adverse effects* | Comments and interactions |
|---|---|---|
| Co-trimoxazole | **Neutropenia, hypersensitivity,** nausea and vomiting | Increases serum levels of phenytoin and warfarin |
| Pentamidine (iv) | **Nephrotoxicity, hyper/hypoglycaemia, severe hypotension (with rapid infusion),** hepatitis, hyperkalaemia, pancreatitis, neutropenia, thrombocytopenia, ventricular arrhythmias | Inhaled pentamidine causes cough and wheeze, but is otherwise relatively free of adverse effects |
| Ganciclovir | **Neutropenia, thrombocytopenia** | Co-administration with imipenem may cause fits |
| Foscarnet | **Nephrotoxicity, hypo/hypercalcaemia, hyperphosphataemia, anaemia, hepatotoxicity,** nausea | Maintain hydration and reduce dose in renal impairment. Administration with pentamidine may cause severe hypocalcaemia |
| Pyrimethamine | **Neutropenia, thrombocytopenia,** rash, raised liver enzymes | Haematological toxicity minimized by giving folinic acid 15 mg daily |
| Sulphadiazine | **Hypersensitivity, crystalluria** | Crystalluria may be avoided by maintaining urine output >3 L/day and alkalinizing urine (sodium bicarbonate, 3 g po 6 hly) |
| Dapsone | **Rash,** methaemoglobinuria | |

* More important adverse effects are highlighted in bold type.

time to respond is 4–6 days, and patients often deteriorate before they improve. Continued worsening at 4 days or failure to improve by 7 days is an indication to change therapy from co-trimoxazole to pentamidine. Alternative regimens include trimethoprim (20 mg/kg/day) and dapsone (100 mg/day) **or** clindamycin (450 mg iv q6h) and primaquine (15 mg oral q24h). Nebulized pentamidine (600 mg q24h) has been used, but is not suitable for patients who are hypoxic. Atovaquone (750 mg q8h) may be used in patients intolerant of other regimens. Following recovery secondary prophylaxis is given (➤155); if, on HAART, CD4 count exceeds 200 for 6 months prophylaxis can be stopped.

**Supportive management:** Steroids improve survival and shorten duration of illness. If $Po_2$ <9.3 kPa, give 80 mg prednisolone daily for 5 days, then 40 mg daily for 5 days and then 20 mg daily for 10 days. High-dose oxygen is given. Fluid overload should be avoided. Mechanical ventilation may be needed.

**Complications: Pneumothorax** is not unusual, and can be very difficult to manage. If the pneumothorax is large or there is suspicion of tension, then a chest drain must be inserted, but bronchopleural fistula formation with continued leakage of air is common. The chest drain should be maintained on low-pressure suction to maintain full inflation. Other methods used to close fistulae, such as tetracycline pleuradhesis or thoracotomy and repair, are not usually successful.

### Desensitization regimen for co-trimoxazole (Table 16.9)

Patients with a history of Stevens–Johnson syndrome should be excluded. The regimen shown in Table 16.9 may be followed. In any desensitization regime there is always a risk of anaphylactic reactions.

### Other pulmonary infections

HIV patients are at increased risk of **bacterial pneumonia** (➤25) usually due to *Streptococcus*

**Table 16.9** Desensitization regimen for co-trimoxazole

| Formulation | Day | Dose |
|---|---|---|
| 1 : 20 dilution of paediatric co-trimoxazole suspension (2.4 mg/mL) | 1 | 1 mL |
| | 2 | 2 mL |
| | 3 | 4 mL |
| | 4 | 8 mL |
| Undiluted paediatric co-trimoxazole suspension (48 mg/mL) | 5 | 0.6 mL |
| | 6 | 1.25 mL |
| | 7 | 2.5 mL |
| | 8 | 5 mL |
| | 9 | 10 mL |
| Co-trimoxazole 480 mg | 10 | 1 tab |
| | 11 | 1 tab |

*pneumoniae, Haemophilus influenzae* or *Staphylococcus aureus*. Recurrent bacterial pneumonia (> two episodes in 12 months) is an AIDS-defining diagnosis. Recurrent acute or chronic **sinusitis** (➤17) due to *Streptococcus pneumoniae, Haemophilus influenzae* or *Pseudomonas aeruginosa* is common. The possibility of rarer organisms, including fungi (➤363) should be considered and material obtained for microscopy and culture if infection persists.

**Pulmonary tuberculosis** occurs with increased frequency in patients with HIV infection (➤167). MDRTB should be suspected in all HIV+ TB patients until proven otherwise. Fungal pneumonia due to *Cryptococcus neoformans* (➤164) usually occurs in the context of disseminated infection.

**Kaposi's sarcoma** (➤168) may affect the lungs, typically with patchy nodular shadowing and pleural effusions. Bacterial superinfection, particularly with *Staphylococcus aureus*, is common.

### Skin disease in HIV-infected patients

### Infections

**Common infections:** see Table 16.10.
With the onset of immunodeficiency, patients may suffer from recurrences of HSV, which can

**Table 16.10** Common skin infections in HIV-infected patients

| Organism | Comments |
|---|---|
| *Staphylococcus aureus* | Folliculitis (➤111), bullous impetigo (➤111), boils (➤111) and cellulitis (➤113) |
| Herpes zoster (➤132) | Occasionally with cutaneous dissemination. May be multidermatomal, prolonged or indolent with atypical crusted appearance in the severely immunodeficient |
| Herpes simplex (➤334) | May cause recurrent oral, genital or perianal ulceration. May also present as chronic non-healing ulcer resembling decubitus ulcer. Culture and biopsy are required for diagnosis |
| Molluscum contagiosum (➤119) | Lesions are larger and more numerous than usual |

be genital, oral, cutaneous or systemic. Recurrent attacks of simple HSV can be controlled by oral aciclovir. Patients without immunodeficiency should be managed as per other patients, i.e. prophylaxis for more than three attacks of genital herpes per year would be reasonable. With the onset of immunodeficiency (e.g. CD4 count <200), it is reasonable to institute prophylaxis for even mild attacks, since experience shows that they will recur and/or worsen in severity.

**Bacillary angiomatosis** is a rare cutaneous infection caused by *Bartonella quintana* and *B. henselae* (previously known as *Rochalimaea* spp. ➤308). It presents with disseminated lesions consisting of friable, vascular eruptions resembling granulation tissue, subcutaneous nodules and cellulitis plaques, which may affect any skin or mucosa. Visceral involvement, particularly of liver and spleen (peliosis hepatis) and osteolytic bone lesions occur. Diagnosis is by histology. Infection may be fatal if untreated, but responds well to erythromycin or doxycycline in standard doses for 8 weeks (cutaneous disease) or 16 weeks (visceral disease). Chronic *Bartonella henselae* bacteraemia has been reported as a cause of malaise, fever and weight loss.

### Hypersensitivity reactions

**Drug reactions** and allergic reactions to insect bites are common. Up to 50% of patients treated with co-trimoxazole for PCP develop a rash (➤156). Many patients develop multiple drug allergies. **Scabies** should be excluded in patients complaining of pruritus. May present with classical burrows or with hyperkeratotic ('Norwegian') scabies, which requires repeated treatment.

### Papulosquamous disorders

Seborrhoeic dermatitis, psoriasis and Reiter's disease with keratoderma blenorrhagica are commoner in patients with HIV. **Seborrhoeic dermatitis** (➤117) causes erythematous plaques with a yellowish, greasy scale on the hairy areas of the face, chest, back and groin. It responds to topical steroids and antifungals, such as miconazole/hydrocortisone cream, although stronger steroids may occasionally be required. **Psoriasis** often begins after HIV infection and may be complicated by arthritis. Topical calcipotriol is a good first-line treatment. Dithranol or coal tar are also used. Short courses of mild topical steroids (e.g. 1% hydrocortisone) may be used, but more potent steroids must only be used under dermatological supervision, because of the risk of precipitating rebound exacerbation or severe pustular psoriasis.

Itchy **folliculitis** may be due to *Staphylococcus aureus* infection, although pustular lesions may not be visible, and systemic flucloxacillin and topical antiseptic emollients may be useful.

In patients with CD4 counts below 200, **eosinophilic folliculitis** is common. This causes pruritic, oedematous papules a few millimetres in diameter, particularly on the trunk, head and arms. Diagnosis can be confirmed by biopsy, but this is rarely performed. Oral antihistamines and topical steroids can help. Try clobetasone (Eumovate) first, then betamethasone (Betnovate) but only give 1% hydrocortisone for the face. Oral high-dose itraconazole (200 or 400 mg) daily is often effective, suggesting that hypersensitivity to fungus is important, as it is in seborrhoeic dermatitis.

The skin is also a common site for **Kaposi's sarcoma** (➤168).

## Oral manifestations of HIV infection
### Candidiasis

Oral *Candida albicans* infection is common and may be the first indication of immunodeficiency.

**Clinical features:** Typical white plaques are usually present, but mucosal erythema without exudate or angular stomatitis may be due to candidiasis.

**Organisms:** *Candida albicans,* other *Candida* spp., including *C. krusei* and *C. dubliniensis.*

**Microbiological investigations:** Culture, microscopy of scrapings. Biopsy may be performed if clinical features are atypical.

**Antibiotic management:** Topical agents such as nystatin or amphotericin lozenges may be effective, but oesophageal and genital candidiasis are indications for systemic therapy. Fluconazole-resistant *Candida albicans* and other *Candida* spp., such as *C. krusei*, which are intrinsically fluconazole-resistant may occur after repeated treatment. Prophylactic use of fluconazole is no longer advised; we recommend high doses (200–400 mg q24h) and minimum duration. Itraconazole has a broader spectrum and is often effective in this situation; intravenous amphotericin is occasionally necessary.

### Gingivitis

Common in advanced immunodeficiency and sometimes severe, with progression to **necrotizing stomatitis**, with rapid progressive loss of gingival tissue. Urgent dental referral for debridement, application of topical antiseptic and systemic treatment with metronidazole or co-amoxiclav is required.

### Oral hairy leukoplakia

Produces white thickening of the buccal mucosa, along the lateral borders of the tongue. It is due to EBV infection (➤339) and is an indicator of poor prognosis.

### Kaposi's sarcoma ( KS ➤168) and lymphoma (➤169)

May both affect the mouth.

## Gastrointestinal disease in HIV-infected patients
### Oesophagitis

May be caused by *Candida albicans*, HSV or CMV. All three cause dysphagia and are clinically indistinguishable, although there may be evidence of oropharyngeal candidiasis. Barium swallow will document oesophagitis (AIDS-defining illness). Differential diagnosis by endoscopy and biopsy. **KS** (➤168) and **lymphoma** (➤169) both affect the oesophagus and stomach.

### Hepatobiliary disease

Right upper quadrant (RUQ) pain and tenderness, abnormal liver function tests and hepatomegaly are common in patients with AIDS, often in the context of previously diagnosed widely disseminated disease such as MAI (➤168) or KS. Sclerosing cholangitis, often secondary to biliary infection by CMV (➤339) or *Cryptosporidium parvum* (➤230) is common, causing RUQ pain and marked elevation of alkaline phosphatase. Diagnosis is by ERCP. Endoscopic sphincterotomy may relieve symptoms if there is papillary stenosis.

## Diarrhoea

Abdominal cramps. weight loss and large-volume diarrhoea are common, and usually indicate infection. Bacterial pathogens such as *Salmonella* spp. (➤279), *Shigella* spp. (➤282) and *Campylobacter jejuni* (➤288), and protozoa such as *Giardia lamblia* (➤218), *Entamoeba histolytica* (➤218), *Cryptosporidium parvum* (➤230), *Isospora* (➤230) and *Microsporidia* (➤231) should be excluded by stool microscopy and culture. Malabsorption with severe weight loss may be due to small-bowel infection by MAI (➤168). Diagnosis is made by stool culture for acid-fast bacilli and small-bowel biopsy. Recurrent salmonella bacteraemia can occur.

**Cryptosporidiosis** is difficult to eradicate in immunodeficient patients. There is no effective specific therapy. Patients with CD4 < 200 are often advised to boil drinking water (tap and bottled).

    💻 www.dwi.detr.gov.uk/crypto/bou001.htm

Diarrhoea with tenesmus, frequent small-volume stools and rectal bleeding suggest colitis. The bacteria listed above should be excluded. Sigmoidoscopy may show changes of **CMV colitis** (submucosal haemorrhages, shallow ulcers in the distal colon). Diagnosis is confirmed by biopsy. Treatment with ganciclovir is usually effective, and may usually be stopped after resolution of colitis. Concurrent CMV retinitis should be excluded. Valganciclovir, an oral prodrug of ganciclovir, is now available and licensed for use in CMV retinitis; it will probably replace iv ganciclovir in CMV colitis (➤166).

No specific pathogens are found in 25–50% of AIDS patients with diarrhoea. If stool examination and sigmoidoscopy are negative, further investigations are unlikely to be helpful.

Diarrhoea in immunocompetent patients is most frequently caused by HAART, esp. PIs. Loperamide is useful.

## Neurological disease in HIV-infected patients

HIV seroconversion (➤145) is frequently associated with neurological symptoms, including meningitis, ataxia and cranial or peripheral neuropathy. Recovery usually occurs over several weeks. During **clinical latency** (➤145), there is an increased frequency of demyelinating neuropathy resembling Guillain–Barré syndrome.

In **advanced disease**, neurological disease is common and may present with a number of clinical syndromes (Table 16.11).

Abnormalities of the CSF, such as mild lymphocytic pleocytosis and moderate elevation of protein, are common in asymptomatic HIV-seropositive patients with relatively intact cellular immunity and preserved CD4 counts.

## HIV encephalopathy (HIVE, syn. AIDS dementia complex, ADC)

HIVE describes a clinical complex of cognitive, motor and behavioural abnormalities. Neuropathological changes correlate to some extent with the clinical picture, affecting in particular the central white matter, basal ganglia and brainstem. The spinal cord is often affected, with vacuolar myelopathy. These changes are thought to be due to the direct effects of HIV infection. Thirty per cent to 50% of patients progressing to severe immunodeficiency develop symptomatic HIVE, although neuropsychological and electrophysiological testing reveals subclinical abnormalities in many more.

**Clinical features:** Early symptoms of **cognitive deficit** are poor concentration and memory loss, with difficulty completing complex tasks. Progression to severe dementia occurs with, in many cases, an eventual almost vegetative end-stage. **Motor abnormalities** usually lag behind cognitive defects. Poor balance, incoordination and clumsiness are frequent early complaints. Generalized hyperreflexia and primitive reflexes (e.g. grasp reflex) may develop. Severe ataxia, leg weakness and incontinence are common in later stages. **Behavioural abnormalities** include apathy and lack of initiative or agitation and hyperactivity. Psychiatric illness, including depression and mania, are also common. Fits may occur.

**Investigations:** The diagnosis is clinical. Neuropsychological and electrophysiological

Table 16.11 Neurological syndromes in HIV+ patients

| Clinical syndrome | Causes |
| --- | --- |
| Diffuse encephalopathy | **AIDS dementia complex** (➢161)<br>CMV encephalitis (➢163)<br>HSV encephalitis (➢163)<br>Hypoxia or metabolic disturbance secondary to sepsis<br>*Toxoplasma gondii* encephalitis (➢163) |
| Focal cerebral disease | ***Toxoplasma gondii* encephalitis** (➢163)<br>**Cerebral lymphoma** (➢169)<br>**Progressive multifocal leucoencephalopathy** (➢163)<br>Tuberculoma (➢167)<br>*Cryptococcus neoformans* abscess (➢164)<br>HSV encephalitis (➢163)<br>VZV encephalitis<br>*Candida albicans* abscess |
| Meningitis | ***Cryptococcus neoformans* meningitis** (➢164)<br>Tuberculous meningitis (➢167)<br>Syphilis (➢165)<br>Metastatic lymphomatous meningitis (➢169) |
| Peripheral neuropathy | **Sensory polyneuropathy**<br>Iatrogenic toxic neuropathy |
| Myelopathy | **Vacuolar myelopathy** (➢165)<br>Acute transverse myelitis due to VZV, lymphoma, toxoplasmosis (➢163), or CMV |

CMV, cytomegalovirus; HSV, herpes simplex virus; VZV, varicella zoster virus.

Table 16.12 Infections associated with injecting drug use

| | Organism | Notes |
| --- | --- | --- |
| Viruses | HIV | (➢143) |
| | Hepatitis A | (➢70) |
| | Hepatitis B and delta virus | (➢70) |
| | Hepatitis C | (➢73) |
| Bacteria* | *Staphylococcus aureus* | Local abscesses (➢249); infective endocarditis (especially right-sided) (➢51) |
| | Streptococci of the '*milleri*' group | Local abscesses (➢259) |
| | *Clostridium novyi* | Local abscesses, myonecrosis and septicaemia (➢319) |
| | *Clostridium botulinum* | (➢316) |
| Fungi | *Candida albicans* and other spp. | Folliculitis, local abscesses and infective endocarditis (➢367) |
| | Zygomycete fungi | Injection abscesses (➢369) |

* Injection abscesses frequently contain mixtures of upper respiratory tract commensals (from saliva) and coliforms, pseudomonads and environmental Gram-negative bacteria (from contaminated water sources, e.g. toilets).

testing confirm and quantitate abnormalities. MRI and CT scan show cerebral atrophy, with wide sulci and enlarged ventricles. MRI reveals white-matter abnormalities, particularly in periventricular areas. CSF is usually non-specifically abnormal, with a moderately elevated protein and a mild lymphocytic pleocytosis.

**Differential diagnosis:** Progressive multifocal leucoencephalopathy (➤163), CMV encephalitis (➤163), HSV encephalitis (➤163), hypoxia or metabolic disturbance secondary to sepsis, *Toxoplasma gondii* encephalitis (➤163).

**Management:** HIVE can be prevented by successful HAART. Once HIVE has become established, there is a variable response to HAART with marked improvement in some patients.

## Cytomegalovirus (CMV) encephalitis

May present in a very similar manner to ADC, although the course is often more rapid. It occurs frequently with concurrent disseminated CMV infection and retinitis. Clinical diagnosis is difficult, but can be confirmed by brain biopsy. Ganciclovir is given, although the response may be disappointing.

## Herpes simplex (HSV) encephalitis

May present typically, with rapid onset of headache, fever, confusion and temporal lobe abnormality, or it may develop subacutely as a non-specific neurological illness indistinguishable from other causes of diffuse encephalopathy listed above. CSF shows elevated protein and a lymphocytic pleocytosis, but culture for HSV is usually negative. PCR for HSV in CSF is helpful if positive, but is often negative. Definitive diagnosis requires brain biopsy, but empirical treatment with aciclovir is often given.

## Progressive multifocal leucoencephalopathy (PML)

PML is caused by reactivation of the polyomavirus JC virus (➤343). Pre-HAART, ≈2% of AIDS patients developed PML, which has also been reported in patients with haematological malignancies or iatrogenic immunosuppression. PML is a disease of patients with advanced immunodeficiency (CD4 count <100 cells/μL).

**Clinical features:** Progressive accumulation of focal neurological deficits, typically including hemiparesis, ataxia or aphasia. Fever is absent and there is no clouding of consciousness. Without HAART, progression is inexorable, over weeks or months, although a relapsing and remitting course has been described rarely. Prognosis is very poor, with a median survival of ≈16 weeks in one series.

**Investigations:** CT and MRI scan shows multiple non-enhancing lesions with no mass effect, scattered throughout the white matter. CSF and EEG are normal or non-specifically abnormal, but JC virus can usually be demonstrated by PCR. Diagnosis is usually made on the basis of the clinical features and characteristic MRI appearances, but brain biopsy is required for definitive diagnosis.

**Differential diagnosis:** Cerebral toxoplasmosis (➤163), cerebral lymphoma (➤169), tuberculoma.

**Management:** Untreated, prognosis is very poor, but progression can often be halted by initiation of HAART. Established neurological deficits do not usually improve. There is no proven specific therapy, but retrospective studies support the use of cidofovir.

## AIDS-associated toxoplasmosis

Toxoplasmosis in AIDS is due to reactivation of cysts of *Toxoplasma gondii* (➤137) which persist in the CNS and multiple extraneural sites after primary infection. In patients with advanced immunodeficiency, cysts reactivate to cause necrotic inflammatory abscesses scattered throughout the cerebral hemispheres. Toxoplasma encephalitis is the commonest cause of focal neurological deficit in AIDS patients.

**Risk factors:** The incidence of toxoplasma encephalitis varies depending on rates of seropositivity against *Toxoplasma gondii*. It is particularly common in France, where adult seroprevalence rates are ≈80%. Some 50% of UK adults are seropositive.

**Clinical features:** Fever, confusion, fits and focal neurological deficit developing over a few days. Sixty per cent have focal neurological signs including hemiparesis, ataxia, aphasia or visual field defect. *Toxoplasma gondii* may also cause **chorioretinitis** (➤108), which may accompany or precede encephalitis. Ophthalmoscopic examination reveals unilateral or bilateral diffuse or focal areas of retinal necrosis and haemorrhage.

**Organisms:** *Toxoplasma gondii* (➤137).

**Microbiological investigations:** Patients are nearly always (97%) seropositive for *Toxoplasma gondii*. Negative serology strongly suggests an alternative diagnosis. Changes in antibody titre and IgM levels are rarely helpful. Serum and/or CSF should be examined for cryptococcal antigen, as *Cryptococcus neoformans* occasionally causes identical CT changes. PCR is available and helpful.

**Other investigations:** CT scan shows multiple hypodense lesions in the cerebral hemispheres, particularly in the basal ganglia and at the hemispheric corticomedullary junction, which develop 'ring enhancement' after injection of iv contrast. Lesions can be solitary and non-enhancing. MRI is more sensitive, and solitary lesions on MRI are unlikely to be due to *Toxoplasma gondii*. Definitive diagnosis is by brain biopsy, but this is rarely performed. A trial of anti-toxoplasma therapy should result in radiological improvement within 2–3 weeks.

**Differential diagnosis:** Cerebral lymphoma (➤169), progressive multifocal leuco-encephalopathy (➤163), fungal abscess, including *Cryptococcus neoformans* (➤164), tuberculoma (➤167).

**Antibiotic management:** Primary therapy is given for at least 6 weeks. Pyrimethamine, loading dose 200 mg, followed by 1–1.5 mg/kg daily as a single oral dose **plus** folinic acid 15 mg daily **plus** sulphadiazine 1 g 6 hly or clindamycin 600 mg 6 hly. Allergies to sulphadiazine and clindamycin are common. Clarithromycin (1 g 12 hly) is an alternative. Sulpha-

diazine causes crystalluria, which presents with flank pain, renal failure and haematuria. To avoid this, maintain urine output >3L/24 h and urine pH >7 (give sodium bicarbonate 3 g, 6 hly, po). Steroids may have to be given for cerebral oedema; dose and duration of course should be as low as possible. Atovaquone 750 mg q6h is an alternative. Anticonvulsants may be required.

After 6 weeks of primary therapy, **maintenance therapy** is commenced: pyrimethamine (25–50 mg 24 hly, po) **plus** folinic acid (15 mg 24 hly) **plus either** sulphadiazine (500 mg 6 hly, po) **or** clindamycin (300 mg 6hly, po) **or** clarithromycin (500 mg 12 hly, po). Secondary prophylaxis may be discontinued if CD4 rises above 200 for >6 months.

**Comments:** Infection of the spinal cord leading to **transverse myelitis** is described. *Toxoplasma gondii* also causes **pneumonitis**. Prophylaxis (Table 16.7).

## Cryptococcal meningitis

*Cryptococcus neoformans* is distributed globally, in contrast to other fungi causing systemic infection, such as histoplasmosis and blastomycosis, which are geographically restricted. *Cryptococcus neoformans* is widespread in the environment in bird droppings, and infection occurs via inhalation. Whilst this organism does cause pneumonia, most AIDS patients with cryptococcal infection have meningitis.

**Risk factors:** Rare in patients with CD4 count >100 cells/μL.

**Clinical features:** Presentation is usually subtle and non-specific, with prolonged fever, headache and malaise. Nausea and vomiting occur in ≈50%, but neck stiffness and photophobia are unusual, occurring in ≈20–30%. Altered mental state is present in ≈10–30% and fits or focal signs in <10%. Many patients have a history of recent chest infection, which may represent cryptococcal pneumonia. Cryptococcal skin sepsis occurs infrequently. Symptomatic cryptococcal infection elsewhere is rare, although isolation of *Cryptococcus neoformans* from blood, urine and GI tract is not uncommon. Persistent asymptomatic genitourinary infection (particularly prostate) is thought to act as a reservoir for relapse after treatment.

**Organisms:** *Cryptococcus neoformans* (➤368).

**Microbiological investigations:** CSF should be negatively stained for capsulate yeasts using **India ink**—positive in ≈70% of cases. Serum and CSF **cryptococcal antigen detection** is sensitive and specific, detecting ≈99% of cases. The titre usually rises after treatment and then falls. It is unusual for it to become negative, even after full clinical response. Routine CSF examination is sometimes normal. Raised opening pressure is common. CSF cell count is < 20 in ≈60%. CSF glucose may be reduced, but is normal in ≈70%, and CSF protein may be elevated but is normal in ≈50%. CSF fungal culture may be positive.

**Other investigations:** CXR shows diffuse or focal interstitial infiltrates if there is concurrent cryptococcal pneumonia. Hilar lymphadenopathy is common. Large nodules and cavities may be seen more rarely. CT head scan is abnormal in 30–50%, but changes seen are non-specific, including cerebral atrophy or occasionally mass lesions with oedema and ring enhancement, indistinguishable from *Toxoplasma gondii* encephalitis.

**Differential diagnosis:** Cerebral lymphoma (➤169), progressive multifocal leucoencephalopathy (➤163), *Toxoplasma gondii* encephalitis (➤163), tuberculoma (➤167).

**Antibiotic management:** Amphotericin (dosing schedule ➤372) ± flucytosine (75–100 mg/kg/day in three divided doses ⚠) until stable, then fluconazole 400 mg po q24h for 10 weeks. Thereafter, lifelong maintenance is required (fluconazole 200 mg q24h).

**Comments:** Prognosis is influenced by the fact that cryptococcal infection occurs in patients with advanced immunodeficiency. Pre-HAART, ≈20% of patients did not survive initial therapy. A very high cryptococcal antigen titre, altered mental state and positive India ink test are associated with worse prognosis.

## Peripheral neuropathy (PN) and myopathy

A sensory polyneuropathy causing glove-and-stocking distribution numbness, paraesthesiae and dysaesthesiae, mainly in the feet and legs, is common. Although it can be a result of HIV *per se*, PN is much more frequently seen as a complication of therapy. Dideoxynucleoside reverse transcriptase inhibitors (didanosine, stavudine, zalcitabine) are particularly likely to cause PN, which is frequently a treatment limiting adverse effect. Tricyclics, analgesics, carbemazepine and gabapentin may relieve symptoms. It usually resolves after stopping treatment, although it may get worse before it improves, and recovery may be prolonged over many months. **CMV infection** causes progressive radiculopathy affecting the sacral and lumbar roots. It occurs in patients with advanced disease and causes flaccid paralysis of the legs, with sacral pain and sphincter disturbance. Concurrent CMV retinitis is common. MRI shows thickened spinal roots and CSF contains neutrophils. CMV is often cultured from blood and CSF; ganciclovir should be given.

**Myopathy** resembling polymyosities may occur. Zidovudine also causes proximal myopathy rarely.

## Syphilis in HIV-infected patients

Syphilis (➤89) and HIV share a number of risk factors and genital ulcer disease, including syphilis, is thought to enhance transmission of HIV. The two infections may therefore co-exist. HIV influences the presentation and management of syphilis in the following ways:

**Clinical features:** Most HIV patients with primary or secondary syphilis have a typical illness, but neurological disease occurring during secondary syphilis ('early neurosyphilis') is commoner in HIV-infected persons. The latent period to the development of meningovascular syphilis may be shortened, and uveitis and sensorineural hearing loss occur more frequently.

**Diagnosis:** False-negative specific serological tests (e.g. TPHA) and false-positive non-specific tests (e.g. VDRL) have been reported. Changes in titre of VDRL are unreliable as indicators of latency or relapse in HIV-infected persons. The CSF abnormalities attributable to HIV infection and described above (➤161) may make diagnosis of neurosyphilis difficult. If syphilis is suspected but cannot be confirmed, it may be appropriate to monitor clinical course and serology, or to treat presumptively.

**Treatment:** Treatment failures and neurological relapse have been reported in HIV patients with standard regimens. It is recommended that patients are treated wherever possible with penicillin. In patients with syphilis of less than 1 yr's duration, and no evidence of neurological involvement, a single dose of benzathine penicillin (2.4 MU im), or procaine penicillin (2.4 MU im daily for 10 days) may be given. In other patients, treatment should be extended (e.g. three doses of benzathine penicillin, 2.4 MU im at weekly intervals, or benzylpenicillin 4 MU 4-hly iv for 14 days). Penicillin-allergic patients may be treated with doxycycline, but erythromycin has been reported to be ineffective in this context.

## Cytomegalovirus (CMV) retinitis

Sight-threatening retinitis is the usual presentation of recurrent CMV disease in HIV+ patients, although it can also present as oesophagitis, colitis, hypoadrenalism, encephalitis, myelitis and/or a painful neuritis. CMV disease usually occurs in the context of severe immunodeficiency (CD4 count < 100 cells/μL), and all patients with advanced HIV disease should have their fundi examined regularly, preferably fully dilated.

**Clinical features:** Unilateral visual field loss, floaters or loss of acuity. Asymptomatic lesions are often discovered at routine fundoscopy. Retinitis appears as fluffy white areas of necrosis and haemorrhage ('cottage cheese and ketchup'). Diagnosis is based on clinical findings and ophthalmoscopic appearances. Without treatment, progression to blindness in both eyes is the rule.

**Microbiological investigations:** CMV viraemia and viruria are common. Patients are usually CMV seropositive, often to high titres. PCR can be used to demonstrate CMV in blood and other body fluids, including aqueous humour.

**Differential diagnosis:** *Toxoplasma gondii* retinitis is usually associated with cerebral toxoplasmosis. The lesions are not usually haemorrhagic. Serology and PCR may contribute to distinguishing these infections.

**Management: Ganciclovir** (5 mg/kg 12 hly iv) is given for 14 days as induction therapy. Some 80% show stabilization of ophthalmoscopic appearances, but visual field defects do not usually resolve. Ganciclovir causes neutropenia. Dose should be reduced if neutrophil count falls below $1000 \times 10^6$/L, and stopped if below $500 \times 10^6$/L. **Foscarnet** is an alternative. Induction dose: 60 mg/kg 8 hly iv, maintenance dose 90 mg/kg daily 5 days/week. Dose must be adjusted for renal function 🖺, and patients require prehydration and concurrent iv fluid adminstration during foscarnet dosing. Adverse effects include nephrotoxicity, metabolic disturbance, particularly hypocalcaemia, but also hypercalcaemia, hypomagnesaemia, hypokalaemia, hyper- and hypophosphataemia. Hypocalcaemia causes vomiting, paraesthesia, tetany, convulsions. Give slow injection of 10 mL calcium gluconate 10% (2.23 mmol) over 2–5 min, and then continue calcium administration. (Dose of calcium gluconate should not exceed 40 mL of 10% solution over 24 h.) Anaemia, thrombophlebitis and penile ulceration (due to irritant effect of excreted drug, indicating too rapid infusion of foscarnet or inadequate saline loading before and during infusions) also occur.

**Cidofovir** is a newer treatment for CMV retinitis which is given at a dose of 5 mg/kg **weekly** for 2 weeks for induction therapy, and fortnightly thereafter. It is given with probenecid, and patients require prehydration 🖺. Main side effects are renal impairment, proteinuria and neutropenia.

**Valganciclovir** is an oral prodrug of ganciclovir which achieves comparable levels to iv ganciclovir and has been shown to be as effective as parenteral treatment in CMV retinitis (usual dose 900 mg q12h). It is also effective as maintenance therapy (900 mg q24h) and has recently been licensed. It is likely that valganciclovir will replace ganciclovir for most indications.

**Maintenance therapy** is required unless successful HAART can be given. IV maintenance ganciclovir is given at 6 mg/kg daily for 5 days/week. Oral ganciclovir (1000 mg q8h) is available and causes fewer haematological side effects, but it is less effective and should not be given to patients with 'zone 1' disease (i.e. affecting the fundus or macula). Valganciclovir will probably become the agent of choice.

**Complications:** Retinal detachment.

## Mycobacterial infection and HIV
### *Mycobacterium* tuberculosis

Tuberculosis (TB, ➤37) is commoner in the presence of HIV infection. In areas of high TB prevalence such as sub-Saharan Africa, >50% of patients dying of AIDS have active TB at post-mortem. HIV infection has led to a very significant increase in the prevalence of TB in these areas. TB in a patient with HIV infection is an AIDS-defining illness.

**Clinical features:** In the developed world, TB occurs at any time during HIV infection. In patients with relatively preserved cellular immunity (e.g. CD4 count >300 cells/µL), clinical features are those of typical reactivated TB, with apical cavitation and fibrosis. In patients with more advanced disease (e.g. CD4 count < 100 cells/µL) pulmonary TB presents atypically with hilar and mediastinal lymphadenopathy and CXR infiltrates in the middle and lower lung fields. Cavitation is rare. Extrapulmonary TB occurs in at least 50%; sites often involved include peripheral lymph nodes, bone marrow, bone, joint, genitourinary tract, liver, spleen, skin and peritoneum. *Mycobacterium tuberculosis* bacteraemia occurs in ≈25%. Central nervous system mass lesions ('tuberculoma') have been described. These lesions cause a wide

range of CT appearances and diagnosis is usually made only at brain biopsy.

**Diagnosis:** Mantoux testing is unhelpful, as false-negatives are common. Diagnosis depends on obtaining appropriate specimens for microscopy and culture. Special blood culture techniques and PCR of blood and body fluids are used. PCR can also be used to demonstrate the presence of antibiotic resistance genes.

**Antibiotic management:** For non-MDRTB, standard treatment regimens are used, although the duration of therapy may be extended. Current UK guidelines (➤42) suggest standard duration of therapy. US guidelines suggest extending therapy for those who respond slowly. Interactions between anti-TB drugs and HAART (particularly between PIs, NNRTIs and rifamycins) make concurrent adminstration very difficult. Extensive dose modifications and drug level monitoring are essential to ensure success of both therapies. Detailed advice at:

  🖳 www.hiv-druginteractions.org/
  🖳 www.cdc.gov/mmwr/preview/
   mmwrhtml/mm4909a4.htm
  🖳 www.cdc.gov/mmwr/preview/
   mmwrhtml/00055357.htm
  🖳 www.hivatis.org

**Isolation:** HIV is associated with MDRTB, and it is our practice to isolate HIV+ patients who are smear-positive as if they have MDRTB, pending the results of sensitivity testing. PCR may be able to provide this information rapidly.

Special precautions should be taken to avoid cross-infection between patients with TB and HIV+ persons (e.g. segregation of outpatients). More rigorous criteria for assessment of non-infectiousness after starting treatment are appropriate if patients are to be discharged to situations where contact with other HIV+ persons is likely; detailed guidance is given in BTS guidelines.

  🖳 www.brit-thoracic.org.uk
  🖳 www.doh.gov.uk/tbguide.htm
  ↪ Thorax 2000; 55: 887–901
  ↪ BTS guidelines, Thorax 1998; 53: 536–48

## *Mycobacterium avium-intracellulare* (MAI)

*Mycobacterium avium-intracellulare* causes disseminated infection in patients with advanced immunodeficiency (CD4 count <100 cells/μL). At least 50% of patients dying of AIDS have post-mortem evidence of MAI, with infection involving bone marrow, lymph nodes and any of the viscera.

**Clinical features:** Fever, malaise, weight loss and anaemia. Diarrhoea and abdominal pain due to colonic infection. Chronic malabsorption with severe weight loss due to small-bowel infection. Extrabiliary obstructive jaundice due to periportal lymphadenopathy. Patients with MAI always have other opportunist infections and/or malignancies, and it is often difficult to attribute symptoms exclusively to one or other pathogen.

**Diagnosis:** MAI bacteraemia occurs in most patients — special media are often used ☎. MAI may be seen in or cultured from other tissues such as lymph node, bone marrow, small bowel or liver biopsy. MAI may be found in stools, although this does not always indicate active infection.

**Antibiotic management:** MAI is resistant to most antituberculous agents. Treatment with rifampicin or rifabutin, plus ethambutol and clarithromycin is recommended pending the results of sensitivity testing. See above for comments on drug interactions with HAART.

**Comments:** Infection with other atypical mycobacteria, such as *Mycobacterium kansasii* or *Mycobacterium xenopi*, has also been reported in AIDS patients.

## Cardiac disease in HIV infection

Myocarditis and dilated cardiomyopathy are common post-mortem findings in AIDS patients, but clinical presentation is rare. Symptomatic pericardial effusion occurs infrequently and is usually infectious, due to mycobacteria or *Cryptococcus neoformans*.

## Haematological abnormalities in HIV infection

A number of factors cause haematological abnormalities in HIV-infected individuals. These include direct suppression of bone marrow by HIV itself, infiltration of bone marrow by opportunist pathogens or malignancies, drug toxicity, nutritional deficiency and immunodysregulation with autoantibody production.

**Anaemia** occurs in the majority of patients with AIDS. Most have normochromic normocytic anaemia, attributable to HIV infection itself and prolonged ill health with recurrent infections. Iron deficiency is less common, and may result from intestinal KS. Severe anaemia may result from infiltration of bone marrow by MAI. AZT causes macrocytosis in most recipients and anaemia in a minority.

**Neutropenia** is common in advanced disease and may be due to drugs (e.g. ganciclovir, pyrimethamine, sulphonamides). Bacteraemia is common if neutrophil count falls below $500 \times 10^6$/L. Granulocyte colony-stimulating factor (G-CSF) may be used to sustain the neutrophil count in patients with severe neutropenia or during chemotherapy, pending response to HAART.

**Thrombocytopenia**, with platelet-associated immunoglobulin, is common. It is characteristically seen early in HIV infection and often resolves with the onset of AIDS. Bleeding is rare. It usually responds to HAART. Dapsone is also helpful. Splenectomy may be required and is usually effective.

## Malignancies associated with HIV infection

KS, non-Hodgkin's lymphoma and cervical carcinoma are AIDS-defining illnesses.

### Kaposi's sarcoma

KS was previously recognized as an unusual indolent tumour endemic in sub-Saharan Africa and among elderly white men of Mediterranean or East European origin, affecting primarily the legs. It was one of the first conditions to be associated with HIV infection. KS has been shown to be associated with coinfection with HIV and HHV-8 (➤341). HHV-8 is commoner in homosexual men, and this accounts for the relative infrequency of KS in other risk groups in Europe and the US.

**Clinical features:** In HIV infection, KS is usually an aggressive multifocal tumour. Skin is most frequently involved, with palpable, firm cutaneous nodules, 0.5–2 cm in diameter. Lesions are usually violaceous, although they may be brown or black in pigmented skin. Head and neck are often involved, particularly the buccal mucosa. Lesions tend to progress with time, becoming larger and more numerous. Visceral disease is common and can involve any organ. Gastrointestinal lesions are common and cause haemorrhage. Pulmonary disease typically causes patchy nodular shadowing and pleural effusions. Bacterial superinfection, particularly with *Staphylococcus aureus*, is common. Lymphoedema results from lymph-node infiltration.

**Diagnosis:** Diagnosis is confirmed by biopsy.

**Management:** Patients with KS have advanced immunodeficiency and require HAART. Specific treatment is not always indicated. Treatment is aimed at palliation and cosmesis. Particular indications include lymphoedema, painful or bulky lesions anywhere, but particularly in the oropharynx, and pulmonary disease, which may progress rapidly. Radiotherapy is the most appropriate therapy for patients with localized disease. Other local therapies include intralesional chemotherapy and cryotherapy. The treatment of choice for systemic chemotherapy is liposomal doxorubicin (Caelyx), which is well tolerated and effective, although very expensive.

### Non-Hodgkin's lymphoma (NHL)

NHL occurs at all stages of HIV infection; ≈30% of patients have CD4 counts >200 cells/µL. It is not clear whether HAART reduces the incidence of extracerebral lymphoma. CNS lymphomas arise almost exclusively in patients with advanced disease and CD4 count <50, and are more rarely seen in the developed world since the implementation of HAART.

**Clinical features:** Widespread extranodal disease is usual, particularly affecting the gastrointestinal tract, CNS, bone marrow and liver. CNS lymphoma presents with gradual onset of confusion, lethargy, cognitive loss, fits and focal signs such as hemiplegia, aphasia and cranial nerve palsies. CT scan usually shows one or two discrete lesions deep in the white matter, which may be hypodense and weakly contrast-enhancing. Differentiation from *Toxoplasma gondii* encephalitis (➤163) can be very difficult on CT grounds alone, and brain biopsy may be required if there is no response to anti-toxoplasma therapy.

**Management:** Chemotherapy is less likely to be successful in HIV-infected individuals than in non-infected patients with similar tumours. Failure to respond, relapse and severe drug toxicity are all more common. Patients with relatively good immune function and no previous AIDS-defining illness are good candidates for chemotherapy and may be cured. Most patients with cerebral lymphoma will die within a few months despite HAART.

### Cervical carcinoma in HIV infection

Human papillomavirus infection (➤342), abnormal cervical cytology and cervical neoplasia are all more common in HIV-infected women, who should have cervical smear or culposcopy performed at least annually. Many clinics offer baseline culposcopy at the time of HIV diagnosis.

# Chapter 17

# Infections in the immunocompromised host

## Congenital immunodeficiency syndromes

Congenital immunodeficiency syndromes affecting all components of the immune system are described. They are all very rare, but have served as 'experiments of nature', allowing elucidation of the function of the normal immune system (Tables 17.1–3). Patients with complement deficiency should receive vaccination against *Streptococcus pneumoniae*, *Haemophilus influenzae* and *Neisseria meningitidis*, although these vaccines may not give their usual levels of protection in these patients.

## Acquired disorders of immunity

In practice, acquired defects of immunity are far commoner than congenital disorders. These may be **local defects**, such as trauma, burns, foreign bodies, anatomical abnormalities or iv lines, or **generalized defects**, such as:

• Malnutrition, advanced age or neoplastic disease.

• Viral infections, e.g. increased susceptibility to bacterial infection during measles, or profound immunodeficiency due to HIV infection (➤143).

• Chronic diseases, e.g. diabetes mellitus, cirrhosis, alcoholism, renal failure.

• Splenectomy

• Iatrogenic, due to radiotherapy, cytotoxic chemotherapy and immunosuppression (e.g. steroids, cyclosporin A, cyclophosphamide).

**Patients with recurrent severe bacterial infections** are common in clinical practice. If the history suggests immunodeficiency but factors listed above are not present, other aspects of the history should be elicited, e.g. allergy, autoimmune phenomena (rash, arthropathy), delayed separation of the umbili-

cal cord, family history of early male deaths (esp. neonatal) and consanguinity (Table 17.4) The following screening tests are indicated: FBC including differential WBC, quantitation of T cell subsets, total immunoglobulin levels and IgG subclass levels, complement levels ($CH_{50}$, C3, C1q, C4). These are best done when the patient is not currently infected. For more specialized tests, referral to a clinical immunologist is required.

### Splenectomy

After splenectomy (whether for haematological malignancy, trauma, or as the result of sickle-cell disease), patients are at risk from a range of infections, particularly acute severe sepsis due to capsulate bacteria: *Streptococcus pneumoniae*, *Haemophilus influenzae* and *Neisseria meningitidis*. Patients are at increased risk of severe malaria and should take optimum prophylaxis if they travel (➤214). They are also at risk of severe infection with *Capnocytophaga canimorsus* after dog bite (➤302) and babesiosis in endemic areas (➤229). Although infection risk remains small (0.4% p.a.), it is overall 12.6 times that of normal people.

The following precautions are recommended:

• Patients must be warned to have a low threshold for presentation. Their family members should be informed of the early signs of septicaemia and meningitis, and patients should be encouraged to wear a medical alert bracelet.

• Patients should receive antibiotic prophylaxis until at least 16 yrs, and for at least the first 2 yrs after splenectomy. Some experts recommend lifelong prophylaxis. Regimens include penicillin V 250 mg q12h (<5 yrs: 125 mg q12h). Erythromycin may be given to penicillin-allergic patients (<2 yrs: 125 mg q24h; 2–8 yrs:

Table 17.1 Congenital disorders affecting non-antigen specific ('natural') immunity

| | Disorder | Common infectious complications |
|---|---|---|
| Neutropenia | Infantile lethal agranulocytosis, autoimmune neutropenia, isoimmune neonatal neutropenia | Recurrent or severe bacterial infection (e.g. staphylococci, streptococci, coliforms, |
| Abnormal neutrophil function (e.g. abnormalities of chemotaxis, adherence, phagocytosis and microbial killing) | Chédiak–Higashi, leucocyte adhesion deficiency, chronic granulomatous disease myeloperoxidase deficiency, hyper-IgE syndrome | *Pseudomonas aeruginosa*, *Haemophilus influenzae*) and fungi (e.g. *Candida albicans*, *Aspergillus* spp.) |
| Complement disorders | Inherited deficiencies of C3, C5, C6, C7, C8, factor I, properdin | Severe recurrent infection with capsulate bacteria |

Table 17.2 Congenital disorders of antigen-specific immunity, 1: disorders affecting humoral immunity

| Disorder | Comments | Common infectious complications |
|---|---|---|
| X-linked hypogammaglobulinaemia ('Bruton's agammaglobulinaemia') | X-linked deficiency of tyrosine kinase, critical for B cell maturation. Regular IVIG is effective Occasionally associated with growth hormone deficiency | Chronic or recurrent bacterial infections Chronic disseminated enteroviral infection |
| Common variable immunodeficiency (CVID) | Heterogeneous group of patients with hypogamma-globulinaemia | Chronic respiratory and GI infection |
| IgA deficiency | Common, affecting 1 in 600 individuals | Frequently asymptomatic. Chronic respiratory and GI infection. Increased incidence of cutaneous, respiratory and GI allergies. Anaphylaxis with IgA-containing blood products may occur. |
| IgG subclass deficiency | Usually affects IgG2 or IgG2 and IgG4 | Infection with encapsulated bacteria. Poor response to some vaccines |
| Hyper-IgM syndrome | Failure of B cells to switch from IgM to IgG production. Usually X-linked due to absence of T-cell ligand for CD40 on B cells | Recurrent pyogenic and opportunistic infections, including *Pneumocystis* and cryptosporidiosis. Lymphoid malignancy |
| Selective IgM deficiency | Very low levels of IgM | Severe systemic bacterial infection |
| Transient hypogammaglobulinaemia of infancy | May persist for many months. Generally benign | Diarrhoea. Otitis media |

**Table 17.3** Congenital disorders of antigen-specific immunity, 2: disorders affecting both cellular and humoral immunity

| Disorder | Comments | Common infectious complications |
|---|---|---|
| Severe combined immunodeficiency (SCID) | Heterogeneous group of patients with deficient cell-mediated and humoral immunity; ≈50% have X-linked mutation in cytokine receptor. Other mutations affecting cytokine receptors (e.g. Jak-3), T and B cell antigen receptor genes ('Swiss-type agammaglobulinaemia') and adenosine deaminase deficiency, purine nucleotide phosphorylase deficiency | Chronic and severe recurrent bacterial, viral, fungal and opportunist infections. Often fatal in infancy. Severe or fatal reactions to live vaccines. Mucocutaneous candidiasis |
| DiGeorge syndrome | Embryopathy of 3rd and 4th pharyngeal pouch, resulting in thymic aplasia, hypoparathyroidism and congenital heart disease | Chronic and recurrent respiratory and GI infections |
| Wiskott–Aldrich syndrome | Thrombocytopenia, eczema and immunodeficiency. X-linked defect in WASP (Wiskott–Aldrich-associated protein), function of which is currently unknown | Bacterial and fungal infections. Lymphoma |
| Ataxia telangiectasia | Cerebellar ataxia, oculocutaneous telengiectasia and immunodeficiency. Autosomal-recessive associated with defective DNA repair mechanisms | Chronic sinopulmonary infection. Lymphoma and lymphatic leukaemia also common |
| Chronic mucocutaneous candidiasis | Frequently associated with endocrinopathies and autoimmune disease | Also more susceptible to bacterial and viral infections |
| X-linked lymphoproliferative syndrome (Duncan syndrome) | Genetic inability to mount immune response to Epstein–Barr virus infection | Chronic Epstein–Barr virus infection with hypogammaglobulinaemia, pancytopenia and lymphoma. Usually fatal |

250 mg q24h; >8 yrs: 500 mg q24h). Amoxicillin or co-amoxiclav may also be used.

• Patients should have a supply of antibiotics at home to commence immediately in the event of fever, before seeking medical advice. Patients on penicillin prophylaxis should take amoxicillin. Those taking erythromycin should increase the dose to a therapeutic level or switch to a broader-spectrum agent.

• Every precaution should be taken to avoid mosquito bites in malaria endemic areas, and they should take **expert** advice on malaria prophylaxis.

• Vaccination against:
  • *Streptococcus pneumoniae* for all >2 yrs, repeated once between 5 and 10 yrs later. Preferably given 2 weeks pre-splenectomy. Children under 2 yrs respond poorly to unconjugated polyvalent pneumococcal vaccine and should receive the new 7-valent conjugated vaccine (Prevenar).
  • *Haemophilus influenzae* (single dose).

**Table 17.4** Forms of immunodeficiency associated with particular organisms

| Pathogen | Clinical details | Deficit | Examples |
|---|---|---|---|
| *Pneumocystis carinii*, *Cryptococcus neoformans*, herpesviruses | Disseminated opportunist infections, persistent viral infections | T cells | Severe combined immunodeficiency, HIV |
| *Haemophilus influenzae*, *Streptococcus pneumoniae*, *Giardia lamblia*, *Campylobacter* spp., enteroviruses | Recurrent respiratory infections with encapsulated organisms, chronic diarrhoea, aseptic meningitis | B cells | Common variable immunodeficiency, X-linked agammaglobulinaemia |
| *Staphylococcus aureus*, *Burkholderia cepacia*, *Serratia marcescens*, *Aspergillus* spp., *Nocardia* spp. | Gingivitis, aphthous ulceration, recurrent pyogenic infections, delayed umbilical stump separation | Phagocytes | Chronic granulomatous disease, Chédiak–Higashi syndrome, leucocyte adhesion deficiency |
| *Staphylococcus aureus*, *Haemophilus influenzae*, *Streptococcus pneumoniae*, *Candida albicans* | Eczema, kyphoscoliosis, bony deformities and fractures, pulmonary and cutaneous infections, mucocutaneous candidiasis | T cells, phagocytes | Hyperimmunoglobulin E and recurrent infections (Job's syndrome) |
| *Mycobacterium avium* complex, BCG | Recurrent, disseminated infections | Macrophages | Interferon-γ receptor 1 deficiency |
| *Neisseria* spp. | Recurrent bacteraemia, meningitis | Complement | Late complement component deficiency |
| *Pseudomonas aeruginosa* | Recurrent pneumonia | Defensins | Cystic fibrosis |

- *Neisseria meningitidis* group C (single dose) (➤417). Travellers abroad should receive A&C vaccine (➤193), although protection is short-lived.
- Influenza (annually).
  - ↪ BMJ 1996; 312: 430. For 2001 update, see: www.bcshguidelines.com/pdf/spleen96.pdf

## Common clinical examples of acquired immunodeficiency

Most patients with severe acquired immunodeficiency fall into one of the following categories:
- Neutropenia
- Post solid organ transplant
- Post bone marrow transplant
- HIV infection.

**The following pages discuss the management of these situations in outline only.** Most such patients will be managed in specialist centres with established protocols for investigation and treatment of possible infection, drawn up in the light of detailed knowledge of local antibiotic sensitivity rates and immunosuppressive practice, which should be consulted whenever possible. HIV and AIDS are discussed elsewhere in this manual (➤143).

(↪ For more detailed reading, we recommend Glauser M, Pizzo P, *Management of Infections in Immunocompromised Patients*, London: Saunders, 2000).

Table 17.5 Pathogens common in neutropenic patients

|  | Common | Less common |
|---|---|---|
| Gram-positive organisms | *Staphylococcus aureus*, coagulase-negative staphylococci, viridans group streptococci, enterococci | *Corynebacterium jeikeium*, *Bacillus* spp., *Clostridium* spp. |
| Gram-negative organisms | *Escherichia coli*, *Klebsiella* spp., *Pseudomonas aeruginosa* | *Serratia* spp., *Enterobacter* spp., *Acinetobacter* spp., *Bacteroides* spp. *Capnocytophaga* spp. |
| Viruses | Herpes simplex | Varicella zoster |
| Fungi | *Aspergillus* spp., *Candida* spp. | *Fusarium* spp., *Trichosporon* spp., *Candida glabrata* |

Patients with impaired immunity are at potential risk from a wide range of opportunist organisms, but in general, the clinical situation and the nature of the immunological defect predicts a reasonably reliable shortlist of likely pathogens. Accurate diagnosis depends critically on obtaining specimens for culture and maintaining close liaison with the microbiology laboratory.

## Neutropenia

Neutropenia occurs in patients with haematological malignancy, HIV infection or bone-marrow infiltration by malignant disease, but it is most frequently a result of cytotoxic chemotherapy. Risk of infection is inversely related to absolute neutrophil count. Below 0.1 $\times 10^9$ cells/L, infection is very common; above 1 $\times 10^9$ cells/L, there is little added risk of infection, and patients should be managed as for normal patients with severe infection ($\blacktriangleright$185). A rapid fall in cell numbers is associated with a higher risk of infection. Neutropenic patients are commonly infected with their own normal flora ('endogenous' or 'autoinfection'), and many centres take precautions to reduce exposure to new colonizing bacteria (e.g. microbiologically clean food). Some centres nurse patients in HEPA-filtered air (reduces *Aspergillus* exposure), and a few use full protective isolation precautions ($\blacktriangleright$8). Gram-positive organisms account for >50% of

microbiologically confirmed cases (Table 17.5). Patients with long-standing iv access (e.g. Hickman catheter) are most commonly infected with coagulase-negative staphylococci.

**Clinical features:** Common sites for focal infection include iv lines, the oral cavity, lungs, skin, sinuses, perineal region and urinary tract. Any of these may be accompanied by bacteraemia, or this may result 'primarily' by direct translocation of bacteria (commonly aerobic Gram-negative rods) across the barriers between the gastrointestinal tract and the bloodstream. Colonization and translocation may be reduced by preservation of the patient's normal anaerobic and Gram-positive gut flora ('colonization resistance'). Classical signs of infection such as purulent sputum and CXR changes may be absent. Patients may present with the features of septic shock ($\blacktriangleright$185). **Neutropenic enterocolitis** (typhlitis) is a serious complication of neutropenia in which the bowel (usually the caecum) becomes ulcerated, oedematous and necrotic. It is associated with *Clostridium septicum*, which may be grown from blood cultures, and *Pseudomonas aeruginosa*. Presents with fever, shock and abdominal pain, usually in the right iliac fossa, and usually requires surgical resection. *Pseudomonas aeruginosa* bacteraemia is associated with **ecthyma gangrenosum**, which develops as dark red or purple cutaneous macules, which may ulcerate to leave a central ulcer surrounded by an erythematous margin. This was previously considered pathognomonic, but can occur with other Gram-negative bacteraemias.

Patients undergoing cycles of chemotherapy (e.g. for chronic leukaemia) tend to suffer repeated episodes of infection, with each episode involving progressively more antibiotic-resistant pathogens, as their normal flora is modified by antibiotic exposure.

**Microbiological investigations:** Cultures from all available sites (blood via peripheral vein and central line, urine, any focal site) should be taken before starting or altering therapy. No infective cause is proven in 50–60% of febrile neutropenic episodes, but 60–80% of them appear to respond to antibacterial therapy.

**Antibiotic management:** The incidence of Gram-negative bacteraemia may be reduced by giving **prophylactic antibiotics**, such as ciprofloxacin or co-trimoxazole, and this is widespread practice. However, improved survival has not been proved, and many units are reviewing their practice in the light of rising resistance rates. **Antifungal prophylaxis** is firmly established in patients undergoing bone-marrow transplantation, but its use in other situations is less well evidenced. Many different regimens to treat sepsis in the neutropenic patient are used in different units, and such regimens allow for planned progression of therapy when initial choices fail ☎. Local protocols are informed by numerous factors, including:
- The nature of the underlying malignancy.
- The chemotherapy regimen used, and the degree of and expected duration of neutropenia.
- The extent of other effects of chemotherapy, such as mucositis.
- A wide variety of infecting organisms, most of which are endogenous and unresponsive to commonly used antibiotics.
- Previous use of prophylaxis.
- Results of surveillance cultures.
- Local knowledge of antibiotic resistance patterns.
- A desire to minimize the use of some agents (particularly vancomycin and antifungals) to avoid production of further antibiotic resistance.

Scoring systems to stratify patients into low-risk (who may be treated with oral antibiotics at home) and high-risk (who require admission and iv therapy) are used in some units to reduce exposure to antibiotic organisms.

Three initial strategies are commonly employed:
- Monotherapy with an anti-pseudomonal penicillin (e.g. piperacillin–tazobactam), a carbapenem (e.g. imi/meropenem) or ceftazidime.
- Dual therapy with one of the above plus gentamicin.
- Vancomycin ± one of the above ± gentamicin.

A recent meta-analysis found that there was no clear benefit from combination therapy including gentamicin compared with single-agent therapy (↦ Furno, Lancet Infect Dis 2002; 2: 231). An initial regimen containing vancomycin might be considered in a patient with clinically suspected catheter-related infection, known colonization with penicillin-resistant pneumococci or MRSA, known Gram-positive bacteraemia, or presenting with septic shock (↦ Feld R, Clin Infect Dis 1999; 29: 503). Metronidazole should be added if there is evidence of perianal sepsis, and considered if there is prominent oral or gastrointestinal mucositis.

Regular and careful reassessment of clinical features, imaging and microbiological data is clearly essential.

Patients who fail to respond after 5 (in some units, 3) days of antibacterials and who have no documented bacterial infection are usually started empirically on amphotericin B. Experimental data demonstrating equivalent efficacy for newer antifungals (itraconazole and voriconazole) are now available, and it is likely that these agents will replace amphotericin in many protocols (≻366, ≻375). Most centres continue antibiotics for documented bacterial infections for 10 days (Gram-positive) or 14 days (Gram-negative), and discontinue agents which are inactive against the isolated organisms. Culture-negative cases are normally treated for 5 days after becoming afebrile. Some centres continue all antibiotics until the patient is no longer neutropenic.

A number of factors clearly influence the

**Table 17.6** Relative risks of invasive fungal infection in neutropenic patients

| | |
|---|---|
| Low risk | Period of neutropenia <10 days |
| | Autologous bone marrow or peripheral stem-cell transplant treated with growth factors |
| Medium risk | Corticosteroid therapy |
| | Period of neutropenia 10–21 days |
| | Treated with purine analogues (e.g. fludarabine) |
| | Severe mucositis |
| | Chronic pulmonary disease |
| High risk | Allogeneic bone-marrow transplant, especially with prolonged neutropenia, mismatched, or graft-versus-host disease |
| | Period of neutropenia >21 days |
| | Bacteraemic during period of neutropenia |
| | Colonized with *Candida tropicalis* |
| | Colonized with *Aspergillus* spp. |
| | Fungal infection during previous neutropenic episode |

likelihood of invasive fungal infection in neutropenic patients, listed in Table 17.6.

These issues are discussed in detail in helpful recent US guidelines (↪ Clin Inf Dis 2002; 34: 730, available at www.journals.uchicago.edu/IDSA/guidelines/).

☎ Close liaison with the microbiology laboratory is essential at every stage. Modification of therapy is often required in the light of antibiotic sensitivity of organisms isolated from blood or surveillance stool cultures. **The importance of the early involvement of local expertise and following locally determined protocols cannot be overemphasized.**

## Infections associated with solid organ transplantation

Patients receiving organ transplants require continuous immunosuppression and are therefore at risk of infection, which remains a leading cause of death at all times after transplantation. All centres therefore have detailed protocols for prophylaxis and management of infections, which should be consulted. Particular infections are likely to occur at predictable times after transplantation, and it is possible to construct a timetable which may direct investigation and presumptive therapy (Table 17.7).

Diagnosis is made more difficult by several features unique to this clinical situation:
- Clinical features may be modified by immunosuppressive therapy.
- Graft rejection may mimic infection, causing fever, myalgia, arthralgia and leucocytosis.
- Similar symptoms may occur as adverse effects of immunosuppressive medication, particularly antilymphocyte globulin.
- Transplant recipients are usually predisposed to local infection associated with their original failed organs (e.g. polycystic kidneys remaining *in situ*; *Burkholderia cepacia* and *Aspergillus* spp. in heart lung recipients with cystic fibrosis).

Risks of some of these infections may be reduced, for example by vaccination presplenectomy, treatment of strongyloidiasis (➤235) and resection of polycystic kidneys.

### CMV IN TRANSPLANT RECIPIENTS
CMV infection is one of the most important infections in solid organ recipients. The risk of clinical disease is highest when infection is acquired by a seronegative recipient from a seropositive donor, although reactivation of infection also occurs in seropositive recipients.

**Table 17.7** Common infections in solid organ transplant recipients

| Time after transplantation | Most common infections |
| --- | --- |
| First month | Nosocomial infections: wound infection, pneumonia, iv catheter infection |
| | Reactivation of pre-existing infection, e.g. tuberculosis (➤37), strongyloidiasis (➤235) |
| 1–6 months | Viral infections, especially CMV, but also hepatitis C (➤73), EBV (➤339) |
| | Opportunist infections: *Pneumocystis carinii* (➤156), *Legionella pneumophila* (➤32), aspergillosis (➤363), *Listeria monocytogenes* (➤266) |
| >6 months | Progressive chronic viral infection, e.g. CMV chorioretinitis, hepatitis B or hepatitis C related chronic active hepatitis |
| | Opportunist infections: *Pneumocystis carinii* (➤156), *Cryptococcus neoformans* (➤368), *Listeria monocytogenes* (➤266), *Nocardia asteroides* (➤271) (particularly if immunosuppression has been increased to treat rejection) |
| | Community-acquired infections, e.g. influenza (➤344), pneumococcal pneumonia (➤25) |

**Clinical features:** During the first 6 months, fever, pneumonia, hepatitis, gastrointestinal ulceration, leucopenia, thrombocytopenia. Encephalitis, transverse myelitis and cutaneous vasculitis occur rarely. After 6 months, progressive chorioretinitis is more common. CMV infection predisposes to superinfection with other opportunist agents especially fungi (➤363) and is associated with graft dysfunction and rejection.

**Prevention:** Measures to prevent CMV disease after transplantation include donor-recipient matching for CMV status, long-term administration of prophylactic oral ganciclovir and surveillance for CMV viraemia followed by pre-emptive ganciclovir therapy.

## Infections associated with bone-marrow transplantation

Bone-marrow transplantation is used to treat haematological malignancy and disorders of haemopoiesis such as aplastic anaemia.

After ablation of their own marrow, patients experience an **initial period** (≈21 days) of profound neutropenia, associated with disruption of anatomical barriers by mucositis of the oropharyngeal and gastrointestinal mucosa and the use of indwelling venous catheters. Bacterial and fungal infections (➤363) are common during this period, and should be managed as in neutropenic patients (➤174). Reactivation of herpes simplex virus infection, sometimes with severe cutaneous ulceration, may occur and aciclovir prophylaxis is widely used to reduce this risk. If there is graft failure or rejection, this period of neutropenia may be extended.

After successful engraftment, **between 21 and 100 days,** the major hazard is acute graft-versus-host disease (GVHD), which causes rash, diarrhoea and hepatic dysfunction and is due to donor T cells reacting against host tissue antigens. Differential diagnosis of GVHD and infection can be very difficult. In the absence of GVHD, opportunist infections due to viruses and protozoa may still occur. Before the routine use of prophylactic regimens, BMT recipients were at high risk of reactivation of CMV, causing fever of unknown origin, interstitial pneumonitis, or enteritis, and less often retinitis, encephalitis, hepatitis, or bone-marrow suppression. Pre-emptive antiviral therapy has significantly reduced the incidence and severity of CMV disease and delayed its onset from a median of 8 weeks to greater than 3 months. *Pneumocystis carinii* is largely prevented by co-trimoxazole prophylaxis. Aspergillosis, adenovirus, HSV and chlamydia are less common causes. Broad-spectrum antibiotics as recommended for neutropenic patients (➤174) should be commenced, and investigations, when possible including bronchoscopy and broncho-alveolar lavage, performed as soon as possible.

Infections occurring **after 100 days** affect patients on long-term immunosuppression for chronic GVHD. Bacterial infections, particularly due to *Streptococcus pneumoniae*, *Haemophilus influenzae*, *Neisseria meningitidis*, *Staphylococcus aureus* and coagulase-negative staphylococci, are common. Fungal, viral and protozoal opportunist infections occur less frequently. Empirical therapy should be as for neutropenic patients (➤174) if the neutrophil count is $<1 \times 10^9$ cells/L, and as for severe infection in normal patients (➤185) if it is $\geq 1 \times 10^9$ cells/L.

# Chapter 18

# Fever

Most patients with fever in hospital or general practice have associated symptoms that make diagnosis straightforward—the majority have viral respiratory infections or uncomplicated bacterial respiratory or urinary infections. Assessment of the acutely ill febrile patient is a familiar problem, and a laborious account is not indicated. However, we emphasize the value of a careful history and a full examination.

If the diagnosis is not immediately obvious, particular attention should be paid to special features of history and examination, listed below under PUO. First-line investigations include full blood count, MSU and CXR.

Antibiotics should never be started until appropriate cultures have been sent. If patients are sufficiently unwell to be referred to hospital with fever, then blood and urine (and sputum if produced) should always be cultured.

Although fever is the hallmark of infectious disease, many illnesses can cause fever, including trauma and surgery, neoplastic disease, myocardial infarct, cerebrovascular accident, venous thrombosis and pulmonary embolism. A number of non-infectious multi-system diseases may present with clinical features suggesting acute infection. The key features of some of these are outlined in Table 18.1, with suggestions for diagnostic tests that may help to confirm or exclude them.

## Prolonged pyrexia of unknown origin (PUO)

PUO has been variably defined by a number of authors reporting large series of patients. These definitions, which specify a duration of 2 or 3 weeks of fever, are nowadays not useful clinically. Advances in culture techniques, serology and imaging have changed the spectrum of diseases that may cause diagnostic delay and con-

fusion. These notes are intended as guidance to the diagnosis of unexplained fever lasting more than a 7–10 days.

> Most patients with PUO have a rare presentation of a common illness, rather than a common presentation of a rare illness; occult malignancy is as common as infection. Patients usually have one rather than multiple causes of fever.

### History and examination

**The history is of central importance.** Apart from the history of the presenting complaint and the patient's previous medical history, direct enquiry should be made about:
- Travel (see also Fever in the returning traveller ➤206).
- Drugs (therapeutic and recreational, including alcohol).
- Sexual history, including risk factors for HIV infection.
- Family history and history of contacts with similar symptoms.
- Occupational exposure, especially animal/agricultural contact.
- Pets.

Drug fever (➤182) usually occurs within 7–10 days of starting treatment although it can begin during long-term treatment with previously well-tolerated drugs. It usually resolves within 12–48 h of discontinuation, although this period may be longer for drugs with long elimination half lives, such as co-trimoxazole. Amp/amoxicillin rash and fever have been reported as occurring up to 3 weeks after the last dose.

**Physical examination** should be repeated at daily intervals in patients in hospital, looking particularly for changing heart murmurs, chest signs and developing lymph nodes. Other areas

**Table 18.1** Non-infectious multisystem illnesses causing acute fever, with or without skin rash

| Condition | Relative frequency (hospital practice) | Clinical features | Useful tests |
|---|---|---|---|
| Temporal (giant cell) arteritis/polymyalgia rheumatica | Common | Age >50, headache, temporal artery tenderness, visual disturbance, myalgia, proximal limb girdle stiffness, jaw claudication | High ESR. Temporal artery biopsy |
| Sarcoidosis | Common | Pulmonary symptoms, erythema nodosum, bilateral hilar lymphadenopathy, arthritis, granulomata in many tissues | Histology showing non-caseating granulomata. Serum ACE |
| Drug reactions, including erythema multiforme (syn. Stevens–Johnson syndrome) | Common | Hypersensitivity to infection or drugs. Widespread maculopapular or pustular rash with oral and conjunctival ulcers | Clinical diagnosis |
| Systemic lupus erythematosus | Common, esp. young women | Facial rash, arthralgia, nephritis, polyserositis, photosensitivity | Clinical diagnosis. Anti-dsDNA antibodies |
| Wegener's granulomatosis | Rare | Sinusitis, nephritis, cavitating pulmonary nodules | Histology. ANCA |
| Polyarteritis nodosa | Rare. Commoner in males | Hypertension, angina, nephritis, abdominal pain, variable skin rash, inc. tender subcutaneous nodules and vasculitis (nailbed and splinter haemorrhages) | Clinical diagnosis. Histology. Angiography |
| Polymyositis/ dermatomyositis | Rare. Sometimes associated with malignancy | Muscle pain, tenderness and weakness. Heliotrope rash on eyelids and extensor surfaces | EMG, raised creatine kinase, muscle biopsy. Specific autoantibody (Jo-1) may be present |
| Adult-onset Still's disease/systemic onset juvenile chronic arthritis | Rare | Evanescent salmon pink rash, worse during high daily fever, arthritis, lymphadenopathy, hepatosplenomegaly | Clinical diagnosis. High serum ferritin. Rheumatoid factor and ANA usually negative |
| Kawasaki disease | Rare. Occurs in infants and young children | Fever, conjunctivitis, lymphadenopathy, oedema and erythema of hands/feet with rash which may desquamate. Oropharyngeal erythema, fissured red lips. Coronary artery vasculitis | Clinical diagnosis |
| Sweet's syndrome | Very rare | Tender discrete red/purple cutaneous plaques, arthralgia, myalgia, neutrophilia | Clinical diagnosis. Histology |
| Familial Mediterranean fever | Very rare in UK. Autosomal recessive inheritance among Jews, Armenians, Arabs, Turks | Recurrent polyserositis: peritonitis, pleurisy, arthritis, skin rash resembling erysipelas invariably on extensor surface of lower leg and dorsum of foot | Clinical diagnosis |

of particular interest, or that tend to be neglected include:
- Temporal arteries and scalp.
- Fundi.
- Sinuses and teeth.
- Skin and nails (rashes, stigmata of IE).
- Orifices (mouth, ears, rectum, vagina).
- Pelvis (gynaecological disease, perirectal abscess, the male genitalia).
- Hidden or forgotten iv lines and other prostheses/foreign bodies.

## Routine investigations

These investigations are likely to have been performed before the label of PUO is applied; it is safer to repeat them, particularly if they were performed early in the course of illness:
- Full blood count, including differential white cell count.
- ESR and C-reactive protein.
- Dipstick testing of urine for blood and protein.
- Midstream urine for microscopy and routine bacterial culture.
- Microscopy of spun urine deposit for casts (not routinely performed by most microbiology labs when processing an MSU).
- Sputum if available for routine culture.
- Blood cultures (send at least 20 mL on three separate occasions).
- Biochemical screen including urea, electrolytes, liver function tests and thyroid function tests.
- Chest X-ray.

In patients at risk for tuberculosis, or in whom it is suspected for any reason:
- Sputum if available for AFBs on three occasions.
- Early morning urine for AFBs (send >150 mL on three occasions in correct container).

## Second-line investigations

Any or all of the following may be indicated, depending on the clinical picture:
- Aspiration or biopsy of any lesions discovered. Samples sent for microbiology should not be fixed in formalin.
- Immunological screen, including rheumatoid factor, anti-nuclear antibodies, organ-specific autoantibodies, anti-neutrophil cytoplasmic antibodies (ANCA), complement levels.
- Immunoglobulin electrophoresis.
- Coagulation screen (including lupus anticoagulant, fibrin degradation products).
- Viral serology, including flu, adenovirus, herpes viruses, mumps, measles and parvovirus.
- Bacterial serology including coxiella, mycoplasma, chlamydia, syphilis, leptospirosis, bartonella, legionella and brucella.
- Protozoal serology, including *Toxoplasma*.
- Fungal serology including *Aspergillus*.

☎ Most microbiology laboratories will select those serological tests which are most appropriate on the basis of the clinical history. A full and detailed summary on the request form, or preferably a telephone discussion with the microbiologist, is essential.

**HIV infection** is an unlikely cause of PUO in the absence of a history of risk behaviour. HIV testing may be appropriate but must only be carried out after the patient has received pretest counselling (➤147).

## Imaging

Advances in imaging have revolutionized the investigation of PUO. We would recommend early ultrasound scan (USS) of the upper abdomen and pelvis in all cases, looking specifically for hepatic, subphrenic and renal lesions (abscess, neoplasm), splenic size, posterior abdominal wall lymph nodes and pelvic sepsis. The following may then be necessary:
- CT or MRI scan of the thorax and abdomen—for fluid collections, solid tumours and lymphadenopathy. Guided aspiration, or preferably biopsy, may be possible.
- Echocardiography may confirm the presence of vegetations in suspected IE, but a normal transthoracic echo does not exclude IE (➤49).
- Radiolabelled white cell and bone scans.

## Causes of PUO (Table 18.2)

Any list of causes is incomplete; most large textbooks of infectious diseases or general medicine have lists and these should be referred to.

**Table 18.2** Some causes of pyrexia of unknown origin (PUO)

| Category | Conditions | |
|---|---|---|
| Infections | **Infective endocarditis** | Partially treated bacterial endocarditis, coxiella, bartonella, nutritionally deficient streptococci, fastidious Gram-negative rods, brucella, legionella, fungi, chlamydia |
| | **Collections of pus** | Subphrenic, intrahepatic, renal, pelvic (including appendix), pleural, bone, sinuses, spleen |
| | Systemic bacterial infections | *Mycoplasma*, syphilis, leptospirosis, Lyme disease, typhoid, coxiella, brucella |
| | **Tuberculosis** | (especially extrapulmonary) |
| | Viral | e.g. CMV, EBV, hepatitis B |
| Malignancy | **Visceral** | e.g. **kidney, liver, pancreas** |
| | Haematological | **Lymphoma**, leukaemia, myeloma |
| Rheumatological disease | Rheumatoid disease, SLE, polyarteritis nodosa, Still's disease, **temporal arteritis** (see also ➤180) | |
| Granulomatous disease | Sarcoidosis, Crohn's disease, granulomatous hepatitis (➤76) | |
| **Drugs** | Penicillins, cephalosporins, para-aminosalicylic acid, amphotericin B, antihistamines, barbiturates, phenytoin, quinidine, sulphonamides, iodides, propylthiouracil, methyldopa, procainamide, hydralazine, isoniazid, phenylbutazone, nitrofurantoin | |
| Hepatic | Cirrhosis, alcoholic hepatitis, chronic active hepatitis, abscess | |
| Factitious fever | Particularly in health-care professionals | |

More frequent causes are indicated in bold type.

**Table 18.4** Causes of lymphadenopathy

| Category | Conditions |
|---|---|
| Local infection | Local suppurative disease (staphylococci, streptococci), tuberculosis, atypical mycobacteria |
| Generalized infection | EBV, CMV, toxoplasmosis, HIV, rubella, secondary syphilis, hepatitis A, malaria, histoplasmosis, coccidioidomycosis, brucellosis, LGV |
| Malignancy | Lymphoma, leukaemia, carcinoma |
| Sarcoidosis | |
| Connective-tissue disease | Rheumatoid disease, systemic lupus erythematosus, dermatomyositis |
| Dermatopathic | Related to local skin disease, particularly eczema |
| Endocrine | Hyperthyroidism, Addison's disease |

**Table 18.3** Causes of fever and rash

| | | | |
|---|---|---|---|
| *Purpura* | | Disseminated herpes simplex | (➤338) |
| Bacterial infection | | Eczema herpeticum | (➤338) |
|   *Neisseria meningitidis* | (➤299) | Rickettsial pox | (➤329) |
|   *Staphylococcus aureus* | (➤249) | Drug hypersensitivity | |
|   *Pseudomonas aeruginosa* | (➤291) | | |
| Infective endocarditis | (➤49) | *Maculopapular* | |
| Enteroviruses | (➤347) | Scarlet fever | (➤135) |
| Rickettsia | | Erythema marginatum | (➤258) |
| (Rocky Mountain spotted fever, typhus) | (➤329) | Staphylococcal toxins | |
| Drug hypersensitivity | |   Toxic epidermal necrolysis | (➤136) |
| Systemic vasculitis | |   Toxic shock syndrome | (➤84) |
| Henoch–Schönlein disease | | Secondary syphilis | (➤89) |
| | | Typhoid | (➤281) |
| *Vesicles or pustules* | | Erythema chronica migrans | (➤323) |
| Staphylococcal toxins | | Viral exanthemata (measles, rubella, EBV, | (➤126) |
|   Toxic epidermal necrolysis | (➤136) | adenovirus, enterovirus, etc.) | |
|   Toxic shock syndrome | (➤84) | Primary HIV infection | (➤145) |
| Enteroviruses | (➤347) | Drug and food hypersensitivity | |
| Herpes virus infections | | Kawasaki disease | (➤180) |
|   Varicella zoster | (➤130) | Systemic lupus erythematosus | (➤180) |

**Table 18.5** Causes of eosinophilia

| Category | Conditions |
|---|---|
| Drugs | Iodides, aspirin, sulphonamides, nitrofurantoin |
| Parasites | Helminths, but excluding *Enterobius vermicularis* |
| Infection | Tuberculosis, (particularly miliary ➤39), cat-scratch disease (➤309) |
| Allergy and atopy | Hay fever, asthma, systemic vasculitis, eczema, pemphigus, Churg–Strauss syndrome |
| Connective-tissue disease | Rheumatoid disease, polyarteritis nodosa, dermatomyositis, eosinophilic fasciitis |
| Malignancy | Carcinomatosis, mycosis fungoides, Hodgkin's disease, chronic myeloid leukaemia, eosinophilic leukaemia |
| Hypereosinophilic syndromes | Loeffler's syndrome (pulmonary eosinophilia) and Loeffler's endocarditis |

## Fever and rash

The presence of a rash in an acutely febrile patient is always useful diagnostically. Many rashes are characteristic, not only in their appearance but also in their distribution and pattern of progression. Table 18.3 lists some of the infectious and non-infectious causes of rash in the acutely febrile patient.

## Fever and lymphadenopathy

Fever and lymphadenopathy are common manifestations of infection, but also occur in other disorders. The nature of lymphadenopathy may be a helpful aid to diagnosis. Firm, rubbery, mobile, non-tender nodes suggest lymphoma. Hard, fixed nodes suggest carcinoma. Tender, asymmetrical, matted or fluctuant nodes suggest infection. Table 18.4 lists some causes of lymphadenopathy which may need to be excluded.

The clinical characteristics mentioned above are not sufficiently reliable to exclude malig-nancy. Lymph nodes which fail to regress over a few weeks merit biopsy.

## Eosinophilia

Causes of eosinophilia are listed in Table 18.5.

# Chapter 19

# Septic shock

**Septic shock**, broadly defined as the development of hypotension and organ failure as a result of severe infection, is an important cause of death in hospital patients, particularly on the intensive-care unit. The diagnosis of septic shock remains a clinical one, confirmed by positive blood cultures in only a proportion of cases. It is useful to have **clinical definitions** which allow identification of patients before they develop positive blood cultures and resistant hypotension. The past decade has seen an ongoing debate about appropriate definitions of terms used in this area, and some of these are listed in Table 19.1.

**Pathogenesis:** Septic shock has in the past been associated with Gram-negative bacteraemia, but Gram-positive organisms have become more common in hospital patients, particularly as result of increased frequency of interventions, indwelling medical devices and more immunocompromised patients. It is not possible to distinguish between Gram-positive and -negative bacteraemia clinically. Shock is the end result of a complex cascade initiated by bacterial infection, which stimulates the release of inflammatory mediators such as tumour necrosis factor (TNF) and interleukin-1 (IL-1) from host leucocytes. These damage vascular endothelial cells, causing increased capillary permeability, abnormal vasomotor activity and activation of the clotting system, resulting in maldistribution of blood flow and damage to multiple organs, including kidneys, lungs, brain, liver and myocardium.

**Risk factors: Sources of sepsis:** Intravascular sources include infected heart valves in IE (➤49), iv cannulae, infected atheromatous plaques or shunts. Extravascular sources include wounds, abscesses, focal infections such as pneumonia, gut perforation or urinary tract infection. Recent trauma or manipulation, such as surgery or IVDU, may be involved. **Host factors:** Severe underlying illness such as diabetes, renal failure or hepatic disease, which may compromise the host immune system or cause loss of integrity of epithelial surfaces. Trauma and malignancy are particularly important in this respect. Anatomical abnormalities such as stones or obstruction in the urinary or biliary tracts may predispose to infection. Patients at either of the extremes of age are at increased risk, as are those with indwelling foreign bodies, in particular intravenous medical devices such as central venous cannulae.

**Clinical features:** There may be a **history of risk factors** as above. **Fever and rigors** commonly occur, but neonatal, elderly, debilitated or immunocompromised patients may not manifest these classical symptoms. **Hypothermia** is common. A **change in mental state**, with apprehension or confusion, may be the first sign of impending sepsis, and a search for infection should be considered in any elderly patient who becomes acutely confused. Stupor and coma occur less often. Cough or disturbance of micturition may indicate a **primary site of infection**. Careful enquiry and examination for sites of skin sepsis such as boils, infected intravenous lines. Patients should be specifically asked about previous splenectomy and rheumatic and congenital cardiac disease.

**On examination,** there may be signs consistent with the definition given above, with or without hypotension (≤90 mmHg). In early shock, there is peripheral vasodilatation, decreased systemic vascular resistance and increased cardiac output. The patient is hypotensive, but warm. Later, there is periph-

**Table 19.1** Definition of terms used to describe severe sepsis and hypotension

| | |
|---|---|
| Bacteraemia | The presence of viable bacteria in the blood |
| Systemic inflammatory response syndrome (SIRS) | A widespread inflammatory response to a variety of severe clinical insults, clinically recognized by the presence of two or more of the following:<br>    Temperature >38°C or <36°C<br>    Heart rate >90 beats/min<br>    Respiratory rate >20 breaths/min or $Paco_2$ <4.3 kPa<br>    WBC >12 000 cells/mm$^3$, <4000 cells/mm$^3$, or >10% immature forms |
| Sepsis | SIRS plus evidence of infection |
| Severe sepsis | Sepsis plus organ dysfunction, hypoperfusion (e.g. lactic acidosis, oliguria, or an acute alteration in mental status) or hypotension (systolic BP <90 mmHg) |
| Septic shock | Sepsis with hypotension despite adequate fluid resuscitation |

↪Bone, Chest 1992; 101: 1644

eral vasoconstriction, increased systemic vascular resistance and reduced cardiac output. As cardiac output falls, the skin becomes cold, cyanotic and mottled.

Auscultation and chest X-ray may reveal pneumonia or evidence of **adult respiratory distress syndrome** (ARDS), characterized by increased alveolar capillary permeability and pulmonary oedema without left atrial hypertension, leading to hypoxia with reduced lung compliance. ARDS occurs in up to 40% of cases, and is associated with a very high mortality.

**Cutaneous manifestations** include the signs referred to above, due to changes in peripheral perfusion, but also cellulitis and, particularly in those who develop disseminated intravascular coagulation, vasculitic skin lesions progressing to gangrene. Meningococcaemia is associated with a rash that is initially petechial, progressing to a purpuric or ecchymotic rash on both limbs and trunk. *Staphylococcus aureus* bacteraemia may cause a very similar rash. *Pseudomonas aeruginosa* bacteraemia is associated with ecthyma gangrenosum, which develops as dark red or purple macules, which may ulcerate to leave a central ulcer surrounded by an erythematous margin. This was previously considered pathognomonic, although it has been reported in association with other Gram-negative bacteraemias.

**Organisms:** Community-acquired sepsis: coliforms, *Streptococcus pneumoniae, Neisseria gonorrhoeae, Neisseria meningitidis, Staphylococcus aureus.* In hospital patients, particularly with indwelling intravenous lines, *Staphylococcus epidermidis* should also be considered, but septic shock is unusual. In patients with malignancy or abdominal sepsis coliforms, enterococci and anaerobic infections, particularly *Bacteroides fragilis.* In patients with neutropenia, *Pseudomonas aeruginosa* and fungi should also be covered (➤174). Splenectomized patients are at particular risk from capsulated organisms (*Streptococcus pneumoniae, Haemophilus influenzae, Neisseria meningitidis*) and *Capnocytophaga* spp., particularly after bites (➤114). Recent manipulations of particular body sites may suggest particular organisms (Table 19.2).

**Microbiological investigations:** Gram stain and culture of urine, pus, sputum or CSF. Blood cultures should be sent as soon as the diagnosis is suspected. At least two venepunctures should be performed in the assessment period and at least 10 and preferably 20 mL of blood should be cultured from each.

**Other investigations:** Neutrophil leucocytosis with 'left shift'. Thrombocytopenia and disseminated intravascular coagulation with prolonged prothrombin and partial throm-

**Table 19.2** Organisms causing bacteraemia associated with particular interventions

| Manipulated site | Organisms |
| --- | --- |
| GU manipulation | Coliforms, enterococci |
| Boils | *Staphylococcus aureus* |
| Septic abortion | Coliforms, anaerobes |
| IVDU | *Staphylococcus aureus*, enterococci, *Pseudomonas aeruginosa* |
| IV lines | *Staphylococcus aureus*, coliforms, *Candida albicans*, *Staphylococcus epidermidis*, enterococci |

boplastin times, reduced plasma fibrinogen and raised fibrin degradation products. Raised serum lactate levels occur in a majority of patients. Most patients with septic shock develop some degree of renal failure, usually due to acute tubular necrosis secondary to hypotension. Abnormal liver function are frequently seen. Chest X-ray may show pneumonia or ARDS. Ultrasound and CT scanning will usually be required to exclude local collections of pus.

**Differential diagnosis:** Specific syndromes causing hypotension and shock include severe pneumonia with hypoxaemia (➤27), anaphylaxis induced by antibiotics, peritonitis, toxic shock syndrome (➤84), mediastinitis (for example after oesophageal surgery or variceal sclerotherapy) and purulent bacterial pericardial effusion.

**Antibiotic management:** Depends on likely infectious cause and local prevalence of resistance. Many different regimens are suitable—it is important to start as soon as cultures have been taken and give large doses intravenously (Table 19.3). Be guided thereafter by microbiology results. For management of neutropenic sepsis ➤174.

**Supportive management:** Careful supportive management is as important as administration of adequate antibiotics. Haemodynamic monitoring and inotropic support in the intensive care unit is often required; a full discussion is beyond the scope of this manual. Recent studies have confirmed the value of early, aggressive optimization of tissue oxygen delivery using a step-wise algorithm combining fluid resuscitation, vasopressors, red cell transfusion, and inotropes (➥Rivers, N Engl J Med 2001; 345: 1368). Monoclonal antibodies against endotoxin and TNF have not been shown to be useful and are not currently used. Steroids are not indicated.

Recent trials have shown that recombinant human activated protein C (drotrecogin alfa) reduces mortality in severe sepsis, particularly in those with more adverse severity scores. Precise indications for this expensive agent remain to be developed.

➥ Bernard, N Engl J Med 2001; 344: 699

## Emergency management of septic shock

**Whilst you wait for help from ITU, proceed as follows:** Make a full assessment of the patient's condition and the likely aetiology as above. Insert a large-bore peripheral venous line and administer saline or colloid. An initial bolus of 1 L of normal saline given over 30 min is appropriate if the patient is hypotensive. Take cultures, then choose and start appropriate antibiotics (Table 19.3). Give supplementary oxygen by face mask. Unless you suspect chronic $CO_2$ retention, give at least 60% $FiO_2$. Volume replacement is a priority, and should be monitored by central venous line, vital signs and urine output. A mixture of two-thirds crystalloid (e.g. two-thirds normal saline and one-

**Table 19.3** Suitable antibiotic regimens in severe sepsis

| Suspected site of infection | Regimen |
| --- | --- |
| Suspected meningococcaemia with rash | High dose parenteral cephalosporin (e.g. ceftriaxone 2 g q12h) |
| Chest | Parenteral cephalosporin + macrolide |
| Urinary tract | Co-amoxiclav or parenteral cephalosporin |
| No obvious source | Ampicillin + gentamicin + metronidazole |
| If *Staphylococcus aureus* suspected (cutaneous sepsis, recent flu epidemic, IVDU, iv line) | Include flucloxacillin or vancomycin in regimen |
| Patients with neutropenia | (➤174) |

third 5% dextrose) and one-third colloid (gelatin or etherified starch) is appropriate for most situations. Avoid dextrans, because they can cause bleeding and interfere with cross-matching and some laboratory tests. Insert a urinary catheter. Observe carefully for fluid overload and be aware of the possibility of acute renal failure.

---

**Emergency inotropic support with epinephrine**

Dilute 6 mg of epinephrine in 100 mL normal saline and start infusion at 1 mL/h (equivalent to 1 microgram/min = approximately 0.015 microgram/kg/min for a 70-kg patient). Infusion rate can be increased up to 10 mL/h depending on response.

---

Insert a central line. If CVP >10 cmH$_2$O, start epinephrine as emergency inotropic support.

'**Source control**': Remove or drain any obvious source of infection such as a boil or infected iv line. Assess the patient carefully for sources of infection that may be amenable to drainage or surgical intervention (e.g. sinuses, empyema, mediastinitis, peritonitis, cholangitis, urinary obstruction, septic arthritis, infective endocarditis).

Repeat assessment daily.

**Complications:** Mortality increases with the number of organ systems involved—if four or more organ systems fail, mortality approaches 100%. In terminal stages, patients become progressively acidotic, with resistant hypotension refractory to treatment with fluids and inotropic drugs.

# Tropical and Travel Medicine

# Chapter 20

# Pre-travel advice

Advice to travellers is based on the countries they intend to visit, location (urban vs. rural), current health status (e.g. pregnancy, immuno-compromise), duration of stay, and previous medical history (e.g. splenectomy). UK Departments of Health have published a detailed handbook, *Health Information for Overseas Travellers* (the 'yellow book'), the full text of which is available at:

🖳 www.the-stationery-office.co.uk/doh/hinfo/index.htm

## Avoiding infection

### Avoiding insect-borne infections
• Sleep in a properly screened room and use a knockdown insecticide spray before retiring, or use a mosquito net which has been impregnated with permethrin.
• Wear long sleeves and trousers after sunset.
• Use an insect repellant containing DEET (*N,N*-diethylmetatoluamide). Preparations containing >50% DEET (20% in children) should be avoided, as neurological toxicity may result from absorption.
• African trypanosomiasis (➤220) is spread by tsetse flies in Africa between 15° N and 20° S. It is very rare in travellers. Those most at risk are travellers to remote rural areas (safari, animal workers). Tsetse flies bite during the day and are attracted to large moving objects and strong dark colours. Wrist- and ankle-length clothing and insect repellant should be worn. Car windows should be kept closed and flies killed with insecticide spray.
• Loiasis (➤241) can be prevented in long-term visitors to endemic areas (Cameroon, Central African Republic, Congo, Equatorial Guinea, Gabon, Ghana, Nigeria and Zaire) by taking diethylcarbamazine 300 mg weekly. This

should **not** be prescribed if acute infection is suspected.

## Avoiding food- and water-borne infections
• Choose foods which have been freshly prepared and thoroughly cooked with a minimum of handling.
• Avoid shellfish, and meat that may be partly cooked.
• Avoid salads, fruit that cannot be peeled, ice and ice cream.
• Drinking water should be boiled or chemically disinfected. Commercially available purification tablets are available and effective unless water is very heavily contaminated. Portable water filters are available but expensive.

### Avoiding schistosomiasis
• Schistosomiasis (for more detailed notes on distribution ➤226) is acquired by bathing in fresh water containing snails. Risk is highest in Nile Valley, Lake Victoria, Lake Malawi, Tigris and Euphrates river systems, in artificial lakes in Africa (e.g. Lake Kariba, Lake Volta) and in some areas of Brazil. Minimize risk by bathing for short periods in flowing rather than still water, avoiding the early and late parts of the day and rubbing down vigorously with a towel after swimming.

### Avoiding blood-borne and sexually transmitted infection
• Condoms reduce but do not abolish risk.
• Procedures involving surgery, injections or blood transfusion may transmit HIV or HBV. Travellers should carry an emergency medical pack containing suture materials, needles and syringes, available from pharmacies and travel clinics.

## Splenectomized travellers (➤170)

Travellers with anatomical or functional asplenia are at high risk of severe or fatal malaria, and optimum antimalarial prophylaxis and bite avoidance are essential. For advice on antibiotic prophylaxis for this group, ➤170. They should receive pneumo-coccal (➤172), meningococcal (➤193) and Hib (➤296) vaccination. They are also at risk of contracting babesiosis (➤229) and fulminant septicaemia due to *Capnocytophaga canimorsus* (➤302) after dog bites.

For travel advice for **immunocompromised patients**, see ↪Conlon C, Hosp Med 2000; 61: 167.

# Immunization for foreign travel

Polio, tetanus and diphtheria immunization should be reviewed, and a course or booster given if required, regardless of destination (➤417). Travellers to areas of poor hygiene usually require immunization against typhoid and hepatitis A. Detailed guidance for the UK is published in *Immunisation against Infectious Disease* (the 'green book'), last published in 1996, and also available at ▣ www.doh.gov.uk/greenbook/. For country-by-country require-ments, consult Table 20.1 at the end of this chapter.

## Typhoid (➤280)

Indicated for travellers to endemic areas (Table 20.1) and laboratory workers who may handle specimens containing *S. typhi*. Two forms of vaccine are available:

**Vi capsular polysaccharide vaccine** (Typhim Vi, Typherix): Single 0.5-mL dose im or deep sc with booster every 3 yrs on continued exposure. Children under 2 yrs may make a suboptimal response. Local reactions occur, and systemic reactions occur in ~8%.

**Oral Ty21a vaccine** (Vivotif): One capsule alternate days for three doses, with three-dose booster course annually. This is a live attenuated vaccine and is contraindicated in the immuno-suppressed, in patients on sulphonamides or other antibiotics and in children under 6 yrs. If mefloquine is being taken, then these two medications should be separated by at least 12 h. It should not be given simultaneously with OPV. The oral vaccine is very sensitive to heat and must be refrigerated and taken with cool liquid only. Side effects include febrile reactions, gastrointestinal symptoms and rarely hypersensitivity, including anaphylaxis.

Both vaccines are contraindicated in acute febrile illness, after previous severe reaction to the same vaccine, or in pregnancy, unless there is a very clear indication.

**Combined typhoid and hepatitis A vaccine preparations** are available (Hepatyrix, ViATIM). These are currently recommended for adults (single 1 mL dose im into deltoid). Boosters are required as for component vac-cines. Some preliminary evidence suggests that ViATIM is more immunogenic than Hepatyrix.

## Hepatitis A (➤70)

**Active vaccination** with formaldehyde-inactivated HAV is now available and is recom-mended for laboratory staff who work with virus, travellers to high-risk areas, individuals at risk because of their sexual behaviour and haemophiliacs with hepatitis B or C or other liver disease. A number of preparations are currently licensed (Avaxim, Havrix Monodose, Vaqta), all of which must be injected into the deltoid (sc an alternative in haemophiliacs). For exact dose schedules, ▣. Dose is reduced in children under 16 yrs (paediatric preparations available). Boosters are required at 6–12 months, and every 10 yrs thereafter. **Con-traindicated** in severe febrile illness. It should only be given in pregnancy if there is a clear indication.

Combination preparations with typhoid vaccine (see above) and hepatitis B vaccine (Twinrix, Twinrix Paediatric: course of 3 injec-tions at 0, 1 and 6 months ▣).

> Some preparations of Vaqta produced during ≈1997–2002 were found to be inadequately immunogenic, and persons immunized with these formulations should be considered non-immune, and receive a further full course if exposure continues.

**Passive immunization** with normal human immunoglobulin has been used in the past to protect against HAV. Immunoglobulin may be given at the same time as HAV vaccine if immediate protection is required. May interfere with the response to live virus vaccines, which should be given at least 3 weeks before or 3 months after an injection of immunoglobulin. This does not apply to yellow fever, since normal immunoglobulin is unlikely to contain antibodies against this virus.

## Yellow fever (➤352)

Live attenuated virus yellow fever virus (17D strain): single dose 0.5 mL sc gives protection for 10 yrs.

Vaccination is a legal requirement for entry to some countries, either for all travellers, or those arriving from endemic areas, and is only given at designated centres. The International Certificate of Vaccination is valid for 10 yrs from 10 days after immunization, or immediately after reimmunisation. See Table 20.1 for countries where vaccination is required.

**Contraindications and cautions:** Vaccine is well tolerated, with few adverse effects; encephalitis (reversible) occurs rarely and has only been reported in children. Risk is highest for very young children, and for this reason vaccination is contraindicated in pregnancy and under 9 months of age unless travel to a high-risk area is unavoidable. Absolutely contraindicated under age 4 months. Vaccine is contraindicated in concurrent febrile illness, immunosuppressed patients, including those on high-dose steroids, chemotherapy, or with haematological malignancy or HIV. Contraindicated in patients allergic to eggs, neomycin or polymyxin. Avoid simultaneous administration with cholera vaccine.

## Meningococcal vaccine (➤299)

**Meningococcal group C conjugate vaccine** (MenC) provides long-lasting immunity against serogroup C infection and since late 1999 has been part of routine immunization in the UK (➤417). Travellers requiring immunization should be vaccinated with meningococcal polysaccharide A & C vaccine, irrespective of whether they have received MenC vaccine.

**Meningococcal polysaccharide A & C** vaccine is indicated for visits >1 month to high-risk areas (Table 20.1), esp. if travelling rough or in close contact with local people. Two preparations are currently available (AC Vax, Mengivac(A + C)). Initial dose for both is 0.5 mL im or deep sc. The efficacy and duration of protection is much lower in infants, and the product literature for these vaccines differ on the lower age limit. Booster dose is required at 1 yr for infants, and between 3 and 5 years for adults 🔖.

**Pilgrims visiting Saudi Arabia for the Hajj** are at particular risk of meningococcal disease, and Saudi authorities currently require all children under 2 yrs to have had 2 doses of A & C vaccine given 3 months apart. All pilgrims >2 yrs old must carry certificate stating use of **ACWY vaccine** (licensed in the UK since late 2001), >9 days and <3 yrs before arrival.

Vaccine is also used in the UK for contacts of group A and C cases (in addition to chemoprophylaxis ➤100), in control of local outbreaks and for patients post splenectomy (➤170) or with complement deficiency (➤171).

**Contraindications and cautions:** Well tolerated. Contraindicated during febrile illness, or if there has been a previous severe reaction to same vaccine. Pregnancy is a relative contraindication.

## Japanese B encephalitis (➤354)

Two unlicensed vaccines are available for named patient use only (Pasteur Merieux, Korean Green Cross). Protection is ≈95%, but does not develop until about 6 weeks after starting immunization. Three doses required, and schedules vary between products 🔖.

**Indications:** Rural travel to infected areas (mainly SE Asia and Indian subcontinent) for >1 month. Risk is highest during May–June, but is present all year in some areas. See Table 20.1 for countries where vaccination is recommended.

**Contraindications and cautions:** Current febrile illness or other infection, heart, kidney or liver disease, diabetes or other hormonal dysfunction, malnutrition, malignancy, hypersensitivity to mouse brain products, pregnancy, history of anaphylaxis or urticaria.

(Pasteur Merieux MSD: ☎ 0500 106410.)

### Rabies (➤357)

Two safe modern killed virus preparations are available (Aventis Pasteur human diploid cell vaccine (HDCV), Rabipur purified chick embryo cell vaccine (PCEC)). Both are given as three doses of 1 mL, im into the deltoid, on days 0, 7 and 21–28 with boosters at 2–5-yr intervals 📄. Although not licensed as such, HDCV is often given as 0.1 mL intradermally. This reduces costs and has been shown to be effective provided a blister is raised. Choroquine reduces the efficacy of the intradermal route — patients already taking chloroquine should receive im vaccination. The efficacy of the intradermal route has not been demonstrated for PCEC.

**Indications:** Travellers to enzootic areas who may be unable to obtain postexposure vaccination, or who are particularly likely to be bitten (animal workers, bat handlers, cyclists). See Table 20.1 for countries where vaccination is recommended.

**Contraindications and cautions:** Local and systemic reactions occur. Anaphylaxis and Guillain–Barré syndrome have been reported.

PCEC is available from MASTA (0113 238 7500).

For postexposure management ➤358.

### Tick-borne encephalitis (➤354)

An unlicensed vaccine is available for named patient use only. Gives protection against all TBE strains occurring in Europe and Asia. Further information and vaccine supplies from Immuno Ltd (01732 458101). Three doses of 0.5 mL im, at day 0, 4–12 weeks and 9–12 months, with a booster at 3-yr intervals.

**Indications:** Walkers and campers in warm, forested parts of Europe and Scandinavia, especially where there is heavy undergrowth and during late spring and summer, are most at risk. TBE occurs in foci throughout the eastern half of Europe, and across Russia, but accurate surveillance data are not available for many coun-

tries. Areas of established risk include SE coastal Sweden, around Stockholm and the island of Gotland, S. Finland around Turku and the Aland Islands, throughout Poland, Germany, the Czech and Slovak Republics, Switzerland, Austria, Hungary, Slovenia, Croatia and Albania. Very rarely reported from Tuscany, Central Italy. Specific immunoglobulin is available from the same supplier for postexposure prophylaxis.

**Contraindications and cautions:** Mild local and systemic reactions occur. Contraindicated in acute febrile illness, and allergy to thiomersal or eggs.

### Tuberculosis (➤37)

Visitors to Asia, Africa, C. & S. America who have not had BCG and who are tuberculin-negative should be offered BCG. Contraindicated in immunosuppressed (including HIV), haematological malignancy, pregnancy and intercurrent fever.

### Cholera (➤285)

Cholera vaccine gives ~50% protection which lasts 3–6 months, and is no longer recommended for protection of individuals. It plays no part in the control of epidemics and is not currently available in the UK.

### Plague (➤305)

Vaccine no longer available because of unreliable efficacy, but new subunit vaccine under development.

### Hepatitis B (➤70)

Hepatitis B vaccination is indicated for healthcare workers and individuals who expect to become resident in endemic areas. For doses ➤73.

## Timing of vaccinations

With the exception of oral polio virus (OPV), live virus vaccines should ideally be separated by at least 3 weeks (Table 20.2). If travellers present late, these spacings should be ignored, but antibody responses may be blunted and consideration should be given to repeating

**Table 20.2** Timing of vaccinations for travellers

| Vaccine | May be administered simultaneously | Interval recommended |
| --- | --- | --- |
| Inactivated vaccines | All other vaccines | |
| Yellow fever (➤193) | OPV, hepatitis B | |
| OPV (➤348) | All live vaccines, immunoglobulin | Oral typhoid—3 weeks |
| Oral typhoid (Ty21a) (➤192) | Yellow fever, immunoglobulin | OPV—3 weeks |
| MMR | OPV | Other live vaccines—4 weeks |
| BCG | OPV, immunoglobulin | Other live vaccines—4 weeks |
| Immunoglobulin | Yellow fever, OPV, all inactivated vaccines | MMR—give 3 weeks before or 3 months after immunoglobulin |

**Table 20.3** Accelerated vaccination schedule

| First visit | Second visit |
| --- | --- |
| Yellow fever | Polio (OPV) booster |
| Typhoid (Vi) | Meningitis |
| Tetanus booster | |
| Hepatitis A vaccine | |

vaccination on return or giving early booster. A single dose of most vaccines will give some protection. Most travellers can be vaccinated at two visits 4 weeks apart (Table 20.3).

## Standby treatment

**Malaria:** Rarely, travellers to remote malarious areas may need to carry a drug for emergency self-treatment; this should not be the same as the prophylactic drug. Malarone (➤217) is the drug of choice when it is not being used for prevention. Alternatives include Fansidar (➤217, only useful in the Indian subcontinent and limited areas of sub-Saharan Africa and not to be taken if allergic to sulfa drugs), or quinine plus doxycycline (➤410). Mefloquine is not recommended for self-treatment, because side effects are much commoner when used for treatment (seizures and/or psychosis in one in 100–1500). Emergency self-treatment is a temporary measure, and medical attention should be sought as soon as possible.

**Travellers' diarrhoea:** Travellers are likely to develop diarrhoea (➤64). Fluid and electrolyte replacement is crucial. Bottled drinks, tea or oral rehydration solution (commercial or home-made ➤62) may be used. Fasting is unnecessary, but milk is best avoided. Anti-diarrhoeal agents reduce frequency of diarrhoea, but do not stop fluid loss into the gut. They should not be given if there is fever, blood in stools, in pregnancy or in children under 12 yrs. Loperamide is the agent of choice (4 mg initially, thereafter 2 mg after each loose stool, up to 16 mg in 24 h).

**Antibiotic treatment** is indicated if diarrhoea is severe or prolonged, or is accompanied by fever, prostration or blood in stools. If diarrhoea fails to respond to ciprofloxacin, 500 mg 12hly for 3 days, it is likely to be protozoal in origin, and metronidazole, 400 mg 8hly for 5 days, should be given. Depending on the level of health care available, it may be appropriate for travellers to carry a supply of loperamide, ciprofloxacin and metronidazole, with instructions on their use. Azithromycin has also been proven effective. Medical advice should be sought as soon as possible.

## Antimalarial prophylaxis (➤214)

Recommendations change as new areas of antimalarial resistance emerge; country-by-country recommendations are shown in Table

20.1. For details of drugs and regimens used ➤215.

# Sources of information for those advising travellers

## Publications
• World Health Organization Weekly Epidemiological Record: ▭www.who.int/wer/
• *Health Advice for Travellers*, published by the Department of Health (0800 555777): ▭www.doh.gov.uk/traveladvice/index.htm
• *Health Information for Overseas Travellers*: ▭www.the-stationery-office.co.uk/doh/hinfo/index.htm
• *British National Formulary*: ▭www.bnf.org/
• *Immunisation against Infectious Disease* (1996), published by the Department of Health—the 'green book'.

⌨ www.doh.gov.uk/greenbook/

## Telephone advice on malaria
Malaria Reference Laboratory
• 09065 508908 (24-h premium-cost helpline)
• 020 7636 3924 (health professionals only, 09:00–16:30)
• PHLS Communicable Disease Surveillance Centre: 0208 8200 6868

## Departments of tropical medicine
Birmingham
    0121 766 6611 ext 4403

Edinburgh
    0131 537 1000 (treatment)
    0131 537 2822 (travel clinic)
Liverpool
    0151 708 9393
London—Hospital for Tropical Diseases:
    020 7387 9300 (treatment)
    020 7388 9600 (prophylaxis)
Manchester
    0161 720 2677
Oxford
    01865 225214

## Resources for professionals
Current UK guidelines on malaria prevention:
↪ Bradley, Commun Dis Public Health 2001; 4: 84
⌨ www.phls.co.uk/advice/
⌨ www.phls.co.uk/publications/CDPHVol4/No%202/malaria%20guidelinesp.pdf
    Comprehensive WHO website:
⌨ www.who.int/ith/

## Websites for patients
⌨ www.fitfortravel.scot.nhs.uk
⌨ www.doh.gov.uk/traveladvice/index.htm
⌨ www.tripprep.com/
⌨ www.masta.org/
⌨ www.cdc.gov/travel/travel.html

**Table 20.1** Country-by-country recommendations for travellers

| Country | Typhoid | Hepatitis A | Rabies | Meningitis A | Yellow fever | Japanese B encephalitis | Tick-borne encephalitis | Malaria prophylaxis (➤214) Comments | Recommended regimen | Alternative regimen |
|---|---|---|---|---|---|---|---|---|---|---|
| Abu Dhabi | S | R | S | | | | | | W | |
| Afghanistan | R | R | S | | | | | Below 2000 m May–Nov | PC | * |
| Albania | S | R | S | | | | S | | | |
| Algeria | R | R | S | | | | | | W | |
| Angola | R | R | S | | R | | | | ME or DO or MON | PC (LP) |
| Antigua/Barbuda | S | R | | | | | | | | |
| Argentina | S | R | S | | | | | Small area in NW only | C | P |
| Armenia | S | R | S | | | | S | June–Oct (no risk in tourist areas) | C | P |
| Austria | | | | | | | S | | | |
| Azerbaijan | R | R | S | | | | S | S border areas, Khachmas June–Oct | C | P |
| Bahamas | S | R | | | | | | | | |
| Bahrain | S | R | S | | | | | | | |
| Bali | R | R | S | | | S | | | W | |
| Bangladesh | R | R | S | | | S | | Chittagong hill tracts | ME or DO or MON | PC |
| | | | | | | | | Elsewhere (no risk in Dhaka City) | PC | * |
| Barbados | S | R | | | | | | | | |
| Belarus | S | R | S | | | | S | | | |
| Belize | R | R | S | | | | | Rural | C | P |
| Benin | R | R | S | S | M | | | | ME or DO or MON | PC (LP) |
| Bermuda | S | S | | | | | | | | |
| Bhutan | R | R | S | | | S | | Southern districts | PC | * |
| Bolivia | R | R | S | | R | | | Amazon basin | ME or DO or MON | PC |
| | | | | | | | | Other rural areas below 2500 m | PC | ME or DO or MON |

(Continued)

Table 20.1 (*Continued*)

| Country | Typhoid | Hepatitis A | Rabies | Meningitis A | Yellow fever | Japanese B encephalitis | Tick-borne encephalitis | Malaria prophylaxis (➤214) Comments | Recommended regimen | Alternative regimen |
|---|---|---|---|---|---|---|---|---|---|---|
| Bosnia | S | R | S | | | | S | | | |
| Botswana | R | R | S | | | | | Northern half, Nov–June | PC | ME or DO or MON |
| Brazil | R | R | S | | R | | | Amazon basin, Mato Grosso & Maranhao | ME or DO or MON | PC |
| | | | | | | | | Elsewhere in Brazil | W | |
| Brunei | R | R | S | | | S | | | | |
| Bulgaria | S | R | S | | | | S | | | |
| Burkina Faso | R | R | S | S | M | | | | ME or DO or MON | PC (LP) |
| Burundi | R | R | S | S | R | | | | ME or DO or MON | PC (LP) |
| Cambodia | R | R | S | | | S | | Phnom Penh | W | * |
| | | | | | | | | Western provinces | DO or MON | * |
| | | | | | | | | Elsewhere | ME or DO or MON | PC (LP) |
| Cameroon | R | R | S | S | M | | | | ME or DO or MON | PC (LP) |
| Canada | | | S | | | | | | | |
| Cape Verde | R | R | S | | | | | | W | |
| Cayman Islands | S | R | | | | | | | | |
| Central African Rep. | R | R | S | S | M | | | | ME or DO or MON | PC (LP) |
| Chad | R | R | S | S | R | | | | ME or DO or MON | PC (LP) |
| Chile | S | R | S | | | | | | | |
| China (Mainland) | R | R | S | | | S | | Main tourist areas | W | |
| | | | | | | | | Yunnan and Hainan | ME or DO or MON | PC |
| | | | | | | | | Remote rural areas | C | P |
| China (Hong Kong) | S | S | | | | | | | | |
| China (Macau) | R | R | | | | | | | | |
| Colombia | R | R | S | | R | S | | Below 800 m | ME or DO or MON | PC |
| Comoros | R | R | | S | | | | | ME or DO or MON | PC (LP) |
| Congo | R | R | S | S | M | | | | ME or DO or MON | PC (LP) |
| Congo Dem. Rep. (Zaire) | R | R | S | S | M | | | | ME or DO or MON | PC (LP) |

| Country | | | | | | | |
|---|---|---|---|---|---|---|---|
| Cook Islands | R | | | | | | |
| Costa Rica | R | S | | | Rural below 500 m | C | P |
| Croatia | S | S | | | | | |
| Cuba | R | S | | | | | |
| Cyprus | S | | | | | | |
| Czech Republic | S | | | | | | |
| Djibouti | R | S | | | | ME or DO or MON | PC (LP) |
| Dominica | R | | | | | | |
| Dominican Republic | R | S | | | | C | P |
| East Timor | R | S | S | | | ME or DO or MON | * |
| Ecuador | R | S | R | | Below 1500 m (no risk in Galapagos Is., Quito) | PC | ME or DO or MON |
| | | | | | Esmereldas province | ME or DO or MON | PC |
| Egypt | R | S | | | | | |
| | | | | | El Faiyum Jun–Oct | C | P |
| | | | | | Elsewhere | W | |
| El Salvador | R | S | | | | C | P |
| Equatorial Guinea | R | S | R | | | ME or DO or MON | PC (LP) |
| Eritrea | R | S | | | No risk in Asmara | ME or DO or MON | PC (LP) |
| Estonia | S | S | | | | | |
| Ethiopia | R | S | R | S | Below 2200 m (no risk in Addis Ababa) | ME or DO or MON | PC (LP) |
| Fiji | R | | | | | | |
| Finland | | | | | | | |
| French Guiana | R | S | M | S | | ME or DO or MON | PC |
| French Polynesia | R | S | | | | | |
| Gabon | R | S | M | S | | ME or DO or MON | PC (LP) |
| Gambia | R | S | R | S | | ME or DO or MON | PC (LP) |
| Georgia | S | S | | | Jul–Oct | C | P |
| Germany | | | | | | | |
| Ghana | R | S | M | S | | ME or DO or MON | PC (LP) |
| Greece | S | | | | | | |
| Greenland | S | | | | | | |
| Grenada | S | S | | | | | |
| Guam | R | | | | | | |
| Guatemala | R | S | | | Below 1500 m | C | P |

*(Continued)*

**Table 20.1** (*Continued*)

| Country | Typhoid | Hepatitis A | Rabies | Meningitis A | Yellow fever | Japanese B encephalitis | Tick-borne encephalitis | Comments | Malaria prophylaxis (>214) Recommended regimen | Alternative regimen |
|---|---|---|---|---|---|---|---|---|---|---|
| Guinea | R | R | S | S | R | | | | ME or DO or MON | PC (LP) |
| Guinea-Bissau | R | R | S | S | R | | | | ME or DO or MON | PC (LP) |
| Guyana | R | R | S | | R | | | | ME or DO or MON | PC |
| Haiti | R | R | S | | | | | | C | P |
| Honduras | R | R | S | | | | | | C | P |
| Hungary | | S | | | | | S | | | |
| India | R | R | S | | | S | | No risk in mountain states | PC | * |
| Indonesia | R | R | S | | | S | | Irian Jaya, Lombok | ME or DO or MON | PC |
| | | | | | | | | Bali and cities, Java | W | |
| | | | | | | | | Elsewhere in Indonesia | PC | |
| Iran | R | R | S | | | | | | PC | ME or DO or MON |
| Iraq | R | R | S | | | | | | PC | * |
| | | | | | | | | Rural north and Basrah Province, May–Nov | C | P |
| Israel | S | R | S | | | | | | | |
| Italy | | S | | | | | | | | |
| Ivory Coast | R | R | S | S | M | | | | ME or DO or MON | PC (LP) |
| Jamaica | S | R | | | | | | | | |
| Japan | | R | | | | S | S | | | |
| Jordan | R | R | S | | | | | | | |
| Kazakhstan | R | R | S | | | S | S | | | |
| Kenya | R | R | S | S | R | | | | ME or DO or MON | PC (LP) |
| Kiribati | R | R | | | | | | | | |
| Korea (N. and S.) | S | R | S | | | S | | | | |
| Kuwait | S | R | | | | | | | | |
| Kyrgyzstan | R | R | S | | | | S | | | |
| Laos | R | R | S | | | S | | Minimal risk in Vientiane | ME or DO or MON | * |
| Latvia | S | R | S | | | | S | | | |
| Lebanon | S | R | | | | | S | | | |

| Country | | | | | | Area / timing | Malaria | |
|---|---|---|---|---|---|---|---|---|
| Lesotho | R | R | S | | | | ME or DO or MON | PC (LP) |
| Liberia | R | R | S | | | | W | |
| Libya | R | R | S | | S | | | |
| Lithuania | S | R | S | | S | | | |
| Macedonia | R | R | S | | | | | |
| Madagascar | R | R | S | | | | ME or DO or MON | PC (LP) |
| Malawi | R | R | S | | | | ME or DO or MON | PC (LP) |
| Malaysia | R | R | S | | S | | ME or DO or MON | PC |
| | | | | | | Sabah | PC | |
| | | | | | | Deep forests of Malaysia | W | |
| | | | | | | Sarawak and elsewhere in Malaysia | | |
| Maldives | R | R | S | M | | | ME or DO or MON | PC (LP) |
| Mali | R | R | S | M | | | ME or DO or MON | |
| Martinique | R | S | S | | | | | |
| Mauritania | R | R | S | M | | All year in S; N Jul–Oct | PC | |
| | | | | | | Rural areas | C | |
| | | | | | | Elsewhere | W | |
| Mauritius | R | R | S | | | | P | |
| Mayotte | R | R | S | | | | ME or DO or MON | PC (LP) |
| | | | | | | Main tourist areas | W | |
| Mexico | R | R | S | | | Rural areas | C | P |
| Moldova | S | R | S | | S | | | |
| Mongolia | R | R | S | | | | | |
| Montenegro | S | R | S | | S | | | |
| Montserrat | R | R | S | | | | | |
| Morocco | R | R | S | | | | W | |
| Mozambique | R | R | S | | | | ME or DO or MON | PC (LP) |
| Myanmar (Burma) | R | R | S | | S | | ME or DO or MON | * |
| Namibia | R | R | S | | S | Northern third only, Nov–Jun; all year along Kavango and Kunene rivers | PC | ME or DO or MON |
| Nauru | R | | | | | | | |
| Nepal | R | R | S | | S | Below 1300 m (no risk in Kathmandu) | PC | * |
| Netherlands, Antilles | S | R | | | | | | |

(Continued)

**Table 20.1** (*Continued*)

| Country | Typhoid | Hepatitis A | Rabies | Meningitis A | Yellow fever | Japanese B encephalitis | Tick-borne encephalitis | Malaria prophylaxis (≥ 214) Comments | Recommended regimen | Alternative regimen |
|---|---|---|---|---|---|---|---|---|---|---|
| New Caledonia | R | R | | | | | | | | |
| Nicaragua | R | R | S | | | | | | C | P |
| Niger | R | R | S | S | M | | | | ME or DO or MON | PC (LP) |
| Nigeria | R | R | S | S | R | | | | ME or DO or MON | PC (LP) |
| Niue | R | R | | | | | | | | |
| Norway | | | | | | | S | | | |
| Oman | R | R | S | | | | | Rural areas only | PC | * |
| Pakistan | R | R | S | | | S | | Below 2000 m | PC | * |
| Panama | R | R | S | | R | | | East of canal | PC | ME or DO or MON |
| | | | | | | | | West of canal | C | P |
| Papua New Guinea | R | R | S | | | S | | Below 1800 m | ME or DO or MON | MPM + C |
| Paraguay | R | R | S | | S | | | Rural areas, Oct–May | C | P |
| Peru | R | R | S | | R | | | Amazon basin | ME or DO or MON | PC |
| | | | | | | | | Other rural areas below 1500 m | PC | ME or DO or MON |
| Philippines | R | R | S | | | S | | Rural areas below 600 m | PC | ME or DO or MON |
| | | | | | | | | Cebu, Leyte, Bohol, Catanduanes and metropolitan Manila | W | |
| Pitcairn Islands | S | R | | | | | | | | |
| Poland | S | S | S | | | | S | | | |
| Portugal | S | S | | | | | | | | |
| Puerto Rico | R | R | S | | | | | | | |
| Qatar | R | R | S | | | | | | | |
| Reunion | R | R | | | | | | | | |
| Romania | S | R | S | | | | S | | | |
| Russian Federation | S | R | S | | S | | S | | | |
| Rwanda | R | R | S | S | M | | | | ME or DO or MON | PC (LP) |

| Country | | | | | | Area | | |
|---|---|---|---|---|---|---|---|---|
| St Helena | S | R | | | | | | |
| St Kitts and Nevis | S | R | | | | | | |
| St Lucia | S | R | | | | | | |
| St Vincent & Grenadines | S | R | | | | | | |
| Samoa | R | R | S | M | | | | |
| São Tomé and Principe | R | R | S | S | | | ME or DO or MON | PC (LP) |
| Saudi Arabia (≥193) | S | R | S/M | | | Western border cities, N, E, central provinces, Asir plateau | W | PC |
| | | | | | | Elsewhere | | * |
| Senegal | R | R | S | R | | | ME or DO or MON | PC (LP) |
| Serbia | S | R | S | | S | | | |
| Seychelles | R | R | S | | | | | |
| Sierra Leone | R | R | S | R | | | ME or DO or MON | PC (LP) |
| Singapore | S | S | S | | | | | |
| Slovakia | S | S | S | | S | | | |
| Slovenia | S | R | S | | S | | | |
| Solomon Islands | R | R | S | | | | ME or DO or MON | MPM+C |
| Somalia | R | R | S | | | | ME or DO or MON | PC (LP) |
| South Africa | R | R | S | R | | NE, low altitude areas of N province and Mpumalanga, and E KwaZulu-Natal down to 100 km N of Durban. Risk present in Kruger National Park | ME or DO or MON | PC (LP) |
| | | | | | | Elsewhere | W | |
| Spain | | | S | | S | | | |
| Sri Lanka | R | R | S | S | | No risk in Colombo | PC | * |
| Sudan | R | R | S | R | | | ME or DO or MON | PC (LP) |
| Surinam | R | R | S | R | | Except Paramaribo and coast | ME or DO or MON | PC |
| Swaziland | R | R | S | | | | ME or DO or MON | PC (LP) |

(Continued)

**Table 20.1** (*Continued*)

| Country | Typhoid | Hepatitis A | Rabies | Meningitis A | Yellow fever | Japanese B encephalitis | Tick-borne encephalitis | Malaria prophylaxis (>214) Comments | Recommended regimen | Alternative regimen |
|---|---|---|---|---|---|---|---|---|---|---|
| Sweden | | | | | | | S | | | |
| Switzerland | | | | | | | S | | | |
| Syria | R | R | S | | | | | Rural N May–Oct | C | P |
| Taiwan | S | R | | | | S | | | | |
| Tajikistan | R | R | S | | | | S | Jun–Oct | C | P |
| Tanzania | R | R | S | S | R | | | | ME or DO or MON | PC (LP) |
| Thailand | R | R | S | | | S | | Bangkok, tourist centres and rural areas away from borders | W | |
| | | | | | | | | Cambodian and Burmese border areas, Ko Chang | DO or MON | * |
| Togo | R | R | S | S | M | | | | ME or DO or MON | PC (LP) |
| Tonga | S | R | S | | | | | | | |
| Trinidad and Tobago | S | R | S | | S | | | | | |
| Tunisia | R | R | S | | | | | | | |
| Turkey | S | R | S | | | | | Antalya, Side, Alanya and east coast, plain around Adana, SE Anatolia, May–Oct (no risk west of Antalya) | C | P |
| Turkmenistan | R | R | S | | | | S | Jun–Oct | C | P |
| Turks and Caicos Islands | | R | | | | | | | | |
| Tuvalu | S | R | | | | | | | | |

| Country | | | | | | Malaria area | Prophylaxis | |
|---|---|---|---|---|---|---|---|---|
| Uganda | R | | S | S | R | | ME or DO or MON | PC (LP) |
| Ukraine | S | R | S | S | | | | |
| United Arab Emirates | S | R | S | | S | Rural N | PC | * |
| Uruguay | S | R | S | | | | | |
| USA | | | | | S | | | |
| Uzbekistan | R | R | S | | | | | |
| Vanuatu | R | R | | | | | ME or DO or MON | MPM + C |
| Venezuela | R | R | S | R | | Amazon basin | ME or DO or MON | PC |
| | | | | | | Rural (no risk in Caracas or Margarita) | PC | ME or DO or MON |
| Vietnam | R | S | R | | S | No risk in cities, Red River delta, coastal plain N of Nha Trang | ME or DO or MON | * |
| Virgin Islands | S | R | | | | | PC | * |
| Yemen | R | R | S | | | | ME or DO or MON | PC (LP) |
| Zambia | R | R | S | S | | | ME or DO or MON | PC (LP) |
| Zimbabwe | R | R | S | S | | Zambezi valley | ME or DO or MON | PC (LP) |
| | | | | | | Elsewhere below 1200 m Nov–Jun | PC | ME or DO or MON |
| | | | | | | Harare and Bulawayo | W | |

➤ Bradley, Communicable Dis Pub Health 2001; 4: 84

▢ www.phls.co.uk/advice/

▢ www.phls.co.uk/publications/CDPHVol4/No%202/malaria%20guidelinesp.pdf

*Immunizations:* M, immunization mandatory; R, immunization recommended; S, immunization recommended sometimes, e.g. >3 visits per year, prolonged stay in rural area, high-risk because of occupation or intended recreational activity, backpackers.

All travellers should have up-to-date immunity against diphtheria, polio and tetanus.

Immunization against hepatitis B (➤72) and BCG vaccination against tuberculosis (➤46) may be indicated in some travellers, depending on intended length and location of stay.

*Malaria prophylaxis:* For discussion of choice of agent, doses, adverse effects and contraindications ➤214. *Seek expert advice. C, chloroquine weekly. DO, doxycycline daily. ME, mefloquine weekly. MON, Malarone (atovaquone/proguanil) daily. MPM, Maloprim (pyrimethamine/dapsone) weekly. MPM + C, Maloprim + chloroquine weekly. P, proguanil daily. PC, proguanil daily, chloroquine weekly. W, No prophylaxis, but be aware of low risk of malaria. (LP) indicates that this alternative regimen gives only limited protection and is only for those who cannot tolerate one of the recommended first-line regimens.

# Chapter 21

# Tropical medicine and the returning traveller

This chapter gives advice on the diagnosis and management of ill health in travellers returning from the tropics, and describes some of the major tropical diseases worldwide. Some of the infections included for discussion are common in returning travellers (e.g. malaria, schistosomiasis). Others are rarely seen, but frequently enter the differential diagnosis of the febrile traveller (e.g. filariasis). Protozoal infections and helminths which occur less often are dealt with in Chapters 22 and 23.

## General approach to illness in the returning traveller

An individual's clinical presentation, the relative likelihood of different infections in the areas they have visited and the timing of their exposure with respect to their presentation must be taken into account when planning investigations and empirical therapy. Surveys suggest that ≈10% of travellers to developing countries suffer from severe, self-limiting diarrhoea, ≈1% catch *Giardia lamblia* or *Entamoeba histolytica*, and ≈0.1% develop malaria on their return. Other tropical protozoal and helminth infections are extremely rare.

### Fever

About 50% of returning travellers from the tropics have a 'conventional' cause and about 50% a tropical diagnosis.

**Malaria** (➤211) is common; *Plasmodium falciparum* infection is particularly likely in travellers from Africa within a few days of return. In non-immune patients, levels of parasitaemia are often low and one negative film is not conclusive. The typical pattern of cyclical fever is often absent early in disease. In general, patterns of fever are neither reliable nor useful aids to diagnosis.

The following **investigations** are recommended in all patients in whom the diagnosis is not clear, provided that there is no possibility of viral haemorrhagic fever (see below): three malaria films, full blood count, liver function tests, CXR, three blood cultures, MSU, stools for culture, cysts and parasites, serology for viral infections and rickettsia, USS or CT liver scan.

Apart from positive malarial films or bacterial cultures, the most useful pieces of information are the peripheral white cell count (WBC) and a detailed travel history, since many rickettsial and viral infections have a short and relatively predictable incubation period.

**Common presentations** (with common diagnoses highlighted in bold type) are shown in Table 21.1.

### Possible viral haemorrhagic fever

Patients who have a feverish illness, rash or sore throat within 3 weeks of having visited rural areas of West or Central Africa may have viral haemorrhagic fever (➤356). The likelihood of this is remote, whereas malaria is very likely and potentially fatal. In the last 20 yrs, there have been ≈10 cases of Lassa fever imported into the UK, with no secondary cases. All units admitting returning travellers should have policies in place to identify patients potentially at risk of VHF, primarily to avoid the possibility of secondary infection of ward staff, patients and particularly laboratory staff. The UK Department of Health have issued detailed guidance on assessment of returning travelers (*Memorandum on the Control of Viral Haemorrhagic Fevers*, 1998; available at

🖥 www.doh.gov.uk/pubs/docs/doh/vhf.pdf).

**Table 21.1** Commoner presentations of infection in the returning tropical traveller

| Diagnosis | Clues |
|---|---|
| **Acute fever with normal or reduced WBC** | |
| Malaria (➤211) | Cyclical high fever, response to quinine, thrombocytopenia |
| Typhoid/paratyphoid (➤280) | Severity of illness, persistent fever |
| Viral infections (e.g. dengue) (➤353) | Biphasic fever, myalgia, rash, thrombocytopenia |
| *Rickettsia* (➤329) | Rash, localized lymphadenopathy, eschar |
| Acute brucellosis (➤303) | Very rare |
| **Acute fever with raised WBC** | |
| Amoebic liver abscess (➤218) | Liver function often normal, hepatic tenderness often minimal —often diagnosed on USS liver scan |
| Leptospirosis (➤327) | Fever, neutrophilia, no localizing signs, conjunctivitis |
| Pyogenic infections (e.g. pneumonia, meningitis, cellulitis) | Localizing signs |
| **Chronic fever with normal/reduced WBC** | |
| Malaria (➤211) | |
| Disseminated tuberculosis (➤37) | |
| Visceral leishmaniasis (➤222) | |
| Brucellosis (➤303) | |
| **Chronic fever with eosinophilia** (➤184) | |
| Schistosomiasis (➤226) | |
| Fascioliasis | |
| Visceral larva migrans | |
| Filariasis | |

## Important clinical features of VHFs

**Incubation period** ranges from a few days to 3 weeks. Patients are not infectious before they develop symptoms. **Early clinical features** do not really help to distinguish VHF from other much more common causes of fever in the returning traveller. They include fever, cough, headache, myalgia, pharyngitis, sometimes with dysphagia and facial or neck oedema, nausea, vomiting, diarrhoea or constipation, abdominal and chest pain, and general weakness. Later symptoms include encephalopathy, hepatitis, haemorrhage and shock. Onset is usually insidious, and most patients are not severely unwell when they present. **Human-to-human transmission** is thought to depend on direct contact with the patient or infected secretions. Aerosol transmission (as opposed to respiratory droplet transmission) is not considered a significant route of transmission.

In the recent outbreak of Ebola in Zaire, transmission in hospital was interrupted by the use of gowns, masks and gloves.

Recovering patients continue to excrete virus in the urine for many weeks.

## Risk assessment

**The diagnosis of VHF should be considered in a patient who has:**
• Returned from tropical Africa or a VHF-endemic country within 3 weeks.
• Has a febrile illness.

All such persons should undergo risk assessment for VHF (Table 21.2)—immediate discussion with a local expert or referral centre is essential (contact your local clinical virologist or infectious diseases specialist first ☎). Lassa is endemic in Nigeria and Sierra Leone and has been reported from Liberia and Côte d'Ivoire,

**Table 21.2** Risk assessment of patients who may have viral haemorrhagic fever

| Risk | Criteria |
| --- | --- |
| Minimum | Not in a *known endemic area* |
| | or |
| | Onset >21 days after leaving endemic area |
| Moderate | In a known endemic area <21 days before onset (and no high-risk features) |
| | or |
| | Not in a known endemic area, but in adjacent area within 21 days and have severe illness with organ failure and/or haemorrhage which could be due to VHF |
| High | In a known endemic area <21 days before onset |
| | **and either** |
| | Stayed in house with case/suspected case |
| | or |
| | Nursed case/suspected case |
| | or |
| | Contact with fluids or body of case/suspected case |
| | or |
| | Lab worker in contact with fluids or body of case/suspected case |
| | or |
| | Were previously moderate-risk, but have developed severe illness with organ failure and/or haemorrhage which could be due to VHF |
| | Have not been in a known endemic area <21 days before onset, but have cared for or had contact with case/suspected case |
| | or |
| | Handled fluids or body of case/suspected case |

but VHF (Lassa or Ebola) has been reported from countries as far west as Sierra Leone and Côte d'Ivoire, and as far south as Gabon and Zaire. Between these limits, distribution is patchy—for example, there has never been a reported case of Lassa from Ghana. Some information on endemic areas can be found at the WHO collaborative information website (🖳 www.who.ch/wer), although at the time of writing there is no reliable Internet source for up-to-date maps of known endemic areas. There is always a chance that a patient will present from a previously unrecognized endemic focus or from a new epidemic.

## Immediate action

**No specimens should be sent from the patient until risk assessment has been completed.** If specimens have already been sent to laborato-ries, then medical staff should immediately inform the labs of the possibility of VHF so that samples may be stored and processed appropriately. In many cases, this will result in sample processing being postponed until risk assessment and malaria film examination have been performed. Staff taking blood samples or carrying out any invasive procedure, or disposing of excreta, must wear disposable gloves, plastic aprons (water-repellent gowns in the case of patients at moderate or high risk), face mask and a visor. Extreme care should be taken with disposal of sharps and contaminated equipment.

Subsequent actions depend on the initial risk assessment and subsequent clinical progress. Table 21.3 gives an indication of the required procedures, but in every case local protocols, based on DoH guidance, should be followed.

**Table 21.3** Summary of immediate action based on VHF risk assessment

| Risk* | Admission | Transport of specimens | Processing of specimens | Transport of patients |
|---|---|---|---|---|
| Minimum | If unwell, to standard isolation (single room, apron, gloves) | Standard procedures for transport; as for other blood-borne viruses | Processing in minimum containment level 2. Specimens should be tracked and their handling audited | Category II |
| Moderate | Isolation in room with controlled ventilation if available | Special precautions for obtaining specimens (gown, gloves, eye and face protection). Rigid packaging for transport to lab | Malaria film only. Processing in minimum containment level 3 | Category III |
| High | Isolation in room with controlled ventilation if available. Consider urgent transfer to high-security isolation unit (Newcastle, Coppetts Wood) | | Arrangements may be in place for preparation and decontamination of a film in containment level 3 facility followed by staining and examination in lower level of containment elsewhere | Category III |

*See Table 21.2.

## Management following initial assessment

Guidelines for subsequent management are outlined in Fig. 21.1. Most patients initially categorized as 'Moderate risk' will have malaria. If they do, they may be recategorized as 'minimum risk' pending a satisfactory response to anti-malarial therapy. If the initial malaria film is negative and the patient remains unwell, serious consideration should be given to urgent transfer to a high-security isolation unit. Patients initially categorized as 'high risk' who have a negative malarial film should be transferred as soon as possible.

Patients who recover clinically, with resolution of fever, who are not known to have VHF and who do not develop any new clinical signs suggestive of VHF such as haemorrhage or organ failure, are deemed non-infectious once they have been afebrile for 48 h.

Patients who do have VHF continue to excrete virus in their urine for many weeks after clinical recovery.

### Presentations to recognize

**Severe pneumonia on return from SE Asia:** Consider melioidosis, due to *Burkholderia pseudomallei* (➤293) esp. in diabetics. Ceftazidime is the agent of choice.

**Cyclical fever 3–6 months after return from malaria-endemic region:** Relapse of benign malaria: primaquine is required to eradicate hypnozoites (➤212).

## Diarrhoea in the returning traveller

About 50% of cases are bacterial. Certain clinical features allow an educated guess at the cause of diarrhoea. Diarrhoea of less than 2 weeks' duration may be due to any of the causes of infectious gastroenteritis (➤57), but may also be an epiphenomenon of malaria. Diarrhoea of greater than 2 weeks' duration with blood indicates a need to exclude *Entamoeba histolytica* (➤218) and schistosomiasis (➤226), as well as non-infectious causes such as inflamma-

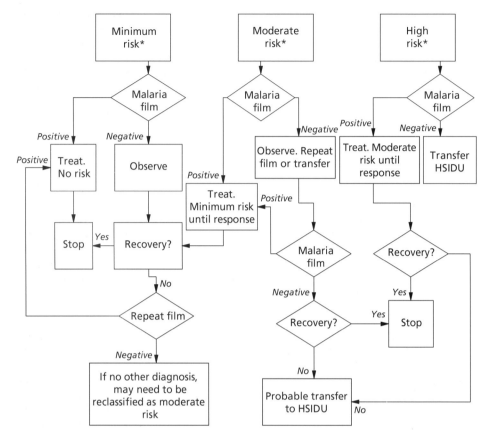

**Figure 21.1** Algorithm for viral haemorrhagic fever (VHF) assessment. *See Table 21.2. HSIDU, high-security infectious diseases unit.

tory bowel disease. Weight loss, with fever or steatorrhoea may indicate *Giardia lamblia* (≻218), sprue, mesenteric tuberculosis (≻40), visceral leishmaniasis (≻222), or other causes of malabsorption unrelated to travel. Diarrhoea and persistent eosinophilia are caused by schistosomiasis (≻226), strongyloidiasis (≻235), capillariasis (≻237), trichuriasis (≻235).

Symptoms of 'irritable bowel disease', with altered bowel habit, cramps and flatulence are common after infectious gastroenteritis, even after stool cultures are negative (e.g. ≈25% of patients at 6 months after salmonellosis), but investigations to exclude non-infectious causes are often indicated.

## Tropical sprue

A syndrome of malabsorption and wasting seen in expatriates resident in the tropics, probably due to bacterial overgrowth in the small intestine.

**Epidemiology:** Occurs in well-defined areas, including Indian subcontinent, SE Asia, northern countries of S. America, Haiti, Puerto Rico, Cuba and Dominican Republic. Rare in Africa.

**Clinical features:** Symptoms develop over months, usually after several years' residence in tropics. Often starts with an attack of acute diarrhoea. Anorexia, weight loss and chronic steatorrhoea. Folate and $B_{12}$ deficiency lead to megaloblastic anaemia. Hypoalbuminaemia may occur. Untreated sprue can persist for decades, even after return to temperate climate.

**Investigations:** Exclusion of other infections, e.g. *Giardia lamblia* (➤218), cryptosporidiosis (➤230) or *Cyclospora* spp. (➤231). Small-bowel biopsy shows minor degree of villous atrophy and submucosal cellular infiltrate.

**Management:** Folic acid 5 mg po daily, $B_{12}$, 1 mg im daily for three doses then monthly, tetracycline 250 mg po 6hly for several months until full recovery. This regimen is usually highly effective. Metronidazole is also often effective.

### Skin lesions
**Fever and a rash immediately on return:** viral infections (e.g. dengue ➤353), meningococcal septicaemia (➤185), other bacteraemias (including *Staphylococcus aureus*), viral haemorrhagic fevers (➤356), tick typhus and other rickettsial infections (➤329).

**Chronic skin lesions** include the ulcer of cutaneous leishmaniasis (➤223) and the serpiginous pruritic track of cutaneous larva migrans (➤236). Both are relatively common. Chronic infection of minor skin lesion by non-sporing anaerobes (esp. *Fusobacterium* spp.) and *Corynebacterium diphtheriae* occur rarely. Cutaneous mycoses are the commonest skin disorders acquired by travellers (➤117), including tinea versicolor, cruris and pedis.

**Cutaneous myiasis** from S. America (*Dermatobia* spp.) and Africa (*Cordylobia* spp., 'Tumbu fly'): adult female flies lay eggs on skin or clothes, following which the larva penetrates and develops under the skin to form a painful boil, in which the maggot-like larva can be felt moving. The larvae depend on air for respiration, and they 'breathe' through spiracles situated on one end, close to the opening of the boil. They can often be removed by occluding the orifice of the boil with petroleum jelly, which suffocates them and allows them to be grasped with forceps when they partially emerge in search of air. The S. American type can be very difficult to remove without resorting to minor surgery; they will eventually emerge spontaneously when mature. Secondary bacterial infection is common.

**Sand fleas** (*Tunga penetrans*, 'jiggers') invade the skin, especially around the toes, and may be removed with forceps.

**Scabies and lice** may be acquired when hygiene is poor.

## Malaria ✉

There are ≈1900 imported cases of malaria p.a. in the UK and ≈10 deaths p.a. Factors contributing to mortality are failure to consider the diagnosis, delay in starting therapy, failure to recognize the onset of severe complications and misplaced trust in the efficacy of prophylaxis and 'negative' blood films. *Plasmodium falciparum* accounts for ≈50% of cases.

🖥 www.malaria.org

**Epidemiology and transmission:** Malaria occurs throughout the tropics and subtropics, although some areas have achieved eradication. WHO estimates >$10^8$ cases/yr worldwide and >$10^6$ child deaths/yr in Africa alone. 90% of cases and deaths occur in sub-Saharan Africa. Four species of *Plasmodium* cause malaria in man (Table 21.4).

**Transmission** occurs by bite of the female *Anopheles* mosquito. Control programmes are aimed principally at eradication of the mosquito vector. Vertical, transfusion and organ-transplant transmission may occur.

**Life cycle:** The mosquito injects *sporozoites*, which rapidly attach to and enter liver cells. An asymptomatic period of 1–2 weeks follows, during which parasites mature and multiply within liver cells, forming *hepatic schizonts* ('exoerythrocytic' forms). These rupture, releasing *merozoites*, which enter RBCs and mature and multiply through *ring* and *trophozoite* forms to become *schizonts*. This process takes 48h (72h for *P. malariae*), following which the schizonts rupture, releasing between 6 and 24 merozoites, depending on the species, which may then infect further RBCs. This cycle repeats, causing the well-recognized pattern

Table 21.4 *Plasmodium* spp. causing malaria in man

| Species | Disease | Areas of greatest prevalence | Key biological/clinical features |
|---|---|---|---|
| P. falciparum<br>Σ ≈ 1050 | Malignant tertian malaria | Worldwide. Predominant species in Africa. Common in SE Asia, S. America | Potentially fatal. Chloroquine resistance common |
| P. vivax<br>Σ ≈ 700 | Benign tertian malaria | Predominant species in Indian subcontinent. Common in Central/South America, SE Asia | Rarely severe. Late relapses can occur due to persistence in liver ('hypnozoites'). Chloroquine resistance previously rare, but chloroquine-resistant strains of P. vivax are emerging in SE Asia |
| P. ovale<br>Σ ≈ 130 | Ovale tertian malaria | Least common species. Mainly African | |
| P. malariae<br>Σ ≈ 20 | Quartan malaria | Widely distributed in Africa | Rarely severe. Causes nephrotic syndrome in children |

Table 21.5 Natural history of untreated malaria

| Species | Natural history of *untreated* infection |
|---|---|
| P. falciparum | If the patient survives the primary attack, there may be recrudescences at increasing intervals due to persistence of blood forms between attacks. These die out after ~1 year unless reinfection occurs |
| P. vivax, P. ovale | Relapses due to dormant liver forms ('hypnozoites') occur for up to 5 years |
| P. malariae | Recurrent fevers for many years (≤ 50 years). Anaemia and hepatosplenomegaly are common |

of cyclical fevers. Some merozoites develop in RBCs into sexual forms, *gametocytes*, which may be taken up by a biting mosquito. Sexual reproduction takes place in the mosquito, and the cycle is completed. Each stage in the life cycle for each species has a characteristic morphology which allows diagnosis and speciation.

*P. vivax* and *P. ovale* have hepatic schizonts which lie dormant in the liver and cause late relapse (*hypnozoites*) (Table 21.5).

**Pathogenesis:** Febrile episodes are related to schizont rupture. Only *P. falciparum* causes severe complications such as cerebral malaria. *P. falciparum* may infect RBCs of all ages (other species are restricted to RBCs at particular stages of development) and can therefore cause very high rates of parasitaemia (>1% of all RBCs). It also causes sequestration of infected RBCs in vascular beds, leading to severe disturbance of microcirculation. Anaemia is due to haemolysis, splenic sequestration and depressed erythropoiesis.

**Partial immunity** develops with repeated attacks but is lost rapidly without exposure (e.g. after emigration). Infection is usually only severe in children, non-immune travellers and pregnant women.

**Clinical features**

**Incubation time:** Primary attack: 7–30 days.

Relapse of *P. vivax* or *P. ovale*: up to 1 yr, typically 38 weeks. Seventy-five per cent of *falciparum* cases present within 1 month of exposure, and 90% within 2 months.

**Symptoms and signs:** There may be a short prodrome mimicking viral infection with malaise and fatigue. Paroxysmal fever is the cardinal symptom. Patients typically notice three stages: shivering with rigors; then flushed and pyrexial for several hours; finally, drenched in sweat as the fever resolves. The typical pattern of cyclical fever takes $\geq 1$ week to develop and is unusual in patients in the UK. Hyperpyrexia may occur, and occasionally patients with severe falciparum malaria may be apyrexial ($\approx 20\%$ in some series). On examination, anaemia and jaundice due to haemolysis may be detectable clinically. Tachycardia with flow murmur, hepatosplenomegaly and abdominal tenderness are common. Respiratory distress has recently been recognized as in important indicator of severity, particularly in children. Many cases have potentially misleading symptoms such as diarrhoea, abdominal pain and cough.

**Complications:** These occur almost exclusively with *P. falciparum* and are common and severe only in non-immune patients, i.e. children, travellers and pregnant women. **Cerebral malaria** presents with disturbed level of consciousness, fits, and less often focal neurological deficits, progressing to coma and death. Mortality is $\approx 20$–$50\%$. It is usually, but not always, associated with heavy parasitaemia. Patients who survive usually have full recovery of neurological function. Pathogenesis is related to sequestration of parasitized RBCs in cerebral circulation, but exact mechanism remains controversial. Cerebral oedema is not a feature and steroids are **not** indicated. **Renal failure** occurs due to acute tubular necrosis secondary to hypovolaemia and shock and occasionally massive haemolysis and haemoglobinuria ('blackwater fever'). **Hypoglycaemia** is common, due to glucose use by parasites, impaired hepatic gluconeogenesis and stimulation of insulin secretion by quinine. It is particularly severe in patients with cerebral malaria or receiving intravenous quinine. **Adult respiratory distress syndrome** presents with tachypnoea and bilateral interstitial shadowing on CXR. Similar appearances may be due to fluid overload and diagnosis and management depend on haemodynamic monitoring of fluid status. **Algid malaria** describes septic shock due to Gram-negative bacteraemia complicating severe malaria. **Thrombocytopenia** is very common, but significant bleeding and disseminated intravascular coagulation occur only rarely.

*P. malariae* causes severe nephrotic syndrome in children, which rarely resolves after antimalarial treatment.

**Malaria in pregnancy** is often more severe, even in patients who would otherwise have partial immunity. Severe haemolytic anaemia may occur and hypoglycaemia is more frequent. There is increased risk of fetal death, small birth weight and prematurity, attributable to placental microcirculatory damage. Mefloquine and halofantrine are relatively contraindicated in pregnancy, but chloroquine and quinine may be given safely. **Congenital malaria** occurs rarely, more often due to *P. vivax* than *P. falciparum*. It presents as progressive haemolytic anaemia, and should be treated as appropriate for the species involved, with the exception that primaquine is not required, because the fetus is infected by blood forms which cannot re-enter the liver.

**Investigations:** Anaemia, thrombocytopenia and leucopenia are common. Prolonged coagulation tests and positive fibrin degradation products suggest DIC, which is often due to secondary Gram-negative septicaemia, probably secondary to gut microvascular damage. Diagnosis of malaria is made by examination of **thick and thin blood films** processed using special stains (Field's, Leishman's, Giemsa).

Thin films comprise a single layer of RBCs; parasite morphology is preserved, so it is possible to determine species reliably, but many high-power fields may have to be examined. Thick films are made by allowing a thick smear of blood to dry. RBCs are then lysed, leaving parasites concentrated in a small area. This allows more rapid diagnosis of malaria, but parasite morphology is damaged and it may not be possible to determine species. If in doubt, *P. falciparum* infection should be assumed. In expert hands, smears done on the first blood sample are 98% sensitive for detecting true cases of malaria. At least three negative films taken at intervals are required to exclude malaria, particularly as levels of parasitaemia fall between febrile paroxysms. New methods of detecting parasites based on immunological and molecular technology are available (e.g. based on detection of histidine-rich protein 2 (HRP-2)), but at present microscopy remains the gold standard and the only method in widespread use. **Serology** is not used for the diagnosis of acute illness, but is sometimes helpful in ex-cluding malaria as a cause of recurrent fever, e.g. in old soldiers.

## Management
## Prevention of malaria

The incidence of malaria is reduced, but not eliminated, by bite avoidance (➤191) and by chemoprophylaxis. Appropriate regimens are shown in Table 21.6 and in the country-by-country guide (see Table 20.1). Individual advice on antimalarial prophylaxis must take into account a wide range of factors beyond the geographical itinerary, including type of trip (e.g. rural vs. urban), standard of accommodation, intended activities, previous medical and psychiatric history, other medications and possible pregnancy. 25% of travellers taking antimalarial prophylaxis report side effects. Backpackers and travellers visiting friends and relations in malarious areas are at particular risk of infection. Consideration should also be given to providing standby medication (➤195). Emigrants to non-malarious areas may not realize they have lost their partial immunity, and it is important for this group to receive guidance on prophylaxis and avoidance of mosquito bites before they return to their countries of origin for short visits.

### ANTIMALARIAL PROPHYLAXIS IN PREGNANCY
Malaria is more severe in pregnancy (➤213), and prophylaxis is essential. Chloroquine and proguanil are safe, but mefloquine, doxycycline and Malarone are contraindicated. Fansidar is relatively contraindicated. **The best advice to a pregnant woman is not to travel to areas of chloroquine resistance.** If proguanil is given, folate supplements should also be given. Maloprim is contraindicated in the first trimester. If used later in pregnancy, give folate supplements.

### ANTIMALARIAL PROPHYLAXIS FOR CHILDREN
Doxycycline and Malarone are not licensed for use in children. Doses for other agents are shown in Table 21.7.

## Treatment of malaria

Chloroquine resistance in *P. falciparum* has been reported from almost all areas except the Middle East and North Africa, and all patients returning to the UK with *P. falciparum* should be assumed to have chloroquine-resistant malaria. The other species are usually susceptible, although there is chloroquine-resistant *P. vivax* in SE Asia. Fansidar resistance is now widespread in Africa and SE Asia.

**Currently available antimalarials** are described in Table 21.8.

**Artemisinins**, derived from the Chinese herbal medicine qinghaosu, are not currently licensed in the UK, although a number of preparations are available worldwide. These preparations are highly effective and well tolerated, and resistance is uncommon so far. WHO has promoted the use of artemisinins in combination with other antimalarials in an effort to prevent development of resistance (artemisinin combination therapy, ACT), although this may be too expensive for widespread use in the developing world. **Lumefantrine** is a novel drug related to halofantrine, and a combination preparation with artemether (coartemether, Riamet) is now available. Artemisinins are only

**Table 21.6** Antimalaria prophylaxis regimens. See Table 20.1 for country-by-country recommendations

| Code | Drug | Dose | Comments |
|------|------|------|----------|
| MON | Malarone (atovaquone 250 mg/ proguanil 100 mg) | One tablet daily | Not licensed for children or for stays over 1 month. Contraindicated in pregnancy. Start 2 days before departure, continue for 7 days after return. Avoid in renal failure |
| ME | Mefloquine 250 mg | One tablet weekly | Significant adverse effects and contraindications (➤217). Contraindicated in pregnancy. Start 3 weeks prior to departure and continue for 4 weeks after return |
| DO | Doxycycline 100 mg | One capsule daily | Not for children under 12 y, in pregnancy, or for stays over 3 months. Start 1 week prior to travel and continue for 4 weeks after return |
| P | Proguanil 200 mg | Two 100 mg tablets daily | Start 1 week prior to travel and continue for 4 weeks after return. GI upset, rarely mouth ulcers. Reduce dose in renal failure 📄 |
| C | Chloroquine 300 mg base | Avloclor (2 × 250 mg) or Nivaquine (2 × 200 mg) weekly | Start 1 week prior to travel and continue for 4 weeks after return |
| PC | Proguanil and choloroquine, both at dose/interval shown above | | Start 1 week prior to travel and continue for 4 weeks after return |
| MPM | Maloprim (pyrimethamine 12.5 mg/dapsone 100 mg) | One tablet weekly | Contraindicated in first trimester of pregnancy (➤214). Start 1 week prior to travel and continue for 4 weeks after return. Skin rash, myelotoxicity |
| MPM+C | Maloprim plus choroquine in doses given above | | Contraindicated in first trimester of pregnancy (➤214). Start 1 week prior to travel and continue for 4 weeks after return |

available in the UK on a named patient basis through national specialist centres (➤196).

**Specific recommendations for treatment:**

**Non-falciparum malaria:** Chloroquine 600 mg oral stat (four tablets of Avloclor or Nivaquine), then 300 mg after 6 h, then 300 mg q24h for 2 days. (Children 10 mg/kg initially, then 5 mg/kg.) If patient unable to swallow, slow iv infusion of 10 mg/kg over 8 h may be given, followed by oral therapy if possible or a further 15 mg/kg iv over 24 h. Failure to clear parasitaemia should raise the question of mixed infection with *P. falciparum* or chloroquine resistance, and quinine should be substituted — see below. After chloroquine treatment for *P. vivax* and *P. ovale*, give primaquine 15 mg 24hly for 15 days (21 days for travellers from SE Asia) to destroy hypnozoites. Check glucose-6-phosphate dehydrogenase (G6PD) levels, as primaquine causes haemolysis in G6PD deficiency. Primaquine is also contraindicated in pregnancy. In pregnancy or G6PD deficiency, give chloroquine 300 mg weekly for 6 months instead of primaquine.

**Uncomplicated falciparum malaria** (see below for definition of 'complicated'): quinine (sulphate, hydrochloride or dihydrochloride) 600 mg 8hly for 7 days (child 10 mg/kg 8hly) fol-

Table 21.7 Doses of antimalarials for **prophylaxis** in children (dose in parentheses indicates standard tablet size)

| Weight (kg) | Chloroquine (150 mg base) Proguanil (100 mg) | Mefloquine (250 mg) | Maloprim (one tablet) | Approximate age |
|---|---|---|---|---|
| <6 | 0.125 adult dose $^1/_4$ tablet | Not recommended | Not recommended | Term to 12 wks |
| 6–9.9 | 0.25 adult dose $^1/_2$ tablet | 0.25 adult dose $^1/_4$ tablet | Not feasible | 3–11 months |
| 10–15.9 | 0.375 adult dose $^3/_4$ tablet | 0.25 adult dose $^1/_4$ tablet | Not feasible | 1–3 yrs |
| 16–24.9 | 0.5 adult dose 1 tablet | 0.5 adult dose $^1/_2$ tablet | 0.5 adult dose $^1/_2$ tablet | 4 to 7 yrs |
| 25–44.9 | 0.75 adult dose $1^1/_2$ tablets | 0.75 adult dose $^3/_4$ tablet | 0.75 adult dose $^3/_4$ tablet | 8–12 yrs |
| >45 | Adult dose 2 tablets | Adult dose 1 tablet | Adult dose 1 tablet | 13 yrs and over |

Weight is the preferred guide to dosage.
Doxycycline is only given >12 yrs; adult dose of 100 mg is given, as capsule cannot be divided.
Malarone is not licensed for use in children.

lowed by doxycycline 200 mg q24h for 7 days. Fansidar (pyrimethamine/sulfadoxine), three tablets stat, is an alternative to doxycycline, particularly for children (see BNF for child doses). Dose of quinine may be reduced to 12hly if side effects (esp. tinnitus) are severe. Serial blood films are recommended to follow response to therapy, although a rise in parasitaemia on the first day of treatment is not uncommon and does not indicate treatment failure.

Alternative regimens: mefloquine 10 mg/kg (max. 700 mg) two doses 6 h apart (child >15 kg and <45 kg, 12.5 mg/kg two doses 6 h apart). Contraindicated in pregnancy, in patients on β-blockers, in neurological disease including epilepsy. **Or** Malarone four tablets q24h for 3 days. Both are contraindicated in pregnancy.

**Complicated falciparum malaria.** This is defined by the presence of one of the following complications: impaired conscious level, renal failure, respiratory distress syndrome, haemorrhage, severe anaemia, shock, haemoglobinuria, hypoglycaemia, fits, prostration, parasitaemia >2%, jaundice, hyperpyrexia or continued vomiting. Quinine dihydrochloride

20 mg/kg (max 1.4 g) loading dose, infused over 4 h, then after 8–12 h, maintenance dose of 10 mg/kg (max 700 mg) infused over 4 h every 8 h until patient can swallow oral quinine **plus** fansidar or doxycycline as above under uncomplicated falciparum malaria. Omit loading dose if patient has received quinine or mefloquine in preceding 24 h.

**Supportive management:** Patients with severe malaria should be monitored as closely as possible, and this usually means transfer to a high-dependency or intensive-therapy unit. Meticulous attention should be paid to fluid balance. Blood glucose should be monitored frequently, because hypoglycaemia is a frequent and serious adverse effect of quinine in this situation. Patients with cerebral malaria should receive prophylactic anticonvulsants (e.g. phenytoin, 10 mg/kg iv over 30 min with ECG monitoring, then 100 mg t.d.s. orally or iv, check levels early). IV diazepam may be necessary if fits occur. ECG should be monitored for rhythm and QT interval. Check $Ca^+$, $Mg^+$, and correct if low, esp. if QT prolonged. Transfusion is not usually required, but may be given if Hb

**Table 21.8** Features of individual antimalarial drugs

| Drug | Chloroquine | Quinine | Mefloquine | Malarone | Fansidar | Primaquine | Halofantrine |
|---|---|---|---|---|---|---|---|
| Formulation | Avloclor (chloroquine phosphate 250 mg ≡155 mg base) Nivaquine (chloroquine sulphate 200 mg ≡150 mg base) | Quinine sulphate 200 mg and 300 mg tablets are usually supplied. Quinine dihydrochloride for iv infusion | 250 mg tablet | Proguanil 100 mg/ atovaquone 250 mg | Pyrimethamine 25 mg/ sulfadoxine 500 mg | 7.5 mg tablet | 250 mg tablet Unlicensed in UK, and not currently recommended |
| **Treatment dose** | | | | | | | |
| Adults | 4 tablets (600 mg base) stat, 2 tablets after 6 h, then 2 tablets q24h for 2 days (➤215) | 600 mg q8h oral for 7 days. iv: 20 mg/kg loading dose, then 10 mg/kg q8h (for cautions ➤216) | 20–25 mg/kg (max 1.5 g) as single-dose or in 2 divided doses 8 h apart | 4 tablets q24h for 3 days | Not recommended for treatment on its own | 15 mg q24h for 14–21 days, after appropriate course of chloroquine | 500 mg q6h for 3 doses. Repeat after 1 week |
| Children | 10 mg/kg initially, then 5 mg/kg at intervals as above | Oral dose = 10 mg/kg iv doses as above | As above | 11–20 kg: 1 tablet 21–30 kg: 2 tablets 31–40 kg: 3 tablets | | 250 µg/kg q24h for 14–21 days | <40 kg: 8 mg/kg q6h as above |
| Important side effects | GI upset, headache, retinal damage and cataracts, rarely myelotoxicity, psychosis | Tinnitus, hypoglycaemia (particularly with iv infusion), headaches, flushing, GI upset, rash, myelotoxicity. Very toxic in overdose | GI upset. Neuropsychiatric effects, including neuropathy, mood disorder, hallucinations, psychosis. Arrhythmia, hypotension. Rash | GI upset, insomnia, rash | Skin rash, myelotoxicity | GI upset, haemolysis, particularly in G6PD deficiency—check status before dosing | GI upset, pruritus, transient elevation of serum transaminases. Serious prolongation of QT, so **must not be coadministered with mefloquine** (leave 28-day gap). |
| Contraindicated in | | | Pregnancy, breast feeding, neurological disease, concurrent β-blocker therapy | Pregnancy, breast feeding | Pregnancy, breast feeding | Pregnancy, breast feeding | Pregnancy, previous cardiac disease, concurrent β-blockers or mefloquine |
| Comments | Resistance is widespread, but still mainly confined to P. falciparum. Not active against dormant hepatic forms ('hypnozoites') of P. vivax and P. ovale | Agent of choice for treatment of chloroquine-resistant or severe P. falciparum malaria | Prophylaxis and treatment of chloroquine-resistant P. falciparum malaria | Not licensed for prophylaxis in children | An alternative to doxycycline for eradication of P. falciparum infection after quinine, e.g. in children | Eradication of dormant hepatic forms ('hypnozoites') of P. vivax and P. ovale | Treatment of uncomplicated P. falciparum infection |

<8 g/dL (adults) or <5 g/dL (children), particularly if there is respiratory distress or metabolic acidosis.

**Exchange transfusion** has been advocated for patients with very heavy parasitaemia (≥10%) but there has been no controlled trial and indications for its use are not yet defined. It should be combined with intensive monitoring, optimal drug therapy, and continued until parasitaemia <5%.

⊶ Winstanley, Lancet Inf Dis 2001; 1: 242

# Intestinal protozoa causing diarrhoea in the returning traveller

## Giardia lamblia

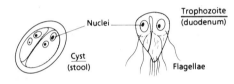

**Epidemiology and transmission:** Worldwide, but much commoner in developing countries. Transmission occurs by contaminated water and food, and by direct person-to-person contact. Mammalian reservoirs are often important in local epidemiology, e.g. by contaminating water supplies. Σ >6000.

**Life cycle:** *Giardia lamblia* has two stages. The flagellated motile trophozoite is fragile and cannot survive outside the host; the chitin-walled cyst is the infective stage, and can survive in the environment, particularly in moist cool conditions. Cysts are highly infectious — the infectious dose is estimated at between 10 and 100 cysts. After ingestion, cysts develop into trophozoites in the duodenum and small intestine, where they adhere to gut epithelial cells and multiply by binary fission. Tissue invasion is very rare, but cholecystitis and granulomatous hepatitis have been reported.

### Clinical features
**Incubation time:** 1–3 weeks.
**Symptoms and signs:** Infection is often asymptomatic. Diarrhoea is the primary symptom, with bulky, pale, offensive stools, but no blood.

Anorexia, nausea, abdominal bloating and low-grade fever may occur. Tiredness may be a prominent feature. Arthralgia, myalgia, urticaria and eosinophilia are rare; 30–50% progress to chronic diarrhoea, of whom ≈50% develop malabsorption, which may be severe, particularly in malnourished or immuno-deficient patients, especially those with hypogammaglobulinaemia.

**Investigations:** Stool microscopy for cysts is positive in ≈80% of patients if three samples are examined. Trophozoites may be seen in duodenal juice or biopsy material obtained at endoscopy. Apart from the presence of trophozoites, duodenal histology is usually normal. In the 'hairy string test', the patient swallows the end of a string which passes into the duodenum, before being pulled back and examined for parasites. Immunological tests for the detection of *Giardia lamblia* antigens in stools are being developed.

**Management:** Metronidazole 2 g 24hly for 3 days or 400 mg 8hly for 5 days. Treatment failure is common (≈10%). The course should be repeated, and reinfection from family members or contaminated water sources excluded. Persistent symptoms may indicate lactose intolerance rather than persistent infection; for true persistent infection, albendazole (400 mg or 22.5 mg/kg oral q24h for 5 days) or mepacrine (100 mg q8h for 7 days) are useful second-line agents.

## Entamoeba histolytica ✉ ②

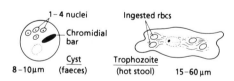

**Epidemiology and transmission:** Worldwide: ≈10% of the world's population are chronically infected, mainly in underdeveloped countries. Infection is unusual in the UK, except in returning travellers, male homosexuals and residents of institutions. Σ ≈1000. Amoebiasis is a relatively rare cause of travellers' diarrhoea, and infection is uncommon in travellers who have spent less than a month in an endemic area.

Life cycle: *Entamoeba histolytica* exists in two forms. The motile trophozoite is responsible for clinical disease, but is incapable of surviving outside the host. Trophozoites develop into cysts in the colon. The cyst form may survive in the environment for weeks and is responsible for transmission. Some 90% of carriage of *Entamoeba histolytica* is asymptomatic, and carriage of morphologically identical non-pathogenic strains of *Entamoeba dispar* is also common; *E. dispar* was previously thought to represent a non-pathogenic strain of *E. histolytica*. These species were initially distinguished by isoenzyme electrophoresis, but molecular methods are now available to confirm that they are genetically distinct. *Entamoeba histolytica* adheres to colonic epithelium and invades it directly, causing lysis of mucosal cells.

### Clinical features

Incubation time: Variable, from a few days to months. Commonly 2–4 weeks.

Symptoms and signs: Infection may be **asymptomatic** or cause only mild diarrhoea and colicky abdominal pain ('non-invasive disease'). Epithelial invasion causes **amoebic dysentery**, an acute rectocolitis with abdominal pain, tenderness and bloody diarrhoea. Constitutional symptoms are few; fever occurs in ≈30%. Immunosuppressed patients, children or pregnant women are at risk of developing **fulminant amoebic colitis**, which may cause perforation or toxic megacolon. Chronic localized invasive disease, usually in the right colon, causes an inflammatory mass, an **amoeboma**, which resembles colonic carcinoma on barium enema, but responds rapidly to amoebicidal therapy. **Amoebic liver abscess** (ALA) presents with weight loss, fever, right upper quadrant pain and tenderness. In returning travellers to the UK, it usually develops 2–5 months after exposure, and there is often no history of dysentery. Symptoms and signs may be minimal, and jaundice is rare. Untreated, ALA grows until it ruptures either through skin, diaphragm, pericardium (rarely) or into peritoneal cavity, causing acute abdominal pain. Metastasis to brain and lung may occur rarely. **Cutaneous amoebiasis** is a rare complication that develops from sites of skin exposure to amoebae, such as ALA rupture site or perianal region, causing progressive destructive and sometimes extensive ulceration.

Investigations: **stool microscopy** for cysts and trophozoites. In amoebic dysentery, stools contain blood but few pus cells. Motile trophozoites containing red blood cells are usually seen. Diarrhoea from other causes (e.g. bacterial dysentery) may accelerate gut transit time, resulting in the presence of amoebae in stools of patients who were previously asymptomatically passing cysts, but the characteristic sign of invasive amoebiasis is ingestion of red blood cells by amoebae. In asymptomatic infection, cysts are seen in ≈30%; at least three samples should be examined to exclude carriage. Examination of stools for cysts is only relevant in patients who have left the endemic area. In ALA, stools are positive for cysts or trophozoites in ≈20%.

**Antigen testing** for detection of *Entamoeba histolytica* in stools is becoming available.

Serology: Many methods exist for demonstrating antibodies; currently in the UK, sera are screened using IFAT, and positive tests confirmed by a cellulose acetate precipitin test (CAP). These are positive in acute dysentery (≈75%), amoeboma and ALA (≈95–100%, often to high titre), and asymptomatic carriage (≈40%). In ALA, blood cultures should be sent (in case abscess is in fact pyogenic ➤67).

Diagnosis of ALA: leucocytosis, fever, anaemia and raised ESR are usual. Mild elevation of alkaline phosphatase is common, but liver function tests are often normal. CXR may show raised hemidiaphragm, right basal shadowing and pleural effusion, even in the absence of diaphragmatic rupture. Diagnosis may be confirmed by USS or CT scanning. Abscesses may be multiple (less commonly than pyogenic liver abscess ➤67) and are most frequently located in the right lobe. Aspiration may be carried out to exclude pyogenic liver abscess, or to prevent rupture. Indications for aspiration are bulging of the rib cage or abdominal wall, a very raised hemidiaphragm, marked local tenderness or oedema or failure to respond to medical therapy. Abscess contents resemble 'anchovy sauce'. Trophozoites are seen on microscopy of pus in only ≈20% of cases. Pus cells are not seen, as the abscess contains only the liquid remains of digested liver cells because amoebic products are leucotoxic. Aspiration to dryness is essential.

**Management:** Dysentery and asymptomatic carriage: metronidazole 800 mg 8hly **followed by** the luminal amoebicide diloxanide furoate, 500 mg 8hly for 5 days to prevent relapse. In severe cases, tetracycline 500 mg 8hly should be added. ALA: metronidazole 800 mg 8hly **followed by** diloxanide furoate, 500 mg 8hly for 10 days. If ALA fails to respond to treatment (see above for indications) diagnostic/therapeutic aspiration should be performed.

## Systemic protozoal infections rarely seen in the returning traveller

Trypanosomiasis and leishmaniasis are important diseases globally, but are very rarely seen in the returning traveller, with the exception of South American cutaneous leishmaniasis.

### Trypanosomiasis

Four species of *Trypanosoma brucei* infect humans (Table 21.9).

### African trypanosomiasis (sleeping sickness)

**Epidemiology and transmission:** Occurs in focal areas of tropical Africa. 10 000–20 000 cases are reported p.a. *T. b. rhodesiense*, found mainly in E. Africa, causes a more severe and rapid illness

than *T. b. gambiense*, which is commoner in W. and Central Africa. Currently, ≈80% of cases globally occur in the Democratic Republic of Congo (prev. Zaire). Transmission is via the bite of the tsetse fly (*Glossinia* sp.) and prevention depends on avoiding being bitten (➤191). Σ ≈ 1.

**Pathogenesis:** In mammals, the parasite is a flagellated organism that circulates extracellularly in blood, lymph and extracellular fluid, replicating by binary fission. Trypanosomes have a glycoprotein surface coat that undergoes spontaneous antigenic variation during infection, thus avoiding host antibodies; each change in antigenic structure is followed by a surge in parasite replication. This mechanism allows the organism to persist for years, eventually entering the CNS.

**Clinical features**

**Incubation time:** The bite may be inconspicuous or may develop after ≈5 days into a painful inflamed nodule (trypanosomal chancre).

**Symptoms and signs:** This is followed by fever, headache, myalgia and lymphadenopathy. Splenomegaly, transient painful cutaneous oedema and generalized pruritus occur, and a circinate erythematous rash is commonly seen in Caucasians. In *T. b. gambiense* infection, CNS invasion occurs after months to years, causing a chronic meningoencephalitis with dementia and behavioural changes, including sleep reversal. Focal signs, tremor and ataxia follow, progressing to coma and death. *T. b. rhodesiense*

Table 21.9 Species of *Trypanosoma* that infect humans

| Species | Disease | Vector | Reservoir |
|---|---|---|---|
| *Trypanosoma brucei rhodesiense* | African trypanosomiasis ('rhodesiense sleeping sickness') | Tsetse fly | Wild mammals, e.g. bushbuck, hartebeest |
| *Trypanosoma brucei gambiense* | African trypanosomiasis ('gambiense sleeping sickness') | Tsetse fly | Mainly other humans, but also domestic animals, e.g. pigs |
| *Trypanosoma cruzi* | South American trypanosomiasis (Chagas' disease) | Reduviid bug | Many wild and domestic mammals |
| *Trypansoma rangeli* | Non-pathogenic | | |

causes a more rapid and severe infection, which is often fatal within weeks. Myocarditis causing congestive heart failure and arrhythmia, and disseminated intravascular coagulation commonly cause death before CNS invasion takes place. Features of CNS disease are similar to *T. b. gambiense* infection, but develop more rapidly.

**Investigations:** Anaemia, lymphocytosis and a marked elevation of total serum IgM are characteristic. In early stages, trypanosomes may be seen on blood films processed as for malaria. Concentration methods are used to detect scanty parasitaemia. Lymph-node puncture or bone-marrow material can also be examined for parasites. CSF is abnormal after CNS invasion has occurred, with raised opening pressure, raised protein and IgM and a lymphocytic pleocytosis. Mott cells ('morula cells') are characteristic plasma cells with intracellular aggregations of IgM, seen in CSF. Organisms are sometimes seen in centrifuged deposit of CSF. Serology (IFAT and card agglutination assays) is also widely used.

**Management:** Treatment with suramin and pentamidine is most effective before CNS invasion has occurred; cases due to *T. b. rhodesiense* are rarely identified before this has happened. After CNS invasion, the trivalent arsenical melarsoprol (Mel B) or eflornithine is given. These agents are all toxic; 1–5% of patients treated with Mel B die of side effects, including encephalopathy. ☎

## South American trypanosomiasis (Chagas' disease)

Chagas' disease, due to infection by *Trypanosoma cruzi*, is a major cause of cardiovascular death and gastrointestinal disease in Central and South America.

**Epidemiology and transmission:** Most prevalent in Brazil, Bolivia, Argentina and Chile. *T. cruzi* infection is associated with poverty. WHO estimates 18 million persons infected worldwide, with ≈50000 deaths p.a. The reduviid bug vector lives in roofs and walls of rural/slum housing and emerges at night to bite the occupants. Bug faeces containing trypanosomes are then rubbed into the bite wound or conjunctiva. Apart from infected humans, many wild and domestic animals act as reservoirs. Congenital and transfusion-related infections also occur. $\Sigma \approx 1$.

**Pathogenesis:** Parasites replicate intracellularly in many cells, especially muscle, macrophages and central and peripheral nervous tissue, causing progressive inflammation and destruction.

**Clinical Features:** Mean age at acquisition 4 yrs. Asymptomatic acute infection is common.

**Incubation time:** About 1–2 weeks after inoculation, unilateral orbital oedema (Romaña's sign) or an area of cutaneous oedema (chagoma) may develop. May reactivate in HIV+.

**Symptoms and signs:** This is associated with fever, malaise and generalized lymphadenopathy. This usually resolves after 4–8 weeks, although 5–10% (usually children) die due to acute myocarditis or meningoencephalitis. After resolution of acute infection there is an asymptomatic period (with persistent parasitaemia) lasting many years, following which ≈10–30% develop evidence of chronic sequelae. These present in early adulthood or middle age and include dilated cardiomyopathy, arrhythmias, heart block and denervation of the gastrointestinal tract presenting as megaoesophagus or megacolon.

**Investigations:** Diagnosis is made by finding *T. cruzi* in blood films, by special blood culture for trypanosomes, or by xenodiagnosis (feeding laboratory reared 'clean' bugs on the patient and examining the bugs for infection 3–4 weeks later) ♟. Serology is also used ☎.

**Management:** Nifurtimox (not currently available) and benznidazole are used for acute infection; they terminate parasitaemia, but do not always eradicate intracellular parasites. It is estimated that ≈50% achieve parasitological cure. They are not helpful once chronic sequelae have developed. ☎

## Leishmaniasis

Visceral and cutaneous leishmaniasis are different diseases best considered separately, but all species cause persistent parasitization of tissue macrophages. Intact T-cell-dependent, cytokine activated macrophage activation crucial in control of infection.

## Visceral leishmaniasis (kala azar, VL)

Caused by *Leishmania donovani* and *Leishmania infantum* (syn. *L. chagasi*) in both Old and New Worlds. *Leishmania mexicana amazonensis* has also been infrequently associated with VL.

**Epidemiology and transmission:** Widely distributed around Mediterranean, in tropical Africa, S. America, E. and Central Asia. Ninety per cent of cases worldwide occur in India, Bangladesh, Brazil and Sudan. Wild and domestic mammals, especially rodents and canines, are reservoirs. Transmitted by bite of sandfly. In the sandfly, parasites are flagellated *promastigotes*; in mammals, they become small non-flagellate intracellular *amastigotes*. Transfusion and person-to-person sexual transmission have been reported rarely. Infection is more likely to progress in the malnourished. In southern Europe, the majority of cases of VL are co-infected with HIV (usually due to *L. infantum*); coinfection is increasingly reported from Africa, Asia and S. America. Rising incidence worldwide associated with land reclamation and population migration. WHO estimate 2 million new cases p.a. $\Sigma \approx 5$. Subclinical 'cryptic' infection is probably commoner than previously thought; e.g. $\approx 50\%$ of discarded syringes from IVDUs in one Spanish city were positive for *Leishmania* DNA by PCR (↪ Cruz, Lancet 2002; 359: 1124).

**Pathogenesis:** A local inflammatory reaction occurs at the site of the bite, and infection can be eradicated at this stage. Dissemination is followed by replication within cells of the reticuloendothelial system.

### Clinical features
Incubation time: 3–18 months.
Symptoms and signs: Reaction at the site of the bite produces a nodule ('leishmanioma'). Dissemination is associated with recurrent fever,

night sweats and weight loss. On examination, cachexia, lymphadenopathy and moderate to massive hepatosplenomegaly with anaemia, hypoalbuminaemia and oedema. Patients are immunocompromised, and secondary bacterial infections and tuberculosis account for $\approx 95\%$ of deaths. Untreated visceral leishmaniasis is fatal in $>95\%$ of cases usually within 2 yrs, although spontaneous recovery is reported. Cirrhosis, glomerulonephritis and amyloidosis are rare complications. The clinical course in HIV coinfected patients is similar, although symptoms may be vaguer, hepatosplenomegaly less pronounced, serology is often negative, and there is a poorer response to therapy.

**Investigations:** Normocytic normochromic anaemia, leucopenia and thrombocytopenia (frequently with haemorrhagic complications, e.g. epistaxis) are usual. Marked polyclonal increase in IgG occurs and underlies the outdated and non-specific formol gel test for leishmaniasis, in which a drop of formalin is added to patient's serum, which then coagulates due to hyperglobulinaemia. Hypoalbuminaemia is common. Diagnosis is made by demonstrating amastigotes by microscopy, culture or animal inoculation. If the spleen is enlarged, splenic puncture is safe in experienced hands and gives the best yield. Bone marrow, liver biopsy and buffy coat may also be examined. Ninety-five per cent of cases of VL have positive serology; newer tests (e.g. K39 ELISA) are more sensitive and specific than older tests, although currently not widely available. Molecular methods (e.g. PCR) and culture can reliably detect and speciate, but are not widely available, particularly in endemic areas.

**Management:** Pentavalent antimony (sodium stibogluconate, Pentostam) remains the drug of choice in most areas (resistance common in parts of India). Important side effects include malaise and arthralgia, disordered liver function tests and cardiotoxicity. Treatment failures and relapses occur. Amphotericin, in particular lipid-based formulations, is widely used and is first-line therapy in India. The relative merits of these agents are still under investigation. Second-line drugs include pentamidine and paromomycin. Miltefosine is an orally active, well-tolerated agent that appears to be effective in VL—trials are ongoing. TB should be excluded in patients who fail to respond to therapy ☎.

**Post-kala azar dermal leishmaniasis:** Following apparent cure of visceral leishmaniasis, relapse may occur in the skin causing disseminated erythematous and hypopigmented nodules and papules, which act as a reservoir of infection, particularly in India, where there is no animal reservoir.

## Cutaneous leishmaniasis (CL)

CL is caused by many *Leishmania* species (Table 21.10). Each is geographically restricted by the distribution of its specific sandfly vector and animal reservoir, and they produce different clinical patterns. CL occurs in travellers returning to the UK, particularly from S. and Central America.

**Epidemiology and transmission:** See VL, ≻222.

**Clinical features:** CL typically presents with a persistent erythematous skin ulcer at the site of the bite, which heals over a number of months. Lesions are solitary and dry or multiple and exudative ('wet CL'). Relapses occur after apparent healing, and occasionally lesions become chronic ('recidivans CL'). Disseminated or 'diffuse CL' is associated with impaired host immunity and causes diffuse or nodular

**Table 21.10** Species of leishmania causing cutaneous leishmaniasis

| Species | Distribution | Diseases | Reservoir |
|---|---|---|---|
| **Old World cutaneous leishmaniasis** | | | |
| *L. tropica* | Middle East, S. Europe, India, China | Old World CL, recidivans CL | Man |
| *L. major* | Middle East, Africa, India, China | Old World CL; multiple sores are frequent | Various desert rodents |
| *L. aethiopica* | Ethiopia, Kenya, Yemen | Old World CL; small number develop disseminated CL (DCL) | Hyrax |
| **New World cutaneous leishmaniasis** | | | |
| *L. viannia braziliensis* | S. America, esp. Amazon basin. As far north as Belize | S. American CL, mucocutaneous leishmaniasis ('espundia') | Forest rodents |
| *L. viannia guyanensis* | Guyanas, and adjacent parts of Venezuela and Brazil | S. American CL ('forest sore' or 'pian bois') | Various sloths |
| *L. viannia panamensis* | Central America | S. American CL, very rarely mucocutaneous leishmaniasis | Sloths and other forest mammals |
| *L. mexicana mexicana* | Central America, esp. Belize | S. American CL, ('chiclero's ear') | Forest rodents |
| *L. mexicana amazonensis* | Brazil, Amazon basin | S. American CL, DCL | Forest rodents |
| *L. mexicana pifanoi* | Venezuela | S. American CL, DCL | Unknown |
| *L. peruviana* | Peruvian Andes, Argentina | Uta | ?Dog |

CL, cutaneous leishmaniasis.

infiltration of skin, with depigmentation but little ulceration.

**Mucocutaneous disease** ('espundia') is a serious destructive complication, usually involving the mucocutaneous junction of the nose and spreading inwards to destroy adjacent tissue over a number of years. It is only seen with *L. viannia* group infections (principally *L. viannia braziliensis*, complicating ≤5% of cases). Secondary bacterial infection may be important and there is significant mortality.

**Investigations:** Diagnosis is by biopsy of the lesions. Biopsy is taken from the edge of the ulcer and impression smears made before it is fixed. Liaison with histology is essential ☎. Serology is available, but is usually negative in returning UK travellers with early disease. Culture of organisms from lesions is possible and allows typing by isoenzyme studies. PCR allows typing directly from biopsy material, but is not widely available.

**Management:** It is essential to treat infection by *L. viannia* group to prevent mucocutaneous disease. Old World CL and *L. mexicana* group infections do not cause mucosal disease and are usually self-limiting. The decision to treat is made on an individual basis. Speciation of *Leishmania* is not usually possible clinically, and information about species prevalent in the area of travel is usually lacking. Thus, many patients suspected to have *L. mexicana* group infections are treated in case they have *L. viannia* infection. Pentavalent antimony is used, the dose depending on the species. Second-line drugs include pentamidine, amphotericin B (➤372) and the imidazoles (➤374) ☎.

# Systemic helminth infections seen in returning travellers

*Strongyloides stercoralis* (➤235) is occasionally encountered in returning travellers; because it can persist it can present many years later, particularly if immune function becomes compromised. Schistosomiasis is frequently acquired by travellers, particularly to sub-Saharan Africa, but clinical disease is relatively uncommon. Lymphatic filariasis is a major global health problem, but is rare in travellers.

## Lymphatic filariasis

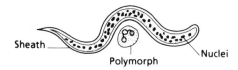

**W. bancrofti** in thick blood smear

Caused by *Wuchereria bancrofti*, *Brugia malayi* and *Brugia timori*. Threadlike adult worms, 4–10 mm long, living in lymphatics.

**Epidemiology:** WHO estimates 120 million infected persons in 73 countries worldwide; 90% have *Wuchereria bancrofti*, which is endemic throughout the tropics. *Brugia malayi* is found in SE Asia and the Indian subcontinent and *Brugia timori* is found in Indonesia. $\Sigma \approx 5$.

**Transmission and life cycle:** Adult worms mate and produce large numbers of larvae (*microfilariae*) which are present in blood and are taken up by biting mosquitos. Human infection is acquired by mosquito bite.

### Clinical features
**Life expectancy of adult worm:** ≈30 yrs.
**Symptoms and signs:** Symptoms usually develop at least 6 months after infection. Microfilaraemia may be asymptomatic or cause recurrent fever, malaise and headache. Recurrent attacks of lymphangitis occur at irregular intervals due to adult worms in lymphatics draining limbs and external genitalia, causing fever, tenderness and redness over lymphatics with temporary lymphoedema, resolving over 2–3 weeks. After repeated attacks, there is persistent damage to lymph drainage, with hydrocoele, chronic peripheral oedema, overgrowth of soft tissue and ultimately elephantiasis of limbs, scrotum, breast or vulva. Secondary bacterial infection is frequent. Chyluria—the presence of chylous lymph in the urine—is due to rupture of dilated lymphatics in the renal pelvis.

**Diagnosis:** Demonstration of microfilariae in blood. Species are distinguished by morphology. Concentration methods (e.g. membrane filtration) are used to demonstrate scanty parasitaemia. Microfilariae show marked nocturnal periodicity, being present in large numbers only during the night (except in Pacific strains, which show 'diurnal periodicity'). These patterns are determined by host sleep patterns and synchronize with vector biting behaviour; blood for microfilariae should be taken at midnight (including in returning travellers in the UK). Card-based antigen test kits are also available, and are at least as sensitive as microscopy. Serology and PCR are also available. USS may show motile adult worms.

**Management:** Diethylcarbamazine (DEC) is widely used. It kills microfilariae and adult worms if given for long enough, but is associated with adverse effects due to release of worm antigens. Ivermectin is a newer, less toxic, agent that effectively abolishes microfilaraemia for months after a single dose, but it does not kill adult worms. Since adult worms are the primary pathogens in filariasis, ivermectin has not replaced DEC in the treatment of individuals, but it plays an important role in mass chemoprophylaxis regimens. Once-yearly single-dose treatment with albendazole and ivermectin is an effective way of controlling filariasis by reducing microfilaraemia and hence transmission. The success of combination therapy (albendazole plus DEC in Asia, and albendazole plus ivermectin in Africa) has raised the possibility that LF may be eradicated, and the WHO has a collaborative programme working towards this.

It has recently been recognized that there is a remarkable degree of reversibility to elephantiasis of the limbs, and that bacterial and fungal superinfection play a major role in exacerbating oedema. Rigorous hygiene and careful management plus antifilarial treatment can result in considerable improvement ☎.

It has been recently recognized that the lymphatic filarial parasites contain rickettsia-like *Wolbachia* endosymbiotic bacteria. Some of the inflammatory manifestations recognized in lymphatic filariasis are probably attributable to these organisms. Initial studies suggest that doxycycline, which has good activity against *Wolbachia*, leads to sterility of adult worms.

### Tropical pulmonary eosinophilia (TPE)
An immune-mediated response to infection by *Wuchereria bancrofti* or *Brugia malayi*, which affects children and young adults, especially in the Indian subcontinent. Gradual onset of low fever, lassitude, cough and wheeze are associated with marked eosinophilia ($\leq 20 \times 10^9$/L), high IgE, and high-titre anti-filarial antibodies. CXR may be normal or show patchy shadows. DEC (2 mg/kg 8hly for 10 days) causes rapid and complete recovery (see also Table 21.14).

**Table 21.11** *Schistosoma* spp. causing disease in man

| Species | Distribution | Location of adult worms | Eggs excreted in | Complications |
|---|---|---|---|---|
| *Schistosoma haematobium* | Africa, Middle East | Vesical plexus | Urine | Obstructive uropathy |
| *S. mansoni* | Africa, Middle East, S. America | Lower mesenteric veins | Faeces | Portal hypertension |
| *S. japonicum* | Asia, Philippines | Lower mesenteric veins | Faeces | Portal hypertension, fits |
| *S. mekongi* | SE Asia | Lower mesenteric veins | Faeces | Portal hypertension |
| *S. intercalatum* | Africa | Lower mesenteric veins | Faeces | Portal hypertension |

Other forms of tissue nematode infection are discussed in Chapter 23.

## Schistosomiasis (bilharzia)

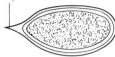

**Ovum _S. haematobium_ (urine, occasionally faeces, rectal biopsy)**

Adult worms 1–2 cm long live in veins draining the bowel or bladder; the female lives in a groove on the ventral surface of the male. Most disease is due to inflammatory response to eggs. Five species of schistosome cause disease in man, although only the first three are common (Table 21.11).

**Epidemiology:** Children are most heavily infected. Infection is acquired by contact with contaminated fresh water containing infected snails, and control efforts have in the past been

**Table 21.12**  Infections associated with exposure to freshwater and freshwater fish

| Infection | Causative organisms and notes |
| --- | --- |
| Skin and soft tissue (➤111) | _Pseudomonas aeruginosa_ dermatitis and folliculitis<br>Otitis externa (➤18)<br>Schistosome dermatitis (➤227)<br>Non-tuberculous mycobacterial infection (_Mycobacterium marinum, fortuitum, chelonae, abscessus_) (➤48)<br>_Aeromonas hydrophila_ and non-halophilic vibrio wound infection (➤114)<br>_Legionella_ (➤32)<br>Algae (_Prototheca_ spp.) |
| Eye (➤104) | Pharyngoconjunctival fever ('swimming-pool conjunctivitis')<br>Amoebic keratitis (_Acanthamoeba_ spp. (➤231)) |
| Upper respiratory tract infection | Acute sinusitis (coliforms, pseudomonads, vibrios etc.) |
| Pulmonary infection | Legionellosis (Legionnaires' disease, Pontiac fever ➤32)<br>Aerobic Gram-negative rod pneumonia (coliforms, pseudomonads, _Aeromonas, Burkholderia pseudomallei_)<br>_Mycobacterium avium_<br>_Aspergillus_ spp. pneumonia<br>_Pseudallescheria boydii_ pneumonia |
| Disseminated infection | _Leptospira_ spp. (➤327)<br>Schistosomiasis (➤226)<br>_Chromobacterium violaceum_ pneumonia and septicaemia<br>Shellfish poisoning (➤60) |
| Enteric infections (➤57) | Amoebic and bacillary dysentery<br>Salmonellosis, paratyphoid and typhoid<br>_Cryptosporidium_ infection<br>_Escherichia coli_ diarrhoeas<br>_Giardia_ infection<br>Hepatitis A<br>Norwalk virus infection<br>Shellfish poisoning (➤60) |
| CNS infection (➤96) | Coxsackievirus meningitis and encephalitis<br>Primary amoebic meningoencephalitis (_Naegleria fowleri_)<br>_Pseudallescheria boydii_ meningitis and brain abscess |

**Table 21.13** Infections associated with exposure to seawater, beaches and seafood

| Infection | Causative organisms and notes |
| --- | --- |
| Skin and soft tissue (➤111) | Otitis externa (➤18) <br> Non-tuberculous mycobacterial infection (*Mycobacterium marinum, fortuitum, chelonae, abscessus*) (➤48) <br> Halophilic vibrio wound infection (➤114) <br> Cutaneous larva migrans (➤236) |
| Upper respiratory tract infection | Acute sinusitis (coliforms, pseudomonads, vibrios, etc.) |
| Pulmonary infection | Aerobic Gram-negative rod pneumonia (coliforms, pseudomonads, vibrios) |
| Disseminated infection | Shellfish poisoning (➤60) <br> Scombroid, ciguatera and puffer fish poisoning (➤60) |
| Enteric infections (➤57) | Amoebic and bacillary dysentery <br> Salmonellosis, paratyphoid and typhoid <br> Cholera <br> *Cryptosporidium* infection <br> *Escherichia coli* diarrhoeas <br> *Giardia* infection <br> Hepatitis A <br> Norwalk virus infection <br> Shellfish poisoning (➤60) <br> Scombroid, ciguatera and puffer fish poisoning (➤60) |
| CNS infection (➤96) | Coxsackievirus meningitis and encephalitis <br> Scombroid, ciguatera and puffer fish poisoning (➤60) |

directed at control of snails. Mass chemo-prophylaxis with praziquantel is now used. $\Sigma \approx 150$.

**Transmission and life cycle:** Female worm lays eggs in terminal venules. Eggs penetrate the vein wall and traverse the wall of the bowel or bladder to be excreted in urine or faeces. Eggs hatch in water and infect particular species of snail. After 2–3 weeks, minute motile *cercariae* are released. These penetrate human skin and become *schistosomula*, which migrate via the lungs and liver to become adults in the vesical or mesenteric veins. Susceptibility to infection and likelihoood of portal hypertension recently linked to specific host genes.

**Practice point**

Schistosomiasis is frequently acquired by travellers, especially backpackers, whilst swimming in Lake Malawi, Lake Karibe and the Zambezi River. Praziquantel is often offered for sale at the lakeside as 'postexposure prophylaxis', but it is ineffective, because it does not kill schistosomula during the first 21 days in the body.

**Clinical features:** Skin penetration may be associated with an itchy papular rash ('swimmer's itch'). Initial illness ('Katayama fever') is usually only recognized in travellers; 2–8 weeks after exposure, they may develop fever, urticaria, eosinophilia, hepatosplenomegaly, diarrhoea,

**Table 21.14** Helminths causing eosinophilia in travellers

| Stage | Conditions |
|---|---|
| In early stages of infection, due to tissue migration | Ascariasis (➤233), hookworms (➤234), strongyloidiasis (➤235), visceral larva migrans (➤236), trichinosis (➤241), schistosomiasis (➤226), fascioliasis (➤243) |
| In established infection | Strongyloidiasis (➤235), visceral larva migrans (➤236), lymphatic filariasis (➤224), tropical pulmonary eosinophilia (➤225), onchocerciasis (➤240), loiasis (➤241), trichinosis (➤241), paragonimiasis (➤244), cysticercosis (➤238), echinococcosis (➤239), angiostrongyliasis (➤237). |

A careful history and examination will eliminate many of these possibilities in an individual patient. For other causes of eosinophilia ➤184.

cough and wheeze. These symptoms resolve spontaneously. Most important sequelae of infection are due to granulomatous reaction to eggs:

*Schistosoma haematobium*: terminal haematuria, dysuria, fibrosis and calcification of the bladder and obstructive uropathy (hydronephrosis, renal failure). Kidney stones and squamous-cell carcinoma of the bladder are late complications. In heavy infections, eggs may reach the lungs via the inferior vena cava, causing pulmonary hypertension and cor pulmonale.

*S. mansoni* and *S. japonicum*: Bloody diarrhoea may occur. Long-standing infection causes periportal fibrosis with portal hypertension, hepatosplenomegaly and oesophageal varices. Hepatocellular function is characteristically well-preserved. Eggs may reach lungs via portocaval anastamoses to cause cor pulmonale.

Adult worms of all species (particularly *S. japonicum*) occasionally migrate into other tissues, such as the spinal cord and brain. Schistosomiasis is also associated with increased prevalence of *Salmonella typhi* urinary carriage (➤281) and recurrent salmonella septicaemia.

**Diagnosis:** Demonstration of eggs in stool or urine, or on rectal biopsy. Eosinophilia is common. ELISA is available but is only useful in travellers and visitors to endemic regions. AXR may show pathognomic ring calcification of the bladder. USS of abdomen useful to define portal hypertension and urinary tract involvement.

**Management:** Praziquantel is the drug of choice for all species. It is free of serious adverse effects. Dose for *Schistosoma japonicum*, *S. mekongi*, 60 mg/kg, in 3 divided doses; other species, 40 mg/kg as a single dose.

---

**Practice point**

Differential diagnosis of a returning traveller with eosinophilia and diarrhoea includes schistosomiasis, strongyloidiasis (➤235), capillariasis (➤237) and trichuriasis (➤235). To exclude schistosomiasis in the returning traveller, check for eosinophilia and send serum for ELISA at 6 and 12 weeks after return. If negative and schistosomiasis is still suspected, send three terminal urine specimens collected at midday and three stool samples for ova, cysts and parasites at least 3 months after exposure.

# Chapter 22

# Protozoa

The taxonomy of protozoan parasites is complex, and includes many non-pathogenic species. For practical purposes, the protozoa of medical importance fall into four groups: flagellates, Sporozoa, Amoebae (including the ciliate protozoan *Balantidium coli*, which causes bloody diarrhoea similar to amoebic dysentery) and Microsporidia (Table 22.1).

## Babesiosis

A tick-borne illness caused by malaria-like parasites that infect red blood cells and cause haemolysis. There are more than 100 species, each with an animal reservoir (typically rodents or cattle). Three species have been definitely associated with human disease: *Babesia divergens* (Europe), *Babesia microti* (USA) and a strain described as WA-1 which has been reported from a handful of cases in Western USA.

**Epidemiology:** Transmitted by the ixodid tick, which is also responsible for transmission of Lyme disease (➤323) and ehrlichiosis (➤302). There have been ≈30 case reports of *B. divergens* infection from Europe, including the UK, almost all associated with immunocompromised hosts, esp. asplenia. Cases in the USA due to *B. microti* have been reported more frequently, and are not restricted to immunocompromised hosts, although disease is typically more severe in older patients, those without spleens, or with other causes of immunodeficiency. Frequently travel-associated. Seroprevalence in coastal areas of New England ≈5%, indicating most cases are subclinical. Recently reported from Sudan in patients suspected of having malaria.

**Incubation period:** 1–3 weeks.

**Clinical features:** Often asymptomatic. May cause non-specific flu-like illness (including headache, meningism and conjunctivitis) in the immunocompetent, and severe disease with massive intravascular haemolysis, shock, renal failure and multi-organ failure in the immunodeficient. Symptoms usually last for several weeks, and may last many months.

In US cases requiring hospital admission, mortality is ≈5%. Mortality in European cases caused by *B. divergens* is higher, ≈40%.

**Investigations:** Anaemia and evidence of haemolysis may suggest the diagnosis, which is confirmed by examination of a blood smear for intra-erythrocytic parasites ('Maltese cross'). Levels of parasitaemia up to 80% have been reported in severe cases. PCR and serology (IFAT) are also available (✈).

**Management:** Combination therapy with either quinine **plus** clindamycin, or atovaquone **plus** azithromycin, is recommended. Treatment failure is common ☎.

## *Sarcocystis* spp.

May cause acute myositis, fever and eosinophilia. Acquired by eating cysts in meat, principally undercooked pork.

## *Dientamoeba fragilis*

**Epidemiology:** Worldwide. True incidence unknown. Status as pathogen previously disputed.

**Clinical features:** Causes diarrhoea, bloating and suggested biliary involvement.

**Diagnosis:** Stool microscopy.

229

**Table 22.1** Protozoa of medical importance

| Species | Ref. |
| --- | --- |
| **Flagellates** | |
| Systemic infection | |
| *Trypanosoma* spp. | ➢220 |
| *Leishmania* spp. | ➢221 |
| GI infection | |
| *Giardia lamblia* | ➢218 |
| *Dientamoeba fragilis* | ➢229 |
| Genital infection | |
| *Trichomonas vaginalis* | ➢92 |
| **Sporozoa** | |
| Systemic infection | |
| *Plasmodium* spp. | ➢211 |
| *Toxoplasma gondii* | ➢137 |
| *Babesia* spp. | ➢229 |
| *Sarcocystis* spp. | ➢229 |
| GI infection | |
| *Isospora belli* | ➢230 |
| *Cryptosporidium parvum* | ➢230 |
| *Cyclospora* spp. | ➢231 |
| **Amoebae and Ciliophora** | |
| GI infection | |
| *Entamoeba histolytica* | ➢218 |
| *Balantidium coli* | ➢231 |
| • *Endolinax nana** | |
| • *Iodamoeba buetschlii** | |
| • *Entamoeba coli** | |
| Free-living amoebae | |
| *Naegleria fowleri* | ➢231 |
| *Acanthamoeba* spp. | ➢231 |
| **Microsporidia** | |
| *Enterocytozoon bieneusi* | ➢231 |
| *Encephalitozoon* spp. | |
| *Pleistophora* spp. | |
| *Trachipleistophora* spp. | |
| *Nosema connori* | |
| *Microsporidium* spp. | |

* Non-pathogenic protozoa found in stools, which may be confused with *E. histolytica*.
*Pneumocystis carinii* is now classified as a fungus (➢364).

**Management:** None proven. Iodoquinol, tetracycline or paromomycin may be effective.

# Intestinal sporozoa

*Isospora belli*, *Cryptosporidium parvum* and *Cyclospora* spp. are sporozoa which cause diarrhoea in humans. All are more severe/persistent in the immunodeficient host. Special stains are required for their detection in stool, so they are unlikely to be detected if 'routine OC&P' is requested. Many UK laboratories perform *Cryptosporidium* smears on all faeces samples.

### Isospora belli

**Epidemiology:** Worldwide. Commoner in subtropics and tropics.

**Clinical features:** Disputed pathogen. Diarrhoea with abdominal cramps and weight loss. Self-limiting in immunocompetent, but may be severe and prolonged in immunodeficient.

**Diagnosis:** Stool microscopy for trophozoites.

**Management:** Co-trimoxazole 960 mg 6hly for 1 week is curative. Iodoquinol has also been used.

### Cryptosporidium parvum (➢161)

Multiplies in association with the cell membrane of villus cells of the small intestine. Infective dose 1–5 oocysts.

**Epidemiology:** Worldwide. Many mammalian hosts. Transmitted human-to-human and via contaminated water. Oocysts highly resistant to disinfectants. Σ 5000.

**Clinical features:** Incubation period 2–14 days. Diarrhoea with abdominal cramps and weight loss. Common in children in UK. Self-limiting in 3–20 days in normal host, but may be severe and prolonged in immunodeficient. Common in AIDS patients, who may also develop cholangitis, cholecystitis and extra-intestinal infection (e.g. pancreatitis, pneumonia, sinusitis).

**Diagnosis:** Stool microscopy: acid-fast and immunofluorescence stains.

**Management:** No reliable therapy. None is required in the normal host. Experimental agents include paromomycin.

### Cyclospora cayetanensis

**Epidemiology:** Worldwide distribution, esp. tropics. True incidence unknown. Transmitted via contaminated food/water. Person-to-person spread unlikely, as oocysts require several days to become infective.

**Clinical features:** Incubation ≈7 days. Diarrhoea with flu-like symptoms and fatigue. May be self-limiting, but prolonged relapsing course is common, esp. in HIV coinfection.

**Diagnosis:** Stool microscopy. Small-bowel biopsy may also show organisms, plus lymphocytic infiltrate, villous atrophy and crypt hyperplasia. HIV patients may need maintenance therapy.

**Management:** Co-trimoxazole 960 mg q12h for 7 days.

## Naegleria fowleri

**Epidemiology:** Free-living amoeba. Acquired by exposure of nasal passages to contaminated fresh water, e.g. swimming.

**Clinical features:** Unusual cause of severe meningoencephalitis, with high mortality. Epidemics may occur related to a common source of contaminated fresh water.

**Diagnosis:** Wet preparation of CSF, culture, serology ☎.

**Management:** Amphotericin B, chloramphenicol, miconazole and rifampicin have been used in various combinations.

## Acanthamoeba spp.

**Epidemiology:** Free-living amoeba. Frequent contaminant of contact lens cases . $\Sigma \approx 60$.

**Clinical features:** Keratitis (➤107). Rare cause of meningoencephalitis.

**Diagnosis:** Conjunctival scrapings (☎ special stain, culture on non-nutrient agar plates sown with *E. coli*). Serology for meningo-encephalitis.

**Management:** (➤108) ☎.

## Balantidium coli

**Epidemiology:** Intestinal parasite of humans, pigs and rodents. Worldwide, wherever humans and pigs associate.

**Clinical features:** Bloody diarrhoea with colonic ulceration. Perforation may occur. Disputed pathogen.

**Diagnosis:** Stool microscopy (thin smear, special stains) ☎.

**Management:** Oxytetracycline **or** metronidazole.

## Microsporidia

Intracellular spore-forming protozoa. Ubiquitous in the environment, infecting a wide range of vertebrate and invertebrate species. Spores are typically oval and 1–2 μm in diameter, are highly resilient and can survive in the environment for months. Spores enter the host via ingestion or inhalation; once within the intestinal or respiratory tract, they are propelled into the host cell by their polar filament. Spores multiply within the cell and then burst out to infect nearby host cells or pass out into the environment. Several species cause infection in humans (Table 22.2).

**Epidemiology and transmission:** Present worldwide; prevalence of infection unknown, but seroprevalence in healthy Dutch blood donors ≈5%. Microsporidia spores have been detected in urine, feces, and respiratory secretions.

**Clinical features:** *Enterocytozoon bieneusi* has been reported as a rare cause of self-limiting diarrhoea in immunocompetent humans, including 'travellers' diarrhoea'. Other species have caused deep stromal infection of the

**Table 22.2** Microsporidia causing disease in humans

| Species | Associated morbidity |
| --- | --- |
| Enterocytozoon bieneusi, E. intestinalis | Diarrhoea, wasting, biliary disease, respiratory tract infection, urinary tract infection |
| Encephalitozoon hellem, E. cuniculi | Disseminated infection, keratoconjunctivitis, respiratory tract infection, urinary tract infection |
| Pleistophora spp. | Myositis |
| Trachipleistophora spp. | Disseminated infection, keratoconjunctivitis, myositis |
| Nosema connori | Disseminated infection |
| Microsporidium africanum, M. ceylonensis | Corneal ulcer |

cornea, but symptomatic infection has typically been described in HIV patients with advanced immunodeficiency. Cases have also been reported in patients with immunosuppression from other causes. In HIV+ patients, *Enterocytozoon bieneusi* and *Encephalitozoon intestinalis* cause chronic diarrhoea, typically non-bloody, watery, and associated with cramps, weight loss, wasting, nausea and vomiting and malabsorption. Fever is rare. Biliary tract involvement is also described, with cholangitis or acalculous cholecystitis. Disseminated infection due to *Encephalitozoon hellem, Encephalitozoon cuniculi*

and *Trachipleistophora* species has also been described, with microsporidia demonstrated in almost all body tissues, including brain.

**Diagnosis:** Stool microscopy, using electron microscopy, or light microscopy using a modified trichrome stain.

**Management:** Albendazole is recommended for *Enterocytozoon bieneusi*, but it has little activity against *Encephalitozoon intestinalis*. Restoration of immunity with HAART is the most useful therapy.

# Chapter 23

# Helminths

Helminths (Table 23.1) are divided into three groups:
- Nematodes (roundworms).
- Trematodes (flatworms or flukes).
- Cestodes (tapeworms).

Although they may produce innumerable larvae or eggs, which may themselves cause disease, adult worms cannot usually reproduce without a period of development outside the body, often involving specific environmental conditions, animal hosts and/or vectors. Therefore the total 'worm burden' cannot increase without constant re-exposure to infection. For this reason, clinically significant helminth infections are very rare in the UK, even in travellers returning from the tropics. Figures given below ($\Sigma$) to indicate relative frequency are usually due to imported infection. The exception is *Enterobius vermicularis*, which is common in the UK because it produces eggs which are directly infective for humans. Lymphatic filariasis and schistosomiasis are discussed in detail in Chapter 21.

For anti-helminth therapy, see Table 23.8 ($\succ$243).

## Soil-transmitted intestinal nematodes

These are all nematode infections that are transmitted from man to man. The egg or larva is not usually infectious when first passed, but must undergo development in the soil. Transmission depends on contamination of soil with faeces, and appropriate environmental conditions. Diagnosis is usually made by identifying characteristic eggs of each species in faeces. The **prepatent period** is the interval between infection and the appearance of eggs in the stool.

## *Ascaris lumbricoides* — the large roundworm

Egg in faeces

Adults: cream-coloured, 15–30 cm, resident in small intestine.

**Epidemiology:** Common worldwide, mainly in tropics. Most prevalent in children. $\Sigma \approx 600$.

**Transmission and life cycle:** Eggs are swallowed and develop into larvae in the intestine. Larvae then migrate through tissues, penetrating gut wall and travelling via circulation to lungs. After penetrating the alveolus, they travel up the trachea and are swallowed. Arriving in the gut a second time, they develop into adult worms, mate and produce eggs, which are passed in faeces.

### Clinical features
Prepatent period: 60–75 days.
Life expectancy of adult worm: $\approx 1$ yr.
Symptoms and signs: *Larval migration* is associated with cough, fever, wheeze, dyspnoea, CXR infiltrates and eosinophilia, occurring 10–14 days after infection and lasting a few days. *Adult worms* usually are asymptomatic or may only cause abdominal discomfort, but may rarely cause intestinal obstruction. They may contribute to malnutrition or cause mechanical damage/inflammation by entering biliary tree, pancreatic duct, appendix. If bowel is opened at surgery, *Ascaris lumbricoides* will disrupt the suture line and enter peritoneum. Prevent

**Table 23.1** Human helminth infections

this by prophylactic or intraoperative antihelminthics.

**Diagnosis:** Stool microscopy for eggs.

**Management:** Levasimole (named-patient basis) 150 mg single dose **or** piperazine 4.5 g single dose **or** mebendazole 100 mg q12h for 3 days (contraindicated in pregnancy). For child doses 📖.

## *Ancylostoma duodenale, Necator americanus* —the hookworms

Adults: 1 cm, attached to jejunal mucosa.

**Epidemiology:** Widespread in tropics and subtropics. $\Sigma \approx 500$.

**Transmission and life cycle:** Eggs passed in faeces develop into infectious larvae in the soil. These penetrate intact skin, e.g. on the feet, and travel via the circulation to the lungs and thence to the gut. Adult worms attach to jejunal mucosa and suck blood, each worm causing the loss of about 0.1 mL/day.

**Clinical features**
**Prepatent period:** 40–100 days.

Life expectancy of adult worm: 1–5 yrs.

**Symptoms and signs:** Itchy papules may develop at the site of larval penetration ('ground itch'). Mild pulmonary symptoms associated with lung migration (compared with severe manifestations associated with *Ascaris lumbricoides*). Hookworm infection is an important cause of **iron-deficiency anaemia**, which may be severe, particularly if dietary iron intake is poor.

**Diagnosis:** Stool microscopy for eggs.

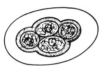

Egg in faeces

**Management:** Levasimole (named-patient basis) 150 mg single dose **or** mebendazole 100 mg q12h for 3 days (contraindicated in pregnancy) **or** albendazole 200 mg q24h for 3 days **or** pyrantel 10 mg/kg single dose. For child doses 📖.

## *Trichuris trichiura* —whipworm

Adults: 2–5 cm long, reside partly buried in the mucosa of the large bowel.

**Epidemiology:** Worldwide, commonest in tropics. $\Sigma \approx 1000$.

**Transmission and life cycle:** Eggs are ingested and develop into adults in the gut. There is no tissue migratory phase.

### Clinical features
Prepatent period: 70–90 days.
Life expectancy of adult worm: 1 yr.
**Symptoms and signs:** Usually asymptomatic. Heavy infection may cause bloody diarrhoea, rectal prolapse, anaemia, wasting and eosinophilia. Worms may be seen on sigmoidoscopy.

**Diagnosis:** Stool microscopy for eggs.

Egg in faeces

**Management:** Mebendazole 100 mg 12hly for 3 days (contraindicated in pregnancy and under 2 yrs) **or** albendazole 400 mg stat.

## *Enterobius vermicularis* — pinworm, threadworm

Adult worms: 5–10 mm long, resident in large bowel. May emerge from anus.

**Epidemiology:** Worldwide, commoner in temperate regions than tropics. The only common helminth infection in the UK. Infection is commonest in children; other members of the same household are often also infected.

**Transmission and life cycle:** Female emerges from anus at night to lay eggs on perianal skin. These become infectious after $\approx 4$ h. After ingestion, they develop into adults, with no tissue migratory phase.

### Clinical features
Prepatent period: $\approx 40$ days.
Life expectancy of adult worm: 8 weeks.
**Symptoms and signs:** Pruritus ani. Very rarely, worms migrate into vagina and uterus, causing endometritis and salpingitis. Appendicitis is a rare complication.

**Diagnosis:** Microscopy of sellotape swab from perianal region.

Egg in sellotape slide

**Management:** Adults and children over 2 yrs: mebendazole 100 mg stat repeated after 1 week. Piperazine is an alternative; for doses, see Table 23.2.

## *Strongyloides stercoralis*

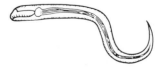

Larva in faeces

**Table 23.2** Doses of piperazine for the treatment of threadworm

| Age | Piperazine citrate elixir 750 mg/5 mL* | Piperazine phosphate† |
| --- | --- | --- |
| Adult/child > 6 yrs | 15 mL q24h for 7 days | 4 g sachet single dose |
| 7–12 yrs | 10 mL q24h for 7 days | 4 g sachet single dose |
| 4–6 yrs | 7.5 mL q24h for 7 days | 1 level 5 mL teaspoon single dose |
| 2–3 yrs | 5 mL q24h for 7 days | 1 level 5 mL teaspoon single dose |
| 1–2 yrs | 0.3–0.5 mL/kg q24h for 7 days | 1 level 5 mL teaspoon single dose |
| 3 months – 1 yrs | 0.3–0.5 mL/kg q24h for 7 days | 1 level 2.5 mL teaspoon single dose |

* Repeated after 1 week if necessary.
† Repeated after 2 weeks.

Adults: 2 mm long, live burrowed into mucosa of small intestine.

**Epidemiology:** Worldwide in tropics and subtropics. $\Sigma \approx 60$.

**Transmission and life cycle:** *Strongyloides stercoralis* is unusual because adults worms can reproduce within one host. Adult females lay eggs, which develop into larvae within the gut. These are normally non-infectious and must undergo development in the soil before penetrating intact skin and travelling via the lungs to the gut, as for hookworm (➤234). Sometimes larvae develop into the infective form before they leave the host, and are then able to penetrate perianal skin or intestinal wall, travelling from there to the lungs. This 'autoinfective cycle' maintains infection for many years in patients who have left the tropics and is responsible for hyperinfection in patients who become immunocompromised. This can occur 50 or more years after infection (e.g. Far East prisoners of war). Larvae may also enter a free-living cycle which can survive in the soil in appropriate tropical conditions.

**Clinical features**
**Prepatent period:** 17–28 days.
**Life expectancy of adult worm:** not known.
**Symptoms and signs:** Occasional pruritus at the site of larval entry, or pulmonary symptoms related to larval migration. Development of adult worms in the gut may cause malabsorption with eosinophilia. Most patients become asymptomatic after a few weeks. If infection is maintained by autoinfection, signs of estab-

lished infection occur. These include intermittent diarrhoea and **larva currens**, a raised serpiginous wheal due to larval migration that appears on the skin usually of the trunk. It is very itchy, migrates at several centimetres/hour and usually resolves within 24 h.

**Hyperinfection** occurs when patients become immunocompromised. It causes diarrhoea and malabsorption, paralytic ileus, peritonitis, secondary Gram-negative bacteraemia, meningitis and pulmonary symptoms. Diagnosis is made by finding larvae in clinical material, particularly stools and sputum. Eosinophilia is rare in hyperinfection.

**Diagnosis:** Stool microscopy for larvae is insensitive, so at least 6 samples should be examined before excluding the diagnosis in likely cases ☎. Microscopy of duodenal string test, duodenal aspirate or jejunal biopsy. Stools may be cultured for larvae—this takes 3 weeks ☠. Filaria ELISA cross reacts in ≈90% of cases—a specific serological test for strongyloides is also available.

**Management:** Thiabendazole 25 mg/kg (max 1.5 g) 12hly for 3 days **or** albendazole 400 mg q12h for 3 days **or** ivermectin 200 µg/kg q24h for 2 days. Often ineffective in hyperinfection. Repeated courses of suppressive treatment may be needed.

There are a number of rarer zoonotic intestinal nematode infections (Table 23.3).

## Larva migrans
**Visceral larva migrans** (VLM) is due to *Toxocara canis* and *T. cati*, the dog and cat round-

**Table 23.3** Rarer zoonotic intestinal nematodes

| Species | Natural host | Most prevalent in | Acquired by | Comments |
|---|---|---|---|---|
| *Trichostrongylus* spp. | Various mammals | Japan, Indonesia, Egypt | Eating vegetables contaminated with larvae | Usually asymptomatic. Abdominal pain, diarrhoea, anaemia |
| *Angiostrongylus costaricensis* | Rats | Costa Rica | Eating vegetables contaminated by slugs or their secretions | Abdominal pain, eosinophilia |
| *Capillaria phillippinensis* | Birds | Philippines, Thailand | Eating undercooked, infected fish | Diarrhoea, malabsorption, wasting, fever, eosinophilia. Severe fatal diarrhoea may occur with heavy infection. Autoinfection occurs |
| *Anisakis* spp. | Sea mammals | Japan | Eating undercooked, infected fish | Eosinophilic gastritis |

worms. $\Sigma \approx 20$. Eggs (from animal faeces) ingested by humans, develop into larvae and migrate through tissues for 1–2 yrs. Heavy infections in children may cause fever, hepatomegaly, eosinophilia and asthma. VLM is usually self-limited, and usually requires no treatment. The drug of choice for severe VLM is diethylcarbamazine (2 mg/kg q8h for 10 days). Alternatives include mebendazole 200 mg q12h for 5 days **or** albendazole 400 mg q12h for 5 days. **Ocular disease** is more important. Larvae trapped in the retina cause a granulomatous reaction, which presents as a solid retinal mass and may cause blindness in the affected eye. Eosinophilia is not usually seen in ocular toxocariasis. Sensitive and specific serology is available. High-titre antibodies in aqueous humour are strongly predictive of infection. Antigen detection and PCR also available: ➤. Steroids (systemic and intraocular) and thiabendazole are used, although antihelminthics have not been shown to influence outcome. Differential diagnosis includes retinoblastoma and other retinal tumours.

**Cutaneous larva migrans** are due to the dog hookworms *Ancylostoma caninum* and *Ancylostoma braziliense*, which are common in N., Central and S. America, including the Caribbean. Larvae penetrate the skin, usually on the buttocks or feet of humans exposed to warm, sandy soil contaminated with dog faeces. Migration of larvae causes **creeping eruption** — a very itchy serpiginous track advancing about 1 mm/day and persisting for several weeks before resolving spontaneously (in contrast to 'larva currens' due to *Strongyloides stercoralis* ➤235). *Ancylostoma caninum* larvae may occasionally reach the bowel, causing eosinophilic enteritis. Systemic treatments include thiabendazole (25 mg/kg daily in divided doses for 5 days repeated after 1 week), albendazole 200 mg q12h for 3 days or ivermectin 200 µg/kg single dose. Topical 10% thiabendazole in petroleum jelly applied daily for 5 days has also been recommended. Individual larvae may be killed by freezing the skin with ethyl chloride spray.

## Tapeworms

### *Taenia saginata*—beef tapeworm

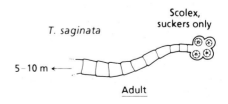

Adult worms: 5–10 m long, resident in small intestine.

**Epidemiology:** Worldwide. $\Sigma \approx 40$.

**Transmission and life cycle:** Humans acquire infection by eating undercooked beef containing encysted larvae. Cysts mature into adult segmented worm in the small intestine, attached to the mucosa by the head. Segments (*proglottids*) full of eggs are shed from the tail end. Proglottids, and eggs from proglottids that rupture in the gut, are shed in faeces and contaminate pastureland, where they infect cattle.

**Clinical features**
Prepatent period: 12 weeks.
Life expectancy of adult worm: ≥30 yrs.
Symptoms and signs: Patients may notice white motile proglottids in stools or emerging from the anus. Otherwise usually asymptomatic.

**Diagnosis:** Stool microscopy for eggs and proglottids.

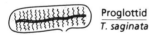
Proglottid
*T. saginata*

**Management:** Niclosamide, 2 doses of 1 g, 1 h apart **or** praziquantel 10 mg/kg stat.

## *Taenia solium* — pork tapeworm and cysticercosis

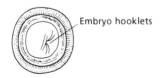
Embryo hooklets

**Egg** of *solium* or *saginata* (**faeces**)

Adult worms 3–5 m long in small intestine.

**Epidemiology:** Worldwide; very rare in the UK. $\Sigma \approx 20$.

**Transmission and life cycle:** As for *Taenia saginata* (pigs substituting for cattle), with the very

important difference that **eggs are infectious for humans**, who may unwittingly act as secondary hosts. Eggs consumed by humans hatch in the gut and develop into *oncospheres*, which enter the circulation and are carried to muscles, CNS and other organs, where they develop into larval cysts — this is called **cysticercosis**.

**Clinical features**
Prepatent period: 3–6 months.

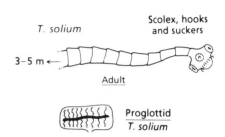
*T. solium*

Scolex, hooks
and suckers

3–5 m ←

Adult

Proglottid
*T. solium*

Life expectancy of adult worm: ≤25 yrs.
Symptoms and signs: Infection by adult worms is usually asymptomatic, except for passage of proglottids. Manifestations of cysticercosis depend on magnitude of infection and location of cysts. Infection is often asymptomatic and diagnosed coincidentally by discovery of spindle-shaped calcified tissue cysts on X-ray. Epilepsy developing 3–5 yrs after infection is the most common presentation; other neurological defects include raised intracranial pressure, without focal signs, due to chronic basal meningitis.

**Diagnosis:** *Adult T. solium:* Stool microscopy for eggs and proglottids. **Cysticercosis:** serology (IFAT), demonstration of cysts in muscle by X-ray or in CNS by CT/MRI. CSF shows lymphocytic pleocytosis, raised protein, eosinophilia (50% of cases) and reduced glucose (25% of cases).

**Management:** **Adult *Taenia solium*:** niclosamide or praziquantel 10 mg/kg stat, as for *Taenia saginatum.* It is usual to give an antiemetic 1 h before and a purgative 1 h after treatment to avoid the risk of autoinfection by eggs released from the dying worm. **Cysticercosis:** Praziquantel and aldendazole have both been used effectively. Anticonvulsants may be required ☎.

### *Echinococcus granulosus* and *Echinococcus multilocularis*

Dog tapeworms, causing **hydatid disease** in sheep, cattle and humans.

**Epidemiology:** Worldwide, associated with sheep and cattle rearing and contact with dogs. Incidence varies widely depending on degree of human contact with dogs and degree to which dogs feed on herbivore carcasses. *Echinococcus granulosus* accounts for most human infections. $\Sigma \approx 25$.

**Transmission and life cycle:** Dogs are the definitive host for the small adult tapeworms. Eggs passed in dog faeces infect secondary host — usually sheep or cattle, where they develop in the intestine, enter the circulation and form cysts in the viscera. Cysts are encapsulated by host fibrous tissue and may continue to grow for many years. Dogs are infected by eating herbivore carcasses containing cysts. Man is infected from dog faeces and acts as a secondary host, developing visceral cysts.

    *E. multilocularis* is associated with wild canines and rodents, and human infection is rare. Unlike *E. granulosus*, cysts are multiloculated, not contained within a capsule and may spread through surrounding tissue like a malignant tumour.

#### Clinical features

Cysts are found in the liver (70%), lungs (25%) and other organs. Hepatic cysts may be very large (e.g. 15 L capacity). Symptoms may occur months to years after infection and are due to mechanical pressure or the release of allergenic cyst contents causing urticaria or anaphylaxis. Ruptured cysts may seed multiple secondary cysts or cause death by anaphylaxis. Cysts may become secondarily bacterially infected.

**Diagnosis:** USS and CT are used to delineate cysts, but diagnostic aspiration is **absolutely contraindicated** because of the risks described above. Serology (ELISA) is helpful to support the clinical and radiological diagnosis. It is sensitive and specific in hepatic and disseminated disease, but less sensitive in pulmonary disease. Eosinophilia occurs (25% of cases).

**Management:** Surgical removal is the treatment of choice and requires the use of specialized techniques to avoid rupture. It is particularly indicated if bacterial superinfection has occurred, or if the cyst is in communication with the biliary tree, or for cysts in brain, heart, kidney, bone or spine. If patients are too unwell to undergo surgery, or if the location of the cysts precludes removal, a regimen of percutaneous puncture, aspiration, instillation of protoscolicide and reaspiration ('PAIR') is used, combined with albendazole. Prolonged treatment with albendazole alone results in resolution of $\approx30\%$ of cysts and shrinkage of a further $\approx30\%$. *E. multilocularis* is usually fatal untreated. Surgical removal is often impossible, and very prolonged albendazole treatment is used.

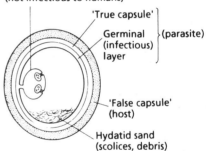

Brood capsule containing scolices
(not infectious to humans)

'True capsule'
Germinal (infectious) layer ⎱(parasite)
'False capsule' (host)
Hydatid sand (scolices, debris)

Hydatid cyst in intermediate host (sheep, man)

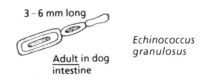

3–6 mm long

*Echinococcus granulosus*

Adult in dog intestine

### Rarer tapeworms

Table 23.4.

## Tissue nematodes

### *Wuchereria bancrofti, Brugia malayi* and *Brugia timori*

Lymphatic filariasis (➤224)

Table 23.4 Minor tapeworms

| Species | Definitive host | Secondary host | Clinical features |
| --- | --- | --- | --- |
| Diphyllobothrium latum | Man | Freshwater fish | Usually asymptomatic. Rare cause of $B_{12}$ deficiency |
| Hymenolepis nana | Man | None | Occasional GI upset |

## Dracunculus medinensis — Guinea worm

Adult worm up to 1 m long, living subcutaneously and emerging through the skin of the leg.

**Epidemiology:** Previously seen throughout Middle East, Africa, Asia and S. America. A vigorous control programme has all but eradicated this parasite, except for an endemic focus in war-torn Sudan.

**Transmission and life cycle:** Man acquires infection by swallowing a small crustacean (*Cyclops*) in contaminated fresh water. *Dracunculus medinensis* eggs hatch in the human gut, and larvae penetrate the intestinal mucosa. They develop into adults in the subcutaneous tissues. After ≈1 yr, the female worm, which may be up to 1 m long, approaches the skin, and a blister forms. On contact of skin with water, the blister bursts and larvae are discharged, escaping to infect *Cyclops* and complete the cycle.

### Clinical features

Incubation period: ≈1 yr.
Life expectancy of adult worm: ≈1 yr.
Localized pain, swelling and itching. Fever and urticaria. The appearance of the ulcer is characteristic with a central pearly loop formed by the worm's uterus. A drop of water placed on the ulcer causes reflex contraction of the uterus and expulsion of larvae. Secondary bacterial infection, localized responses to dead worms and arthritis, which may either be immune mediated or due to worms migrating through joint spaces, may all occur.

**Management:** The ulcer is bathed for several days to deplete larvae, then the end of the worm is attached to a small stick and removed by carefully winding it out, over the course of 10–14 days.

## Onchocerca volvulus — onchocerciasis, 'river blindness'

Adult worms (males 4 cm, females 50 cm) live free in subcutaneous tissues or in fibrous subcutaneous nodules.

**Epidemiology:** Focally distributed across Equatorial Africa. Also found in some areas of C. America and Yemen. Foci of infection are located near fast-flowing rivers, which are breeding areas of the blackfly vector. $\Sigma \approx 10$.

**Transmission and life cycle:** Infection is acquired by the bite of the blackfly (*Simulium* spp.). Adult worms live free in subcutaneous tissues unless they are contained by fibrous nodules. Large numbers of motile larvae (*microfilariae*) are produced; it is the inflammatory response to the microfilariae which is responsible for most clinical features.

### Clinical features

Incubation period: ≈1 yr.
Life expectancy of adult worm: ≈20 yrs.

**Symptoms and signs:** Nodules (2–5 cm) tend to occur over bony prominences and it is postulated that the worms become trapped between bone and skin, allowing host defence mechanisms to trap them. Symptoms due to microfilariae include a papular rash and severe pruritus (which may affect normal looking skin) and excoriation, which is often secondarily infected by bacteria. These eventually progress to depigmentation, loss of elasticity and severe premature ageing of the skin. These changes and inguinal lymphadenopathy give rise to the 'hanging groin' appearance. There may be

**Table 23.5** *Trichinella* spp.

| Species | Source of human infection | Distribution |
| --- | --- | --- |
| *Trichinella spiralis spiralis* | Domestic pigs | USA, Europe |
| *Trichinella spiralis nelsoni* | Wild pigs | Africa, S. Europe |
| *Trichinella spiralis nativa* | Wild mammals (bear, walrus, seal) | Arctic |

minor elephantiasis of the legs or scrotum. Migration of microfilariae into the eye cause severe keratitis, iritis and retinitis eventually leading to blindness.

**Diagnosis:** By finding microfilariae in skin snips taken from pruritic areas.

**Management:** A vigorous effort has been made to eradicate onchocerciasis, initially with vector control programmes and lately with mass chemoprophylaxis with ivermectin, which kills microfilariae, thus preventing transmission and removing the cause of the symptoms. Ivermectin is also used for treatment of individual cases. Global eradication is a real possibility. Palpable nodules represent only some of the adult worms, so removal is not logical, except for nodules on the head, which should be removed because of the increased risk of ocular damage. (Microfilariae density is highest close to nodules.)

### *Loa loa* — loiasis, Calabar swelling
Adults 3–7 cm long live free in subcutaneous tissues.

**Epidemiology:** Forest areas of Western and Central Africa. $\Sigma \approx 10$.

**Transmission and life cycle:** Transmitted by the biting fly, *Chrysops*. Adult worms take about 1 yr to develop before mating to produce microfilariae; these are found in the circulation (showing diurnal periodicity) and are taken up by the fly.

**Clinical features**
**Incubation period:** 1 yr.
**Life expectancy of adult worm:** ≥20 yrs.

**Symptoms and signs:** Usually asymptomatic. Sudden painful itchy subcutaneous swellings ('Calabar swellings') occur, often related to minor trauma. Occasionally, worms may be seen crossing the conjunctiva — this is associated with intense irritation and periorbital swelling. Eosinophilia is common.

**Diagnosis:** By detection of microfilariae in the blood, or by seeing the worm under the conjunctiva.

**Management:** DEC kills microfilariae and adult worms, but reactions to treatment are common, including fever, headache, tender subcutaneous swellings around dead worms, very high eosinophilia and encephalitis. Reactions are less severe if DEC is introduced gradually (often with steroids). Ivermectin kills microfilariae with fewer adverse effects, but can also cause encephalopathy. Albendazole is partially macrofilaricidal, and is sometimes used to reduce microfilaria levels before treatment with DEC.

### *Trichinella spiralis*

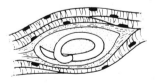

Cyst within skeletal muscle

**Epidemiology:** Worldwide, particularly in Europe and the USA. Recent outbreaks in E. European sausages. $\Sigma \approx 5$. Three species cause disease in man (Table 23.5).

**Transmission and life cycle:** Infection is acquired by eating undercooked meat containing encysted larvae. These hatch in the gut and mature in the small intestine. After mating, larvae are produced, which migrate to striated muscle where they encyst. Transmission continues when the new host is eaten. Encysted larvae are killed by thorough cooking, or by freezing (<15°C for >3 weeks). Meat inspection.

**Clinical features:** Usually asymptomatic; ≈1 week after ingestion, GI disturbance associated with intestinal development of worms may occur. After 2–8 weeks, there may be fever, headache and cough, with muscle tenderness and swelling. Periorbital oedema and conjunctivitis are common. Splinter haemorrhages may occur. Neurological signs (deafness, encephalitis, fits, focal signs), myocarditis and pneumonitis occur rarely. Severe cases may be fatal but most recover spontaneously.

**Diagnosis:** Suspected in any patient with fever, eosinophilia, myositis and periorbital oedema, who has recently eaten pork. Leucocytosis and raised creatine phosphokinase are common. Serology becomes positive 3–4 weeks into illness, at which time larvae may be demonstrated on muscle biopsy.

**Management:** During the GI phase, mebendazole 7.5 mg/kg 12hly for 3 days. During muscle migration phase, mebendazole 5 mg/kg 12hly for 10–13 days (no proof of therapeutic efficacy). Steroids and aspirin are also given in severe cases (prednisolone 40–60 mg 24hly).

## Minor tissue helminths
See Table 23.6.

## Helminths causing eosinophilic meningitis
See Tables 23.7, 23.8.

**Table 23.6** Minor tissue nematodes

| Species | Distribution | Vector | Site of adult worms | Clinical features |
|---------|-------------|--------|--------------------|--------------------|
| Mansonella* perstans | Tropical Africa, S. America | Midges | Peritoneum | Serositis; usually asymptomatic |
| Mansonella* streptocerca | W. Africa | Midges | Dermis | Pruritus, hypopigmented macules |
| Mansonella* ozzardi | S. & C. America | Midges, blackflies | Peritoneum | Usually asymptomatic |
| Dirofilaria immitis ('dog heartworm') | Worldwide, esp. Mediterranean | Mosquito | Lung | Usually asymptomatic. Can cause coin lesion on CXR |

* Formerly *Dipetalonema* spp.

**Table 23.7** Nematodes causing eosinophilic meningitis

| Species | Distribution | Host | Acquired from | Clinical features |
|---------|-------------|------|---------------|--------------------|
| Angiostrongylus cantonensis | SE Asia, Japan, India, Oceania | Rat | Ingestion of infected molluscs on vegetables or undercooked | Eosinophilic meningitis |
| Gnathostoma spinigerum | SE Asia | Cats and dogs | Fish | Larva migrans with cutaneous swellings, creeping eruption. Eosinophilic meningitis |

# Flukes (trematodes)

## Schistosomiasis (➤226)

### Intestinal flukes (Table 23.9)

Diagnosis: Stool microscopy for eggs (sputum microscopy for lung flukes) ☎. Serology is also available.

Management: Praziquantel, 25 mg/kg 8hly for 3 days.

Comments: A large number of other flukes normally parasitic on other mammals may rarely infect humans.

**Table 23.8** Antihelminthic drugs

| Drug | Common indications | Important adverse effects |
|------|-------------------|---------------------------|
| Mebendazole | Threadworm, roundworm, whipworm, hookworm | Diarrhoea, rash. Contraindicated in pregnancy and children < 2 yrs |
| Piperazine | Threadworm, roundworm | GI disturbance, rash, bronchospasm. rarely, dizziness, ataxia, drowsiness, convulsions. Contraindicated in first trimester, epilepsy |
| Pyrantel | Threadworm, roundworm, hookworm | GI disturbance, rash, headache |
| Levamisole | Roundworm, whipworm | GI disturbance |
| Niclosamide | Intestinal tapeworms | GI disturbance, pruritus |
| Albendazole | Threadworm, roundworm, whipworm, hookworm, strongyloidiasis, hydatid disease, cysticercosis | GI disturbance, rash, fever, headache. Abnormal liver function tests. Myelotoxicity |
| Praziquantel | Trematodes, cestodes | Mild dizziness. Contraindicated in ocular cysticercosis |
| Diethylcarbamazine (DEC) | Filariasis, *Loa loa* | Headache, dizziness, nausea, fever, allergic reactions to death of worms |
| Ivermectin | Onchocerciasis, strongyloides, *Loa loa* | Fever, pruritus, rash (all mild) |
| Thiabendazole | Strongyloidiasis, larva migrans, trichinosis | GI disturbance, headache, rash; rarely, tinnitus, collapse, hepatitis |

Table 23.9 Intestinal flukes

| Species | Acquired from | Secondary host | Distribution | Size (mm) | Clinical features |
|---|---|---|---|---|---|
| **Liver flukes—adults resident in human biliary tree** | | | | | |
| Clonorchis sinensis | Freshwater fish | Snail | China, SE Asia | 15 × 3 | Abdominal pain, pancreatitis, cholangitis, cholangiocarcinoma; often asymptomatic |
| Opisthorchis fileneus | | | Eastern Europe | 10 × 2 | |
| Opisthorchis viverrini | | | Thailand | 10 × 2 | |
| Fasciola hepatica | Freshwater plants | Snail | Worldwide | 25 × 18 | Eosinophilia, hepatitis, biliary colic, obstructive jaundice |
| **Lung fluke—adults resident in human lung** | | | | | |
| Paragonimus westermani | Freshwater crabs, crayfish | Snail | Far East, SE Asia | 10 × 5 | Cough, haemoptysis, chest pain, fever. CXR shadowing with cavitation. Flukes may rarely migrate to many other organs, including CNS |
| **Intestinal flukes—adults resident in human intestine** | | | | | |
| Fasciolopsis buski | Edible water plants | Snail | SE Asia | 30 × 12 | Usually asymptomatic. Heavy infection may cause abdominal pain and diarrhoea |
| Heterophyes heterophyes | Fish | Snail | China, Japan, Egypt | 1.5 × 0.5 | |
| Metagonimus yokogawai | Fish | Snail | Far East | 1 × 0.5 | |

# Section IV

# Microbiology

# Bacteria

## Classification of medically important bacteria

In the following chapters we have used this classification, which provides a practical, memorable and clinically relevant structure for the major bacterial pathogens.

| Group | | Most important species | Chapter |
|---|---|---|---|
| **Gram-positive aerobes** | Cocci | *Staphylococcus* spp. | 24 (➤249) |
| | | *Streptococcus* spp. | 25 (➤254) |
| | Rods | *Bacillus* spp. | 26 (➤263) |
| | | *Listeria* spp. | |
| | | *Corynebacterium* spp. | |
| **Gram-negative aerobic rods** | Coliforms (Enterobacteriacae) | *Escherichia* spp. | 27 (➤273) |
| | | *Klebsiella* spp. | |
| | | *Proteus* spp. | |
| | | *Salmonella* spp. | |
| | | *Shigella* spp. | |
| | Vibrios | *Vibrio* spp. | 28 (➤285) |
| | Campylobacters | *Campylobacter* spp. | 29 (➤288) |
| | | *Helicobacter* spp. | |
| | Pseudomonads | *Pseudomonas* spp. | 30 (➤291) |
| **Fastidious Gram-negative organisms** | | *Haemophilus* spp. | 31 (➤296) |
| | | *Neisseria* spp. | |
| | | *Legionella* spp. | |
| | | *Bordetella* spp. | |
| **Anaerobes** | Spore-forming | *Clostridium* spp. | 32 (➤312) |
| | Non-sporing | *Bacteroides* spp. | |
| | | *Fusobacterium* spp. | |
| | Spirochaetes | *Treponema* spp. | 33 (➤322) |
| | | *Borrelia* spp. | |
| | | *Leptospira* spp. | |
| **Mycobacteria** | | *Mycobacterium* spp. | 4 (➤37) |
| **Mycoplasma** | | *Mycoplasma* spp. | 34 (➤329) |
| | | *Ureaplasma* spp. | |
| **Chlamydia** | | *Chlamydia* spp. | 34 (➤329) |
| **Rickettsia** | | *Rickettsia* spp. | 34 (➤329) |
| | | *Coxiella* spp. | |

# Chapter 24

# Staphylococci

Staphylococci ('bunch of grapes') are members of the family *Micrococcaceae*—round, Gram-positive organisms arranged in clumps or packets. All are commensals of human skin. *Staphylococcus aureus* ('golden' colonies) is a major pathogen, causing pyogenic and toxin-mediated infections in humans. More recently, coagulase-negative staphylococci (CNSt) have emerged as important pathogens, especially as opportunists in hospitalized patients and in the urinary tract.

## Classification (Table 24.1)

All CNSt used to be grouped as '*Staphylococcus albus*'. Many laboratories now use '*Staphylococcus epidermidis*' to refer to all CNSt and micrococci, and we have adopted this for convenience. Identification (other than as *epidermidis* and *saprophyticus*, when needed) is best done with commercial biochemical test kits.

## *Staphylococcus aureus*

**Pathogenesis:** Produces a wide variety of extra-cellular enzymes and other products. Some are superantigens (also known as 'pyrogenic toxin superantigens', marked * below), some of which may also be produced by *Streptococcus pyogenes* (➤254). Large quantities may activate T lymphocytes, bypassing standard antigen-presenting mechanisms → cytokine release → fever, rash, vomiting, diarrhoea, multi-organ failure, desquamation. Also direct endothelial cytotoxicity → DIC, thrombocytopenia, tissue haemorrhage; macrophage cytotoxicity → failure to clear Gram-negative endotoxin → hypotension.

Almost **all** strains secrete: haemolysins, staphylokinase, lipase, phospholipase (cell membrane damage), clumping factor, coagulase (converts fibrinogen to fibrin), protein A (immunoglobulin Fc region-binding), collagen-binding protein, fibronectin-binding protein (adhesion), deoxyribonuclease, proteases, collagenase, hyaluronidase.

**Some** strains secrete one or more of the following:
- Epidermolytic toxins causing staphylococcal scalded-skin syndrome (syn. Ritter's disease, toxic epidermal necrolysis, Lyell's syndrome) (➤136).
- Exfoliative toxins* (ETA and ETB).
- Toxic shock syndrome toxin-1 (TSST-1*; also called enterotoxin F and staphylococcal pyrogenic exotoxin C) (➤84).
- Enterotoxins* types A–E (recently named SEA–E, and newly recognized SEG, SEH and SEI) cause food poisoning (➤58)—one or more produced by 40% of *Staphylococcus aureus* strains.
- Leucocidin.

**Epidemiology:** Regularly carried by 20–30% normal people in anterior nares, usually a single strain carried for long periods; ~50% of the remainder carry different strains intermittently. Sometimes carried heavily on axillary and/or perineal skin, but 98% of these individuals also positive in anterior nares. New strains are acquired by direct contact (e.g. hands of health-care workers) and airborne exposure (e.g. from clouds of staphylococci dispersed during bed-making). Acquisition enhanced by prior antibiotic therapy. A single nose swab detects 80%

**Table 24.1** Classification of staphylococci

| Genus | Species | Notes |
|---|---|---|
| Coagulase + | | |
| *Staphylococcus* | *aureus* | Human pathogen |
| | *intermedius* | Animal pathogen, occasionally infects bites |
| Coagulase – | | |
| *Staphylococcus* | *epidermidis* | Human opportunist |
| | *saprophyticus* | UTI |
| | (*capitis, hominis, lugdunensis, schleiferi, xylosus, haemolyticus, auricularis, warneri, simulans, cohnii, saccharolyticus,* etc.) | Occasional opportunists |
| (*Micrococcus* | *luteus, roseus,* etc.) | Rare opportunists |
| (*Kocuria* | *varians, kristinae*) | Previously *Micrococcus* spp. |
| (*Kytococcus* | *sedentarius*) | |
| (*Stomatococcus* | *mucilaginosus*) | Mucoid colonies |
| *Peptococcus* | *niger* (➤313) | 'Anaerobic staph.' |

of carriers. Staphylococci mainly spread from anterior nares to hands to skin to squames to air; very few directly from anterior nares to air. Frequent and heavy skin carriage in insulin-dependent diabetics, haemodialysis, iv drug misusers (all with repeated skin puncture), HIV+ persons. Bacteriophage ('phage') typing of strains by patterns of lysis by bank of bacteriophages now often replaced by typing by cell wall protein patterns after electrophoresis on agarose gel ('PAGE') or gel electrophoresis of DNA cleaved by endonucleases ➤.

**Spectrum of disease (Fig. 24.1):** Hallmark of local sepsis is **abscess** formation (➤111). **Impetigo, paronychia, sycosis barbae, cellulitis** (➤113). **Conjunctivitis** (➤105).

Deep sepsis: **septicaemia** (➤185), **osteomyelitis** and **septic arthritis** (➤120), **infective endocarditis** (➤49), **pneumonia** (➤25).

In hospital: **iv line infection, surgical wound** and **site infection, ventilator-associated pneumonia** (➤33).

**Toxic shock syndrome** (TSS) (➤84).

**Bacteraemia** ($\Sigma$ ~11 000) may be **hospital-acquired**, most commonly from iv catheter infection, usually short-lasting with easily treatable focus. Frequently auto-infections derived from nasal carriage. Uncommonly associated with metastatic infection.

**Community-acquired bacteraemia** is often long-lasting, sometimes presenting with shock, purpuric rash, meningism. Common metastatic infection, including acute endocarditis (➤49).

**Laboratory diagnosis:** Clumps of Gram-positive cocci readily seen in pus, but indistinguishable from coagulase-negative staphylococci. Rapid (24 h) growth on common media → rapid-slide coagulase test (confirm by 4 h tube coagulase test). If bacteraemic, 24–48 h growth from aerobic and anaerobic blood culture bottles. Diagnosis of **TSS** is made by clinical criteria plus isolation of *Staphylococcus aureus* from local site (TSST-1 production confirmed by ➤).

**Treatment:** Drain pus, remove foreign bodies whenever possible. More than 90% are penicillin-resistant ($\beta$-lactamase production) in and out of hospital; locally variable erythromycin and tetracycline resistance rates ~3–15%. **Flucloxacillin** drug of choice: 5–7 days' therapy for mild infections. Co-amoxiclav is a broad-spectrum alternative. Meropenem and most cephalosporins give adequate 'cover'. For **severe infection**: strong evidence for necessary duration is not available, but often given flucloxacillin for (2–)4–6 weeks, initially iv: consider combining with gentamicin or oral

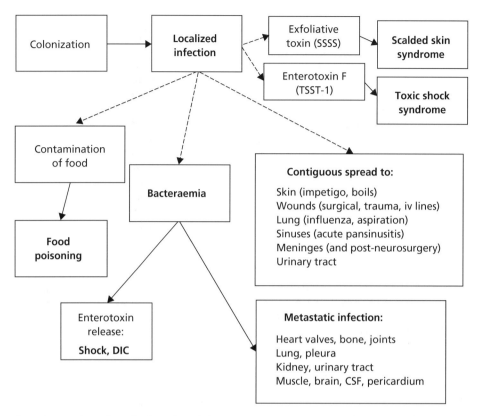

**Figure 24.1** Pathogenic mechanisms of *Staphylococcus aureus*.

fusidic acid or rifampicin especially for initial therapy (if penicillin-allergic, consider substituting erythromycin, vancomycin or parenteral cephalosporin for flucloxacillin).

**Osteomyelitis:** 4–12 weeks (vertebral ⩾8 weeks). Vancomycin and (especially) teicoplanin less effective than flucloxacillin in animal models and clinical studies of severe human infection. **Bacteraemia:** 10–14 days' therapy if short-lasting, e.g. hospital-acquired with removable source (iv line); 4–6 weeks if long-lasting and endocarditis possible (repeat blood cultures during first few days of therapy). Follow-up to exclude metastatic infection (enquire regularly about symptoms; follow ESR, CRP, WBC): seen in up to a third of cases in some series. Consider later switch to oral therapy after initial clinical response. **TSS:** support circulation; identify site of infection and drain if possible; flucloxacillin.

## Methicillin-resistant *Staphylococcus aureus* (MRSA) ①

**Mechanisms:** Resistant to **all** current β-lactam antibiotics (*mecA* gene codes for penicillin-binding protein PBP 2′, which binds β-lactams poorly). Probably arisen by transfer of *mecA* gene from CNSt to multiple strains of susceptible *Staphylococcus aureus* over many years, but great majority of patients acquire MRSA by cross-infection from already colonized patients in hospital.

**Epidemiology:** Many distinct strains, all spread between hospitals by movement of colonized or infected patients and staff. Some apparently have enhanced abilities to spread in hospitals (e.g. 'EMRSA-15' and '-16' currently epidemic in England and Wales), but mechanisms underlying this are unknown. Heavy, persistent colonization associated with chronic skin lesions (e.g. leg ulcers, iv line sites) and in upper airways with antibiotic use.

Rising prevalence since early 1990s in hospitals in the UK and many countries: now endemic in many UK hospitals. Rising prevalence of carriers in long-term care facilities in England and Wales (introduced by patients admitted from local hospitals); occasionally also in some community groups (e.g. iv drug users in US cities): carriage otherwise still rare in general population, but reports of clusters of community-acquired cases are rising.

**Clinical features:** Most MRSA are as virulent as methicillin-sensitive strains. Costs and lengths of stay higher for MRSA-infected patients than matched patients with sensitive *Staphylococcus aureus* infections. Sepsis occurs in 5–60% of those colonized—more frequently in ICU or surgical patients. Currently 43% *Staphylococcus aureus* bacteraemias are MRSA in England and Wales, risen from 2% in 1992 and 22% in 1996 (reporting of MSSA and MRSA bacteraemia by hospitals was made mandatory from April 2001). This rise in MRSA bacteraemias has not been accompanied by a reciprocal fall in methicillin-susceptible *Staphylococcus aureus* bacteraemia, hence the overall prevalence of invasive staphylococcal sepsis has increased.

🖳 www.phls.co.uk

**Antibiotic management:** Often multiply resistant (erythromycin, gentamicin, ciprofloxacin; occasionally rifampicin, fusidic acid, mupirocin).

Vancomycin or teicoplanin the only fully reliable agents. Tetracycline resistance rate locally variable, but may be useful for oral therapy especially in domiciliary practice. Trimethoprim, clindamycin sometimes used.

**New agents:** Quinupristin-dalfopristin (Synercid—iv only) and Linezolid (oral and iv) occasionally useful, but very expensive, innate activity low, side effects troublesome and clinical experience limited (➤412).

**Prevention and control:** Low-prevalence hospitals are recommended to take stringent measures to detect and eradicate MRSA, with isolation of carriers and closure of wards to new admissions when judged clinically worthwhile. High-prevalence units concentrate measures on high-risk areas (e.g. cardiac, vascular and orthopaedic surgery) and rely on 'cohorting' (➤8). Uniform application of stringent measures may be effective at the national level if resources are adequate, e.g. Dutch experience. Consider:

• Surveillance swabbing of high-risk units and isolation (➤8) of high-risk admissions (ICU, interhospital transfers, recent hospital stays abroad and in high-prevalence units, previously positive). Swab nose, throat, 'manipulated sites' and areas of damaged skin (wounds, iv catheter sites, etc.). Results take 3–5 days by culture; rapid molecular methods (e.g. *mecA* detection) under development. Typing of isolates when epidemiologically indicated ➤. Staff now rarely swabbed unless long-term carriage suggested by epidemiological studies.

• Hand hygiene by staff after each patient contact, especially with alcoholic antiseptic handrub.

• Control of antibiotic use. Consider expensive substitution of vancomycin for flucloxacillin for high-risk surgical prophylaxis (➤386).

Control of transmission most successful in specialized isolation unit. Consider 'cohorting' of colonized patients, and closure of wards to new admissions when prevalence of infection high. Risks of transmission greatest when nursing staff workload high.

**Clearance of carriers:** Topical mupirocin and antiseptics; may require systemic antibiotic therapy ☎. Clearance may be necessary to reduce MRSA bacteraemia rates. Most laboratories require three negative weekly screens to designate a once-positive patient clear, but relapse (or reinfection) after this is not rare.

Guidelines for the control of MRSA have been published in the UK and USA:

↦ J Hosp Infect 1998; 39: 253
↦ Am J Infect Control 1998; 26: 102

## 'Vancomycin-resistant' *Staphylococcus aureus*

Emergence in 1997 in Japan of MRSA with

raised glycopeptide MICs giving **intermediate resistance** ('VISA' or 'GISA' strains) in patients given prolonged glycopeptide therapy. Strains with higher-level, stable resistance associated with failure of glycopeptide therapy (vancomycin MIC ~8 mg/L). Mechanism perhaps related to binding of glycopeptide to excess peptidoglycan produced in cell wall. Also reported in other countries, including the USA and UK, and often missed by conventional susceptibility test methods.

The first report of **fully glycopeptide-resistant MRSA** (vancomycin MIC >128 mg/L, teicoplanin 32 mg/L) came in mid-2002 from Michigan, USA. The patient had received several courses of vancomycin for infected foot ulcers, and had chronic renal failure and diabetes. The isolate came from a dialysis catheter and foot ulcer swab, and contained the *vanA* vancomycin resistance gene from enterococci (➤262), and *mecA*. It was susceptible to chloramphenicol, linezolid, minocycline, quinupristin/dalfopristin, tetracycline, and trimethoprim/sulfamethoxazole. No spread to other patients or health-care workers was demonstrated. A second isolate has been reported from Pennsylvania.

## Staphylococcus epidermidis

**Pathogenesis:** Few potential virulence factors; electrostatic attraction to surfaces. Glycocalyx ('slime') production by some strains aids persistent adhesion to medical devices and avoidance of defence mechanisms (by producing 'biofilm').

**Epidemiology:** Resident normal flora of skin, nasopharynx, lower urogenital tract. Most infections are endogenous, but also acquired by hospital cross-infection (especially multiply resistant strains). Outbreaks have been recognized: phage-, bio- and other typing methods available ✈.

**Spectrum of disease:** Predilection for foreign-body infection: iv and ia catheters, pacemakers, heart valve and arterial prostheses, haemodialysis shunts (all causing bacteraemia); Spitz–Holter valves and CSF shunts (➤101); CAPD catheters (➤66); joint prostheses (➤121). Isolation from any site without an implant suggests **contamination**. Also: hospital-associated UTI in elderly males (➤79); neonatal septicaemia and meningitis (often iv catheter-associated) (➤139); rare native valve endocarditis (➤49). Other coagulase-negative staphylococci occasionally isolated from similar infections, but more often contaminants. *Staphylococcus lugdunensis* is associated with endocarditis.

**Laboratory diagnosis:** Clumps of Gram-positive cocci readily seen in pus (indistinguishable from *Staphylococcus aureus*). Rapid (24-h) growth on common media → negative rapid slide coagulase test (confirm by 4-h tube coagulase test). Not usually identified to species level (often reported as 'coagulase-negative staphylococcus'). If bacteraemic, 24–48 h growth from aerobic and anaerobic blood culture bottles. Isolates are more likely to be significant if foreign body present, if multiple bottles from several blood cultures positive, if all cultures positive within 48 h and if same strain (e.g. same sensitivity pattern) isolated from all cultures.

**Treatment:** Often multiply resistant, and vancomycin is the only fully reliable agent for systemic infections (occasional strains teicoplanin-resistant); await susceptibility testing results before choosing alternatives. Removal of foreign body often essential, and may be all that is required in iv catheter infection. If treatment is attempted without device removal (e.g. Hickman line infection), the best choice is vancomycin.

## Staphylococcus saprophyticus

Common cause of lower UTI in sexually active women (➤77). Usually susceptible to trimethoprim, nitrofurantoin, flucloxacillin, oral cephalosporins.

## Stomatococcus mucilaginosus

Oral commensal; mucoid colonies; similar pathogenicity to CNSt.

# Chapter 25

# Streptococci and their relatives

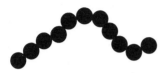

Streptococci are round or oval Gram-positive organisms that tend to form chains, especially in the tissues and in liquid culture. They are commensals of the mouth, nasopharynx, colon and lower urogenital tract, and several species are major pathogens. Penicillin remains the drug of choice for most streptococcal infections, but problems of antibiotic resistance have become increasingly common recently.

## Classification methods (Table 25.1)

**Lancefield grouping:** Classification of cell-wall carbohydrate antigens into groups A–V; originally used only for β-haemolytic strains, now used for many streptococcal species. Colonies are tested by latex agglutination kits; rapid grouping of organisms seen in blood culture broths often possible before growth on solid media.

**Haemolysis:** Classification based on effects of bacterial colonies on blood agar plates:
- **α-Haemolytic:** partial lysis of erythrocytes and haemoglobin breakdown → green pigment (hence 'viridans' group streptococci).
- **β-Haemolytic:** complete haemolysis → clear zones around colonies.
- **Non-haemolytic** (sometimes called 'γ-haemolytic'): no effects.
(N.b. Strains of many bacterial species produce haemolysis on blood agar).

**Identification:** Commercial biochemical kits are now commonly used to identify some groups of streptococci (e.g. 'viridans' group) to species level when necessary.

## Streptococcus pyogenes (Gp A β-haemolytic streptococci, GAS) ①

**Pathogenesis:** Exclusively a human pathogen; many structural and extracellular products with few defined roles (Table 25.2).

**Epidemiology:** Found in nose/throat swabs of 10% normal people; occasionally carried on perineum alone. Minor septic lesions and nasal carriage → heavy airborne dispersal. Also spread by respiratory secretions and hands. Frequent direct transmission between household and close physical contacts; very rarely acquired via fomites. Occasional food- and milk-borne outbreaks. Typing by cell-wall proteins (M, T and R antigens; ✈); some types associated with particular diseases (e.g. outbreaks of acute glomerulonephritis type 49, rheumatic fever type 5).

### Spectrum of disease
**Skin sepsis:** Cardinal sign is cellulitis (➤113). Often blistering → serous discharge. Lymphangitis. Frequently mixed infection with *Staphylococcus aureus*. Important syndromes: impetigo (localized crusting ➤111); erysipelas (well-demarcated cellulitis, especially of face ➤113); necrotizing fasciitis (necrosis of skin and subcutaneous tissues ➤115); streptococcal myositis (80–100% mortality). Nowadays surgical wound infection and puerperal sepsis are rare (and both now most commonly autoinfections).
　　**Pharyngitis and tonsillitis:** (➤19).
　　**Acute otitis media:** (➤17).
　　**Vaginitis:** (➤82).

**Table 25.1** Classification of streptococci

| Genus | Species | Notes |
|---|---|---|
| *Streptococcus* | *pyogenes* | Lancefield Gp A β-haemolytic streptococcus (GAS) |
| | (*dysgalactiae* ssp. *equisimilis*) | Lancefield Gp C β-haemolytic streptococci, Lancefield Gp G β-haemolytic streptococci; previously '*Streptococcus equisimilis*', '*zooepidemicus*' and '*equi*' |
| | (*iniae*) | Rare cause of septicaemia and local septic lesions acquired from contact with pigs |
| | *agalactiae* | Lancefield Gp B β-haemolytic streptococcus |
| | '*milleri*' group | Lancefield Gp A, C, F, G or none; β- or non-haemolytic. Includes *constellatus*, *anginosus* and *intermedius* |
| | (*mutans, oralis, sanguis I* and *II, mitis, salivarius, mitior, sobrinus*, etc.) | 'Viridans' group; many are α-haemolytic. |
| | (*bovis, gallolyticus*) | Previously *bovis* types I and II, respectively; Lancefield Gp D |
| | *pneumoniae* | 'Pneumococci'; α-haemolytic |
| | (*suis*) | Lancefield Gp R (➤260) |
| (*Abiotropha* | *adiacens, defectiva, elegans*) | 'Nutritionally variant' streptococci; formerly '*Streptococcus defectivus*' |
| *Enterococcus* | *faecalis, faecium* (*durans, avium, casseliflavus\*, gallinarum\*, cecorum, dispar, flavescens, hirae*, etc.) | Lancefield Gp D |
| *Peptostreptococcus* | *anaerobius, asaccharolyticus, magnus, micros, prevotii*, etc. | 'Anaerobic streptococci' (➤313). Many previously in '*Peptococcus*' genus. |
| (*Aerococcus* | *viridans\*, urinae*) | Commensals of mucosal surfaces, rarely pathogenic. They have caused endocarditis and meningitis, and various opportunistic infections. |
| (*Leuconostoc\** | *cremoris, citreum*, etc.) | |
| (*Pediococcus\** | *acidilactici, equinus, damnosus*, etc.) | |
| (*Gemella* | *haemolysans\*, morbillorum*, etc.) | |
| (*Lactococcus* | *lactis\*, garvieae*) | |

\* Frequently naturally vancomycin resistant.

**Bacteraemia:** Uncommonly accompanies severe tissue infection; mortality >20%. Occasional 'toxic shock'-like syndrome with high mortality, associated with necrotizing fasciitis (➤115). (Σ 845 bacteraemias.)

**Indirect sequelae** (all uncommon in developed world):

- **Scarlet fever** (➤135).
- **Rheumatic fever** (➤257).
- **Glomerulonephritis** (➤256).

**Laboratory diagnosis:** Ready growth on blood agar in 24 h → dry colonies with wide haemolysis zone. Confirmed by rapid Lancefield grouping. Rising ASO (especially throat infections) and anti-DNAase B (especially skin infections) titres useful for confirming diagnosis of indirect sequelae. Immunoassay kits for direct detection in throat swabs are rapid, but expensive and less sensitive than culture (which should be performed in addition) (➤19).

**Table 25.2** Group A streptococcal products contributing to pathogenicity

| Factor | Role |
|---|---|
| M cell-wall protein | Fimbriae-associated; antiphagocytic, anticomplement and epithelial adhesion roles. Specific antibodies are protective |
| Hyaluronic acid capsule | Antiphagocytic; strains with mucoid colonies produce more capsule and may be more pathogenic |
| DNAases A, B, C, D | Basis of anti-DNAase B assay |
| Streptolysins O and S | Haemolytic, cytotoxic; basis of antistreptolysin O (ASO) assay |
| Hyaluronidase, streptokinase | ? Involved in spread through tissues |
| Erythrogenic toxins | Produced by some strains after phage lysogeny. Rash, fever, cytotoxic effects 'scarlet fever' |

Others include pyrogenic exotoxin, NADase, serum opacity factor. F1 invasin present on surface of epithelial invasive strains. Nephritogenic strains probably share antigens with human glomerular basement membrane.

**Treatment:** Invariably benzylpenicillin-sensitive, but up to 14.4 g/day sometimes needed for clinical response in serious infection (especially with arterial insufficiency). Add clindamycin 600–1200 mg 6-hourly if necrotizing infection suspected; surgical debridement essential (➤115). Combine with flucloxacillin for known or suspected mixed infection with *Staphylococcus aureus* (mild–moderate infections can be managed on flucloxacillin alone). Erythromycin (3–8% resistance, geographically variable) or oral cephalosporin are alternative choices in penicillin allergy. Tetracycline resistance common in some areas; co-trimoxazole or trimethoprim poorly effective. β-Lactamase production by throat commensals may reduce penicillin activity, therefore co-amoxiclav or erythromycin may be preferable. To clear throat carriage, 10 days' therapy required. Topical agents adequate for impetigo in domiciliary practice (➤111). In hospital, isolate patients with *Streptococcus pyogenes* and consider screening contacts (nose, throat, perineum, skin lesions).

## Clinical Syndromes

**Important definitions**
**Rheumatic fever** is an immunological reaction to infection by GAS.

**Rheumatic heart disease** describes the cardiac damage resulting from a previous attack of rheumatic fever. It does not imply ongoing infection. Valvular scarring may continue in the absence of infection, due in part to disturbed blood flow through damaged valves.

**Infective endocarditis** (syn. subacute bacterial endocarditis) is infection of the heart valves. It is particularly likely to occur on valves previously damaged by rheumatic fever. Infection is commonly due to α-haemolytic 'viridans' streptococci.

**POSTSTREPTOCOCCAL GLOMERULONEPHRITIS (PSGN)**
Immune complex-mediated glomerulonephritis may follow pharyngeal or skin/soft tissue infection by some strains (M-type 12 in the UK) of GAS. It is now rare in the UK.

*(continued...)*

**Clinical features:** Asymptomatic episodes of nephritis are common. Patients develop haematuria, proteinuria, hypertension, uraemia and oedema 1–2 weeks after a streptococcal pharyngitis (2–3 weeks after skin infection). Nephrotic syndrome occurs occasionally. Approximately 30% do not recall an antecedent infection. Prognosis in children is very good, with <1% progressing to chronic renal failure. In adults, up to 30% may have long-standing renal damage and ultimate renal failure.

**Microbiological investigations:** Throat/lesion swab may grow GAS. Serology (➤19).

**Other investigations:** ESR is elevated. Renal biopsy is rarely indicated, but shows diffuse proliferative glomerulonephritis.

**Antibiotic management:** Prompt antibiotic treatment of streptococcal pharyngitis reduces the risk of PSGN. Treatment should be given for 10 days with penicillin V, amoxicillin or erythromycin. Antibiotics do not abort established PSGN.

**Supportive management:** Renal failure may require specific management.

**Differential diagnosis:** IgA nephropathy presents with haematuria at the same time as upper respiratory tract infection.

RHEUMATIC FEVER (RF)
RF is an immunologically mediated hypersensitivity response following pharyngeal infection by particular strains of GAS which do not cause skin infection. Incidence has declined dramatically in the developed world, but is increasing in the developing countries. Extremely rare in the UK. Outbreaks reported in the USA among military personnel.

**Risk factors:** Previous and recurrent exposure to infection by GAS predisposes to development of RF. Once RF is acquired, it may easily be reactivated by subsequent streptococcal infections; ≈50% of

GAS infections occurring in the first year after an attack of RF are followed by a second attack.

**Clinical features:** Onset occurs ≈3 weeks (range 1–5) after streptococcal pharyngitis, which may not be recalled by the patient. Diagnosis is made on the basis of modified Jones criteria (see Table 25.3)—RF is suggested by the presence of two major criteria or one major and two minor criteria, plus evidence of recent streptococcal infection. Pleurisy and abdominal pain also occur frequently. Normochromic, normocytic anaemia is common.

**Prognosis:** Immediate mortality is 5%. About 50% develop rheumatic heart disease (RHD) 10 years after RF. Mitral regurgitation and mitral stenosis are the commonest lesions; aortic stenosis and regurgitation and tricuspid lesions also occur, but pulmonary valve lesions are uncommon. Valvular damage may progress in the absence of recurrent RF. Following an attack of RF, patients should receive continuous antibiotic prophylaxis to prevent recurrences—see below. Patients with RHD or a history of RF are also at risk for infective endocarditis and should receive antibiotic prophylaxis prior to dental and other procedures (➤53).

**Microbiological investigations:** Throat swab. Serology (➤19).

**Antibiotic management:** Penicillin should be given to eradicate persistent GAS infection. Aspirin (6–9 g/day) and steroids (prednisolone 40–60 mg daily initially, reducing over ≈6 weeks) may be given to control carditis and arthritis. Secondary prophylaxis must be given to prevent recurrences. Penicillin V 250 mg 12-hly po, erythromycin if penicillin-allergic. Prophylaxis should be continued into adult life in all patients, and many recommend indefinite treatment especially after proven carditis. Primary prophylaxis may also be used to prevent infection in closed communities such as military barracks.
  Strict bedrest for at least 2 weeks is usually advised.

**Table 25.3** Modified Jones criteria for diagnosis of RF

| Major criteria | Comments |
| --- | --- |
| Carditis | 'Pancarditis': Endocarditis causing valvular damage with murmur of mitral regurgitation and, less often, apical mid-diastolic murmur (Carey–Coombs murmur) and aortic regurgitation. Pericarditis (5–10%). Congestive cardiac failure (5–10%). Arrhythmia and heart block rare |
| Arthritis | Large joints mainly affected. Frequently migratory |
| Chorea ('St Vitus's dance') | Abrupt erratic purposeless movements and emotional lability. After puberty, chorea occurs exclusively in women. It is rare after adolescence. Usually lasts 2–4 months |
| Subcutaneous nodules | Painless subcutaneous nodules (0.5–2 cm) over bony prominences and tendons. Often symmetrical and occurring in crops. Not attached to skin, which is mobile and not inflamed |
| Erythema marginatum | Bright pink, blanching, non-indurated, non-pruritic, non-painful, serpiginous 'smoke ring' rash. May persist for several weeks after recovery |
| Minor criteria | Fever, arthralgia, previous rheumatic fever or rheumatic heart disease, raised ESR or CRP, prolonged P–R interval |

# Lancefield Gp C and G streptococci

Release many of the same extracellular products as *Streptococcus pyogenes*, and can cause most of the same diseases; more commonly they behave as commensals, or cause milder illness. Gp C are mainly animal pathogens. Gp G infections associated with underlying malignancy; 11–12% are erythromycin resistant. (Bacteraemia: Σ 528 Gp G; Σ 158 Gp C.)

## *Streptococcus agalactiae* (Lancefield Gp B)

Lancefield Gp B β-haemolytic streptococcus.

**Pathogenesis:** Largely unknown mechanisms; shares sialic acid capsular antigen with K1 *Escherichia coli* (➤279). Low neonatal/maternal capsular antibody titres correlate with infection. Distinct strains cause bovine mastitis. Risk associated with diabetes may be due to high serum glucose concentrations interfering with specific streptococcus-host cell interactions.

**Epidemiology:** Faecal commensal in ≈30% people, colonizing vagina in 10–30%. If maternal vagina positive, neonate has higher risk of premature delivery and 70% become colonized (➤140). Disease commoner with prolonged rupture of membranes, prematurity, heavy vaginal carriage, certain racial groups. Rising incidence for past 30 yrs, but intrapartum prophylaxis has reduced incidence in N. America and Australia. Typing by carbohydrate and protein antigens (➤). (Σ 905 bacteraemias: 1.77/100 000 population.)

### Spectrum of disease
**Neonatal sepsis:** Causes 30% cases: Σ 0.66 per 1000 live births (➤139).
• **Early onset** (first few days): septicaemic systemic infection with meningitis and pneumonia, acquired during passage through maternal vagina. Mortality previously 15–50%, but <10% in 1990s with improved recognition and prompt treatment.
• **Late onset** (after 7 days): meningitis (occasionally other sites, e.g. skin sepsis, osteomyelitis). Less common, better prognosis. Usually acquired by cross-infection in nursery and not associated with prematurity, etc.
**Puerperal sepsis** (➤83): Infected retained products, endometritis, pelvic sepsis, occasional bacteraemia. Often mixed infections with vaginal non-sporing anaerobes, *Strepto-*

coccus 'milleri', Gardnerella vaginalis, Mycoplasma hominis, coliforms, etc.

**Adult infections:** Frequently colonizes bed-sores, varicose ulcers, etc.; UTI; occasional cellulitis of ischaemic limbs (usually mixed infections ➤125), bacteraemia, pneumonia, endocarditis (all associated with old age, diabetes, cirrhosis, renal failure, stroke, malignancy).

**Laboratory diagnosis:** Septic infants: send blood culture, two surface swabs (e.g. ear + umbilicus), maternal HVS. Rapid (24-h) growth on blood agar, forming moist colonies with narrow haemolysis zone. Lancefield grouping of colonies by latex agglutination.

**Treatment:** Less penicillin-sensitive than *Streptococcus pyogenes*; add gentamicin for severe illness for improved bactericidal effect. Parenteral cephalosporin, erythromycin (5–16% resistance) and vancomycin (no resistance reported, but little clinical experience) are alternatives. Evacuation of retained products of conception plus antibiotics (e.g. parenteral cephalosporin + metronidazole) for puerperal sepsis.

**Prevention:** (➤140).

## Streptococcus 'milleri'

A group of related species causing similar clinical syndromes; mucosal commensals requiring raised $CO_2$ and humidity for growth on blood agar.

**Pathogenesis:** Unknown virulence factors.

**Epidemiology:** Normal flora of mouth, upper respiratory tract, colon and lower urogenital tract. Cause endogenous infections, often mixed with other local mucosal commensals (especially non-sporing anaerobes; also coliforms, coagulase-negative staphylococci, coryneforms). $\Sigma$ 428 bacteraemias.

**Spectrum of disease:** Hallmark is **abscess formation** ± associated bacteraemia; includes intra-abdominal (e.g. perforated diverticulum, appendix abscess, puerperal sepsis), liver (portal pyaemia), lung (aspiration pneumonia, empyema), brain. Also chronic sinusitis, occasionally endocarditis.

**Laboratory diagnosis:** Tiny Gram-positive cocci in chains, often grow best with anaerobic incubation → minute colonies (48 h) on blood agar, smelling of toffee. Lancefield grouping of colonies by latex agglutination (most commonly group F; may be A, C, G or none).

**Treatment:** Hunt for and drain abscesses; broad-spectrum therapy for mixed infections, e.g. iv benzylpenicillin + gentamicin + metronidazole, meropenem, or oral co-amoxiclav.

## 'Viridans' and 'non-haemolytic' streptococci

These group names are preferred to 'Streptococcus viridans', which is not a true species.

**Pathogenesis:** No recognized toxins; strains causing IE often produce complex carbohydrates (dextrans), aiding adhesion to teeth and heart valves.

**Epidemiology:** Mucosal commensals of mouth, upper respiratory tract; some strains bind to teeth. Replaced at these sites by coliforms, pseudomonads, *Staphylococcus aureus* and *Candida* spp. after antibiotic treatment or prolonged tracheal intubation.

### Spectrum of disease

Infective endocarditis (➤49).
**Gum sepsis, dental caries:** Especially *Streptococcus mutans*.
**Bacteraemia:** With pulmonary symptoms and signs (especially *Streptococcus mitis* in neutropenic patients with oral ulceration, and neonates).

**Laboratory diagnosis:** Often long chains in broth cultures. Rapid (24-h) growth on blood agar to form tiny α- or non-haemolytic colonies. In IE, 24–48 h growth from aerobic and anaerobic blood culture bottles. Sometimes carry a variety of Lancefield group antigens.

**Treatment:** Mostly penicillin-sensitive, unless patient given penicillin in past month. Combination with gentamicin improves cidal effect in IE treatment/prophylaxis unless high-level aminoglycoside resistant (➢402).

## *Streptococcus bovis*

Colonic commensal carrying Lancefield Gp D antigen, but bacteriologically very similar to 'viridans' streptococci. Causes IE associated with colonic adenocarcinoma (screen cases with barium enema). Σ 158 bacteraemias.

## Nutritionally variant streptococci (*Abiotropha* spp.)

Rare strains nutritionally dependent (pyridoxal/cysteine) for growth on solid agars: satellite around *Staphylococcus aureus* colonies (☎). Reportedly isolated from 4% streptococcal IE; associated with higher rate of failure, relapse and mortality (➢49). Most appear tolerant to penicillin, and clinical response to penicillin–gentamicin combinations not consistent. Vancomycin effective in animal models. Σ 2 bacteraemias.

## *Streptococcus suis* (Lancefield Gp R)

Commensal and pathogen in pigs: occupationally acquired by farmers, butchers, food handlers causing meningitis and septicaemia. Penicillin-susceptible, but some strains reported tolerant (consider adding gentamicin). Σ 2 bacteraemias.

## *Streptococcus pneumoniae* (syn. pneumococcus)

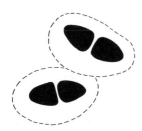

**Pathogenesis:** Pneumonia and invasive infection follow nasopharyngeal colonization. Produces various extracellular toxins, but carbohydrate capsule the most important virulence factor (non-toxic, but antiphagocytic). Heavily capsulate strains form mucoid colonies; those of low serotype (especially types 3, 7 and 1) associated with highest mortality. Protection needs type-specific antibodies (especially $IgG_2$) and intact phagocytic system. Alcoholics, HIV antibody-positive, elderly, very young, post-splenectomy, post-influenza have greatest risk. Other factors include skull fracture, blocked Eustachian tube, smoking, COPD, reduced vascular perfusion (e.g. sickle-cell disease, congestive cardiac failure), C2 and C3 deficiency. Highly toxic polysaccharide cell wall, containing phosphorylcholine (attaches to activated endothelial cells during invasion).

**Epidemiology:** In normal population, 10–30% nasopharyngeal carriage rate. Typing by capsular swelling with specific antibodies (Quellung reaction; 90 serotypes ✈).

**Spectrum of disease**
**Community-acquired pneumonia:** Commonest cause, 50–80% overall; frequently lobar pattern. Bacteraemia occurs in 15–25% patients (➢25). Σ 3585 bacteraemias.

    **Acute exacerbations of COPD:** Often mixed with *Haemophilus influenzae*, *Moraxella catarrhalis* (➢24).

    **Sinusitis and otitis media** (➢17).

    **Meningitis** (➢96).

    **'Occult' bacteraemia:** In febrile children (➢139).

    **Rare others:** acute endocarditis, cellulitis, haemolytic–uraemic syndrome (➢277).

**Laboratory diagnosis:** Direct antigen detection in sputum, serum, CSF or urine sometimes useful (detect capsular polysaccharide or common 'C' antigen). Characteristic 'lanceolate' diplococci on sputum Gram stain, but not specific unless sample is well taken (if >25 pus cells and <10 epithelial cells per high power field, sensitivity is 62% and specificity 85%). In 24–48 h produce α-haemolytic 'draughtsman' colonies (from zonal autolysis) on blood agar.

Differentiate from 'viridans' streptococci by optochin sensitivity and bile solubility. May autolyse in blood culture broths (try antigen detection on the broth ☎).

**Treatment:** Classically, benzylpenicillin is the drug of choice; erythromycin resistance 5–15%. Avoid tetracycline, trimethoprim (resistance up to 20%). Intermediate (IPR: MIC 0.1–1 mg/L) and full (FPR: MIC ≥2 mg/L) penicillin resistance patchily distributed in the UK: higher in inner city areas and after recent antibiotic therapy (see Table 25.4). Meningitis and otitis media caused by IPR strains require alternative treatment (➤96, ➤17, see below), but other infections normally treatable by high doses of benzylpenicillin or other β-lactams (e.g. cefotaxime or ceftriaxone). Recent evidence suggests outcome may be worse for severe pneumonia with IPR. High prevalence (30–50%) of IPR/FPR strains in Spain, E. Europe, S. Africa, S. America, SE Asia: especially types 9, 14, 19, 23 and commoner in children. Outbreaks of infection in Spain, South Africa, New Guinea with multiply-resistant FPR strains—also resistant to erythromycin, tetracycline, chloramphenicol; combinations of cefotaxime, rifampicin and vancomycin have been used (isolation for these strains ①). Optimal empirical therapy depends on local prevalence of penicillin and cefotaxime resistance (☎), severity of illness, prior antibiotic therapy: e.g. cefotaxime + vancomycin recommended in the UK for meningitis with pre-admission antibiotics (➤98). Beware of IPR and FPR in returning travellers from high-prevalence areas. Some β-lactams have poor activity against IPR and FPR strains (e.g. ceftazidime).

**Prevention:** Polysaccharide vaccine available for at-risk groups; includes 23 capsular serotypes which cause >90% invasive infections, including common multiply-resistant serotypes. Poorly effective under age 2. A polyvalent (7-valent) conjugated polysaccharide vaccine has recently been introduced for children between 2 months and 2 yrs of age who are at particular risk. Combine with penicillin prophylaxis after splenectomy (➤170).

# Enterococci

*Enterococcus faecalis* and *faecium* (and rare others).

**Pathogenesis:** Various putative virulence factors, including adhesins and enzymes. Commonly superinfect patients receiving cephalosporins.

**Epidemiology:** Normal flora of colon. Resistant strains spread in hospital by hands and equipment; survive well on surfaces in the environment. Hospital-acquired infections increasingly common, especially catheter-associated UTI, bacteraemia.

### Spectrum of disease
**Urinary tract infection** (➤77).
**Infective endocarditis** (➤49). IE must be excluded whenever enterococci are grown from blood cultures: may present only with fever + metastatic infection (e.g. enterococcal osteomyelitis or mycotic aneurysm) in an elderly patient, and the murmur may be thought to be aortic sclerosis.
**IV catheter infection:** Also joint and heart valve prostheses and other foreign bodies.
**Wound colonization/infection:** Mixed with other faecal flora in wounds, ulcers, abdominal abscesses, bedsores. Not usually clinically significant and may resolve with drainage and treatment of other components of the infection.

**Laboratory diagnosis:** Tolerant of heat, bile salts

**Table 25.4** Rising UK pneumococcal resistance rates (%)

| Antibiotic | 1990 | 1995 | 1997 |
|---|---|---|---|
| Penicillin (intermediate) | 0.9 | 1.9 ⎫ | 7.4 |
| Penicillin (full) | 0.6 | 2.0 ⎬ | |
| Cefotaxime (intermediate) | 1.1 | 2.2 | |
| Cefotaxime (full) | 0 | 0.7 | |
| Erythromycin | 2.8 | 8.6 | 11.8 |
| Tetracycline | 5.0 | 5.1 | |

and high salt concentrations. Ready (24-h) growth on many media to form small, shiny colonies. Some strains α- or β-haemolytic. Lancefield grouping of colonies by latex agglutination.

**Treatment:** Colonization and minor infection are common: serious infection is rare, and iv line-related bacteraemia often responds to simple line removal. Benzylpenicillin the drug of choice, but enterococci are naturally among the most penicillin-resistant streptococci (especially *Enterococcus faecium*). Not killed by penicillin or vancomycin alone, hence add gentamicin for synergistic bactericidal effect in infective endocarditis (➤49) and serious infection. Balance risks of prolonged gentamicin therapy carefully against likelihood of patient having IE in uncertain cases (☎). More sensitive *in vitro* to amp/amoxicillin than benzylpenicillin, but larger doses of benzylpenicillin can be given so difference clinically insignificant. Sensitive to vancomycin, teicoplanin; innately resistant to flucloxacillin, trimethoprim, most cephalosporins; most quinolones only weakly active.

Rising prevalence of 'ampicillin-' and '**high-level gentamicin-resistant**' (**HLGR**) *Enterococcus faecalis* and *faecium* in the 1990s rendered treatment of serious infection difficult because of inability to achieve a cidal effect (☎). Over 50% bacteraemic strains in some hospitals now ampicillin- and/or high-level gentamicin-resistant (some of these remain streptomycin susceptible). Recent emergence of **vancomycin-resistant enterococci (VRE, also known as 'glycopeptide-resistant enterococci', GRE.** Isolation ①): associated with extended-spectrum cephalosporins, but apparently not with glycopeptide use. Some strains have epidemic potential in hospitals (spread on staff hands, and survive well on dry surfaces), and others may be acquired in human faecal flora from animals given glycopeptide growth promoters. Discuss need for antibiotic therapy and choice of agents with ☎ — clinical significance often dubious except in liver transplantation, haematological malignancy, prosthesis infection. Some strains may be treatable by teicoplanin, but roles of quinupristin–dalfopristin (Synercid usually inactive against *Enterococcus faecalis* ➤412) and linezolid (➤412) remain to be established. Possible alternatives include chloramphenicol, rifampicin, tetracyclines, new quinolones.

| **Practice point** |
| :--- |
| Enterococci are innately resistant to all cephalosporins. |

# Chapter 26

# Aerobic Gram-positive rods

A mixed bag of mainly facultative anaerobes. Although obligately anaerobic, *Propionibacterium* spp. cause similar clinical syndromes to the coryneforms, and are therefore considered here. Some of these organisms are associated with specific invasive or toxin-associated infections, including *Bacillus anthracis, Listeria monocytogenes* and *Corynebacterium diphtheriae*. Others are opportunist pathogens. Usage is inconsistent, but we shall use 'coryneforms' and 'diphtheroids' interchangeably for small Gram-positive rods that stain variably, tend to be arranged in angled pairs or palisades, are non-branching, and share various biochemical features. Coryneforms include a number of *Corynebacterium* spp. (e.g. *striatum, renale*) and *Listeria* spp., together with a few non-human pathogens.

## *Bacillus* spp.

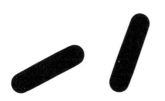

Large, spore-forming Gram-positive rods. Most are obligate aerobes and, with the exception of *Bacillus anthracis*, are common environmental organisms in the UK. Thus they frequently contaminate clinical specimens, and true infection must be carefully distinguished. Considerable colonial, staining (frequently appearing Gram-negative), biochemical and antigenic variation is present within this genus; *Bacillus* spp. are often difficult to identify to species level (✈) and are readily mistaken for other organisms. Σ ≈ 150 bacteraemias.

## *Bacillus anthracis* ✉

**Pathogenesis:** Depends on polypeptide capsule (prevents phagocytosis) and plasmid-encoded protein toxins (bind to cell surfaces and block adenyl cyclase → increased vascular permeability → shock).

**Epidemiology:** *Bacillus anthracis* forms spores which may remain infective in soil for decades. Economically important domesticated animal pathogen in many countries of Africa, Asia and Indian subcontinent. Occasional incidents in UK cattle. Acquired by humans from infected herbivore carcasses. Occupational disease in the UK (mainly hide and wool workers—'woolsorter's disease'; average 1 report p.a. in the UK for past 7 yrs). Last deaths in the UK in 1974, associated with bone-meal exposure. In the past, anthrax has been associated with tanneries and textile industries in which humans come into contact with animal hide or hair. Vaccination of livestock and industrial disinfection procedures have largely eradicated this form of disease in the developed world. In the developing world, anthrax still occurs, also associated with animal herding.

Important **bioterrorism agent** (✈415), especially when milled to fine dust ('weapons-grade'), promoting aerosol dispersal. One deep breath of such preparations may contain $10^5$ spores.

🖥 www.bt.cdc.gov/DocumentsApp/
FactsAbout/FactsAbout.asp

**Spectrum of disease:** Causes anthrax.

**Laboratory diagnosis:** One of the few non-motile *Bacillus* spp.; capsule demonstrable by McFadyean's stain. Grows readily (24 h) on most media to large, grey, non-haemolytic colonies with wavy margins ('Medusa head',

**Table 26.1** Classification of aerobic Gram-positive rods

| Genus | Species | Notes |
|---|---|---|
| *Bacillus* | *anthracis* | Causes anthrax (➢263) |
| | *cereus* | Causes food poisoning (➢266) |
| | (*subtilis, thuringiensis, pumilis, licheniformis, circulans, megaterium,* etc.) | Uncommon opportunistic infections. Environmental organisms, frequently contaminate clinical specimens |
| *Listeria* | *monocytogenes* | Grows at low temperature; tumbling motility (➢266) |
| | (*grayi, ivanovii\*, innocua, seeligeri\*, welshmeri*) | Not human pathogens (*1–6 cases of human infection reported for each) |
| *Corynebacterium* | *diphtheriae* | Causes diphtheria (➢268) |
| | *jeikeium* | Multiply antibiotic-resistant (➢269) |
| | *minutissimum* | Causes erythrasma (➢270) |
| | *urealyticum* | Urinary tract pathogen (➢270) |
| | (*renale, striatum, ulcerans, xerosis, pseudotuberculosis, auris, accolens, pseudodiphtheriticum, amycolatum, afermentans, aquaticum,* CDC coryneform groups (ANF-1, ANF-3, F2, G-1, I2, 6), etc.) | Skin and upper respiratory commensals, rare pathogens. *C. amycolatum* newly described: previously misidentified as *minutissimum* or *striatum* |
| *Propionibacterium* | *acnes,* etc. | Obligate anaerobes |
| (*Rhodococcus*) | (*equi*) | Horse and rare human pathogen (➢270). Some other *Rhodococcus* spp. now known as *Gordona* and *Tsukamurella* spp. |
| *Arcanobacterium* | *haemolyticum* (*pyogenes*) | Causes sore throat with rash (➢19, 270) |
| *Lactobacillus* spp. | | Large group of uncommon pathogens |
| *Erysipelothrix* | *rhusiopathiae* | Causes erysipeloid (➢271) |
| *Nocardia* | *asteroides* (*brasiliensis, otitidiscaviarum, 'caviae',* etc.) | Weakly acid-fast, aerobic |
| (*Tropheryma*) | (*whipplei*) | Previously '*T. whippelii*'. Causes Whipple's disease (➢272) |
| *Gardnerella* | *vaginalis* | Associated with bacterial vaginosis (➢82, 302) |

*Rothia denticarosa, Kurthia* spp., *Bifidobacterium bifidum, Oerskovia* spp., *Arthrobacter* spp., *Aureobacterium* spp., *Brevibacterium* spp., *Cellulomonas* spp., *Dermabacter* spp., *Microbacterium* spp., *Paenibacillus* spp., *Streptomyces* spp., *Tsukamurella* spp., *Turicella* spp. and members of other CDC Groups (A-1, A-2, A-3, A-4, A-5, B-1, B-3, E, 1, 2, 3, 5) are generally human and animal mucosal commensals and very rare causes of local septic lesions in humans. Increasingly they are represented in commercial identification systems (e.g. API (RAPID) Coryne). The rapidly-growing mycobacteria are close relatives.

'bees-eye'); ✦. Serology available for epidemiological investigations (✦).

**Prevention:** Investigation of animal deaths, incineration, isolation, animal vaccination (live, attenuated strain); disinfection of imported animal products; immunization of exposed workers and vets (repeated toxoid injections; some concerns over safety of live vaccine). Extremely rare person → person spread, mainly because sporulation does not occur in the body; secondary aerosols of spores may arise from environmental contamination. Single-room isolation not recommended in the UK, but standard universal precautions should be employed (gloves, plastic aprons, hand hygiene). Decontamination of exposed persons by showering prior to hospital admission. Prophylaxis (see below). Environmental decontamination of small areas can be done with 5000 ppm hypochlorite (1:9 dilution of household bleach).

🖥 www.phls.co.uk/topics_az/
anthrax/guidelines.pdf

## Clinical syndrome

### Anthrax ✉

**Clinical features:** Cutaneous anthrax (syn. 'malignant pustule') accounts for most cases. Infection is acquired by inoculation of spores into an abrasion in the skin. After 3–10 days, a painless pruritic papule develops, which then vesiculates and ulcerates over 1–2 days, leaving a necrotic ulcer ('eschar'), which may be surrounded by a ring of vesicles. Painful regional lymphadenopathy and marked local oedema are usual. Malaise, fever and leucocytosis occur in 50% of patients. Untreated mortality is 5–20%, usually as a result of bacteraemia. Differential diagnoses include boils (➤111), orf (➤119), erysipeloid (➤113) and syphilitic chancre (➤89).

Inhalational anthrax is much rarer. It occurs in industry or as a result of BT following inhalation of large numbers of spores (ID$_{50}$ ≈10$^4$), and causes haemorrhage in mediastinal lymph nodes. Patients present with a few days' history of upper respiratory symptoms, followed by rapid deterioration, with dyspnoea, cyanosis, *(continued...)*

shock and death. Incubation period usually 2–7 days, but can be up to 6 weeks. CXR (abnormal in all BT-associated pulmonary cases) shows mediastinal widening, pulmonary infiltrates and pleural/pericardial effusion. Mediastinal lymph-node enlargement well shown on chest CT scans; pulmonary infiltrates often minimal (🖥 http://anthrax.radpath.org). Blood cultures were positive in all 7 BT-associated pulmonary anthrax cases in 2001 who had not received prior antibiotics.

For advice on distinguishing influenza-like illness from inhalational anthrax and guidelines for investigation of and response to *Bacillus anthracis* exposures:

↦ MMWR 2001; 50: 984–990.

**Gastrointestinal anthrax** is extremely rare. It occurs 1–7 d after eating raw or undercooked meat heavily contaminated with spores, causing abdominal pain and haemorrhagic diarrhoea. Case fatality rate 25–60%.

**Bacteraemia** is a terminal event common to all these syndromes.

**Microbiological investigations:** Aspirate fluid from vesicles surrounding pustule, swab under eschar and send sputum (low yield) and blood cultures (**warn lab!** ☎). Skin biopsy at eschar edge useful for culture, PCR or histochemistry. Nasal swab cultures may be useful in investigating possible airborne *B. anthracis* exposure, but not for diagnosing clinical cases or as a guide to need for prophylaxis (☎ before taking).

**Antibiotic management:** Antibiotics do not speed healing of cutaneous lesions, but prevent death due to bacteraemic spread. Penicillin the classical drug of choice—iv benzylpenicillin 2.4 g 4-hly. Tetracyclines and erythromycin also affective, and ciprofloxacin recommended in the USA as therapy (400 mg iv bd) and prophylaxis after deliberate release of Iowa strain (produces β-lactamases). Because of persistence of spores in lungs, ciprofloxacin (500 mg bd) or doxycycline (100 mg bd) **prophylaxis** for 60 days given in the USA to ≈10 000 persons exposed to aerosolized *B. anthracis* (always ☎ for advice): ≈20% have reported side effects of the prophylaxis. Over 20 000 more started courses that were curtailed when their exposure confirmed as unlikely. Seven days' therapy recommended for cutaneous anthrax.

### Bacillus cereus

**Pathogenesis:** Strains causing food poisoning (➢58) either produce heat-stable peptides (emetic syndrome from reheated rice) or enterotoxin (diarrhoea associated with a variety of foods). Production of enterotoxin and haemolysin (cereolysin) may be associated with pathogenesis of other infections; produce dermonecrosis in rabbit model. All strains produce phospholipase, which is not believed to have a pathogenic role.

**Epidemiology:** Widespread in the environment, and present in many foods. Serotyping available (✈). Σ≈130 (food poisoning).

**Spectrum of disease:** Short-lasting food poisoning (1–6h incubation vomiting, or 10–15h incubation diarrhoeal syndromes). May be isolated from clinical specimens, frequently as a contaminant (especially from samples taken from drainage bags, e.g. bilary or wound drainage), but occasionally cause opportunist infections in traumatic wounds contaminated with soil, and in the immunocompromised and IVDUs (also burn wounds, iv catheters, bacteraemia, meningitis, CSF shunt infection). Occasional endophthalmitis (post-surgical or post-traumatic, also metastatic following bacteraemia).

**Laboratory diagnosis:** Motile and noncapsulate. Ready (24-h) growth to colonies resembling *Bacillus anthracis*; selective medium available, relying on lecithinase production. Readily isolated, in high numbers, from food vehicles of food poisoning if available (✈ for confirmation of toxigenicity and typing).

**Treatment:** Food poisoning, usually selflimiting. Antibiotic sensitivity unpredictable: often resistant to most β-lactam antibiotics; most strains sensitive to gentamicin, erythromycin and vancomycin.

**Prevention:** Cold storage and thorough reheating of cooked rice.

Other *Bacillus* spp. have been isolated from cases of food poisoning, and occasionally from opportunist infections, but are more commonly contaminants. *Bacillus* spp. spores survive washing temperatures, hence they are frequently found in hospital linen, whence patients and specimens (e.g. blood culture broths) may be contaminated.

## Listeria monocytogenes and other Listeria spp.

Short Gram-positive rods. Only *Listeria monocytogenes* is a frequent human pathogen.

**Pathogenesis:** Usually acquired by ingestion. Infective dose uncertain ($10^2$ to $10^6$ cells/g food), but likelihood of infection is dose-related. Most cases acquired by ingestion → penetration of bowel (occasional gastrointestinal symptoms) → multiplication in hepatocytes → haematogenous dissemination after 20–30 days. Listeriolysin O (resembles streptolysin O ➢256) may aid escape from phagosomes. Various toxins, including cytolysin and cell penetration factor (an invasin, implicated in internalization by epithelial and endothelial cells and hepatocytes). Resistance to infection depends on cell-mediated immunity.

**Epidemiology:** All *Listeria* spp. are widespread in domestic animal faeces, in the environment and in many foods (meats, dairy produce, vegetables); can multiply at low temperature (from 4°C) to reach high numbers. About 5% faecal carriage rate in normal adults, normally transient following ingestion. May also be transmitted transplacentally, perinatally or by direct contact with infected animals or birds. Some cases/outbreaks have proven source (e.g. coleslaw, pâté, soft cheese, milk), but most are sporadic (plus rare cross-infection in hospital). Rise in UK cases in 1980s, now falling, probably as a result of control measures aimed at pâté and soft cheeses (currently Σ≈60). Serotyping (✈) shows most UK cases type 4b, with a few type

1/2a or b. No reliable evidence that persistent *Listeria* infection causes recurrent abortion.

**Laboratory diagnosis:** Grows readily (24 h) on many laboratory media; selective media useful for isolation from mixed flora (e.g. foods, faeces). Colonies of *Listeria monocytogenes* and a few others are haemolytic and resemble Gp B β-haemolytic streptococci. Differentiation of species reliable by rapid (24 h) commercial biochemical test kits (✛ confirmation for important isolates), but this is only needed from food and environment. Blood culture the most sensitive and specific test for all infections, but may be negative in late neonatal infection (LNI). Gram stain positive in only ≈30% CSFs that grow Listeria. Culture of conception products positive in early neonatal infection, often negative in LNI. Culture of maternal faeces, urine and HVS rarely (and serology never) helpful.

## Clinical syndrome

### Listeriosis

**Clinical features:** Most infections occur in three well-defined risk groups: pregnant women, neonates (➢139) and immunocompromised or elderly adults.

**Pregnancy-associated infection:** Of proven infections, 25% cause abortion and stillbirth, 70% neonatal sepsis (➢140) and 5% maternal infection without fetus being affected. Probably many others go unrecognized in mother; may cause flu-like illness alone, 2–14 days before miscarriage.

**Early neonatal infections** (ENI: birth–4 days old) usually present with severe systemic sepsis, bacteraemia, meningitis, pneumonia, abscesses: associated with prematurity, maternal fever, obstetric complications (mortality ≈50%; frequent hydrocephalus and psychomotor retardation in survivors). **Late neonatal infections** (LNI: from 5 days) less common and milder (mortality ≈10%), frequently presenting with meningitis and fever alone.

**Adults and the immunocompromised:** Meningitis in 55–70% (occasional cerebritis, 'rhombencephalitis' or cerebral abscess with raised CSF white cells but negative culture; cellular reaction

*(continued...)*

may be predominantly lymphocytic) and bacteraemia; rare IE (native and prosthetic valves), myocarditis, arteritis, pneumonia, arthritis, hepatitis, cholecystitis, peritonitis, localized abscesses etc. Associated with malignancy, HIV and other immunosuppression, organ transplants, chronic liver and renal disease, but 10–15% cases have no predisposing illness. Mortality up to 50% with associated medical conditions; ≈25% overall. Primary cutaneous infection seen in farmers and vets after direct contact with genital tract or placenta of infected cows.

**Microbiological investigations:** Isolation of organisms from blood, CSF or other normally sterile site such as joint fluid (see above). In meningitis the CSF findings are indistinguishable from other causes of bacterial meningitis. CSF Gram stain positive in ≈30% that subsequently grow *Listeria monocytogenes* from blood or CSF.

**Treatment:** Benzylpenicillin or ampicillin/amoxicillin (+gentamicin for improved cidal effect for first 7–10 days for serious infections). Trimethoprim is an alternative, but chloramphenicol is less effective. Tetracycline and erythromycin are also effective. Treatment should be given for 2 weeks, extended to 3 weeks in severe infection such as parenchymal CNS infection, and to 4–6 weeks for endocarditis. *Listeria* is always resistant to cephalosporins, hence cephalosporin + benzylpenicillin best used for empirical therapy of neonatal meningitis/septicaemia when Gram stain of CSF negative and *Listeria* a possibility. *Listeria* is sufficiently common as a cause of meningitis to merit empirical treatment in patients aged over 50 yrs (➢98).

**Prevention of listeriosis:** The Department of Health has issued a booklet detailing guidelines to help prevent listeriosis in vulnerable groups. This is also available in a number of ethnic minority languages, and every pregnant woman should be given a copy. Guidelines are summarized below.

Vulnerable groups are defined as pregnant women, neonates and immunocompromised individuals. They should avoid the following

*(continued...)*

high-risk foods: soft ripened cheeses (e.g. brie, camembert, blue cheese), all forms of pâté and cooked chilled meals and ready-to-eat poultry unless thoroughly reheated until piping hot before being eaten.

Advice on food storage and handling:

- Keep foods for as short a time as possible, follow storage instructions and observe 'best-by' and 'eat-by' dates.
- Do not eat undercooked poultry or meat products. Reheat cooked chilled meals thoroughly according to instructions on the label. Wash salads, fruit and vegetables that will be eaten raw.
- Make sure refrigerator is working properly and keeping food cold.
- Store cooked foods in the refrigerator separately from raw foods and cheeses.
- When reheating food, make sure it is heated until piping hot all the way through and do not reheat more than once.
- When using a microwave oven, observe the standing times recommended by the manufacturers to ensure an even distribution of heat before the food is eaten.
- Throw away left-over reheated food. Cooked food which is not to be eaten straight away should be cooled as rapidly as possible and then stored in a refrigerator.

Pregnant women should also avoid contact with sheep at lambing time, and should not handle silage.

## *Corynebacterium diphtheriae*
✉①

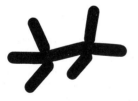

Small, pleomorphic Gram-positive rods, arranged in 'Chinese letters'.

**Pathogenesis:** Diphtheria toxin coded on *tox* gene inserted into chromosome by lysogenic phage. Iron restriction increases toxin production. Exotoxin is a heat-stable protein consisting of two fragments. Fragment B binds to membrane receptors on target cells in the myocardium, nerves and kidneys. Fragment A enters the cell and abolishes protein synthesis by preventing polypeptide chain elongation at the ribosome. Local mucosal necrosis ('pseudomembrane'), and systemic absorption → neuro- and myocardiotoxicity (especially with pharyngeal, rare with skin infection). Laryngeal diphtheria most commonly → respiratory obstruction because of restricted size and rigidity of air passage. No systemic invasion.

**Epidemiology:** Widespread in the developing world, especially tropics; current major outbreak in CIS and other ex-USSR states. Occasional spread in developed world (e.g. among IVDUs in US cities). Usually spread from case or carrier by nasopharyngeal secretions. Nasal carriers shed the most bacilli and are usually only mildly unwell. Skin infection important in tropics, where it often causes mild local inflammation only and establishes immunity. Since the advent of immunization, diphtheria is rare in the UK ($\Sigma$ 5–10 clinical cases, 1–5 toxigenic isolates, virtually all imported; frequently infections of cutaneous ulcers acquired in Indian subcontinent). Rise in non-toxigenic isolates in the UK since surveillance enhanced in 1995. No animal reservoir. The organism survives in dust and transmission by fomites occurs.

**Spectrum of disease:** Causes diphtheria (➤269).

**Cutaneous infection:** ('veld sore', 'desert sore') may occur, usually in tropical environments with poor hygiene. Lesions start as tender pustules which break down to leave a punched out ulcer with a grey sloughy base. Sores are highly infectious, but systemic toxicity is usually less severe than in pharyngeal infection. Immunized individuals may present just with chronic, indolent, sloughy skin sore.

**Laboratory diagnosis:** Ready growth (24–48 h) on media containing serum to form greyish colonies which are black on tellurite medium. Commercial biochemical test kits reliable for differentiation from commensal coryneforms (further 24 h). Toxigenicity determined by immunoprecipitation in agar (Elek test); this takes only 24 h, but is technically demanding for laboratories performing it irregularly, ✛ for EIA and molecular testing (PCR for 'A' portion of *tox*). Three main biotypes (*mitis, intermedius* or *gravis*) by staining and colonial appearances; all may contain the phage and be toxigenic, but *mitis* less commonly than the others. Biotype *belfanti* is non-toxigenic.

**Prevention:** Has been achieved in the developed world by widespread immunization with toxoid (➤417). This has also abolished asymptomatic carriage of the organism, although the reason remains unclear. Isolation/prophylaxis of cases and contacts. Patients with non-toxigenic strains should receive antibiotic treatment, and limited screening measures should be considered because contacts may carry toxigenic variants. Discuss therapeutic, diagnostic and public health measures for suspected cases early (☎).

### Clinical syndrome

**Diphtheria** ✉ ①
A severe pharyngeal infection caused by toxigenic strains of *Corynebacterium diphtheriae*. Death occurs from laryngeal obstruction or the systemic effects of diphtheria exotoxin.

CLINICAL FEATURES
**Incubation time:** Two to six days.

**Symptoms and signs:** Malaise, fever and fatigue. Sore throat (often mild). Thick adherent green-black pseudomembrane on tonsils extending on to the soft palate and uvula. Local lymphadenopathy and oedema ('bull neck'). Nasal infection also occurs, with purulent nasal discharge. Exotoxin causes local pharyngeal paralysis and systemic effects, including myocarditis with signs of heart failure and arrhythmia. Neurological signs include external ophthalmoplegia, dysphagia and peripheral neuritis causing paralysis (Fig. 26.1).

**Investigations:** Diagnosis depends on clinical suspicion and culture of the organism from the
*(continued...)*

pharynx or wound. Take swabs of nose, throat and any skin lesions (if present, swab under any membrane) ☎. Always list appropriate travel history and other clinical details on request cards for cases of pharyngitis and skin infection so that appropriate selective indicator media will be inoculated. Some laboratories will inoculate all throat swabs to appropriate media, but others do so only on special request. Supportive investigations include ECG, which may show abnormality in the absence of clinical evidence or cardiac involvement. ST–T wave changes and 1° heart block are common. Progression to 2° and 3° block are poor prognostic signs.

For guidelines on control measures in the community:

💻 www.phls.co.uk/advice/Dipguidelines.pdf.
↦ For further details on clinical investigations:
Efstratiou, Commun Dis
Public Health 1999; 2: 250

**Management:** Antibiotic treatment with benzylpenicillin or erythromycin. Antitoxin (raised in horses) should be given as soon as the diagnosis is seriously suspected. Mortality increases with delay between the onset of symptoms and the administration of antitoxin. Isolation ①. Supportive care for respiratory obstruction and systemic effects of exotoxin.

**Immunity:** Clinical infection does not always induce adequate antibody response against toxin. Patients should be immunized during the recovery phase. The Schick test is a skin test for immunity—it is not routinely used.

## Other *Corynebacterium* spp.

### *Corynebacterium jeikeium* (previously 'JK coryneforms')

An uncommon skin and bowel commensal causing outbreaks of bacteraemia ($\Sigma \approx 200$) secondary to medical-device and wound infection in haematological malignancy wards. Occasionally also on cardiac surgery (causing endocarditis) and neurosurgery (meningitis) wards. Highly antibiotic-resistant; usually sensitive only to vancomycin and teicoplanin (Linezolid and quinupristin–dalfopristin may be active).

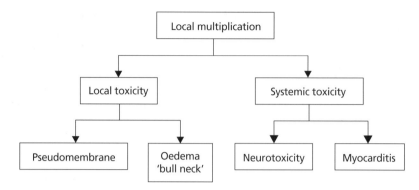

**Figure 26.1** Pathogenesis of diphtheria.

### Corynebacterium minutissimum

Causes an infection of the stratum corneum of the groins, axillae and toe webs (erythrasma ➢117). These areas fluoresce red under Wood's light. Culture is possible from biopsies (lipid-supplemented media), but unnecessary.

### Corynebacterium urealyticum (CDC Group D2)

Recently recognized in association with chronic encrusted cystitis in immunocompromised and elderly patients, catheter- and stone-associated infection, and pyelonephritis in renal transplant patients. Rare bacteraemia. Slow-growing, lipophilic, frequently multiply antibiotic-resistant.

### Corynebacterium ulcerans

Causes bovine mastitis, and human pharyngitis and minor skin sepsis (from direct human or animal contact or milk), usually without systemic toxic effects. Also associated with overseas travel. Rare strains produce diphtheria toxin and can cause diphtheria-like illnesses ($\Sigma$4–6 toxigenic isolates, mostly not acquired abroad).

### Corynebacterium CDC groups M and G2

Rarely associated with endophthalmitis and other infections.

### Corynebacterium pseudotuberculosis

Pathogen of sheep causing human axillary or cervical lymphadenitis after occupational exposure (especially in Australia).

Most of the above, and many other commensal corynebacteria (including *xerosis, bovis,* etc.) are capable of causing bacteraemia and iv catheter and CSF shunt infection, and occasional IE, especially of prosthetic valves. Many isolates are sensitive to penicillin or erythromycin (linezolid and quinupristin–dalfopristin may also be useful), but vancomycin (or teicoplanin) is the only generally reliable agent while awaiting sensitivity results.

## Propionibacterium acnes

Commensal of the skin, mouth, gut and vagina, and is implicated in acne (➢116). It is a rare cause of iv catheter and prosthetic material infection, and very rarely causes IE of prosthetic and native valves. It is a common blood culture contaminant.

## Rhodococcus equi

Pink, mucoid colonies. Very rare cause of necrotizing pneumonia and bacteraemia in immunocompromised patients, which usually responds to erythromycin + gentamicin.

## Arcanobacterium haemolyticum

Causes acute pharyngitis in young adults, often associated with a scarlatiniform rash, occasionally with quinsy. Rarely IE or skin sepsis. Responds to erythromycin or oral penicillin.

## Lactobacillus spp.

Long Gram-positive rods. Commensals of the gastrointestinal tract and vagina that generally prefer low pH for optimal growth. Some are obligate anaerobes. They may grow to form tiny non- or α-haemolytic colonies on blood agar (24–48 h). Very rare isolates from significant infections—blood culture, pelvic abscess mixed with other local flora. Dubious role in lower UTI. Occasionally vancomycin and teicoplanin resistant.

## Erysipelothrix rhusiopathiae

Pathogen of mammals and fish, and causes skin ulcers (rare bacteraemia, IE), especially in butchers and fishmongers (➤113). Usually sensitive to erythromycin or penicillin.

## Nocardia asteroides and other spp.

Branched, filamentous, slow-growing Gram-positive rods, most of which are weakly acid-fast. Aerobic counterpart of *Actinomyces israelii* (➤321) (but most commonly cause invasive infections in the immunocompromised from external sources, rather than focal sepsis from commensal flora of normal individuals).

**Pathogenesis:** Common in the environment. Inhalation route, occasionally direct inoculation. Virulent strains inhibit lysozome activity and oxidative killing in phagocytes, and cell wall glycolipids important in pathogenesis, but other virulence factors unknown.

**Epidemiology:** Infection by *Nocardia asteroides* almost entirely restricted to patients receiving steroids and other immunosuppressive agents for transplants (reduced incidence with modern immunosuppressive regimens), haematological malignancy and autoimmune diseases; also HIV (but incidence may be reduced by co-trimoxazole prophylaxis). Pulmonary nocardiosis sometimes seen in COPD, bronchiectasis, anthracosilicosis, etc., without generalized immunosuppression. Nosocomial outbreaks occasionally associated with building work and environmental contamination. Rare traumatic inoculation to normal patients (usually *Nocardia brasiliensis* or *otitidiscaviarum*); one cause of 'Madura foot' reported from the tropics (especially *Nocardia madurae*).

**Spectrum of disease:** Local inoculation → tissue abscesses (can be sporotrichoid, with local node involvement), keratitis, periodontal infection. Local lung multiplication → progressive pulmonary abscesses, empyema → haematogenous abscesses in brain, liver, mediastinum, bones, joints, retina etc. in ≈30%). A differential diagnosis of tuberculosis in immunocompromised individuals.

**Laboratory diagnosis:** Warn laboratory of chronic nature of infection in compromised patient so cultures are prolonged (☎). Culture of invasive specimens (tissue biopsy, BAL) much more sensitive than sputum or pus alone. Branching, beaded filaments may be seen in stains (Gram, ZN), but culture more sensitive. Strict aerobes, with often slow and scanty growth on blood, Sabouraud's and other agars (2–21 days) to waxy, yellowish colonies: ➤. Sometimes isolated fortuitously on Lowenstein–Jensen media inoculated for mycobacteria, and from lysis-centrifugation blood culture systems. Rarely colonizes skin or respiratory tract, but virtually all isolates should be treated, especially in the immunocompromised.

**Treatment:** Susceptibility testing difficult because of slow growth. Co-trimoxazole the most established agent, but patients with AIDS and co-trimoxazole intolerance have responded to various combinations of minocycline, imipenem, co-amoxiclav, cefotaxime/ceftriaxone and amikacin (☎). Non-immunocompromised patients may require 6–12 months' therapy, and immunocompromised patients at least 12 months; oral treatment may follow initial 3–6 weeks parenteral. Surgical resection of mass lesions may be important.

## *Tropheryma whipplei* (*Gr.* 'nourishment barrier')

Gram-positive rod with unusual trilaminar cell wall, related by 16S ribosomal RNA homology to aerobic actinomycetes. Normal reservoir may be soil, and has been demonstrated in sewage. Not cultivable on laboratory media, but has been propagated in cell culture. Recently established as cause of Whipple's disease (WD).

Consider Whipple's disease as part of the differential diagnosis of the following conditions when more common causes have been excluded: unexplained malabsorption with systemic disease; sarcoid-like systemic granulomatous disease; neurological disease with myoclonus, dementia and supranuclear ophthalmoplegia; culture-negative endocarditis; unexplained uveitis.

**Pathogenesis:** Virulence factors and route of acquisition unknown, but found in environment. Large macrophages in lamina propria of gut → lymphatic blockage.

**Epidemiology:** Annual incidence of WD estimated 10 yrs ago at 12 cases worldwide, but modern diagnostic testing by PCR suggests a higher rate. Affects especially elderly white males, but may occur in children; 30% are HLA-B27 positive.

**Spectrum of disease:** WD presents non-specifically with arthropathy (in over 90%, often preceding other lesions by many years), steatorrhoea (➤64), malabsorption, protein-losing enteropathy. Low-grade fever. Heart valve, eye and CNS lesions; chronic dry cough; lymphadenopathy; hyperpigmentation of skin. Associated immune deficit remains unproven.

**Laboratory diagnosis:** Often delayed. Characteristic histopathological appearances; PAS and silver stain positive bacteria in macrophages in all affected organs (e.g. duodenal biopsy ☎). Differentiate from *Mycobacterium avium-intracellulare* and *Rhodococcus equi* by AFB staining. PCR on fresh or fixed biopsies (even when histologically normal), blood and CSF (✈).

**Treatment:** Response reported within 1–2 weeks to penicillin (+ streptomycin), tetracycline, co-trimoxazole and chloramphenicol. Fewest relapses may follow use of oral co-trimoxazole 160/800 mg bd for at least 1 yr; CSF penetration may be important. Ceftriaxone 2 g od iv for first 2 weeks useful in critically ill patients, and some have recommended it for all with neurological signs. Follow-up by PCR of gastrointestinal biopsy and blood is recommended; relapse reported overall in ≈25%.

# Chapter 27

# Coliforms (syn. enterobacteria, *Enterobacteriaceae*)

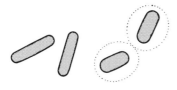

Robust Gram-negative, rod-shaped, facultatively anaerobic organisms that colonize the large bowel of mammals. None produces the enzyme indophenol oxidase, and most reduce nitrate to nitrite and are motile by flagella. Nowadays most laboratories identify members of this group by commercial biochemical test kits (results take 24 h), but some species are confirmed by antigen content (e.g. agglutination for *Salmonella* spp.). Many different virulence factors can be possessed by members of this group, which is reflected in the wide range of diseases that they can produce, but virtually all are capable of causing UTI and wound infection (Table 27.1).

Coliforms rapidly replace the normal largely Gram-positive and non-sporing anaerobic flora of mucosal surfaces of ill patients and those receiving broad-spectrum antibiotics. Granulating surfaces are also frequently colonized. Coliforms are most commonly isolated from these sites in hospitalized patients (including sputum, throat swabs, leg ulcers), and careful clinical assessment is necessary to detect the occasional significant infection amid the abundant cases of colonization.

Resistance to ampicillin/amoxicillin is now too widespread to recommend these agents for empirical treatment of any coliform, and trimethoprim resistance is rising. Co-amoxiclav and oral cephalosporins remain generally reliable for 'easy' coliforms (see below); resistance to parenteral or broad-spectrum cephalosporins is uncommon, and resistance to aminoglycosides, mero/imipenem and quinolones is still rare overall in *Enterobacteriaceae* from outside hospital in the UK. In contrast, resistance rates in isolates from patients who have been in hospital for more than a few days, especially on intensive care units, are much higher: mero/imipenem is generally the most reliable choice.

## 'Hard' and 'easy' coliforms

Coliforms may be considered in two groups—'hard' and 'easy'—reflecting their usual pattern of sensitivity to antibiotics, in particular the likelihood they will be or can become cephalosporin-resistant. '**Hard**' coliforms include *Enterobacter* spp., *Serratia* spp., *Citrobacter* spp., *Proteus vulgaris*, *Providencia* spp. and their relatives. '**Easy**' coliforms include *Escherichia coli*, *Proteus mirabilis* and most *Klebsiella* spp.

---

**Lipopolysaccharide/endotoxin and septic shock**

Bacterial lipopolysaccharide (LPS or endotoxin: see Fig. 27.1) is found within the outer cell membrane of most Gram-negative bacteria, and its release plays a major role in infections caused by coliforms, *Neisseria meningitidis*, *Pseudomonas aeruginosa* and *Bacteroides fragilis*. LPS may reach the circulation from bacteria present within the bloodstream (bacteraemia), or be absorbed from abscesses and other local infections (blood cultures negative). It consists of a hydrophobic **lipid** moiety ('lipid A' which is buried within the membrane and is highly conserved between different species), a more variable polysaccharide core, and a hydrophilic, highly variable polysaccharide **outer region** (O

*(continued...)*

**Table 27.1** Classification of coliforms (syn. enterobacteria, *Enterobacteriaceae*)

| Genus | Species | Notes |
|---|---|---|
| *Escherichia* | *coli* | Many strains now recognized and given acronyms (➤275) |
| | (*fergusonii, hermannii, vulneris*) etc. | Rare human pathogens |
| *Klebsiella* | Sometimes divided into controversial 'species': *oxytoca, planticola, pneumoniae, aerogenes, ozaenae, rhinoscleromatis*, etc. (➤279) | |
| *Proteus* | *mirabilis, penneri, vulgaris* | *Proteus vulgaris* is a 'hard' coliform (➤279), clinically similar to *Citrobacter* and *Enterobacter* spp. (➤283) |
| *Salmonella* | *typhi, paratyphi* A, B and C | 'Enteric' salmonellae. Non-lactose-fermenters (➤279) |
| | '*enteritidis* gp' | Food poisoning salmonellae. Over 2200 'species' classified by antigen content; often grouped 1–6. Gut commensals and pathogens, many with broad host range. Non-lactose-fermenters (➤281). Sometimes called '*Salmonella enterica*' |
| *Shigella* | *boydii, dysenteriae, flexneri, sonnei* | Exclusively human pathogens. Non-motile. Non-lactose-fermenters (➤282) |
| *Citrobacter* | *amalonaticus, braakii, diversus, freundii, koseri* etc. | Related groups. Frequently colonize hospitalized patients and occasionally cause nosocomial infections. *E. sakazakii* is yellow-pigmented. 'Hard' coliforms (➤283) |
| *Enterobacter* | *aerogenes, amnigenus, cloacae* (*asburiae, cancerogenus, gergoviae, hormaechei, intermedius, kobei, sakazakii, 'agglomerans'*) etc. | |
| *Morganella* | *morganii* | Microbiologically related to *Proteus* spp.; cause similar infections to *Citrobacter* and *Enterobacter* spp. 'Hard' coliforms (➤273) |
| *Providencia* | *alcalifaciens, rettgeri, rustigianii, stuartii* | |
| *Serratia* | *liquifaciens, marcescens* (*ficaria, fonticola, grimesii, odorifera, plymuthica, rubidaea* etc.) | Some strains red-pigmented. 'Hard' coliforms (➤273) |
| *Yersinia* | *pestis* | Cause of plague; see under 'fastidious Gram-negative organisms (➤305) |
| | *enterocolitica, pseudotuberculosis* (*aldovae, bercovieri, frederiksenii, intermedia, kristensenii, mollaretii, rohdei* etc.) | Cause uncommon gastrointestinal infections (➤284) |
| (*Erwinia*) | (*herbicola*) | Also called *Enterobacter agglomerans*. Yellow-pigmented |
| (*Hafnia*) | (*alvei*) | Normal gut commensal, very rare pathogen |

Other coliforms include *Buttiauxella agrestis* and *noackiae, Cedecea davisiae, neteri* and *lapagei, Edwardsiella hoshinae* and *tarda, Ewingella americana, Kluyvera ascorbata, cryocrescens,* and *georgiana, Leclercia adecarboxylata, Leminorella* spp., *Moellerella wisconsinsis, Pantoea* spp., *Rahnella aquatilis, Tatumella ptyseos, Trabulsiella guamensis, Yokenella regensburgei*; most have been isolated from the environment and occasionally from animal and human clinical material.

antigen). O antigens are often used to serotype coliform species. Most of the physiological activity of LPS resides in the lipid A; measurable responses follow parenteral administration of minute quantities. Chemical and immunological antagonists of LPS and of the reactions it induces (e.g. TNF and other cytokine release) are under assessment as possible adjuvant treatments for bacterial septic shock; however, the mainstays of all such treatment will remain **circulatory support** and **rapid bacterial killing** by antibiotics. LPS has not been found consistently in the bloodstream of patients presenting with sepsis syndrome (➤185), suggesting that intermittent local or only early release is important.

## *Escherichia coli*

Ubiquitous colonist of the normal colon, and the commonest Gram-negative human pathogen.

Best considered as a group of distinct organisms, some possessing virulence factors that enable them to cause specific diarrhoeal diseases, urinary tract and systemic infections. Names and abbreviations for these organisms proliferate (Table 27.2). All grow rapidly on common laboratory media, most ferment lactose. Typable by somatic 'O', capsular 'K' and flagellar 'H' antigens (➤); some types are associated with possession of particular virulence factors (toxins, epithelial adhesins), and probing for these genes gives specific diagnostic confirmation (➤). Adherence to urinary, intestinal and other epithelia via surface filaments (fimbriae; colonization factors) is fundamental to pathogenesis.

### Enterotoxigenic *Escherichia coli* (ETEC)

**Pathogenesis:** Three groups of virulence factors:
- **Heat-labile** toxin (LT). Closely related to cholera toxin (➤285).
- **Heat-stable** toxin (ST). At least two types, $ST_A$ (acts via cGMP) and $ST_B$ (uncertain mechanism).
- **Colonization factors** (CFA I–IV, etc.), adhering to ileum and jejunum. Mannose-resistant haemagglutinins.

ETEC produce a CFA plus one or both of LT and ST.

**Epidemiology:** Major causes of **diarrhoea in children** <5 yrs in the developing world; travellers' diarrhoea (causes up to 75%; ➤64). Mainly water-borne spread, from faecal contamination. Uncommon in the developed world. Rare outbreaks in neonatal units, spread on staff hands and in feeds.

**Spectrum of disease:** Non-inflammatory acute diarrhoea, sometimes resembling cholera.

## Structure of bacterial lipopolysaccharide

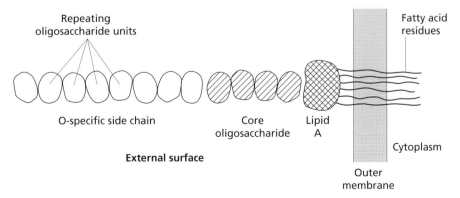

**Figure 27.1** Lipopolysaccharide

**Table 27.2** *E. coli* acronyms

| Type | Acronym or abbreviation | Syndrome |
|---|---|---|
| Enterotoxigenic | ETEC | Secretory diarrhoea in children in developing world and traveller's diarrhoea |
| Verocytotoxic (enterohaemorrhagic) | VTEC, EHEC, 'O157' | Invasive diarrhoea, haemolytic uraemic syndrome |
| Enteroinvasive | EIEC | Invasive diarrhoea |
| Enteropathogenic | EPEC | Secretory diarrhoea infants in developing world |
| Enteroaggregative | EAggEC | Longlasting diarrhoea in children and travellers |
| Diffusely adherent | DAEC | Childhood diarrhoea in tropics |

Incubation period 1–2 days; lasts up to 3 weeks in malnourished children.

**Laboratory diagnosis:** Diagnostic investigations not routinely performed nowadays, but variety of tests available for epidemiological research (cytopathic effects in cell culture, immuno-assay, DNA probes and PCR, animal tests ➤).

**Treatment:** Symptoms are self-limiting, but duration and severity reduced by ciprofloxacin or trimethoprim. Trimethoprim resistance increasing.

**Prevention:** Improve sanitation. Breast-feeding is protective. Boil suspect water.

## Verocytotoxic *Escherichia coli* (VTEC)

Sometimes called enterohaemorrhagic *Escherichia coli* (EHEC).

**Pathogenesis:** Small infecting dose ($\approx 50$ organisms); relatively resistant to drying and stomach acid. 'Attachment–effacement' to terminal ileum and colon. Produce one or both Vero toxins VT1 and VT2 (also called SLT-I and SLT-II)—very similar to Shiga toxin (*Shigella dysenteriae* type 1 ➤282). This is a ricin-like enzyme with five B subunits which bind to an enterocyte receptor and internalize the single toxic A subunit, which inhibits protein synthesis by inactivating the 60S ribosomal subunit.

VT is encoded on a plasmid which is frequently present in type O157 strains (especially O157:H7; occasionally others, e.g. O1:NM, O5:NM, O26:H11, O111:NM, O111:H-). VT also causes vascular endothelial damage especially to cell beds in gut, kidney and brain, leading to DIC and microangiopathic haemolytic anaemia: haemolytic uraemic syndrome (HUS, ➤277). Rare strains of *Citrobacter freundii* and *Enterobacter cloacae* produce Shiga toxin and have been isolated from clinical cases of HUS.

**Epidemiology:** Incidence increased in England and Wales during 1990s ($\Sigma$ 473 in 1992, 792 in 1995, 890 in 1998, 768 in 2001). Commonest in children <5 yrs and the elderly, but affects any age. Found in calf and cattle faeces especially in summer (in 1–16% of UK animals): widespread outbreaks associated with undercooked beef-burgers, cooked and sliced meat, unpasteurised milk, dairy produce, salads and apple juice. Occasional outbreaks in child day care and elderly nursing care centres, probably transmitted on staff hands; also swimming pools and contaminated drinking water. Phage-typing available (➤).

**Spectrum of disease:** Range from mild, loose stool to haemorrhagic colitis and, in children and adolescents, HUS with acute renal failure, microangiopathic haemolytic anaemia and thrombocytopenia. Under 30% are febrile at presentation. Thrombotic thrombocytopenic purpura (TTP) in the elderly with prominent neurological symptoms. Of culture-positive cases, 38% hospitalized, 21% develop HUS and 3% die. Specialist paediatric renal referral is required. Incubation period of diarrhoea ≈ 4 days (can be up to 14 days), duration 2–9 days.

**Laboratory diagnosis:** Inform laboratory of haemorrhagic nature of diarrhoea or HUS (☎); risk of laboratory-acquired infection, so work performed in category 3 accommodation; faeces inoculated to sorbitol–MacConkey agar. Sorbitol non-fermenting colonies are tested for agglutination with O157 antiserum after 24 h (95% non-O157 *Escherichia coli* do ferment; most O157 do not). Cytotoxicity assays and faecal/colony DNA probes/PCR are available (✈) and should be performed in clinically likely cases if only sorbitol-positive and non-O157 antiserum positive colonies are isolated. Rapid reduction in numbers of VTEC in faeces over first 4 days, and diarrhoeal prodrome may be finished when HUS appears, so serology for O157 antibodies may be useful retrospectively (✈).

**Treatment:** Supportive; anti-motility agents and, possibly, antibiotics worsen outcomes in HUS, perhaps by increasing toxin release in gut; plasma exchange has been used.

**Prevention:** Food hygiene and thorough cooking, isolation ②.

➻ Guidelines for the control of VTEC, Commun Dis Public Health 2000; 3: 14

💻 www.phls.co.uk

**Haemolytic–uraemic syndrome (HUS)/thrombotic thrombocytopaenic purpura (TTP) and VTEC**

HUS/TTP is characterized by microangiopathic anaemia, (↑ LDH, fragments on blood film), renal impairment, thrombocytopenia and sometimes neurological features.

**Risk factors:** Age is most important; <5 yrs or
*(continued...)*

>65 yrs ⇒ 20% incidence HUS/TTP, between 5 and 65 yrs ⇒ <5% incidence.

**Clinical features:** The earliest and most significant laboratory predictor of HUS/TTP is **neutrophilia** (often >15 × 10⁹/L) which is often evident within 48 h of the onset of diarrhoea. Five per cent of HUS/TTP cases will never mount a neutrophil response and neutrophilia occurs in 20% of uncomplicated *E. coli* O157 cases. The complete HUS/TTP syndrome is usually established 7 days (range 2–14 days) from the onset of diarrhoea; however, progressive abnormalities of haematology and biochemistry are likely to be identified at an earlier stage.

**Monitoring guidelines:** Children, the elderly, and patients of all ages with hypochlorhydria, immunosuppression or clinical evidence of severe infection presenting with bloody diarrhoea or other suspicion of *E. coli* O157, should have FBC, blood film, urea and electrolytes and LDH. If there is neutrophilia, evidence of red cell haemolysis, abnormal renal function or thrombocytopaenia repeat all bloods within 48 h. The interval for further monitoring is dictated by the trend in abnormalities. Monitoring should continue for at least 7 days or until all abnormalities, including neutrophilia, are clearly reversing.

Cases with normal blood results on first presentation should have them repeated if clinically indicated.

## Enteroinvasive *Escherichia coli* (EIEC)

**Pathogenesis:** Very similar to *Shigella* spp. and contain Shiga-like toxins (➤282). Lipopolysaccharide capsule aids survival in stomach acid and small-bowel enzymes. Penetrate and multiply in colonic epithelial cells ⇨ tissue destruction. Virulent strains can penetrate cells in culture.

**Epidemiology:** Appears to be exclusively a human disease. Faecal–oral spread, but large infective dose (10⁸ bacteria). Occasional outbreaks in developed world in closed communities (e.g. residential homes) with poor hygiene.

**Spectrum of disease:** Bacillary dysentery-like. Incubation 2–4 days. Occasional penetration to bloodstream in the immunocompromised.

**Laboratory diagnosis:** Usually non-motile and do not produce gas from glucose fermentation (i.e. like *Shigella* spp.). Ready (24 h) growth on MacConkey agar, then test non-lactose-fermenting colonies with battery of antisera (e.g. O124, O164). Confirm by DNA probes, cell culture penetration tests (✈).

**Treatment:** Supportive; consider trimethoprim or ciprofloxacin if severe.

## Enteropathogenic *Escherichia coli* (EPEC)

**Pathogenesis:** Originally a heterogeneous group. No toxins consistently produced (some 'EPEC' strains produce LT, ST or VT). 'EPEC' should now be reserved for strains that 'attach–efface' to jejunal/ileal epithelial cells, causing microvillar damage, and adhere to Hep-2 cells by non-fimbrial adhesins. Antibodies to these adhesins are protective. Loss of epithelial disaccharidases ⇨ osmotic diarrhoea.

**Epidemiology:** Now rare in developed world, and many laboratories no longer screen routinely for EPEC (Σ <1000 now); remains commonest cause of infantile diarrhoea in the tropics. Occasional outbreaks in hospitals, spread on hands of staff and in contaminated infant feeds. Large infective dose (up to $10^{10}$). Isolation ②.

**Spectrum of disease:** Non-inflammatory, watery infantile enteritis. Incubation 8–60 h. Can be long-lasting.

**Laboratory diagnosis:** Discuss investigations with a microbiologist (☎). Associated (but not specifically) with certain serotypes (e.g. O26, O55, O128ab); after 24 h incubation on MacConkey agar plates, screen lactose-fermenting colonies with agglutinating antisera. Adhesion in cell culture, probes for adhesins (✈).

**Treatment:** Supportive measures; uncertain value of antibiotics (e.g. trimethoprim, ciprofloxacin). Isolation ②.

## Other *Escherichia coli* diarrhoeas

Evidence is growing to support these strains' roles, but little information yet available on management:

• **Enteroaggregative *Escherichia coli* (EAggEC):** a cause of probably common, long-lasting inflammatory diarrhoea in children and travellers. EAggEC adhere to colonic mucosa in a 'stacked-brick' pattern, causing haemorrhagic necrosis of villus tips. DNA probes available (✈).

• **Diffusely adherent *Escherichia coli* (DAEC)** are associated with childhood diarrhoea in the tropics. DNA probe available (✈).

## Uropathogenic *Escherichia coli*

Compared with strains colonizing the gut, most strains causing cystitis and pyelonephritis (≻77) are positive when probed for Gal-Gal adhesins and P-fimbriae (which adhere to uroepithelium), and they also produce α-haemolysin, belong to only a few O serogroups and demonstrate mannose-resistant haemagglutination. Invasive urinary strains (causing pyelonephritis) belong to a narrower group of O types and additionally are resistant to the killing powers of serum ('serum-resistant'). Severe bacteraemic infections, especially if treatment delayed in elderly patients, may progress to meningitis.

**Treatment:** Approximate UK community resistance rates (mainly from UTI) currently: 40% ampicillin/amoxicillin; 20–30% trimethoprim; 8-10% oral cephalosporins, co-amoxiclav, nitrofurantoin; 0–5% aminoglycosides, parenteral or broad-spectrum cephalosporins, quinolones, mero/imipenem.

## *Escherichia coli* causing wound infection and bacteraemia

These strains are usually serum-resistant. Commonest Gram-negative cause of bacteraemia (Σ ≈11 000 ≻185). UK bacteraemic isolates reported resistance rates (2001): amoxi/ampicillin 55%; cefuroxime 8%; cefotaxime 2%;

ciprofloxacin 6%; gentamicin 3%. Surprisingly rare cause of iv catheter infection, endocarditis and pneumonia.

### *Escherichia coli* causing neonatal meningitis

Generally carry the K1 capsular antigen, shared with Gp B β-haemolytic streptococcus (➤258).

## *Klebsiella* spp.

Non-motile, Gram-negative rods. Classification into species is disputed within this genus, so '*Klebsiella* spp.' is the best term.

**Pathogenesis:** Strains causing primary pneumonia (Friedländer's bacillus) usually produce large quantities of antiphagocytic polysaccharide capsular material of serotype 3, and give mucoid colonies on solid media. Some strains from human infections carry plasmid encoded pili and iron-scavenging systems.

**Epidemiology:** Many strains are normal commensals of human bowel. Strains associated with hospital outbreaks seem capable of prolonged survival on skin of hands. Capsular serotyping available (➤).

**Spectrum of disease:** Nosocomial infections, including outbreaks of **UTI** (➤140), **wound and iv catheter infection, bacteraemia** (Σ ≈3000), **ventilator-associated pneumonia, meningitis and septicaemia in neonates.** Occasional **lower UTI** in normal females. Rare community-acquired **primary pneumonia** (Friedländer's, ➤26). **Rhinoscleroma:** distinct strains causing chronic upper respiratory infection.

**Laboratory diagnosis:** Ready growth (24h) on most laboratory media; identity confirmed by biochemical tests (24h).

**Treatment:** Normally 'easy' coliforms (➤273), but always ampicillin/amoxicillin-resistant, and *Klebsiella* is the commonest coliform to be clinically resistant to aminoglycosides or quinolones. Nosocomial outbreaks with parenteral or broad-spectrum cephalosporin-resistant strains (by mutated or induced

β-lactamase production) increasingly recognized in the UK.

## *Proteus, Morganella* and *Providencia* spp.

Motile, Gram-negative rods producing the enzyme urease. Many strains show 'swarming' of colonies on solid media.

**Pathogenesis:** No specific virulence factors known. Urease may encourage deposition of urinary calculi.

**Epidemiology:** *Proteus mirabilis* is a common faecal commensal; other members of the group usually acquired in hospital. Variety of typing schemes available (➤).

**Spectrum of disease:** UTI (➤77): *Proteus mirabilis* is a common isolate from lower UTI in young females; other members of the group commoner in the abnormal urinary tract, usually acquired in hospital. Sometimes cause pyelonephritis, septicaemia. Wound and iv catheter infection and secondary septicaemia. *Proteus mirabilis* Σ ≈1200 bacteraemias, *vulgaris* Σ ≈60, *Morganella morganii* Σ ≈270, *Providencia* spp. Σ ≈70.

**Laboratory diagnosis:** Ready growth in 24h on most solid media; swarming strains easily recognized, but can swamp other organisms. Confirm identity by biochemical tests (24h).

**Treatment:** All are nitrofurantoin-resistant. *Proteus mirabilis* is an 'easy' coliform (➤273). Reported UK resistance rates for bacteraemic isolates (2001): amoxi/ampicillin 31%; cefuroxime 1.4%; cefotaxime 1%; ciprofloxacin 3%; gentamicin 2%. *Proteus vulgaris, Morganella morganii* and *Providencia* spp. are 'hard' coliforms (➤273) and *Providencia* spp. are frequently resistant to aminoglycosides; a quinolone or imi/meropenem may be required.

## *Salmonella* spp.

Motile, Gram-negative rods; non-lactose fermenters. 'Speciation' within this genus is

Table 27.3 Clinical syndromes associated with *Salmonella* spp. infection

| Syndrome | Features | Species |
|---|---|---|
| Enteric fever | Severe systemic infection | *Salmonella typhi, Salmonella paratyphi* A, B and C |
| Salmonella gastroenteritis | Usually due to multiplication of organisms in food prior to ingestion. Incubation 8–48 h; duration short and self-limited. Vomiting, diarrhoea, abdominal cramps and fever | Many zoonotic 'non-typhoidal' species, particularly *Salmonella enteritidis* |
| Bacteraemia with metastatic infection | A constant feature of enteric fever, but transient bacteraemia is probably not uncommon in patients with salmonella gastroenteritis. Metastatic infection may occur in bone/joint (recent joint prosthesis or sickle-cell anaemia predispose), meninges, or very rarely atherosclerotic plaques of large blood vessels and heart valves | All species |
| Asymptomatic carriage | At 5 weeks, 50% still excrete organism in stools; 9% at 9 weeks. Chronic carriage refers to duration of >1 yr, which may follow clinical disease or asymptomatic infection | All species |

according to possession of somatic 'O' and flagellar 'H' antigens (over 2200 named species). Not normal human commensals (Table 27.3).

## *Salmonella typhi* and *paratyphi* A, B and C

Enteric salmonellae; exclusive human pathogens causing septicaemic illnesses (*paratyphi* B is rarely isolated from animals).

**Pathogenesis:** Infective dose depends upon production of stomach acid, and food vehicle, but usually $10^8$–$10^9$ organisms. Mannose-sensitive adhesins involved in attachment to microvilli of ileum. Epithelium penetrated, and multiplication occurs in epithelial and reticuloendothelial cells ⇨ bacteraemic seeding of many organs (in first 7 days; often asymptomatic). Organisms later released to circulation ⇨ septicaemic presentation, 3 days–6 weeks after ingestion. Gut secondarily infected ⇨ hypersensitivity reaction in Peyer's patches ⇨ ulceration, haemorrhage, perforation.

**Epidemiology and transmission:** Distributed worldwide. Common in developing countries but rare in developed countries such as the UK, due to provision of clean water supply and education of food handlers. Transmission is faeco–oral, either by water (endemic areas) or by contamination of food (non-endemic areas). Risk factors for acquisition of the organism include infancy, hypochlorhydria, abnormal bowel motility and disturbance of bowel flora as occurs following surgery or antibiotic therapy. In contrast to non-typhoidal salmonella infections, asymptomatic carriers are a very important source of infection. *Salmonella typhi:* Σ ≈150, *S. paratyphi* A: Σ ≈160, *S. paratyphi* B: Σ ≈30 (imported, especially *typhi* and *paratyphi* A from Indian subcontinent).

**Spectrum of disease: Typhoid and paratyphoid (enteric fever).**

**Laboratory diagnosis:** Ready growth (24 h) on most solid and blood culture media; a variety of selective media are used for isolation from stool (e.g. desoxycholate-citrate (DCA) or xylose-lysine desoxycholate (XLD) agars; these rely on growth in presence of bile salts, and biochemical reactions giving coloured colonies).

Selective broth enrichment of stool for detection of carriers. Agglutination of colonies by specific antisera (e.g. *Salmonella typhi* carries O antigens 9 and 12, H antigen d, and usually also the surface polysaccharide Vi antigen); commercial biochemical test kits are useful (rapid screening of suspect colonies in 4 h, more reliable tests take further 24 h) ➤. Widal serological test only ever useful for epidemiological studies in high-risk populations.

**Prevention:** Improve sanitation and hygiene; vaccination (➤192). Isolation ②.

---

### Clinical Syndrome

**Typhoid and paratyphoid (enteric fever)**
Typhoid and paratyphoid, collectively referred to as enteric fever, are systemic, potentially fatal, febrile illnesses due to *Salmonella typhi* and *Salmonella paratyphi* types A, B and C. Paratyphoid is generally a milder illness than typhoid. Rarely, other 'non-typhoidal salmonellae' can produce a similar illness.

**Incubation time:** One to 3 weeks; shorter with larger infecting inoculum.

**Clinical features:** Insidious onset of fever, myalgia, abdominal pain and severe headache. Classically, fever rises in a stepwise fashion. Cough, constipation and deafness are common. Diarrhoea occurs in <40% of patients. On examination there may be relative bradycardia, hepatosplenomegaly and rose spots, which are faint, salmon-coloured maculopapular lesions on the trunk, which blanch on pressure. Rose spots occur during the first few days of illness and are easily overlooked. Untreated, fever persists for several weeks. Mortality untreated is ≈20%, with death mainly due to intestinal perforation or haemorrhage. Less common complications include psychosis, hepatitis, cholecystitis, pneumonia, pericarditis and meningitis.

**Investigations:** Leucopenia and abnormal liver function tests are usual. Anaemia occurs secondary to bleeding and due to haemolysis in patients with G6PD deficiency. Diagnosis is confirmed by
*(continued...)*

culture of the organism from blood, stools, urine or bone marrow. Serology (Widal test) is not useful in the diagnosis of the acute attack.

**Management:** Antibiotic therapy reduces the mortality to <1%. Chloramphenicol is the drug of choice for developing countries, although resistance has been widely reported, particularly from India, SE Asia and the Middle East. For travellers returning to the UK, ciprofloxacin 750 mg 12-hly po should be given. Alternative agents are amoxicillin and co-trimoxazole. Treatment should be given for 10–14 days; response is typically slow, with resolution of fever over 2–5 days.

**Comments:** **Chronic carriage** follows enteric fever in ≈5% of cases. Prolonged treatment with ciprofloxacin (750 mg 12-hly po for 1 month) may be successful. Chloramphenicol and amoxicillin may be required, particularly if there are gallstones.
**Vaccine** produces partial immunity (➤192).

## 'Salmonella enteritidis' group

Food-poisoning salmonellae, causing gastroenteritis in humans and many other animal species. Certain salmonellae are associated with particular animals (e.g. *Salmonella enteritidis* PT4 and chickens, *dublin* and cattle); others have wider host associations (e.g. *Salmonella virchow* and *typhimurium*).

**Pathogenesis:** Infective dose depends upon species, production of stomach acid, and food vehicle, but can be $<10^2-10^9$ organisms. Mannose-sensitive adhesins involved in attachment to microvilli of ileum. Epithelium penetrated, and multiplication occurs in epithelial and reticuloendothelial cells. Incubation period 8–48 h; duration of acute illness 48–96 h.

**Epidemiology:** Often transmitted to animals in their feed and spread between them during processing for food (e.g. commercial frozen chicken preparation results in >50% carcasses positive). Human sporadic cases and common-source outbreaks are zoonoses and originate from inadequately cooked meat, contamination of food eaten without further cooking, or occasional acquisition directly from colonized animal (e.g. pet reptiles). Salmonellae can readily multiply in food at environmental temperatures. Rising reported human cases in England and Wales in past 30 yrs ($\Sigma$ 30 654 in 1993, 32 596 in 1997); especially brisk increase after 1985 in *Salmonella enteritidis* phage type 4, associated with chicken meat and eggs ($\Sigma$ 17 258 in 1993). Prevalence has fallen since (all enteric salmonellas $\Sigma$ 16 465 in 2001), with rise seen in wider variety of other serotypes and phage types, more commonly travel-associated. Rising numbers also of *Salmonella typhimurium* DT104, often multiply antibiotic resistant (e.g. to ampicillin, chloramphenicol, streptomycin, sulphonamides, spectinomycin, tetracycline and trimethoprim). Total bacteraemias currently $\Sigma \approx 420$.

Different species and phage types are common in other countries. Human infection from human case or carrier is uncommon. Phage-typing is available for the common species ($\rightarrow$).

**Spectrum of disease: Gastroenteritis** ($\succ$57) ✉, sometimes associated with **bacteraemia**, more commonly in the immunocompromised (especially AIDS). 80% patients with salmonella bacteraemia but no diarrhoea have underlying immunosuppression (e.g. HIV infection). By 9 weeks, 90% cases are faecal culture-negative. Prolonged carriage (>1 yr in $\approx$1%) in bile or urine associated with biliary or urinary tract abnormality and with immunodeficiency. Osteomyelitis especially in sickle-cell disease. Rare other focal infections, including arterial aneurysm (especially in males >60 yrs of age), joint prostheses. Neonates in developing world may suffer meningitis, osteomyelitis (especially with sickle cell disease).

**Laboratory diagnosis:** Ready growth (24 h) on most solid and blood culture media; variety of selective media used for isolation from stool (e.g. DCA and XLD) ($\succ$280). Selective broth enrichment of stool for detection of carriers. Agglutination of colonies by specific antisera (e.g. *Salmonella enteritidis* carries O antigens 1, 9 and 12, H antigen g); commercial biochemical test kits are useful (rapid screening of suspect

colonies in 4 h, more reliable tests take further 24 h) $\rightarrow$.

**Treatment:** *Salmonella* gastroenteritis does not need antibiotic therapy unless patient is systemically ill and bacteraemia is suspected. However, mortality in patients >60 yrs of age with non-typhoidal extra-intestinal salmonellosis is 28%. Salmonellae are frequently fully antibiotic-sensitive in the UK, and extraintestinal infections commonly respond well to many antibiotics active against other 'easy' coliforms ($\succ$273); however, intracellular persistence may lead to incomplete response or later recrudescence. The most reliable agents are quinolones or chloramphenicol.

**Prevention:** Eradication of salmonellae from farm animals; improved catering practices. Isolation ②.

## *Shigella* spp.

Non-motile, Gram-negative rods that generally do not produce gas from glucose fermentation. All are non-lactose-fermenters except for *Shigella sonnei*, which may do so at 24 h.

**Pathogenesis:** Small infecting dose (minimum 10–100 organisms). Attachment, then invasion of colonic mucosa; a large plasmid codes for several outer membrane proteins associated with invasion. Escape from phagocytic vacuole by haemolysin activity. Sloughing of necrotic epithelium follows, with underlying inflammation and capillary thrombosis. *Shigella dysenteriae* type 1 produces largest amount per cell of Shiga toxin ($\succ$276) and causes the most severe disease, but other shigellae also release it. Incubation period usually 1–3 days; duration of *sonnei* dysentery usually 48 h with loose stool for several more days. Other species usually more prolonged.

**Epidemiology:** Worldwide distribution, but only *Shigella sonnei* commonly acquired in the UK (fall in reported cases in England and Wales in late 1990s; 17 000 in 1992, 897 in 2001). The majority of *flexneri* cases are imported ($\Sigma \approx 250$), as are all *boydii* ($\Sigma \approx 50$) and *dysente-*

*riae* cases ($\Sigma \approx 35$). Faecal-oral spread in areas of poor hygiene (especially direct spread and via contaminated surfaces in infant and junior schools in the UK). Household contacts have high attack rate. Flying insects important in transmission (via food) in developing world. Human long-term carriers are rare, and rarely proven to transmit infection, but 75% cases still culture-positive after 7 weeks. Typing by phage susceptibility and antigen content available (✈).

**Spectrum of disease: Bacillary dysentery** (➤57) ✉. *Shigella sonnei* tends to produce **mild** disease, often asymptomatic. Systemic spread beyond gut is rare, but commoner in immunodeficiency. *Shigella dysenteriae* type 1 associated with HUS (➤277).

**Laboratory diagnosis:** Ready growth (24 h) on most solid media; variety of selective media used for isolation from stool (e.g. DCA and XLD ➤280). Selective broth enrichment of stool useful for convalescent cases. Commercial biochemical test kits are useful (rapid screening of suspect colonies in 4 h, more reliable tests take further 24 h); agglutination of colonies by specific antisera allows grouping of non-*sonnei* isolates (✈).

**Treatment:** Antibiotics not generally indicated for the individual unless immunocompromised or severely ill with non-*sonnei* dysentery (e.g. ciprofloxacin; 70% resistance to trimethoprim and ampicillin in developing world); their value for curtailing outbreaks is disputed. Outbreak control usually involves excluding symptomatic cases, emphasizing lavatory hygiene, and (only rarely) school closure ☎.

**Prevention:** Improve sanitation. Isolation ②.

# *Citrobacter* spp. and *Enterobacter* spp.

Motile, Gram-negative rods.

**Pathogenesis:** No specific virulence factors known.

**Epidemiology:** Mostly nosocomial pathogens causing opportunist infections sporadically and in small outbreaks; spread on staff hands and occasionally on contaminated wet equipment. Frequently colonize patients given cephalosporins. Various typing schemes available (✈).

**Spectrum of disease:** Hospital-acquired **wound infection**/colonization, **UTI**, **iv catheter infection**; occasional **bacteraemia** secondary to these (*Citrobacter* spp. $\Sigma \approx 420$; *Enterobacter* $\Sigma \approx 1600$ bacteraemias). Rare **ventilator-associated pneumonia** (➤33) frequently colonize respiratory secretions). *Citrobacter koseri* associated with outbreaks of meningitis on neonatal ICUs. *Enterobacter agglomerans* (also called *Erwinia herbicola*) is a frequent environmental commensal (e.g. toilet water), causing occasional opportunist infections of iv catheters, wounds; also bacteraemia and endocarditis in IVDU.

**Laboratory diagnosis:** Ready growth (24 h) on most laboratory media; confirm identity by commercial biochemical test kits (further 24 h).

**Treatment:** 'Hard' coliforms (➤273). Many resistant to ampicillin/amoxicillin; often also to trimethoprim, co-amoxiclav. Often carry genetic elements coding for parenteral or broad-spectrum cephalosporinases. Resistance in initially sensitive strains therefore sometimes emerges on treatment, by derepression of class 1 cephalosporinase production or selection for strains that produce large amounts of the enzymes. Aminoglycosides, imi/meropenem, aztreonam, cefpirome and quinolones are more reliable.

---

**Practice point**

Avoid most cephalosporins in patients infected with 'hard coliforms' (➤273) i.e. *Citrobacter* spp., *Enterobacter* spp., *Proteus vulgaris*, *Providencia* sp. and *Serratia* spp., even if reported as susceptible by the laboratory.

## *Serratia* spp.

Motile, Gram-negative rods. Many produce striking red-pigmented colonies. Clinically similar to *Enterobacter* and *Citrobacter* spp.; especially associated with outbreaks of bacteraemia, meningitis and ophthalmia on neonatal ICUs, where they are spread on staff hands or via contaminated feeds and medical equipment. Bacteraemias $\Sigma \approx 600$ in all ages. Strains that test aminoglycoside susceptible in the laboratory may be induced to resistance if exposed to these antibiotics—meropenem and quinolones more reliable.

## *Yersinia* spp.

### *Yersinia pestis*
Causes **plague** (➤305).

### *Yersinia enterocolitica*
Small, Gram-negative coccobacillus.

**Pathogenesis:** Oral ingestion. Variety of plasmid-associated virulence factors identified, including 'invasin' protein. Invasion of epithelium overlying Peyer's patches ⇨ multiplication in lymphoid follicles ⇨ hyperplasia; can mimic appendicitis. Iron overload increases invasiveness.

**Epidemiology:** Variety of serotypes associated with pigs, cows, etc.; types 3 and 9 commonest in Europe (✈). Outbreaks associated with milk, ice-cream, pork products. Falling incidence ($\Sigma$ 404 in 1991, 23 in 2001; probably greatly under-reported). Will multiply slowly at refrigerator temperatures.

**Spectrum of disease:** Ranges from acute gastroenteritis to invasive colitis and enteritis with inflammatory diarrhoeas (➤59) lasting a mean of 2 weeks. Mesenteric adenitis in young children and adults. Rare bacteraemia and metastatic spread (osteomyelitis, IE) in the immunocompromised, especially those with diseases of iron accumulation. **Reactive arthritis** (➤122) in 2%, HLA-B27-associated; also Reiter's syndrome and erythema nodosum (➤118).

**Laboratory diagnosis:** Ready growth (24h) on many media, but best to use selective medium (CIN agar) incubated at 25°C for isolation from faeces or tissue if diagnosis is suspected (☎). Identified in commercial biochemical kits, incubated at low temperature. Serology useful to confirm cause of recent rheumatological complications (✈).

**Treatment:** No evidence that course of gastrointestinal illness modified by antibiotics. Usually resistant to ampicillin/amoxicillin; trimethoprim, parenteral or broad-spectrum cephalosporins and quinolones have been used for systemic and focal infections.

### *Yersinia pseudotuberculosis*
Causes mesenteric adenitis with a more chronic picture than *Yersinia enterocolitica*, especially in children and teenagers ($\Sigma$ <10). Serotype 1 causes most human infections. Diagnosis as for *Yersinia enterocolitica*. Commonly associated with septicaemic illnesses in many animals and birds, and taxonomically very closely related to *Yersinia pestis*, the cause of plague (➤305). There are various other *Yersinia* species which have been isolated from the environment and animals.

# Chapter 28

# Vibrios

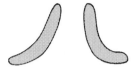

Vibrios and their relatives are mostly curved, Gram-negative rods, tolerant of high salt ('halophilic vibrios' require high salt containing media for optimal isolation) and alkalinity, producing indophenol oxidase. Most can cause both diarrhoea and tissue infections, with the species differing in their tendency to cause one more commonly than the other (Table 28.1). *Aeromonas hydrophila* and other members of the genus are straight Gram-negative rods, fermentative and indophenol oxidase positive; they also may cause wound infection and diarrhoea, but are found in fresh waters.

## *Vibrio* spp.

### *Vibrio cholerae* ✉②
Curved, motile, Gram-negative rods.

**Pathogenesis:** Flagellae involved in adhesion to enterocyte. Cholera toxin (enterotoxin) present in O1 strains (also in a few non-O1 strains); comprises one A and five B peptide subunits (related to *Escherichia coli* LT toxin (➤275). B subunits bind to GM1 ganglioside on enterocyte membrane, and the A subunit is passed through to cytoplasm ⇨ irreversible activation of adenyl cyclase ⇨ inhibition of sodium and chloride uptake and excretion of chloride and bicarbonate ions accompanied by water ⇨ secretory diarrhoea. Both O1 and non-O1 strains produce a variety of other toxins, including mucinase, LT and ST enterotoxins, cytotoxins (Shiga-like) and cytolysins.

**Epidemiology:** Cholera always an imported infection in most of developed world ($\Sigma \approx 5$) Acquired from faecally contaminated water, vegetables, seafood; direct person-to-person spread rarely proved. O1 strains divided into classical and eltor biotypes and serologically into O antigen types Inaba, Ogawa and Hikojima. Current seventh cholera O1 pandemic began 1961 in Indonesia—biotype eltor, serotype Inaba. At present cholera is restricted to SE Asia, Indian subcontinent, Middle East, parts of CIS, Africa and South America. Rare indigenous cases reported Texas and Louisiana (Gulf Coast), Yugoslavia, Italy, Spain; acquired from vibrios multiplying in surface waters. Non-O1 cases are usually sporadic or small, common-source outbreaks, but new epidemic O139 strain (cholera toxin-positive) has swept through Indian subcontinent since 1992. Serotyping available (✈).

**Spectrum of disease:** O1 strains typically cause **acute-onset profuse watery diarrhoea** with infection confined to gut (see below). Wide range of severity of illness, with >90% clinically indistinguishable from other acute diarrhoeal illnesses, and asymptomatic infection common. Non-O1 strains cause spectrum of illness from mild gastroenteritis to fulminant diarrhoea; also rarely associated with **tissue infection**, especially in patients with underlying diseases (e.g. diabetes, arterial insufficiency).

**Laboratory diagnosis:** Inform laboratory of travel history so appropriate media are inoculated (thiosulphate–citrate–bile salt (TCBS) agar, plus alkaline peptone water enrichment for 5–6h). Rapid (24h) production of large yellow colonies on TCBS in acute diarrhoea; sometimes isolated after enrichment when convalescent. Test for indophenol oxidase, and

**Table 28.1** Classification of *Vibrio* spp.

| Genus | Species | Notes |
|---|---|---|
| *Vibrio* | cholerae | Strains carrying the O1 antigen cause cholera; others ('non-O1' strains) may cause diarrhoea and wound infection |
| | vulnificus, damsela (*alginolyticus*, etc.) | Wound infection, seawater/shellfish-associated. Rare diarrhoea, seafood-associated (➤114) |
| | parahaemolyticus, fluvialis, hollisae, mimicus (*furnissii*) | Diarrhoea, seafood-associated. Rare wound infection, seawater-associated (➤59) |
| *Aeromonas* | hydrophila, sobria, caviae (*salmonicida, schubertii, trota, veronii*, etc.) | Wound infection, fresh water-associated. Probably also rare causes of diarrhoea (➤114) |
| (*Plesiomonas*) | (*shigelloides*) | Antigenically related to *Shigella* spp.; may cause diarrhoea |

agglutination by O1 antiserum (➤). Commercial biochemical test kits are reliable for *Vibrio cholerae* identification (further 24 h).

**Prevention:** Clean food and water. Chemoprophylaxis (tetracycline 250 mg 6-hly, or ciprofloxacin) should be reserved for household contacts. Vaccination has no role in prevention or control of epidemics (➤194).

### Clinical syndrome

#### Cholera
Severe secretory diarrhoea caused by *Vibrio cholerae*.

**Incubation time:** Two to 3 days (range <1–5).

**Clinical features:** Sudden onset of profuse painless watery diarrhoea ('rice-water stools') with vomiting. Fever is unusual, except in children. Rapid severe dehydration and circulatory collapse can occur within hours. Fluid loss may be up to 1 L/h, and severely ill patients may lose up to 10% of their body weight in fluid. Mortality (50% in severe untreated cases) is due to fluid loss, and is reduced to <1% if adequate fluid replacement is given. Complication include

(continued...)

metabolic acidosis and renal failure. Asymptomatic and mild cases are common—there may be 10 such cases for every severe case in an epidemic situation.

**Investigations:** Diagnosis may be confirmed by stool culture. Stool microscopy may be helpful during epidemics.

**Management:** Rapid aggressive rehydration, either by oral rehydration fluid (➤62), in mild cases, or iv, in severe cases. Slightly hypotonic alkaline solutions containing potassium are favoured for iv use; Ringer's lactate solution or WHO iv diarrhoea treatment solution both conform to this specification. If these are not available, normal saline and 1.26% sodium bicarbonate in a ratio of 2:1 (both with potassium 10 mmol/L) should be given. Up to 4 L/h may be required initially. Once fluid deficit has been corrected patients should receive daily (orally or iv) the previous day's output (urine + stool volumes + 500 mL). Tetracycline, ampicillin and trimethoprim/co-trimoxazole resistance uncommon but increasing in incidence in Africa and Asia; ciprofloxacin reliably active (500 mg single dose treats cases, but does not reduce secondary household transmission; 250 mg od for 3 d proven effective for both).

## Vibrio parahaemolyticus

Curved, motile, Gram-negative rods.

**Pathogenesis:** Adhesion linked to flagella and haemagglutinin; virtually all pathogenic strains are haemolytic on human blood/mannitol agar (Kanagawa phenomenon) (✦). Also cytotoxin (Shiga), mucinase.

**Epidemiology:** Associated with seafood; common in Japan, Singapore. Σ ≈ 20. Serotyping available (✦).

**Spectrum of disease:** Acute diarrhoea (c. 3 days' duration), rarely fulminant (➤59). Rare extra-gastrointestinal infections associated with local trauma and contamination with seawater/seafood (e.g. wound infection, cellulitis, endophthalmitis).

**Laboratory diagnosis:** Grows on TCBS agar; requires high salt concentration (halophilic). Inform laboratory of seafood/travel association and culture suspect foodstuffs. Commercial identification test kits normally reliable with added salt, but confirm by ✦.

**Treatment:** Antibiotics not normally required for diarrhoea. Usually resistant to ampicillin, antipseudomonal penicillins and oral cephalosporins. For tissue infections use gentamicin or parenteral cephalosporin.

*Vibrio fluvialis, hollisae* and *mimicus* (perhaps also *furnissii*) cause clinical illnesses similar to *parahaemolyticus*, but have biochemical differences.

## Vibrio vulnificus and damsela

Curved, motile, Gram-negative rods.

**Pathogenesis:** *Vibrio vulnificus* has acidic poly-saccharide capsule and is serum-resistant. Also cytolysin (heat-labile), protease, collagenase, iron-binding siderophore.

**Epidemiology and spectrum of disease:** Tissue infections (sometimes severe, necrotizing, bac-teraemic), often following local trauma and contamination with seawater/seafood, especially from warm waters (➤114). Commoner in those with diseases of iron accumulation. Rare diarrhoea.

**Laboratory diagnosis:** Send swabs, tissue, blood culture. Inform laboratory of seawater association. Grow well on TCBS agar; prefer high salt concentration (halophilic), but will grow on blood and MacConkey agars and in blood culture broths. Commercial identification test kits normally reliable with added salt, but confirm by ✦.

**Treatment:** Often resistant to ampicillin, antipseudomonal penicillins and oral cephalosporins. For tissue infections use gentamicin or parenteral cephalosporin. Debride necrotic tissue.

## Vibrio alginolyticus

Halophilic vibrio occasionally isolated from minor septic wounds and ear infections after seawater contact.

# Aeromonas hydrophila, sobria, caviae and others

Motile, Gram-negative, indophenol oxidase-positive rods with ubiquitous distribution in fresh waters. Wound infection (sometimes severe, necrotising, bacteraemic, Σ ≈ 75 bacter-aemias) and other sepsis often associated with freshwater contamination (➤114). Probably also cause diarrhoea, sometimes bloody, some-times travel-associated. Other *Aeromonas* spp. are fish and animal pathogens. Aeromonads can penetrate cells in culture, and possess a range of cytotoxins, adhesins and haemolysins with as yet undefined roles. Most are resistant to ampi-cillin/amoxicillin and antipseudomonal peni-cillins, and rare strains produce β-lactamases active against parenteral or broad-spectrum cephalosporins; generally reliable agents include aminoglycosides, quinolones and trimethoprim.

# Chapter 29

# Campylobacters

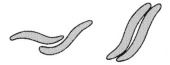

Curved or spiral, motile Gram-negative rods that generally do not grow in conventional culture conditions: require low $O_2$ and high $CO_2$ concentrations, and incorporation of whole blood, haemin, charcoal, etc. in isolation media (Table 29.1). Produce indophenol oxidase; usually identified by colonial appearance on selective medium, Gram stain, plus a few simple tests.

## Campylobacter jejuni and coli

Curved, motile, Gram-negative rods.

**Pathogenesis:** Infective dose low; dependent on host factors (especially gastric acid production), but has followed ingestion of 500 organisms. Disease probably involves toxin production (an enterotoxin very similar to cholera toxin, and a cytotoxin), multiplication within jejunal and ileal enterocytes, and penetration of mucosa. Also mesenteric lymph nodes enlarged; acute inflammation of rectal and lower colonic mucosa.

**Epidemiology:** Commonest proven cause of diarrhoea in England and Wales ($\approx 39\,000$ in 1993, 56 500 in 2001). Many additional cases go unreported (estimated 10 × as many). In the UK, >90% of cases are due to *Campylobacter jejuni* (mainly found in poultry/birds), <10% *coli* (pigs). A zoonosis, with sporadic cases or common-source outbreaks from ingested food (>60% chicken carcasses are culture-positive; less commonly acquired from other meat,

contaminated/unpasteurized milk, untreated water). Do not multiply in food. Rarely transmitted person-to-person, except infant to infant or carers; 39× higher rate of infection in patients with AIDS. Rare cause of outbreaks of meningitis and septicaemia in neonatal ICUs. Typing available by O and surface/flagellar antigens ($\blacktriangleright$). Rare bacteraemia $\Sigma \approx 100$, commoner in the immunocompromised.

**Spectrum of disease:** Incubation period 1–7 days $\Rightarrow$ acute enteritis lasting 2–7 days ($\blacktriangleright 59$). Excretion of organisms continues for about 3 weeks; prolonged carriage very rare in immunocompetent people. Persistent or recurrent diarrhoea sometimes seen in the immunocompromised. Occasional reactive arthritis, rash or Guillain–Barré syndrome 1–2 weeks after diarrhoea.

**Laboratory diagnosis:** Appropriate selective/nutritive media are routinely inoculated with faeces by laboratories; grows in 48 h.

**Treatment:** Normally the diarrhoea is self-limiting, but early treatment with erythromycin may shorten illness. Erythromycin and ciprofloxacin resistance rising in some countries (e.g. Thailand); alternatives include tetracycline, amoxicillin or co-amoxiclav. *Campylobacter coli* more commonly erythromycin-resistant; ciprofloxacin is an alternative.

**Prevention:** Kitchen hygiene. Isolation of neonates and parturient mothers with diarrhoea.

*Campylobacter hyointestinalis, lari* and *upsaliensis* were first described in patients with AIDS as 'Campylobacter-like organisms' (CLO), and are uncommon causes of similar diarrhoeal

**Table 29.1** Classifcation of campylobacters

| Genus | Species | Notes |
|---|---|---|
| Campylobacter | jejuni, coli (hyointestinalis, lari, upsaliensis, etc.) | Primarily cause intestinal infections. Most grow selectively well at high temperature (42°C) |
| | fetus | Causes rare septicaemia in immunocompromised patients |
| Helicobacter | pylori | Causes gastritis and duodenal ulceration |
| | (cinaedi, fennelliae, etc.) | Isolated from proctocolitis and occasional bacteraemia in homosexual men. Asymptomatic carriage also reported |

illnesses in healthy and immunocompromised hosts. Rarely isolated by conventional methods because of demanding cultural requirements (☎).

*Campylobacter concisus* and *sputorum* have been isolated rarely from a variety of soft tissue, oral and gastrointestinal infections.

*Campylobacter fetus* is uncommonly isolated from blood cultures in immunocompromised patients, and causes abortion in sheep and cattle. It carries an antiphagocytic protein 'microcapsule'.

## Helicobacter pylori

Small curved or spiral, highly motile, Gram-negative rod. Typing scheme based on genomic methods used as research tool (✦).

**Pathogenesis:** Colonizes gastroduodenal mucosa. Intense urease production ⇨ local rise in pH, allowing periepithelial survival in stomach. Lipopolysaccharide, cytotoxin-associated gene A and vacuolating cytotoxin virulence factors.

**Spectrum of disease:** Causes chronic active gastritis and is dominant cofactor in duodenal ulceration; carriage associated with gastric ulceration and gastric cancer (the main risk factor). Mucosa-Associated Lymphoid Tissue lymphoma (MALT); 10–15% infected individuals will develop peptic ulcer disease in 20 yrs of follow-up, but at any one time >70% infected people asymptomatic.

**Laboratory diagnosis:** Will grow in low $O_2$, high $CO_2$ in 3–5 days on media enriched with horse serum. Culture available in an increasing number of centres (☎) enabling susceptibility testing to be performed, but it is technically demanding and plates frequently become overgrown.

---

### Clinical syndrome

**Gastritis, duodenal ulcers and *Helicobacter pylori***
*Helicobacter pylori* is found in mucus lining the stomach and in areas of gastric metaplasia in the duodenum. Its presence explains nearly all duodenal ulcers and most gastric ulcers not associated with NSAIDs. Pangastritis may be commoner if carriage occurs at an early age. **Antral gastritis** ⇨ loss of regulatory feedback ⇨ gastric hypersecretion ⇨ reactive duodenal gastric metaplasia ⇨ colonization with *Helicobacter pylori* ⇨ duodenitis and ulceration, and slightly increased risk of gastric cancer. **Pangastritis** ⇨ gastric atrophy and intestinal metaplasia ⇨ loss of acid secretion and increased risk of gastric ulceration and cancer.

*(continued...)*

*Helicobacter pylori* infection may account for 60% of risk for gastric adenocarcinoma.

Carriage rate in UK adults >50yrs is >50%. Rate increases with age and commoner in developing world and with low socio-economic status. Multiple strains often carried. Probably acquired from close household contacts via oral route; faecal–oral route may be important if sanitation poor. Occupation risk for endoscopists. Found in ≈90% of patients with *duodenal* ulceration or antral gastritis. Eradication of organism during/after standard ulcer healing therapy reduces relapse rate from ≈85% to <20%.

**Diagnosis:** The organism may be visualized in and cultured from **endoscopic biopsies**, but distribution of organisms may be patchy so multiple biopsies of antrum and corpus for histology plus one for another diagnostic method are recommended. It may also be detected by subjecting biopsies to the rapid urease test (e.g. CLO test), which may be more sensitive than other diagnostic methods and can be performed by the endoscopist. In the $^{14}$C-**labelled urea breath test**, *Helicobacter pylori* in the stomach cleave labelled urea, liberating $^{14}CO_2$ which is detected in breath. $^{13}$C is used by some departments as it is non-radioactive and is safe for use in children and women of child-bearing age; a mass spectrometer is required to detect it, and commercially available kits include cost of detection at an appropriate lab. **Serological** assays detect IgG responses, but there is variation in performance among different *Helicobacter pylori* strains and human racial groups, and assays require local validation. Titres fall only slowly after successful eradication hence serology is not useful to demonstrate cure. Faecal antigen detection assays and PCR-based tests are under development.

**Management:** Clinically effective investigation/treatment strategies are still being investigated and debated (e.g. 'serology and treat', 'serology and endoscope'), and patient's age import-

ant because risk of gastric cancer is low below age 45.

**Management:** Eradication is indicated in patients with duodenal or gastric ulcer, gastritis and gastric lymphoma. The value of eradication in non-ulcer dyspepsia and oesophagitis is debated.

Seven-day therapy with a proton pump inhibitor (PPI), clarithromycin and either amoxicillin or metronidazole ('triple therapy') eradicates the organism in ≥90%. Fourteen days therapy achieves a higher eradication rate but with higher cost/side effects. Suitable regimens include omeprazole 20 mg q12h, plus two of the following: clarithromycin 500mg q12h, amoxicillin 1g q12h, metronidazole 400mg q12h. In patients with DU, eradication leads to rapid healing and there is usually no need to continue antiacid therapy, unless there has been perforation or haemorrhage. If symptoms persist 4 weeks after therapy, persistent infection should be sought using urea breath test, and if positive, treatment with an alternative regimen should be given. Patients with GU and complicated DU require more careful follow-up, usually with repeat endoscopy.

Failure of eradication may indicate antibiotic resistance, but it is disputed whether *in vitro* resistance tests correlate with clinical outcome and these are not routinely available.

Metronidazole resistance is common (20% of UK strains; 50% across Europe; 90% in developing countries), but of uncertain significance because the drug is highly active in the stomach's acidic environment. Clarithromycin resistance is less frequent (below 10% in Europe) and amoxicillin and tetracycline resistance is very rare. Pre-treatment resistance to clarithromycin reduces effectiveness of triple therapy by 55%. Two-week regimens including bismuth subcitrate plus two antibiotics have been used for primary treatment failure.

Carbon-labelled urea breath tests suitable as tests of cure (98% sensitive and 97% specific if done >4 weeks after finishing treatment).

www.sign.ac.uk/pdf/sign7.pdf

# Chapter 30

# Pseudomonads

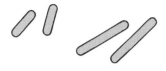

## *Pseudomonas* spp. and their relatives (Table 30.1)

Often called 'non-fermenters' because, unlike coliforms, they usually derive their energy by oxidative metabolism and fail to ferment glucose. Most are environmental saprophytes, are strict aerobes and produce the enzyme indophenol oxidase. A few are primary pathogens, but most cause opportunist infections in the locally or generally compromised host. Most isolates from this group represent colonization rather than infection, and antibiotic treatment must not be commenced lightly; careful clinical assessment is indicated. Many have unusual antibiotic sensitivity patterns, and are resistant to common antibiotics and antiseptics. Commercial biochemical test kits are now fairly reliable at identifying pseudomonads, but important isolates should be sent for confirmation to a reference laboratory.

### *Pseudomonas aeruginosa*

Motile, slim Gram-negative rods.

**Pathogenicity:** Produce an enormous range of enzymes and other putative virulence factors. Those associated with specific diseases include: alginate-like polysaccharide with antiphagocytic and antibiotic-trapping properties, and protease-induced mucosal damage in cystic fibrosis; proteases in corneal ulceration and ecthyma gangrenosum; exotoxins and proteases in significant burn infection.

**Epidemiology:** Found commonly in moist environmental sites and on raw fruit and vegetables. Occasionally isolated from normal faeces (<10%), but widespread colonization rapidly emerges on hospital admission and after antibiotic treatment. Barring occasional common-source outbreaks (e.g. from contaminated antiseptics) and deficient staff aseptic technique, nosocomial infections are usually shown to be with patients' own strains. Hand-borne spread important, especially on neonatal ICU and burns units. Colonization of large-volume, refilled antiseptic containers (e.g. contact-lens solutions) always likely. A variety of typing methods are available, including serological and pyocine typing (➤).

**Spectrum of disease:** Frequently colonizes moist lesions (e.g. leg ulcers, bedsores, oozing surgical incisions) and the upper airways, especially after antibiotic treatment; occasional progression to superinfection. In the normal patient: external otitis (➤18) and folliculitis and tender skin nodules (➤111) (both from exposure to contaminated water, e.g. poorly maintained whirlpool baths, swimming pools). Nosocomial **wound and burn infection, iv catheter sepsis, UTI, ventilator-associated pneumonia and secondary bacteraemia. Primary bacteraemia** (Σ1800) in neutropenic patients following gastrointestinal colonization (➤174). May be associated with necrotic skin lesions—ecthyma gangrenosum (➤174). **Pulmonary colonization/infection** in patients with cystic fibrosis (CF). **Malignant otitis externa** in diabetics (➤18). **Corneal ulceration** with contaminated contact-lens solutions, and aggressive pan-ophthalmitis after penetrating injury (➤109).

**Laboratory diagnosis:** Ready (24-h) growth on many solid media to form characteristic

**Table 30.1** Classification of pseudomonads

| Genus | Species | Notes |
|---|---|---|
| *Pseudomonas* | *aeruginosa* | Green/blue pigmented, 'beaten copper' colonies (➤291) |
| | (*putida, fluorescens, stutzeri, paucimobilis*, etc.) | 'Miscellaneous' group, rarely isolated from significant infections. Commoner in the immunocompromised. Some strains pigmented (➤294) |
| *Burkholderia* | *cepacia* (*gladioli*) | Lung infection in cystic fibrosis (➤293) |
| | *pseudomallei, mallei* | Primary pathogens, causing infections in the tropics (➤293) |
| *Acinetobacter* | *baumannii* (and '*baumanii* complex') | Cause outbreaks on ICUs. May be highly antibiotic resistant. Used to be called '*Acinetobacter anitratus*' (➤294) |
| | *calcoaceticus, junii, lwoffii, johnsonii, radioresistans* | Common skin commensals and food spoilage bacteria. Occasionally cause small outbreaks in hospital (➤294) |
| | (Others, including some currently classified as *calcoaceticus* and *johnsonii*) | Found in soil and waste waters |
| *Stenotrophomonas* | *maltophilia* | Previously in *Pseudomonas*, then *Xanthomonas* genera. Nosocomial infection in ICU and the immunocompromised (➤294) |
| (*Moraxella*) | (*atlantae, lacunata, osloensis, phenylpyruvica, nonliquifaciens*, etc.) | *Moraxella* (*Branhamella*) *catarrhalis* is considered under fastidious Gram-negative rods (➤302) |

Other pseudomonads include *Chryseobacterium* spp. (some strains formerly *Flavobacterium* spp.), *Alkaligenes* spp., *Achromobacter* spp., *Acidovorax* spp., *Agrobacterium* spp., *Brevundimonas* spp., *Chromobacterium violaceum*, *Comamonas* spp., *Flavimonas* spp., *Methylbacterium* spp., *Ochrobactrum anthropi*, *Oligella* spp., *Ralstonia pickettii*, *Roseomonas* spp., *Shewanella* spp., *Sphingobacterium* spp., *Sphingomonas* spp., etc., which behave as 'miscellaneous' pseudomonads. *Weeksella zoohelcum* has been isolated from cases of septicaemia and bite-associated infection.

colonies with ammoniacal odour. Mucoid strains from CF may take 48 h to produce only tiny colonies. Antiseptics (e.g. cetrimide) added to solid agar make useful selective media. Positive indophenol oxidase test gives rapid presumptive diagnosis, with confirmation in further 24 h, usually by commercial test kits.

**Treatment:** Intrinsically resistant (by broad-spectrum β-lactamase production and impermeable outer cell membrane) to many first-line antibiotics. Generally reliable agents include antipseudomonal penicillins, aminoglycosides, ceftazidime, high-dose ciprofloxacin, imi/meropenem and aztreonam but wide geo-graphic variation. In European ICUs recently reported resistance rates: ceftazidime, 19–29%; ciprofloxacin, 27–40%; gentamicin, 26–44%; meropenem, 22–38%. Ciprofloxacin is the most active quinolone against *Pseudomonas aeruginosa*, and is the only available oral agent, but resistant variants frequently emerge if ciprofloxacin is used alone.

**Prevention:** Neutropenic patients should receive bacteriologically clean food. Perform hand hygiene between every patient contact. Avoid antibiotic usage unless clinically necessary. Supply antiseptics in small-volume, disposable containers; alcoholic agents are intrinsically resistant to contamination. Decontaminate medical equipment between each use, and store it dry.

## Burkholderia cepacia

Formerly *Pseudomonas cepacia*. A colonist of wet environments and a plant pathogen, distinguishable from the 'miscellaneous pseudomonad' group by its propensity to colonize the damaged respiratory tracts of patients with cystic fibrosis. A complex of related organisms, comprising at least six 'genomovars' (by nucleotide sequencing of *recA* gene) for which individual species names have been proposed. Various typing schemes available; genomovar 3 most commonly isolated from CF, most persistent, and transmission among patients most frequently demonstrated (✈). Pathogenesis unknown, but the organism secretes many enzymes and carries pili which adhere to mucus. Some patients suffer few ill effects, but others develop progressive deterioration of respiratory function, and necrotizing pneumonia is seen in 20%. Spread by cross-infection in hospital, clinics and summer camps for CF patients; careful disinfection of respiratory equipment is indicated, and some CF units segregate patients carrying *Burkholderia cepacia*, especially strains from 'pathogenic' genomovars (i.e. 3). Frequently multiply antibiotic-resistant; some units recommend temocillin plus amikacin, or temocillin plus ceftazidime.

## Burkholderia pseudomallei

Causes melioidosis (see below). Formerly called *Pseudomonas pseudomallei*.

**Pathogenesis:** Many putative toxins and enzymes produced; survives in reticuloendothelial cells.

**Laboratory diagnosis:** Gram-negative rods seen in exudates and infected tissue. Culture is not difficult (forms rugose, non-pigmented colonies on many media in 24–48 h), but differentiation from other pseudomonads (including ones that may cause nosocomial infection) may take time (✈) and the organism is a cause of laboratory-acquired infection. Variety of serological tests available (✈).

### Clinical syndrome

**Melioidosis**

A potentially fatal infection caused by *Burkholderia pseudomallei*. Latent infection with recrudescence after many years can occur. Melioidosis is extremely rare as an imported disease in the UK, but recognition is important as correct antibiotic therapy significantly reduces mortality.

**Epidemiology and transmission:** Endemic in SE Asia, Oceania and N. Australia, where *Burkholderia pseudomallei* is widely distributed in soil and water. An important cause of community-acquired pneumonia in SE Asia. Individuals may harbour the organism for many years and develop melioidosis during intercurrent illness or after surgery. This has occurred in many US servicemen returning form Vietnam. Commoner in patients with minor abnormalities of immune function, especially diabetes mellitus, and renal or hepatic disease.

**Clinical features:** Asymptomatic infection is common and can be demonstrated by serology. **Pneumonia** may be severe and acute, with upper-lobe consolidation progressing to cavitation. Chronic presentations also occur and may be mistaken for tuberculosis. **Acute septicaemic melioidosis** presents as a severe septicaemic illness without focal signs, with high fever, constitutional symptoms, hepatomegaly and diarrhoea. Secondary lung involvement is common. **Localized suppurative disease** also occurs, with abscesses in skin, lymph nodes, viscera or brain.

**Investigations:** Diagnosis is made by culture of the organism from blood, sputum or other infected sites. Tell laboratory about relevant travel and predisposing medical history so isolates are not discarded as mucosal colonization by non-pathogenic pseudomonads (☎). Serology not useful in diagnosis of acute cases in endemic regions, but may be helpful, particularly in retrospect, in patients from non-endemic areas.

**Management:** Ceftazidime as initial therapy (with or without co-trimoxazole) is superior to previous multidrug regimens. Meropenem also

*(continued...)*

proven effective. Other antibiotics clinically inferior despite *in vitro* susceptibility results. Continuation treatment (which may be oral) must be
given for several months to prevent relapse.
Mortality of acute septicaemic melioidosis
remains ~30% despite optimum therapy.

### Burkholderia mallei

Cause of glanders, a respiratory tract and lymphangitic infection of horses in Asia, Africa and
the Middle East. Humans may acquire infection
via traumatic skin lesions, resulting in a febrile
illness with lymphadenopathy. Visceral
abscesses may develop. Microbiologically
similar to *Pseudomonas pseudomallei*. Potential
bioterrorism agent (➤415). Combinations of
imi/meropenem, doxycycline and azithromycin
have been used; treatment may need to be prolonged for months to prevent relapse.

### 'Miscellaneous' Pseudomonas spp. and 'other' pseudomonads

Generally colonizers of moist environments
(e.g. sink traps, flower vases). They uncommonly colonize patients, and rarely cause
opportunist infections. Isolation of these
species or *Burkholderia cepacia* from blood cultures suggests either 'pseudobacteraemia' (contamination of the blood culture system from an
environmental source) or iatrogenic infection
of the patient (for example, infusion of a contaminated fluid). *Chryseobacterium* spp. (some
strains formerly *Flavobacterium* spp.: yellow or
colourless colonies) have caused outbreaks of
bacteraemia and meningitis on neonatal ICUs
and neurosurgery units.

### Acinetobacter calcoaceticus, baumannii, 'lwoffii' and 'anitratus'

Plump, non-motile, indophenol oxidase-
negative Gram-negative rods.

**Pathogenesis:** Unknown mechanisms.

**Epidemiology:** See Table 30.1. Members of this
genus include strains that are commensals of

moist skin, food spoilage organisms, and environmental bacteria. Nosocomial infections
commoner in hot countries (especially S.
Europe and SE and E. Asia). Spread in hospital
on staff hands and contaminated equipment.
Variety of typing methods available (➤).

**Spectrum of disease:** Most commonly isolated
as colonists of the mucosae of ill, hospitalized
patients. All may, like other skin commensals,
be opportunist pathogens on prosthetic materials and iv catheters; nosocomial UTI, ventilator-
associated pneumonia, etc. common on some
units; rare community-acquired pneumonia. Σ
911 bacteraemias.

**Laboratory diagnosis:** In Gram stains may be
mistaken for *Neisseria* spp. Ready growth (24 h)
on many media to form small, non-pigmented
colonies.

**Treatment:** Community-acquired strains are
often resistant only to trimethoprim; nosocomial isolates are often multiply resistant with
unpredictable sensitivity patterns (☏). May
produce metallo-β-lactamases with activity
against imi/meropenem. UK resistance rates
in 2000: gentamicin 43%, amikacin 21%,
ciprofloxacin 46%, piperacillin–tazobactam
39%, cefotaxime 96%, ceftazidime 89%.
Imi/meropenem is the most reliable empirical
choice in the UK (2% resistance), but 80–90%
resistant in some S. European ICUs. Other therapeutic possibilities include sulbactam (12%),
colistin (2%) and rifampicin (4%). Combination therapy is often used.

### Stenotrophomonas maltophilia

Motile, Gram-negative rods. Formerly '*Xan-
thomonas*' or '*Pseudomonas maltophilia*'.

**Pathogenesis:** Unknown virulence factors, but
versatile antibiotic resistance mechanisms equip
this organism well for superinfection of ICU
patients receiving modern antibiotic therapy,
especially quinolones or imi/meropenem.

**Epidemiology:** Environmental colonizer of
moist areas. Increasingly recognized to cause

outbreaks in ICUs, spread by staff hands and contaminated equipment. Variety of typing methods available (➜).

**Spectrum of disease:** Most commonly only causes colonization, but may cause iv catheter infection and secondary bacteraemia, and a variety of infections in immunocompromised patients. Σ500 bacteraemias.

**Laboratory diagnosis:** Slim Gram-negative rod. Ready growth (24–48 h) on many media; green/yellow or non-pigmented colonies smelling strongly of ammonia; usually slowly indophenol oxidase-positive.

**Treatment:** Often startlingly antibiotic-resistant, including quinolones, amino-glycosides and imi/meropenem; further resistances commonly emerge during therapy.

Co-trimoxazole and colistin have been tried for systemic therapy with apparent success. Other combinations chosen to inhibit chromosomally-encoded β-lactamases include ticarcillin–clavulanic acid, and co-amoxiclav plus aztreonam ☎.

## *Moraxella catarrhalis* (➤302)

## *Moraxella lacunata, osloensis, phenylpyruvica,* non-*liquifaciens,* etc.

Small Gram-negative coccobacilli that colonize oronasopharyngeal mucosae. Indophenol oxidase-positive, and often initially mistaken for *Neisseria* spp. *Moraxella lacunata* sometimes isolated from corneal ulcers; the other species occasionally cause opportunist nosocomial infections. Generally quite antibiotic-sensitive.

# Chapter 31

# Fastidious Gram-negative organisms

Gram-negative rods and cocci which share the need for special culture conditions (e.g. nutritative co-factors, blood, serum, $CO_2$, moisture) and often colonize the mucosae of humans and animals (Table 31.1). With a few notable exceptions (such as *Haemophilus influenzae* from sputum and blood cultures), optimal culture will often not routinely be performed for these organisms, so inform the laboratory if a patient falls into an appropriate risk group (☎).

## *Haemophilus* spp.

### *Haemophilus influenzae*
Small, pleomorphic Gram-negative rods.

**Pathogenesis:** Invasive strains have polysaccharide capsule which resists phagocytosis unless opsonized; commonly type b (polyribosylribitol phosphate), rarely a, very rarely c–f. Other virulence factors unproven, but include IgA protease, adhesion pili and toxicity for mucosal cilia. Entry to bloodstream occurs from nasopharyngeal invasion.

**Epidemiology:** Ubiquitous commensals of the upper respiratory tract; capsulate strains carried by up to 5% normal adults and children, and up to 60% in childhood contacts of invasive infections. Childhood infections with type b strains much rarer since introduction of Hib vaccine (➤417). Some reports of clusters of type a infections since introduction of Hib, but no rise yet seen in nationally reported data. Rare overwhelming infections in patients with asplenia. Capsular typing by agglutination. Σ 286 type b bacteraemias in 1992, compared with 14 in 1999: non-type b bacteraemias unchanged ≈280.

**Spectrum of disease:** Capsulate strains cause meningitis (➤96), epiglottitis (➤21), osteo-myelitis (➤123), septic arthritis (➤120), cellulitis (including orbital and periorbital, ➤109), and secondary bacteraemia in children <6yrs old (peak incidence 4 months to 2 years). Rare in adults. Non-capsulate strains associated with exacerbations of chronic bronchitis (often mixed infections with *Streptococcus pneumoniae* and *Moraxella catarrhalis* (➤24), sinusitis and otitis media (➤17). Rare cellulitis, meningitis, endocarditis and pneumonia (especially post-influenza) in adults, commoner in the immunocompromised; bacteraemic pneumonia especially common in HIV infection. Invasive strains in adults usually non-capsulate.

**Laboratory diagnosis:** Poor growth on blood agar; much better (24–48h) on heated blood ('chocolate') agar, which has greater available X and V factors. Identification 24h later by test for X and V factor dependence or negative porphyrin production. Direct antigen detection for b-capsulate strains widely available.

**Treatment:** Ampicillin/amoxicillin resistance (β-lactamase production) currently 12% overall in the UK, higher in type b. Much higher rates in the USA (≈32%). Resistance rare (<2%) to co-amoxiclav, azithromycin, ciprofloxacin and cefuroxime. Most commonly used empirical choices are oral tetracycline, trimethoprim, co-amoxiclav, cefaclor, cefixime or ciprofloxacin; parenteral cephalosporin (chloramphenicol is an alternative). Other oral cephalosporins have less activity. Frequently erythromycin resistant.

**Prevention:** Hib vaccine (but weak response in those <2yrs and the immunocompromised); rifampicin prophylaxis for household contacts of invasive infections (➤100).

**Table 31.1** Fastidious Gram-negative organisms

| Genus | Species | Notes |
|---|---|---|
| **Environmental source** | | |
| *Legionella* | ***pneumophila*** (*birminghamensis, bozemanii, cincinnatiensis, feeleii, gormanii, jordanesis, longbeachae, micdadei, oakridgensis, tucsonensis, wadsworthii* and others have caused human disease. Some have been classified in the genera *Tatlockia* and *Fluoribacter*) (➤301) | |
| **Human source** | | |
| *Haemophilus* | ***influenzae*** (*parainfluenzae, haemolyticus, parahaemolyticus, haemoglobinophilus, 'aegyptius'*, etc., and see HACEK group below) | Satellitism around *Staphylococcus aureus* colonies on blood agar; require X factor (porphyrins, eg haemin) and V factor (coenzyme 1; NAD or NADP) for growth on nutrient agar. 'Para' species require only V factor (➤296) |
| | *ducreyi* | Causes chancroid (➤93, 298) |
| *Neisseria* | ***meningitidis*** | Meningococcus (➤299) |
| | ***gonorrhoeae*** | Gonococcus (➤300) |
| | (*sicca, flava, perflava, subflava, lactamica,* etc.) | *Neisseria lactamica* sometimes mistaken for *meningitidis* |
| *Bordetella* | *pertussis* (*parapertussis, bronchiseptica*) | Human respiratory tract infection (➤301) |
| *Moraxella* | *catarrhalis* | Human respiratory tract infection (➤302). Used to be in the genus *Branhamella* |
| | (*canis, lacunata, lincolnii, nonliquefaciens, osloensis, phenylpyruvica*) | Occasionally isolated from human infections, especially keratitis (➤295) |
| *Gardnerella* | *vaginalis* | Has belonged to *Haemophilus* and *Corynebacterium* genera. Gram-variable staining (➤264, 302) |
| (*Calymmatobacterium*) | (*granulomatis*) | Granuloma inguinale in tropical countries. Genital ulceration (➤94) |
| (*Anaerobiospirillum*) | (*succiniproducens*) | Spiral organism, rarely isolated from blood or faeces |
| (DF-3) | | Causes chronic diarrhoea in the immunocompromised |
| *Capnocytophaga* | *ochracea* | Human oral and systemic sepsis (➤302) |
| 'HACEK' or 'herbie' group | | *Haemophilus aphrophilus* and *paraphrophilus* and related organisms (➤306) |
| **Zoonoses** | | |
| *Capnocytophaga* | *canimorsus* | Zoonotic wound and systemic sepsis (➤302) |
| (*Ehrlichia*) | (*canis, chaffeensis, sennetsu* and relatives) | Causes human granulocytic and monocytic ehrlichiosis (➤302) |

Table 31.1 (Continued)

| Genus | Species | Notes |
|---|---|---|
| Pasteurella | multocida (canis, gallinarum) | Zoonotic wound and systemic sepsis (➢303) |
| | (pneumotropica, ureae) | Rare respiratory tract infections |
| Yersinia | pestis | Zoonotic plague; BT (➢305, 415) |
| | (enterocolitica, pseudotuberculosis) | (➢284) |
| (Francisella) | (tularensis) | Zoonotic respiratory, wound or systemic infections; BT (➢307, 415) |
| (Streptobacillus) | (moniliformis) | Causes rat bite fever (➢306) |
| Brucella* | abortus, melitensis, suis, ovis, canis, etc. | Systemic sepsis; BT (➢303) |
| (Bartonella)* | (bacilliformis) | Oroya fever and verruga peruana (➢308) |
| | (henselae) | Causes cat scratch disease, bacillary angiomatosis, chronic bacteraemia and infective endocarditis (➢308) |
| | (quintana) | Causes trench fever, bacillary angiomatosis, chronic bacteraemia and infective endocarditis (➢308) |
| | (elizabethae, clarridgeiae) | Very rare human isolates (➢308) |
| (Afipia)* | (felis) | May cause some cases of cat-scratch disease (➢309) |

Other related genera include *Arcobacter* ssp. and *Suttonella* sp.
* Closely related genera.

## Haemophilus aegyptius (Koch–Weeks bacillus)

Subtype of *influenzae* associated with epidemic conjunctivitis, which may progress to systemic sepsis (Brazilian purpuric fever). Ampicillin plus chloramphenicol has been used for therapy.

## Haemophilus parainfluenzae

Occasionally causes similar infections to non-capsulate strains of *Haemophilus influenzae*.

## Haemophilus ducreyi

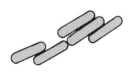

Small Gram-negative rods.

**Pathogenesis:** Largely unknown.

**Epidemiology:** Most common in parts of Africa and Asia.

**Spectrum of disease:** Causes **chancroid** (➢93) or 'soft sore'; painful genital ulceration and regional lymphadenitis. May progress to phimosis and urethral fistula.

**Laboratory diagnosis:** 'Shoal of fish' arrangement of bacilli in smears from undermined edge of ulcers. Can be isolated with difficulty on selective medium containing serum ☎.

**Treatment:** Effective new antibiotics include co-trimoxazole, co-amoxiclav and ciprofloxacin;

older, cheaper regimens included sulphonamides, streptomycin, erythromycin and tetracyclines.

## Neisseria spp.

### Neisseria meningitidis ✉①

Small, Gram-negative, oval diplococci.

**Pathogenesis:** Surface pili involved in mucosal adhesion; also produces IgA protease. Polysaccharide capsule essential to avoid phagocytosis; serum antibodies may be protective, and carriage of *Neisseria lactamica* may raise cross-protective antibody in childhood against outer membrane proteins and capsule. Penetration of mucosa ⇨ bloodstream ⇨ meninges. Possible direct spread through cribriform plate. Host factors then determine whether lipopolysaccharide triggers sepsis syndrome (➤185). Mortality associated with high meningococcal DNA copy number in circulation. Death in fulminant septicaemia (Waterhouse–Friedrichsen syndrome) is from microcirculatory damage and multiorgan failure, not from loss of adrenal function; indeed, circulating corticosteroid levels are usually high.

**Epidemiology:** Σ ≈2200, with ≈800 bacteraemias. In normal nasopharynx 5–20% carriage rate, mostly non-capsulate strains outside outbreaks. Carriage commoner in closed communities (e.g. barracks, boarding schools), and up to 80% during outbreaks. Spread by droplets or direct mucosal contact; household contacts of cases have up to 800× increased risk of infection. Acquisition of new virulent strain ⇨ highest risk of invasive disease in first week. Two-thirds of cases occur in first 5 yrs of life, with smaller peak in late teens. Serogrouping by capsular polysaccharide, subtyping by outer membrane proteins (✛). Group A strains cause only 2% cases in the UK, but associated with epidemics, as seen in sub-Saharan Africa every 5–10 yrs. Groups B and C cause 60% and 35% of UK cases, respectively, as in most of Europe. Others include W135 and Y; associated with higher rate of extra-meningeal focal disease. Serogroup Y now commonest in the USA and rising. International transfer of group A strains with returnees from Hajj in Mecca now controlled with immunization plus antibiotic prophylaxis campaign in Saudi Arabia, but similar problems seen in past 2 yrs with W135 strains (need multivalent vaccine) (➤193).

**Spectrum of disease:** Although there is a gradation of presentations between the two, the commonest systemic manifestations can be divided into **meningitis**, making up two-thirds of cases (➤96), and **septicaemia** in one-third of cases, with multiple organ failure and purpuric rash (➤185). **Rare presentations** include conjunctivitis (➤105), IE (➤49), arthritis (➤120), pericarditis (➤55), vulvovaginitis in children, urethritis, proctitis, pharyngitis, pneumonia. These may occur in isolation or accompany meningitis or bacteraemia, or occasionally fulminant septicaemia. **Chronic meningococcal septicaemia**, with joint involvement and purulent skin lesions, occurs rarely (30% such patients have complement deficiencies — unable to form terminal attack complex). Mortality (treated) approaches 100% in fulminant septicaemia, up to 50% in meningitis with septicaemia and rash, and <5% in meningitis and other sites alone. Sequelae of invasive disease include hearing impairment (8%), visual loss (4%), seizures (2%), cognitive impairment (2%), loss of digits or limbs (4%), scarring/major skin loss (4%), renal impairment (3%).

**Laboratory diagnosis:** CSF Gram stain is the mainstay of rapid species diagnosis. Meningococci often seen inside polymorphs in CSF, blood smears or pus ('intracellular diplococci'). Gram stains of purpuric skin smears allow rapid confirmation, and differentiation from *Staphylococcus aureus* (➤249). Rapid capsular antigen detection rarely any more useful than Gram stain of CSF. Neisserias are sensitive to drying. Require $CO_2$, moisture, serum/heated blood (e.g. 'chocolate' agar) for optimal growth ⇨ tiny, indophenol oxidase-positive colonies at 24 h, larger at 48 h. Sensitive to liquoid (anticoagulant and anticomplement; added to many blood culture systems); therefore some laboratories supply 'meningitis bottle' optimized for neisserias. Confirmation by biochemical tests (rapid (4h) commercial kits available) and antigen content, but biochemically atypical strains are not rare and will need confirmation ✛.

**Treatment:** Benzylpenicillin remains the drug of choice; cefotaxime or ceftriaxone are as effective, are usefully broad-spectrum when the diagnosis is uncertain, and they retain activity against the currently very rare penicillin-resistant meningococci (reported largely from Spain). Steroid therapy of additional benefit in children only. Eradicate carriage from cases with rifampicin, ciprofloxacin or ceftriaxone (➤100).

**Prevention:** Closure of meningeal defects; rational use of antibiotic prophylaxis and meningococcal vaccine in asplenia and close contacts of cases (➤100). No vaccine currently effective against group B strains (unstable, non-immunogenic capsule), but several at trial stage including one derived from *Neisseria lactamica*.

### *Neisseria lactamica*

Biochemically and antigenically similar to meningococcus, but ferments lactose slowly. Rarely causes focal infections, as may the other commensal neisserias.

### *Neisseria gonorrhoeae*

Small, Gram-negative, oval diplococci.

**Pathogenesis:** Piliated strains more virulent (increased adhesion to urethral epithelium and resistance to killing by serum). Also produce a variety of proteases, including IgA protease.

**Epidemiology:** Only spread by direct mucosal contact; risk of transmission depends on frequency and duration of intercourse. Infected females and those with rectal or pharyngeal infections are often asymptomatic. Typing possible by PCR, outer-membrane proteins or biochemistry ('auxotyping' ✛); certain auxotypes associated with invasive disease. Neonate infected during passage through cervix. Incidence rose in the UK, 1960s–1980s, then fell, probably because of increased use of barrier contraception with appearance of HIV. However, this trend reversed after 1994. Between 1999 and 2000, diagnoses of uncomplicated gonorrhoea rose by 31% (to 14 350) in males and 26% (to 6313) in females, and mean age has fallen. Resurgence probably due to increase in unsafe sex practices, particularly in young heterosexuals and homo/bisexual men. Σ ≈300 β-lactamase-producing isolates.

**Spectrum of disease:** Mucosal infection of urethra, uterine endocervix and sometimes rectum or pharynx (➤86); vulvovaginitis (prepubertal). Ophthalmia neonatorum (➤107). Secondary local spread, including epididymitis, salpingitis, peritonitis. Most with the Fitz-Hugh–Curtis syndrome (perihepatitis) are co-infected with *Chlamydia trachomatis*. Metastatic spread, causing acute or chronic bacteraemia, arthritis (➤120), skin pustules, rare endocarditis or meningitis.

**Laboratory diagnosis:** Intracellular Gram-negative diplococci seen in urethral swab of male with urethritis is highly sensitive and specific for gonorrhoea; this is not true for other sites because of their normal flora which contains many similar-looking organisms (commensal neisserias and meningococci, *Acinetobacter* spp., etc.). A delicate, strictly aerobic organism; ideally inoculate selective, nutritive medium (e.g. vancomycin–colistin–nystatin–trimethoprim (VCNT) agar, with lysed blood) with charcoal swabs directly in the clinic; otherwise use transport medium containing charcoal. Forms small colonies in (24–)48h. In the female, culture of endocervical swab more sensitive than HVS. Bacteriologically very similar to the meningococcus (see above), but differentiated by biochemical reactions and antigen content.

**Treatment:** (➤87).

**Prevention:** Barrier contraception or abstinence. Contact tracing and treatment. Silver nitrate prophylaxis to neonatal eyes in high-prevalence areas.

## *Legionella pneumophila* and other legionellas

Slim Gram-negative bacilli.

**Pathogenesis:** Inhalation of aerosol containing bacteria ⇨ pneumonia ⇨ bacteraemia in severe cases. Legionella protease involved in pathogenesis. Survive within macrophages. Pathogenesis of Pontiac fever not understood.

**Epidemiology:** Live in water, especially if warm, often in symbiosis with amoebae; frequently colonize piped water systems and evaporative condensers of air-conditioning cooling towers. Large inocula may be released as aerosols, to be inhaled by susceptible people. Pneumonic infection commoner with immunosuppression, age > 60, chronic chest disease, smoking. 3–4× commoner in males than females. In ≈50% UK cases, there is an association with travel, especially Spain, Balearics, Greece, Turkey, USA. No human-to-human transmission; the only bacteria (other than *Coxiella burnetii*) to cause outbreaks of pneumonia out of hospital. Various typing methods for the major species are available (✈): *Legionella pneumophila* causes >95% cases, and serogroup 1 comprises the majority of these.

**Spectrum of disease: Legionnaire's disease**—pneumonia ± bacteraemia, with 2–10-day incubation period. Σ ≈175 with ≈25 deaths; 2–4% proved nosocomial; now representing up to 5% pneumonias admitted to hospital. Mortality worldwide reported 10–85% (mean 15%) depending on underlying illness (➢32). **Pontiac fever**—minor influenza-like illness with high attack rate in normal people. Σ 10 in 1994. Incubation 24–48h, duration 48–96h. Rare **localized infection**, e.g. IE (usually of prosthetic valves), haemodialysis shunt infection, hepatitis, peritonitis, sinusitis, wound infection, etc.

**Laboratory diagnosis:** May be difficult to see in Gram stains of clinical material. Immunofluorescent stains available for rapid direct visualization in sputum, but sensitivity low and interpretation technically demanding (hence ✈). **Urinary ELISA** is highly specific and sensitive within first 5–7 days of presentation, but only available for serogroup 1. Will not grow on conventional culture media. Readily isolated if sputum, lung/pleural aspirates are inoculated to buffered charcoal–yeast-extract agar (BCYE), which contains iron and cysteine. Forms 'cut-glass' colonies in 48h–5 days (occasionally up to 10 days). Blood culture broths can be inoculated to BCYE after 3–5 days' incubation in suspected bacteraemic cases (☎). Confirm in reference laboratory by antigen content (✈). Serum antibodies vs. *Legionella pneumophila* serogroup 1 detectable by FAT, RMAT or ELISA and usually develop during second week of illness, but up to 20% seroconversions take >1 month (diagnosis requires fourfold rise, or isolated high titre). Serology not widely available for most other serogroups and species (✈), hence attempts to isolate the organism are important.

**Treatment:** Erythromycin iv 1g 6-hly; *in vitro* and animal experiments suggest addition of rifampicin or ciprofloxacin may be synergistic in severe infection. Clarithromycin and azithromycin assumed (but not proven) to be effective; other antibiotics clinically inactive.

**Prevention:** Regular maintenance/disinfection of water systems will reduce (but rarely eliminate) contamination. *Legionella* multiplication reduced by keeping water <20°C or >60°C.

## *Bordetella pertussis*

Small, Gram-negative rods.

**Pathogenesis:** Causes superficial infection of respiratory mucosae. Various recognized virulence factors: three major fimbrial agglutinins (adhesin role, important vaccine components, and useful in typing), 'pertussis toxin' (like diphtheria toxin), adenylate cyclase toxin, tracheal cytotoxin, lymphocytosis factor, endotoxin (differs from usual Gram-negative lipopolysaccharide), filamentous haemagglutinin.

**Epidemiology:** Not a normal commensal. Child-to-child respiratory droplet transmission. Rarely infects adults, but commoner in unvaccinated populations. Highest mortality in children <1 yr. $\Sigma \approx 1100$, with 2 deaths in 1999. Vaccine uptake in UK now $\approx 95\%$. Case fatality rate $\approx 1:200$ under 2 months of age, $\approx 1:15\,000$ in 1–4-yr age group.

**Spectrum of disease:** Whooping cough (➢136).

**Laboratory diagnosis:** Best yield from pernasal swab without transport medium. No growth on conventional media—needs high blood content with antibiotics (e.g. Bordet–Gengou or charcoal medium) and grows slowly to tiny, glistening colonies (72 h or more). Biochemically non-reactive—identified by specific antiserum.

*Bordetella parapertussis* and *bronchiseptica* are less fastidious in their growth requirements, and rarely cause respiratory illness.

## *Moraxella catarrhalis* (formerly *Branhamella catarrhalis*)

Small, Gram-negative diplococci which colonize and probably infect the respiratory tract; colonization commonest in children. Disputed pathogen; may cause exacerbations of chronic bronchitis (➢24) but frequently ($\approx 50\%$) isolated in mixed culture with *Haemophilus influenzae* and the pneumococcus. Sometimes isolated from tracheitis in children, otitis media, sinusitis, and rarely alone from severe bacteraemic pneumonia, endocarditis and meningitis, especially in the immunocompromised ($\Sigma \approx 80$ bacteraemias). More than 90% isolates now produce β-lactamase, which may inactivate ampicillin/amoxicillin used to treat the mixed infection; usually trimethoprim-resistant. Usually reliable agents include co-amoxiclav, erythro/clarithromycin, tetracycline, oral cephalosporins, 4-quinolones.

## *Gardnerella vaginalis*

Small Gram-variable rod. Vaginal and occasional urethral commensal, usually in small numbers. Adheres to squamous epithelial cells ('clue cells') in bacterial vaginosis (➢82, 264),

and occasionally isolated from mixed pelvic and puerperal sepsis (➢83), rarely bacteraemic. Facultative anaerobe, but metronidazole-sensitive.

## *Capnocytophaga* spp.

Small, thin, Gram-negative rods with pointed ends. Slow, $CO_2$-dependent growth (2–5 days) to form small, yellowish colonies with 'gliding' motility. Generally antibiotic-sensitive except to aminoglycosides and trimethoprim.

### *Capnocytophaga ochracea*

Used to be called DF-1 (dysgonic fermenter—ferments carbohydrates to mainly acetate and succinate). Human oral commensal. Opportunist infections, isolated from mixed bacterial periodontitis in those with disorders of neutrophil chemotaxis, and causes oral ulceration and occasional bacteraemia in neutropenic patients. Very rare empyema, endocarditis, osteomyelitis and various abscesses in the normal host.

### *Capnocytophaga canimorsus*

Used to be called DF-2. Oral commensal of many animals, especially cats and dogs. Important cause of bite wound infection in normal patients (➢114), which may progress to overwhelming septicaemia in asplenics (➢170), alcoholics and the immunocompromised.

## *Ehrlichia* spp.

*Ehrlichia chaffeensis* and *sennetsu* are coccobacilli causing **human monocytic ehrlichiosis** in eastern and Midwestern USA and Japan; spread by Lone Star tick. Other *Ehrlichia* spp. cause **human granulocytic ehrlichiosis** in Midwestern and north-eastern USA; spread by *Ixodes* and *Dermacentor* ticks (may also transmit Lyme disease ➢323). Horse and ruminant reservoirs.

**Pathogenesis:** Intracellular parasites of mononuclear cells.

**Clinical syndromes:** Indistinguishable; incubation period up to 4 weeks. Acute fever, myalgia, headache, thrombocytopenia, leucopenia, hepatitis. Occasional renal failure and neurological involvement. Resembles 'spotless' Rocky Mountain spotted fever (➤329).

**Treatment:** Tetracycline or doxycycline for at least 7 days.

**Prevention:** Insect repellent, long sleeves and trousers, examine skin for ticks after walking in woods and fields. Antibiotic prophylaxis not recommended.

## Pasteurella multocida

Small, pleomorphic, Gram-negative coccobacilli.

**Pathogenesis:** Capsulate, and contains lipopolysaccharide, but detailed mechanisms unknown.

**Epidemiology:** Naso-oropharyngeal commensal of many animals, some suffering similar infections to those seen in humans. Serotyping available (✦).

**Spectrum of disease:** Important cause of **bite** wound infections (➤114), including local abscesses, cellulitis and lymphangitis pressing to bacteraemia. Rare pneumonia, empyema.

**Laboratory diagnosis:** Ready growth (24 h) on usual primary culture media to form small, shiny, indophenol oxidase-positive colonies. Usually confirmed by commercial biochemical test kit (further 24 h).

**Treatment:** Usually sensitive to penicillin and tetracycline, and resistant to erythromycin; ➤114 for management of bites.

## Brucella spp.

Small Gram-negative coccobacilli and bacilli.

**Pathogenesis:** Ingested in milk or by handling infected carcasses (must survive stomach acid); inhaled close to aborting animals; occasional direct inoculation from animal contact, or of vaccine strain. Spread via lymphatics and bloodstream, then localization in reticuloendothelial system, causing granulomas.

**Epidemiology:** Animal pathogens, causing abortion and prolonged excretion in milk. Cause zoonotic infections in a few, clearly defined circumstances. Distributed worldwide. Particularly common in Mediterranean countries such as Spain, Greece and the Middle East and in S. America. **Rarely seen in the UK (Σ 15)**, but commonly suspected; the diagnosis can often be ruled out by taking an accurate history. Transmission occurs by eating infected produce, direct contact with infected tissues and by aerosol inhalation, e.g. in abattoir. Person-to-person spread does not occur. *Brucella melitensis* is associated with goats and sheep. Infection is acquired primarily via goat's milk and cheese, occurs at all ages and affects both sexes equally. *Brucella abortus* is associated with cattle. Infection is an occupational disease of farmers, vets and butchers and therefore affects mainly males. *Brucella suis* is associated with pigs, almost exclusively in the USA. Biotyping available (✦).

**Spectrum of disease:** Varied presenting features (see below). *Brucella melitensis* is associated with more severe acute infection and more frequent complications than other species. Subclinical infection, which is the usual form taken by *Brucella abortus*, is rare.

**Laboratory diagnosis:** Slow growth on solid media (48–96 h) to small, shiny colonies, and can take >3 weeks even in modern blood culture systems (prolonged incubation ☗ ☎; but reaches ≈70% positivity given optimal techniques). Grow best in serum- and glucose-enriched media, and *abortus* needs added $CO_2$. Cultures from patients suspected to have brucellosis and further tests on possible *Brucella* isolates must be performed in Category 3 containment facilities. Confirm identity in ✦. Serology needs expert interpretation, especially in those exposed in the past (standard agglutination test, mercaptoethanol test, CFT, anti-human-globulin test; confirm by ✦). Worth repeating if negative in clinically strongly suspected cases because seroconversion often late.

**Prevention: Vaccination** of young cattle; pasteurization of milk and milk products; testing of herds (milk ring test) and slaughter of positive animals.

## Clinical syndrome

### Brucellosis (undulant fever, Malta fever)

A disease of variable severity and duration acquired from domestic animals and caused by *Brucella melitensis*, *Brucella abortus* and *Brucella suis*.

**Clinical features:** The **incubation** period is variable and difficult to ascertain—usually 5–60 days but often several months. **Asymptomatic or mild disease** occurs, but is unusual. **Acute brucellosis** presents with rapid onset of high fever, constitutional symptoms, arthralgia, myalgia, headache, back pain, anorexia, constipation, weight loss, rigors and prostration. Fever (≈98%), leucopenia, bone and joint signs (≈20%), lymphadenopathy (≈10%), neurological signs (≈10%), hepatomegaly (≈40%) and splenomegaly (≈20%) are often found. A transient non-specific skin rash is seen in ≈5% and relative bradycardia in ≈20% cases. The differential diagnosis of fever, prostration and leucopenia in a returning traveller also includes typhoid, malaria and viral infection, which are much commoner in the UK (➤206). Symptoms may resolve after a few weeks, but a relapsing/remitting course often follows. This clinical picture is referred to as **subacute brucellosis or undulant fever**. During this phase, arthralgia, fatigue, low-grade fever and depression are common. Physical examination may be normal or reveal moderate splenomegaly. This form of brucellosis may also develop insidiously, with no preceding acute febrile illness. Suppurative and immune-mediated complications are most likely to occur during this stage. Most patients recover within 1 yr.

**Chronic brucellosis** describes patients who have been unwell for more than a year. The status of this diagnosis remains controversial. Some of these patients have had inadequate

*(continued...)*

antibiotic therapy or have local suppurative complications, but chronic brucellosis has been used in the past to describe a group of patients, usually at occupational risk of acquiring brucellosis, with chronic fatigue but no evidence of ongoing infection. If clinical examination, blood, urine and bone-marrow culture, liver biopsy, radiology and serology all show no evidence of brucellosis, then the diagnosis of chronic brucellosis should not be made, but serology should be repeated over a period of several months.

**Complications: Arthritis** becomes more common as duration of disease increases. Sacroiliitis, acute monoarthritis (usually affecting the hip, knee or ankle) or a polyarticular rheumatoid-like arthritis have been described. **Vertebral osteomyelitis** (predominantly lumbar) occurs occasionally and may be associated with paravertebral abscess. Characteristic radiological changes with lateral osteophyte growth ('parrot's beak sign') are described. Various **skin and soft tissue abscesses** and **thrombophlebitis** have been reported. **Haematological abnormalities** include anaemia. leucopenia and thrombocytopenia, which may be severe, leading to purpura. **Meningitis** and **endophthalmitis** occur occasionally. The CSF shows a lymphocytic pleocytosis, with raised protein and normal or slightly reduced glucose. **Uveitis** occurs. **Pulmonary involvement** is usually restricted to cough with CXR infiltrates, although pleural effusion has been reported. **Brucella endocarditis** is rare and affects primarily the aortic valve. Most patients have pre-existing valve damage. Endocarditis accounts for most of the mortality associated with brucellosis. **Granulomatous hepatitis, cholecystitis, hepatic or splenic abscesses** also occur. Granulomatous disease affecting the **kidney, ureter or bladder** may cause urinary symptoms or obstructive uropathy and **epididymo-orchitis** may be seen.

**Investigations:** Diagnosis is usually suspected on epidemiological grounds and is unequivocally confirmed by isolation of organism from blood, bone marrow or focal lesions. This requires special techniques and prolonged culture—a hazard to laboratory staff ☎. Culture any available biopsies and aspirates of local lesions (warn

*(continued...)*

laboratory of suspected diagnosis), and take two or three blood cultures. Culture is positive in the majority of cases of acute brucellosis, but the yield is lower in subacute infection. Serological tests are more widely used, but are never worth requesting without a history of contact or travel—over 90% of patients give an appropriate exposure history. Persistent negative serology reliably excludes acute brucellosis; the interpretation of low-titre positive results in patients with equivocal chronic disease requires discussion with reference laboratory ☎. In this situation, bone-marrow aspiration and culture are recommended by some authors.

**Management:** Doxycycline 200 mg daily + rifampicin 600–900 mg/day for 6 weeks. Rifampicin + co-trimoxazole or doxycycline + streptomycin are alternatives. Prolonged treatment may be necessary for focal suppurative disease. Overall mortality <1%, but relapse in 3–4%. Patients with brucella endocarditis almost always need valve replacement.

## *Yersinia pestis*

Pleomorphic, bipolar-staining Gram-negative coccobacillus.

**Pathogenesis:** Antiphagocytic capsule, lipopolysaccharide and various other toxins involved.

**Epidemiology and transmission:** Transmitted to humans and animals by flea bites, by direct contact with infected animals (for example, by handling infected animal tissues) or by aerosol from humans or animals with pneumonic plague. Major plague pandemics have occurred throughout history (e.g. the Black Death); the most recent started in China in mid-nineteenth century and peaked in early part of last century. *Yersinia pestis* maintained in geographically restricted enzootic foci throughout all continents. Worldwide ≈5000 cases p.a. reported to WHO, notably western USA (≈15 cases p.a. in USA), S. America, Africa, Central and SE Asia (particularly Burma, Vietnam and Indonesia). Human disease may be sporadic or epidemic. Sporadic cases occur when humans intrude to enzootic areas, following an epizootic or when rodents and fleas enter houses. Epidemic disease is usually associated with poor living conditions, rodent and flea infestation and overcrowding. Person-to-person respiratory spread causing primary plague pneumonia is particularly likely to establish a chain of epidemic spread. Potential BT agent via aerosol release (➤415).

**Spectrum of disease:** **Bubonic** and **pneumonic** plague.

**Laboratory diagnosis:** Aspirate buboes, collect sputum and blood cultures ☎; Hazard Group 3 pathogen, hence work performed in containment level 3 facility in class 1 protective cabinet ☠. Fluorescent antibody staining used in endemic areas. Methylene blue bipolar-stained bacilli. Capsules visible in tissue smears (send heat-fixed smears to ✈) and after culture at 37°C. Best growth on blood agar anaerobically and at low temperature (24–48 h at 27°C). Inoculation to MacConkey and *Yersinia* CIN agars useful for heavily-contaminated samples. Acute and convalescent serology, direct immunofluorescence for F1 antigen, phage lysis and PCR also available (✈).

**Prevention:** Depends on rodent and flea control. Contacts of cases should be disinfested of fleas. Contacts of suspected plague pneumonia should be given chemoprophylaxis (ciprofloxacin 500 mg bd or doxycycline 100 mg bd for 1 week). International quarantine regulations apply to passengers arriving from a plague-endemic area. Vaccine no longer available because of unreliable efficacy, but new subunit vaccine under development (➤194). *Yersinia pestis* is killed by exposure to sunlight for 4 h, but survives longer in dried blood and secretions. Isolation ① during first 72 h of treatment for cases with pneumonia; possible transmission by aerosol or inoculation injury.

## Clinical syndrome

**Plague (syn. Bubonic plague)** ✉ ①
A disease of rodents caused by *Yersinia pestis*.

**Incubation period:** 2–6 days (1–3 (–6) days for primary plague pneumonia).

**Clinical features: Bubonic plague** results from percutaneous inoculation of *Yersinia pestis* by flea bite or contamination of wound by infected material. Presents with sudden onset of fever, rigors, headache, myalgia, prostration, GI upset and abdominal pain, and painfully enlarged regional lymph nodes ('bubo'). Overlying skin is reddened and adherent. Untreated, **secondary septicaemia, meningitis and pneumonia** occur by haematogenous spread. In 10–20% cases **secondary plague septicaemia** occurs, without primary regional lymphadenopathy but with high concentrations of bacteria in the blood. Symptoms are similar to bubonic plague, but recognition is difficult. Mortality is very high, as all may progress to secondary plague pneumonia with septic shock and DIC. **Primary plague pneumonia** follows respiratory transmission. After an incubation period (often as short as 24 h) patients develop fever, cough, bloody sputum, headache, rigors and prostration. Death may supervene rapidly, and secondary transmission may occur by respiratory secretions. **Pharyngeal plague** is very rare and may result from inhalation or ingestion of the organism. There is tonsillar swelling, anterior cervical lymphadenopathy and swelling of the parotid area.

**Investigations:** Warn laboratories of the possibility of the diagnosis ☎. Often suspected on epidemiological grounds. Aspirated material from bubo, sputum or CSF may show characteristic bipolar staining Gram-negative coccobacilli on microscopy; culture of blood, sputum, bubo material, scrapings from skin lesions or tissue biopsy. Immunological methods for rapid identification of organisms are available ✈. Acute and convalescent serology ✈. In primary and secondary plague pneumonia, physical signs in the lungs may be minimal, but multilobar consolidation or bronchopneumonic appearances common on CXR.

*(continued...)*

**Management:** Untreated, mortality is high, 100% in plague pneumonia if antibiotics delayed for over 24 h. Treatment with streptomycin (1 g im bd for adults), doxycycline (100 mg bd po) or chloramphenicol highly effective if started within hours of presentation (overall 8% mortality in WHO reports since 1983, ≈5% in uncomplicated bubonic plague, ≈33% if septicaemic). **Gentamicin** (in standard dosage for severe sepsis) is the current first line recommendation. **Ciprofloxacin** (400 mg iv bd, or 500 mg po bd) very effective for treatment and prophylaxis in animal models; parenteral cephalosporins less effective. Penicillin ineffective. Chloramphenicol (25 mg/kg/day in four divided doses) still recommended for plague meningitis because of good CSF penetration. Cases and suspected cases of plague pneumonia, and those with bubonic plague with cough or CXR changes, should be nursed under standard isolation precautions until 72 h after start of antibiotic therapy. Isolation with drainage/secretion precautions is adequate for cases of bubonic plague.

**Prevention:** Consider antibiotic prophylaxis for health-care workers looking after patients with plague.

## *Streptobacillus moniliformis*

Highly pleomorphic Gram-negative rod; one cause of **rat-bite fever**. Upper respiratory commensal of rats causing infections of rat bites and of contaminated skin lesions, also epidemics of systemic illness associated with consumption of contaminated milk (**Haverhill fever**). Usually causes severe systemic symptoms with fever, polyarthritis and rashes; rare local sepsis unassociated with bites, also IE and pneumonia. Untreated mortality ≈10%. Grows readily in blood cultures, and on blood agar with added $CO_2$, in 48 h to form small, grey colonies; ✈. Sensitive to benzylpenicillin.

## HACEK or 'herbie' group

*Haemophilus aphrophilus* and *paraphrophilus*, *Actinobacillus actinomycetemcomitans*, *Cardiobacterium hominis*, *Eikenella corrodens* and

*Kingella kingae* and *denitrificans*—sometimes known as the '**HACEK**', 'HB' or 'herbie' (a patient's name) group—are bacteriologically related, rod-shaped human oropharyngeal commensals. *Eikenella* colonies pit solid agar surfaces.

Occasionally isolated from oropharyngeal, lung, pleural and brain abscesses, metastatic osteomyelitis and bite wounds, sometimes in mixed culture with other oral commensals. Rare causes of IE; isolation from blood cultures may require prolonged incubation. Variably benzylpenicillin-sensitive, but co-amoxiclav or parenteral or broad-spectrum cephalosporins are more reliable, with ampicillin plus gentamicin used for IE.

## Francisella tularensis

Causes tularaemia. Pleomorphic, capsulate, Gram-negative bacillus. Type A strains (subspecies *tularensis*) cause serious clinical infection in N. America; type B (*palearctica*) cause mainly subclinical infection in Europe. Potential BT agent (➤415): high risk of laboratory-acquired infection ☎ ⚡.

---

### Clinical syndrome

**Tularaemia ① (syn. rabbit fever, lemming fever, deerfly fever, wild hare disease, Ohara disease, Yato-byo)**
Infection with *Francisella tularensis* usually acquired from rabbits or hares. It causes a variety of clinical syndromes depending on the strain involved and the route of transmission, and is readily confused clinically with many other infections.

**Epidemiology and transmission:** Widespread throughout the Northern hemisphere with the exception of the UK: particularly N. America, Scandinavia, CIS, China and Japan. Many wild animals, including mammals and birds, are infected. Infection maintained in the wild by animal-tick, -fly and -mosquito cycles. Human infection acquired by contact with carcasses (hunters), tick or mosquito bite, consuming inadequately cooked infected meat or contaminated

*(continued...)*

water, or inhalation of dust from soil, grain or hay. Laboratory cases occur readily via inhalation (further tests on possible *Francisella* isolates must be performed in Category 3 containment facilities). Person-to-person spread very rare.

**Pathogenesis:** Facultative intracellular parasite; inhibits macrophage phagosome fusion. Inoculation (infective dose as low as 10 colony-forming-units) ⇨ local nodes ⇨ haematogenous spread.

**Incubation period:** Usually 3–15 days (can be 1–21).

**Clinical features:** Depend on route of acquisition (see Table 31.2). Severe constitutional symptoms (fever, headache, myalgia, cough, sore throat, abdominal pain, vomiting) may accompany all forms, preceding lymphadenopathy. Hepatosplenomegaly may be seen later. Illness typically lasts 2–3 weeks. Untreated mortality overall 30% type A, 2% type B, also depending on presentation.

**Investigations:** Warn laboratories of possibility of diagnosis ☎. Leucocytosis, sterile pyuria and abnormal LFTs are common. Serological confirmation possible ➤. Requires cysteine for growth; BCYE agar (used for *Legionella* culture) is a readily-available selective medium, with growth in 3–5 days. Avoid attempts at identification in local laboratories ➤.

**Management:** Classically treated with 10 days streptomycin, but gentamicin (7 mg/kg single daily dosing) is a more practicable alternative. Ten days ciprofloxacin effective in animal studies (human dose 500 mg bd). Higher relapse rate with 14 days doxycycline 100 mg bd; clinical failures seen with cephalosporins.

**Prevention:** Live vaccine not used clinically because of side effects; only protects against inhalational exposure. Avoid insect bites. Oral antibiotic prophylaxis effective, but not recommended for secondary contacts.

**Table 31.2** Clinical features of tularaemia

| Route | Incidence | Clinical form | Clinical features |
|-------|-----------|---------------|-------------------|
| Percutaneous | ≈50% | Ulceroglandular | Indolent skin ulcer, regional lymphadenopathy. Pharyngitis, CXR infiltrates, pleural effusion. Differential diagnosis includes cutaneous anthrax, plague, lymphogranuloma venereum, granuloma inguinale and cat-scratch fever |
| | ≈25% | Glandular | As above, without ulcer |
| Conjunctiva | <5% | Oculoglandular | Blepharitis, severe conjunctivitis with small, yellowish nodules and ulcers. Regional lymphadenopathy |
| Inhalation | <5% | Typhoidal | Severe sepsis & DIC without localizing features. Frequent diarrhoea and secondary *Francisella* pneumonia |
| | <5% | Pneumonic | Dry cough, chest pain, pleurisy, dyspnoea. CXR shows hilar lymphadenopathy or infiltrates |
| Food-borne | <5% | Oropharyngeal | Commoner in children. Pharyngitis and cervical lymphadenopathy |

**Table 31.3** Human *Bartonella* infections

| Species | Reservoir | Vector | Distribution | Clinical associations |
|---------|-----------|--------|--------------|-----------------------|
| *B. bacilliformis* | Unknown; ?rats, ?convalescent human cases | Sandfly | Andes | **Oroya fever, verruga peruana (Carrión's disease)** |
| *B. quintana* | Unknown | Louse | Global | **Bacteraemia, endocarditis, trench fever,** bacillary angiomatosis in HIV patients. Cat-scratch disease |
| *B. henselae* | Cats | Cat flea* | Global | **Cat-scratch disease,** bacillary angiomatosis in HIV patients, bacteraemia, endocarditis, trench fever |
| *B. elizabethiae* | ?Rats | Unknown | Unknown | Very rare human isolates reported |
| *B. clarridgeiae* | Cats | Unknown | Unknown | |

* Implicated in cat-to-cat transmission. Cat-to-human transmission is probably by direct inoculation.

## *Bartonella* spp.

Intracellular Gram-negative pathogens, some of which used to be called *Rochalimaea* spp. These genera were amalgamated in 1993 on the basis of 16S ribosomal RNA sequencing. Fourteen species currently described, primarily infections of non-human animals. *Bartonella henselae* causes chronic bacteraemia in healthy cats and is transmitted among feline hosts by cat fleas. Only five species have been isolated from humans (Table 31.3). Aminoglycosides (e.g. gentamicin) may be the only anti-*Bartonella* agents with bactericidal activity.

**Serological diagnosis** of *Bartonella* infections is best performed in specialist laboratories (✈). IgM antibodies are species specific and appear early during infection and fall later. The IgG response cross-reacts with both *henselae* and *quintana* and is long-lasting, hence a repeat sample 10–21 days after the first is important to observe rising titres. Serology should be repeated after 10–21 days in suspected cases if initial titres are low.

## Practice point

CSD should be considered in all patients with persistent (3 weeks or more) lymphadenopathy. Less common causes include bacterial adenitis, infectious mononucleosis, benign or malignant neoplasm and toxoplasmosis. Rare causes include lymphogranuloma venereum, tuberculosis and MOTT, tularaemia, brucellosis, histoplasmosis, coccidioidomycosis, cryptococcosis, and sarcoidosis.

## Clinical syndromes associated with bartonella infection

### Cat-scratch disease (CSD)

Most cases caused by *Bartonella henselae*; some may involve *Bartonella clarridgeiae* or *quintana*, or *Afipia felis*.

**Epidemiology and transmission:** Commonest cause of regional lymphadenitis in children and adolescents; 24 000 cases per annum in USA; 60–80% of patients are under age 20. Probably ≈50% of cases are unrecognized. Exposure to cats, especially newly-acquired flea-infested kittens (relative risk in household members increased 29-fold; only 15-fold if the kittens are free of fleas). About 30% patients with CSD deny being bitten or scratched, but some cat contact recalled in ≈95%. Transmission may involve inoculation of infected flea faeces.

**Incubation period:** ≈3 weeks after cat scratch.

**Clinical features:** Local suppurative lymphadenopathy, often preceded by papule or pustule at site of inoculation 3–10 days after exposure. Fever (in 30%), malaise (30%), anorexia (15%), sore throat, headache and arthralgia may occur; 2–14% (commoner in the immunocompromised) develop complications, including CNS (encephalopathy, fits, retinitis), splenic, lung, bone and skin involvement, and granulomatous hepatitis. In 2% of CSD cases (after conjunctival exposure), Parinaud's oculoglandular syndrome occurs (granulomatous conjunctivitis and preauricular lymphadenopathy). Isolated fever, presenting as PUO without other signs, has been reported in children (➤179).

**Investigations:** Diagnosis is clinical, but biopsy may be necessary to exclude lymphoma or benign causes. Characteristic histology, with granulomata, multinucleate giant cells and stellate necrosis. Small numbers of organisms sometimes visible on Warthin–Starry silver staining of lesion biopsies. Culture (lesions, blood) possible but not usually attempted because it demands nutritative media and prolonged incubation. Serology available by ELISA and EIA, and expert interpretation is required because of cross reactions with *Coxiella* and *Chlamydia* antigens ➤. PCR, and skin testing with CSD antigen, available in some specialist centers ➤. Eosinophilia is common.

**Management:** Normally resolves without treatment in 2–4 months, one attack generally conferring lifelong immunity. Suppurating lymph nodes should be aspirated, repeatedly if necessary, but resection is to be avoided because a sinus persisting for 6–12 months may result. Antibiotic therapy not generally indicated, but rifampicin, ciprofloxacin, erythromycin, co-trimoxazole and gentamicin have been used; azithromycin has been shown to hasten resolution of lymphadenopathy. Disseminated disease has been treated with doxycycline plus rifampicin, ciprofloxacin (10–15 mg/kg bd for 2–3 weeks) and azithromycin (5–12 mg/kg/day for 2 weeks), among other regimens. Use or addition of parenteral gentamicin recommended for initial therapy of severely ill patients.

**Prevention:** Suspected source cat need not be destroyed, because risk of further cases very small. Flea control. Some have recommended declawing or nail clipping of kittens, keeping cats outdoors, and covering skin lesions before and performing hand hygiene after cat contact.

**Bacteraemia, endocarditis, trench fever, 'persistent or relapsing fever with bacteraemia' (PRFB)**

Mostly caused by *Bartonella quintana*.

**Epidemiology and transmission: Trench fever** transmitted by scratching infected louse faeces to skin lesions. Epidemics occasionally seen worldwide during times of overcrowding when hygiene and sanitation poor and body lice common, e.g. among soldiers in Europe during World War I. **Bacteraemia and endocarditis** recently reported among homeless people and alcoholics in the USA and Europe ('urban trench fever'). Body louse not proven to be the vector. Some cases involve *Bartonella henselae*.

**Incubation period:** Trench fever 3–38 days.

**Clinical features: Trench fever** is a relapsing febrile illness with headache, transient macular rash, splenomegaly. Shin pain is reported to be characteristic. Fatalities rarely reported. *Bartonella quintana* and *henselae* now recognized among the numerous possible causes of **'culture-negative' endocarditis** (➢ 50).

**Investigations:** PCR and serology are available. Serological cross-reactions with *Chlamydia* spp. (especially *pneumoniae*) have led to diagnostic confusion.

**Management:** Antibiotic therapy of **trench fever** is poorly evidenced. Macrolides and tetracyclines are believed to be effective and are usually given for 4–6 weeks. **Endocarditis** often requires valve replacement and 9–12 months' macrolide therapy.

**Prevention:** Improve sanitation, reduce overcrowding, kill lice.

**Bacillary angiomatosis** (➢ 159).
A variety of angiogenic lesions caused by *Bartonella henselae* and *quintana* mainly in immunocompromised patients. Most cases reported in HIV-positive patients with CD4 counts below 100/mm$^3$. Seventy-five per cent of cases give history of cat exposure, and may be acquired via flea vectors.

**Pathogenesis:** Outer membrane adhesin binds endothelial cells. Bacterial angiogenic factor induces proliferation of poorly-formed blood vessels into lobules surrounded by oedema, mucin and fibrosis.

**Clinical features:** Cutaneous lesions in ~50% cases. Characteristic erythematous papules (few mm—few cm in size) with surrounding scaling; singly or in clusters of lesions. Occasional hyperkeratotic plaques. Differential dermatological diagnosis includes Kaposi's sarcoma (➢ 168), benign haemangioma and pyogenic granuloma. Without treatment, usually progresses to generalized infection with fever, abdominal pain and anorexia. *Bartonella henselae* tends to affect lymph nodes, liver and spleen (bacillary peliosis—blood-filled cystic spaces—with prominent abdominal pain and fever); *quintana* associated with lesions of bone (lytic lesions, frequent periosteal reaction) and subcutaneous tissues. Cerebral lesions occur.

**Investigations:** Histology of skin lesion biopsy. Generally, numerous bacilli are seen on silver stained sections. In peliosis hepatis thrombo/pancytopenia and raised alkaline phosphatase are common, and CT scan shows hepatomegaly with multiple hypodense areas. Culture and serology not generally available.

**Management:** Prompt response usually seen to erythromycin 500 mg qds or doxycycline 100 mg bd for 8 weeks. Azithromycin has also been used.

**Prevention:** Immunocompromised patients may be advised to avoid contact with cats (and especially kittens under 1 yr), to avoid cat scratches, to keep their cats free of fleas, to wash hands after any animal contact and to clean and cover any skin abrasions.

**Oroya fever, verruga peruana (Carrión's disease)**

Caused by *Bartonella bacilliformis*; infects erythrocytes to cause acute haemolytic anaemia.

**Epidemiology and transmission:** endemic in certain Andean regions of Peru, Columbia and Ecuador over 3000 feet (the 'verruga zone'). Transmitted by sandflies.

*(continued...)*

**Clinical features:** Biphasic illness. Oroya fever is the acute bacteraemic phase followed by the chronic phase, verruga peruana. Manifestations of Oroya fever range from a mild, self-limiting febrile illness to severe infection with profound anaemia and multi-organ system failure. Untreated mortality up to 40%. Coinfection with other organisms, e.g. *Salmonella* spp. is common and increases mortality; 20% of the survivors develop verruga peruana (Carrión's disease) with painless subcutaneous nodules all over body which grow rapidly, may ulcerate and are histologically similar to those of bacillary angiomatosis.

**Investigations:** Blood cultures are usually positive during the acute febrile stage. Serology and biopsy are also used.

**Management:** Antibiotic therapy rapidly terminates the febrile phase. Chloramphenicol is the drug of choice, but penicillins, streptomycin, macrolides and tetracycline are also effective. Cephalosporins are less reliable.

# Anaerobes

Obligate anaerobes require a reduced oxygen tension for growth, failing to grow on the surface of solid media in 10% $CO_2$ in air (which contains 18% oxygen). They are divided into **sporing** anaerobic (SA: including only *Clostridium* spp.) and **non-sporing anaerobic** (NSA) genera.

## Classification of clinically important anaerobes

Nomenclature of the *Bacteroides* genus has been revised according to the footnotes in Table 32.1 (but most clinical diagnostic laboratories have not yet adopted it).

## Properties common to obligate anaerobes

**Pathogenesis and epidemiology:** Many anaerobes are important components of the commensal mucosal flora of humans and animals (Table 32.2); *Clostridium* spp. vegetative forms and spores are also common in the environment.

**Laboratory diagnosis:** Clinical suspicion of anaerobic infection is supported by:
• Putrid pus.
• Characteristic Gram stain appearances (mixed and 'bizarre' organisms in NSA infections; brick-shaped Gram-positive rods with few pus cells in gas gangrene).
• Brick-red fluorescence under long-wave UV light (especially *B. asaccharolyticus*).
• Gas–liquid chromatography of pus (for short-chain fatty-acid products of anaerobic fermentation).

Anaerobic involvement should be considered, especially when patients do not respond to empirical therapy with limited anti-anaerobic spectra (e.g. parenteral or broad-spectrum cephalosporins, aminoglycosides, most quinolones), and when pus is reported 'culture-negative' (especially if dry swabs were submitted).

Most obligate anaerobes are killed by oxygen; hence liaison between clinician and laboratory (with careful specimen collection and rapid transport, and use of controlled anaerobic atmospheres with nutritive selective media) is essential for their reliable isolation (☎). Send pus in sterile universal container if available, but modern swab transport systems with gel preservation media are effective at preserving anaerobes for 6–48 h.

Appropriate incubation of all specimens where anaerobes may be clinically relevant is performed routinely nowadays by diagnostic laboratories. Some species are aerotolerant (some surface growth on freshly prepared solid media in air—e.g. *Clostridium tertium*) which often leads to mis-identification as *Bacillus* spp.

Most clinically important species grow in 48–72 h; full identification can take much longer but, with some important exceptions, this is of dubious clinical relevance. Many clinical laboratories, therefore, report 'anaerobes isolated' from sites where speciation is not useful. Commercial biochemical test kits are now quite reliable for commonly encountered anaerobes (important isolates ✈). Direct detection of toxin is used for some *Clostridium* infections (*difficile, botulinum*).

**Treatment: Drainage/debridement** is often the mainstay of therapy, and antibiotic therapy usually needs to cover both anaerobic and aerobic components of mixed infections. Of the clinically relevant anaerobes, only *Actinomyces* spp. and *Propionibacterium* spp. are normally

**Table 32.1** Classification of anaerobes

| Gram-positive | Bacilli | Spore-forming | *Clostridium perfringens* ('*welchii*'), *septicum, novyi* ('*oedematiens*'), *tetani, botulinum, difficile*, plus many other non-pathogens |
|---|---|---|---|
| | | Non-spore-forming | *Actinomyces israelii* and other spp. (➤321) *Propionibacterium* spp. (➤270) *Arachnia propionica* *Bifidobacterium* spp. *Eubacterium* spp. *Lactobacillus* spp. *Mobiluncus curtisii* frequently found in bacterial vaginosis (➤82) |
| | Cocci | | *Peptococcus niger* ('anaerobic staphylococcus') *Peptostreptococcus anaerobius, asaccharolyticus, magnus, micros* and many other spp. ('anaerobic streptococci') |
| Gram-negative | Bacilli | | *Bacteroides* spp. Gut-associated '*fragilis*' group (*distasonis, fragilis, ovatus, stercoris, thetaiotaomicron, vulgatus*, etc.) |
| | | | 'Pigmented' group (*melaninogenicus,* * *asaccharolyticus,*† *gingivalis,*† *intermedius,** etc.). 'Other' group (*buccae,** *capillosus, oralis,* * *bivius,** *disiens,* * *urealyticus* etc.). *Fusobacterium nucleatum, necrophorum, ulcerans, varium*, etc. Many others, including *Anaerobiospirillum* spp., *Leptotrichia buccalis, Selenomonas* spp., *Sutterella wadsworthensis* occasionally identified from clinical material, usually in mixed culture |
| | Cocci | | *Veillonella* spp. and others |
| Spirochaetes and other spiral anaerobes | (➤322) | | |

\* Transferred to *Prevotella* genus; † transferred to *Porphyromonas* genus.

resistant to metronidazole (resistance very rare in other genera), but resistance to formerly useful antibiotics, such as tetracycline, erythromycin and most β-lactams, is rising. **Co-amoxiclav, imi/meropenem and piperacillin–tazobactam** are usually reliable, but aminoglycosides and most currently available quinolones have no useful anti-anaerobic activity. **Clindamycin** is sometimes useful for common focal infections with mixed anaerobic and Gram-positive facultative bacteria (e.g. lower limb infections in diabetics, chronic sinusitis). **Cefoxitin** is the only cephalosporin with useful activity.

**Table 32.2** Anaerobes as normal flora

| Anaerobe group | Skin | | Mouth, nasopharynx | Vagina, urethra | Colon |
| | Above umbilicus | Below umbilicus | | | |
| --- | --- | --- | --- | --- | --- |
| *Clostridium* spp. | | + | | | +++ |
| *Actinomyces* spp. | | | + | + | ++ |
| *Propionibacterium* spp. | ++ | ++ | | | |
| 'Fragilis' (gut) bacteroides | | | | | +++ |
| 'Pigmented' bacteroides | ±* | ±* | ++ | + | + |
| 'Other' bacteroides | ±* | ±* | ++ | + | + |
| *Fusobacterium* spp. | | | + | + | + |
| Gram-positive cocci | + | + | ++ | + | ++ |

* Especially in skin follicles of axillae and perineum.

## Spectrum of disease due to anaerobes

Anaerobes cause three types of disease:
- **Toxin-associated**, sometimes with toxic effects remote from the site of bacterial multiplication (e.g. *Clostridium* spp.).
- **Local sepsis involving mixed bacteria** derived from the local mucosal flora (caused by all anaerobic genera). Sometimes 'synergistic' (e.g. *Bacteroides fragilis* + *Escherichia coli* causing more serious sepsis when present together than separately, as shown in rat peritonitis model).
- **Invasive infections associated with specific pathogens** (e.g. *Clostridium perfringens* causing gas gangrene, *Fusobacterium necrophorum* causing necrobacillosis).

## Toxin-associated anaerobic infections

### *Clostridium perfringens*
(Used to be called *Clostridium welchii*).

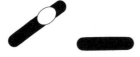

Brick-shaped Gram-positive rod.

**Pathogenesis:** Lecithinase (α-toxin, produced by all strains; the main virulence factor causing tissue damage in gas gangrene), enterotoxin (type A strains, causing food poisoning; damages intestinal mucosa), β-toxin (type C strains, causing enteritis necroticans) and many others. Predominantly releases saccharolytic enzymes, but some proteases including collagenase, hyaluronidase. Inoculation of spores to damaged tissues with compromised blood supply ⇨ sporulation ⇨ α-toxin release ⇨ myonecrosis with gas production.

**Epidemiology:** Gut commensal of humans and animals, and common on human skin and in soil, hence many opportunities for contamination of wounds and foods. Gas gangrene commoner in old age, diabetics and after lower limb surgery in arteriopaths. Five types A to E (typed by toxin production), and subtyping available serologically (➔).

**Spectrum of disease, diagnosis and treatment:** Most commonly isolated from traumatic or surgical wounds contaminated with faeces or soil; sometimes contributes to local tissue infection with mixed flora (i.e. **not** causing gas gangrene). Occasionally grown from blood cultures, usually from skin contamination or as terminal event in dying patient (systemic spread from gut).

Gas gangrene (➤115): Invasive infection, primarily due to α-toxin effects. Patient invariably systemically toxic with severe local pain. Rare cases caused by *Clostridium novyi* (type A strains), *septicum*, *histolyticum* and *sordellii*. Diagnosis is primarily clinical, but Gram stain can be helpful (often mixed with other bacteria, with scant pus cells). Spores rarely seen in clinical material. Blood cultures positive in severe cases ⇨ massive haemolysis. Readily isolated on anaerobic blood agar (24 h), forming large, shiny, clear colonies. Confirm by Nagler reaction (further 24 h): lecithinase (α-toxin) activity on egg-yolk medium, with specific inhibition by antitoxin. Treatment is surgical debridement (plus penicillin or metronidazole). Hyperbaric oxygen may give additional benefit, but gas gangrene antiserum no longer recommended. **Prevention** by surgical toilet of traumatic wounds, antibiotic prophylaxis and careful skin disinfection (esp. before lower limb amputation).

**Food poisoning:** ⊠ Distinct strains, commonly found in human and animal faeces and in meat; highly heat-resistant spores. Partly heat-resistant enterotoxin preformed in food; especially with high protein content (e.g. meat stews). Sporulation and growth (hence toxin release in food) encouraged by storage at room temperature; additional toxin released in gut by sporulation after passage through stomach. $\Sigma \approx 1000$. Mainly diarrhoea + abdominal pain, may be initial vomiting; 6–12-h incubation, illness lasting 12–48 h. Supportive treatment (➤58). No exclusion from work indicated once asymptomatic, because carriage of toxigenic strains is normally common. Outbreak investigation by typing of isolates from faeces and food (✈).

**Necrotizing jejunitis:** 'Enteritis necroticans' or 'pig-bel' in New Guinea. Type C strain contaminating partly cooked meat in pig feasts. When eaten with vegetable containing trypsin inhibitor (or by malnourished people), the β-toxin ⇨ small intestinal necrosis with 50% mortality.

**Nosocomial toxin-associated diarrhoea:** Usually antibiotic-associated in elderly patients following overgrowth in gut of *Clostridium perfringens*; different genotype from that causing food poisoning. Toxigenicity demonstrated in cell culture (as used for *Clostridium difficile*). Therapy supportive + metronidazole if severe; usually self-limiting in $\approx$ 24 h.

## *Clostridium tetani* ⊠

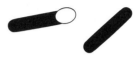

Slender, Gram-positive rod, with terminal spores.

**Pathogenesis:** Many extracellular products, but virulence factor is tetanospasmin (protein with heavy and light polypeptide chains) released by germination of spores in hypoxic tissues. Little or no local invasion needed for toxin release ⇨ axonal transport via motor neurons to CNS, and systemic spread by bloodstream. Inhibits the release of neurotransmitters, including glycine and γ-aminobutyric acid (GABA), resulting in muscle spasms, hyper-reflexia, seizures and autonomic dysfunction.

**Epidemiology:** Commensal of the gut of humans and animals, and frequently found in environment, especially manured soil. $\Sigma$ 2–7, fallen from $\approx$ 20, 30 yrs ago. Mainly in the elderly (unimmunized, and may have more fragile skin allowing penetration of, for example, rose thorns). Immigrants from developing countries and UK residents born before 1961 may not have been vaccinated routinely. Males may have been immunized during military service. Common in developing world, especially in neonates (from umbilical anointment with animal faeces). Rare cases and small outbreaks associated with unsterile surgical catgut or contaminated theatre ventilation systems.

**Spectrum of disease:** Tetanus (see below).

**Laboratory diagnosis:** Swarming colonies on selective anaerobic blood agar in 24–48 h (often only a film of growth, easily missed).

## Clinical syndrome

### Tetanus

A neurological syndrome characterized by tonic muscle spasms and hyperreflexia, caused by the exotoxin of *Clostridium tetani*.

**Clinical features:** Incubation period is typically 3–21 days, partially depending on the distance between the site of infection and the CNS. In many cases, the antecedent wound is trivial or not found. Tetanus may be generalized, localized, cephalic or neonatal.

  **Generalized tetanus** is most common. Trismus (spasm of the masseter muscle causing lockjaw) is the commonest presenting symptom (≈75% of cases), causing the *risus sardonicus* ('sardonic smile'). Restlessness, irritability, dysphagia, opisthotonus and seizures occur. Painful reflex spasms, often triggered by nose, light or touch, may be severe enough to cause fractures or rhabdomyolysis.

  **Localized tetanus** is a rare form of tetanus affecting one extremity with a contaminated bite. It may progress to generalized tetanus but the prognosis is good.

  **Cephalic tetanus** occurs in association with head injury or middle ear infection. The incubation period is typically short (1–2 days) and the prognosis is very poor. Isolated cranial lesions (esp. VII), progressing to generalized tetanus, are common.

  **Neonatal tetanus** is widespread in the developing world. It follows infection of the umbilical cord and presents with spasms between 3 and 10 days of age.

**Microbiological investigations:** Diagnosis made on clinical criteria. Gram stain of swab or pus from lesion rarely useful. Culture worth attempting for confirmation; CSF is normal.

**Management:** Anti-tetanus immunoglobulin 150 IU/kg im at multiple sites. Surgical excision/debridement of the wound if practical. Benzylpenicillin 2 MU 4-hourly for 10 days. Alternatives include metronidazole. **Intensive care** is usually required. Benzodiazepines may ameliorate spasms and prevent seizures. Paralysis and ventilation may be required. Despite full modern intensive care, the mortality remains 25–50%.
*(continued...)*

Patients who recover may require ventilation for 3–6 weeks.

**Prevention of tetanus: Primary prevention** is achieved by immunization with three doses of tetanus toxoid (➤417). A booster is required every 10 yrs until five doses have been given.

**Management of wounds (Table 32.3):** All wounds should be carefully cleaned. Wounds or burns considered 'tetanus-prone' are:

• All wounds sustained >6 h before adequate surgical toilet is carried out.
• Wounds with significant amounts of devitalized tissue.
• Puncture wounds.
• Wounds contaminated with soil or manure.
• Wounds with clinical evidence of sepsis.

### *Clostridium botulinum* ⊠

Gram-positive rod with subterminal spores.

**Pathogenesis:** Spores of *Clostridium botulinum* are ubiquitous in soil and marine sediment. Germination and toxin production take place when appropriate anaerobic conditions are provided within preserved food. **Spores** can survive boiling at 100°C for several hours, but are killed at autoclave temperatures (121°C) after 5 min. **Toxin** is heat-labile and is destroyed by heating to 85°C for 1 min. Botulism is now extremely rare in the UK because home canning of vegetables is rare. Acid fruits may be bottled safely as low pH inhibits growth. Clostridia producing type E toxin are adapted to low-temperature environments; the spores are less heat-resistant than other types, but toxin production may take place as low as 3°C. They are usually associated with a marine source such as fish or seal meat and are prevalent in Arctic regions.

  **Botulinum toxin** is internalized and binds irreversibly to peripheral neurons. It blocks acetylcholine release at the neuromuscular junction and within the autonomic nervous system via peptidase activity on proteins on neurotransmitter vesicles which blocks their exocytosis. Lethal dose ≈1 μg. Destroyed by

**Table 32.3** Anti-tetanus prophylaxis

| Immunization status | Clean wound | Tetanus prone wound |
| --- | --- | --- |
| Full course and booster within last 10 yrs | Nil | Nil (a booster dose of toxoid may be given if the risk is thought to be very high, e.g. contamination with stable manure) |
| Full course and booster greater than 10 yrs ago | Booster dose of toxoid | Booster dose of toxoid **plus** a dose of anti-tetanus immunoglobulin (250 IU*) |
| Not immunized or immunization history not known with certainty | Full course of toxoid | Full course of toxoid **plus** a dose of anti-tetanus immunoglobulin (250 IU*) in a different site |

* Increased to 500 IU if >24 h have elapsed since injury, if there is heavy contamination, or following burns.

chlorination of water and thorough cooking, and within a few days in surface waters.

**Epidemiology:** *Clostridium botulinum* widespread in intestines of humans and animals, plants, soil. Eight serotypes, but only types A, B, E and rarely F associated with disease in humans. Botulism is usually associated with meat (Latin *botulus* = sausage), fish and, most frequently during this century, with home-preserved vegetables. Last outbreak in the UK (1989) of toxin type B botulism from inadequately heat-treated canned hazelnut puree added to yoghurt; 27 patients affected, 12 needing ICU care, one death. In Europe, most commonly reported from France, Germany, Italy and Spain (7–40 cases p.a. each). Has been associated with injecting drug use, possibly from contaminated heroin, and also with contaminated infant milk formula. Rare strains of *Clostridium butyricum* and *baratii* are toxin-positive and have caused clinical botulism. Potential bioterrorism agent by aerosolization or ingestion of toxin (➤415).

**Spectrum of disease: Botulism** (see below).

**Laboratory diagnosis:** ☎ Toxin detection and typing in vomit, food, blood, faeces, stomach contents, pus or swab, bronchiolar lavage, tissue biopsy etc. (send immediately via refrigerated transport to ✈). Take 10 mL serum before anti-toxin administered. All pathogenic strains produce lipase (detected on egg-yolk agar).

**Clinical syndrome**

**Botulism**
An acute, descending, symmetrical, paralytic illness affecting primarily cranial and autonomic nerves, due to exotoxin produced by *Clostridium botulinum*.

**Clinical features:** Botulism is usually **food-borne**—the result of consumption of preformed toxin in contaminated food. Incubation period is 12–72 h (can be 2 h–8 days) depending on the dose. Presenting symptoms include blurred vision, diplopia, dysphagia, generalized weakness, GI upset particularly vomiting, dysphonia, vertigo and urinary retention or incontinence. On examination, patients usually have evidence of depressed ventilatory function, specific muscle weakness or paralysis, and ophthalmoplegia. A characteristic picture is of a **descending, symmetrical, flaccid paralysis in an afebrile patient** (Table 32.4). Autonomic involvement may cause ptosis, dry mouth, fixed dilated pupils and constipation. Higher mental functions and sensation are intact—the patient remains fully alert—and there is no fever. More rarely **wound botulism** occurs, in which contamination of a wound is followed by endogenous production of toxin, in a similar manner to tetanus

*(continued...)*

**Table 32.4** Some differential diagnoses of botulism

| Diagnosis | Notes |
|---|---|
| Guillain–Barré syndrome | Antecedent febrile illness, paraesthesiae, often ascending paralysis, early loss of reflexes, increased CSF protein, EMG findings |
| Myasthenia gravis | Recurrent, sustained response to anti-cholinesterase therapy, EMG findings |
| Stroke | Often asymmetrical paralysis, abnormal CT scan |
| Intoxication/poisoning | e.g. CO, organophosphate, mushrooms, drugs |
| Tick paralysis | Paraesthesia, ascending paralysis, tick attached to skin (➢325) |
| Poliomyelitis | Antecedent febrile illness, asymmetrical paralysis, CSF changes (➢348) |
| CNS infections | Changed mental status, fever, CSF and EEG changes (➢96) |

(➢315). Symptoms and signs are the same as for food-borne disease. **Infant botulism** is due to colonization of the infant gut by *Clostridium botulinum*. It affects children under the age of 1 yr, and has been associated with the consumption of honey, which may contain spores, and occasionally soil and dust. Presenting signs include weakness, hypotonia, listlessness, constipation, failure to feed and respiratory failure. It is thought to account for a small percentage of cases of sudden infant death syndrome. Gastrointestinal botulism occurs extremely rarely in adults with anatomical abnormalities of the gut.

**Microbiological investigations:** Diagnosis is based on clinical signs; suspicion is often aroused because of multiple cases in persons who have all eaten the same contaminated food. Confirmation is by demonstration of toxin in food, serum or stools of patients, or culture of the organism from stools (or wound in the case of wound botulism). Culture of the organism from food is supportive evidence only, as spores are ubiquitous. These investigations may be negative in many cases. In infant botulism, however, the diagnosis may be ruled out if two stool samples obtained during the acute episode are negative for toxin and culture.

**Antibiotic management:** Antibiotics are often given (benzylpenicillin or metronidazole) although there is no evidence that they influence outcome. They may be more useful in wound botulism, but most authorities do not recommend them for infant botulism because they may lead to lysis of organisms in the gut and release of further toxin.

**Supportive management:** Untreated mortality ≈100%: may be reduced to ≈15% by expert intensive care, and ventilation for several weeks is usually required. Death usually due to the complications of prolonged paralysis and ventilation. Recovery may take many months. Trivalent (types A, B and E) botulism antitoxin, prepared in horses, is available (via CDSC) and should be given to suspected cases. It should not be given to infants because there is no evidence of efficacy and may cause sensitization. Hypersensitivity is common and package instructions relating to test dose and administration must be followed. Antitoxin may be given as a single dose (20 mL im) prophylactically to patients who are suspected of having consumed contaminated food. For patients with established disease, repeated doses are given (20 mL by slow iv infusion, followed by 10 mL 2–4 h later, and further doses at 12–24 h intervals). Antitoxin does not affect toxin already bound to neurones, and is ineffective in infant botulism. Guanidine has been used experimentally to counteract the effects of toxin at the neuromuscular junction. Avoid aminoglycosides in proven or suspected infant botulism because of effects on the neuromuscular junction. Discuss cases of infant botulism with an expert paediatrician (e.g. St Mary's Hospital, Paddington in the UK).

**Prevention of botulism:** Careful control of commercial canning processes. Preserved vegetables should be boiled for 3 min, with stirring prior to use. Infected food may or may not show signs of spoilage. Cans which have 'blown' should never be opened; canned food which smells 'off' should never be tasted, as sufficient toxin to cause disease may be present in very small amounts of food. Honey has been implicated as a source of spores in infant botulism—it should not be fed to children under the age of 1 yr.

## Clostridium difficile

Gram-positive rod with subterminal, oval spores.

**Pathogenesis:** Overgrowth of *Clostridium difficile* in gut of patients during or after antibiotic therapy ⇨ toxin release. Two main toxins: A (enterotoxin ⇨ damages villus tips ⇨ 'leaky' gut barrier) and B (cytotoxin ⇨ damages cytoskeleton and cell–cell junctions of enterocytes). Production of both toxins associated with more severe disease. Non-toxigenic strains do not cause diarrhoea. Neonatal enterocytes may lack toxin A receptors; specific antitoxin B IgA in the gut and antitoxin A IgG systemically may be protective.

**Epidemiology:** Normal faecal commensal of neonates and frequent in young children, but rare in adults out of hospital who have not received recent antibiotics. Spores contaminate surroundings of infected (esp. incontinent) patients and survive in environment ⇨ colonize new patients by faecal–oral route; also transmitted on staff hands and unsterile equipment (e.g. sigmoidoscopes). Pseudomembranous colitis (PMC) rarely associated with cytotoxic therapy or gut surgery in the absence of antibiotics. Rising incidence of reported cases in England and Wales in past 15 yrs, Σ ≈3000 in 1993, ≈15 000 in 2000; ≈15% from antibiotic usage out of hospital. Available typing methods include cell-wall protein electrophoresis, PCR ribotyping and DNA restriction fragment polymorphism analysis (➤). About 50% relapses are reinfections with different strains. True relapses probably due to persistence of spores in gut (but may be reinfections with same strain). Total health-care costs of each case estimated £4000 in 1996.

**Spectrum of disease: Antibiotic-associated diarrhoea** (➤63). Occasionally isolated from wound infections in mixed culture, and rarely from blood cultures.

**Laboratory diagnosis:** Detection of cytotoxin B in stool by cell culture and antitoxin neutralization (24 h; highly sensitive ≈10 pg), or variety of immunoassays (for toxins A, B or both; 4–24 h; sensitivity 100–1000 pg, resulting in 10–20% false-negative rate). Some laboratories culture and identify the organism, which is slower (48+ h on selective medium), expensive and not diagnostically specific, but allows typing for outbreak investigation. Some laboratories test for toxin in all faecal samples, others only when requested or when patients said to be on antibiotics.

> *Clostridium noyvi* (type A), well described as an animal pathogen and a very rare cause of human 'gas gangrene', was isolated from local septic lesions and blood cultures from about 40 injecting drug users in England and Wales and Dublin in mid-2000. Over half the cases were fatal, and a wide variety of other bacteria were also isolated from individual cases. Contaminated heroin was believed to be the source, and subcutaneous injection was a risk factor.

## Local purulent infections involving mixed bacteria

(Table 32.5)

These are autoinfections derived from mucosal normal flora by direct or haematogenous spread, and involve 'non-sporing anaerobes' with local aerobes such as streptococci, coliforms and staphylococci. *Streptococcus 'milleri'* is a frequent companion (➤259).

Very common overall. They present to many clinical specialities, and involvement of anaerobes is often suspected late. Knowledge of normal human anaerobic flora allows the primary source of haematogenously disseminated infections to be inferred (e.g. *Bacteroides* of *fragilis* group = gut source). Little evidence for special 'pathogenicity' for most NSA in this type of infection, except *Bacteroides fragilis* (toxic capsule) and suspected for *Bacteroides asaccharolyticus* (common isolate, but unknown virulence factors).

Surgical drainage is often a keystone of treatment, and antibiotic therapy should cover aerobic and anaerobic components. Suitable empirical regimens include: **oral** co-amoxiclav; amoxicillin + metronidazole; clindamycin: **parenteral** penicillin + gentamicin + metronidazole; parenteral cephalosporin + metronidazole; imi/meropenem.

**Table 32.5** Infections commonly involving non-sporing anaerobes

| Region | Condition | |
|---|---|---|
| Head, neck, oropharynx | Vincent's infection (necrotizing gingivitis) | ➤18 |
| | Dental sepsis, periodontal disease | |
| | Chronic sinusitis | |
| | Tonsillar and peritonsillar abscess | |
| | Brain abscess (sinus-associated) | ➤103 |
| Pleuropulmonary | Aspiration pneumonia | ➤28 |
| | Lung abscess (bronchial obstruction, aspiration) | |
| | Empyema | |
| | Bronchiectasis (putrid sputum) | |
| Intra-abdominal | All large-bowel perforations | ➤67 |
| | Appendicitis, diverticulitis, etc. | |
| | Pyogenic liver abscess | |
| | Wound infection after colonic surgery | |
| | Long-standing cholangiostasis, biliary fistulae | |
| Perirectal | Anorectal abscess (isolation of 'gut' flora is predictive of fistula in ano, 'skin' flora is not) | |
| | Necrotizing fasciitis, 'synergistic gangrene' | ➤115 |
| Genital tract (female) | Bacterial vaginosis | ➤82 |
| | Bartholin's abscess | |
| | Tubo-ovarian abscess | |
| | Septic abortion, retained products, episiotomy infections | |
| | Postsurgical infection (e.g. post-hysterectomy) | |
| Genital tract (male) | Scrotal abscess, prostatic abscess | ➤79 |
| | Balanoposthitis | |
| Bone and joint | Osteomyelitis (from faecal contamination, especially after lower limb open fractures) | ➤122 |
| | Diabetic lower limbs | |
| Skin and soft tissue | Ulcers (venous, pressure, diabetic; ulcerating cancers; Meleney's synergistic gangrene) | ➤111 |
| | Infected sebaceous cysts | |
| | Axillary/groin abscesses (including hydradenitis suppurativa) | |
| | Recurrent breast abscess (not puerperal, which usually involve *Staphylococcus aureus*) | |
| | Paronychia | |
| | Bites (human and animal) | |

**Infections rarely involving anaerobes** include UTI; infective endocarditis; infections of prostheses, iv catheters and CNS shunts (but may involve *Propionibacterium* sp.); community-acquired diarrhoea in the UK; pneumonia with no history of aspiration. Empirical therapy of these infections does not need to include metronidazole.

## Invasive, specific pathogen-associated anaerobic infections

These are uncommon, but often serious infections with characteristic clinical signs affecting particular patient groups.

## Gas gangrene (➤115, ➤315)

### Clostridium septicum

Produces a cytotoxic and haemolytic α-toxin. Causes 'neutropenic enterocolitis'—presents as abdominal pain + fever during episode of neutropenia. Severe, necrotizing colitis (sometimes bacteraemic, and metastatic spread with high mortality). Organism isolatable from blood, necrotic bowel wall or faeces (selection for spore-forming bacteria by heat or alcohol shock). Early colectomy plus antibiotics can be curative (e.g. metronidazole added to a standard regimen for fever in neutropenic patients, ➤174). Occasionally also causes bacteraemia in patients with colonic carcinoma, and has been rarely associated with gas gangrene-like illnesses.

### Clostridium tertium

Causes bacteraemia in neutropenic patients, from gut or iv catheter source. Aerotolerant organism, which may grow on aerobic culture plates and be misidentified as a *Bacillus* sp. (hence thought to be a contaminant). Usually treated with vancomycin; consider gut resection if necrosis suspected.

### Fusobacterium necrophorum

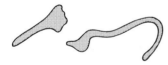

Causes 'necrobacillosis' or 'anaerobic tonsillitis' (Lemierre's syndrome ➤20). Young, previously healthy adults presenting with severe sore throat ⇨ septicaemia ⇨ secondary abscesses (liver, lungs, pleura, bone, joints, brain). Also quinsy and internal jugular vein thrombosis from local spread; ultrasound, CT with contrast or (especially) MRI scanning helpful diagnostically. *Fusobacterium* spp. Σ75 bacteraemias, with ≈20 confirmed cases of necrobacillosis p.a. Grown from blood or pus: bizarrely shaped Gram-negative bacilli. Carry polysaccharide capsule, which may be virulence factor. About one-third of cases are mixed with *Streptococcus 'milleri'* and other respiratory tract flora. Sensitive to erythromycin (85%), penicillin (98%: β-lactamase production may be becoming more prevalent), or metronidazole, co-amoxiclav, imi/meropenem or clindamycin (100%). Prolonged therapy is often recommended (e.g. 6 weeks, the latter stages of which may be oral), especially in cases with endovascular thrombosis and embolism.

## Actinomycosis

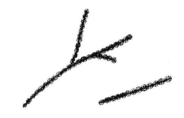

A clinical term describing chronic abscesses and sinuses discharging granular pus ('sulphur granules') containing characteristic microcolonies of Gram-positive branching rods (*Actinomyces israelii*). Begins as a local purulent infection involving mixed bacteria, in which *Actinomyces israelii* attains later predominance: optimal culture will usually isolate several additional organisms even in late stages. Commonest sites include: **oral and neck** (associated with dental disease); **abdominal** (RIF, colon after appendicitis, perforated diverticulum, etc.); **dacrocystitis; IUCD and pelvic infection**. Treatment: penicillin/amoxicillin (plus metronidazole for the commonly associated non-sporing anaerobes), or co-amoxiclav for ≈6 weeks. Alternatives include meropenem, tetracycline, erythromycin, clindamycin or fusidic acid. Drainage/debridement often needed.

*Arachnia propionica* is bacteriologically similar to *Actinomyces israelii* and occasionally causes dacrocystitis.

## Chapter 33

# Spirochaetes

Slender spiral anaerobic rods (Table 33.1). Actively motile with several flagella enclosed within the bacterial outer cell membrane, attached at either end of the cell and wrapping round the cell body. Virulence factors unknown. Lipid-rich outer membrane contributes to sensitivity to detergents and desiccation, and hence only venereal or insect-borne transmission for many species of spirochaete. Pathogenic spirochaetes cannot be cultivated *in vitro* but can be visualized (e.g. dark-ground microscopy of material from syphilitic chancre, or detection of *Borrelia* or *Leptospira* in blood). Serology is important in most spirochaete-associated diseases (often ✈ for expert interpretation).

## Non-venereal treponematoses

Non-venereal infections due to spirochaetes closely related to *Treponema pallidum* occur where environmental conditions allow transmission (Table 33.2). These organisms are morphologically identical to *T. pallidum*, and show only minor antigenic differences. They all cause positive serological tests for syphilis (➤90). All are treated with benzylpenicillin. Mass eradication programmes were mounted against yaws in the 1950s–1960s, and it is now less prevalent.

**Table 33.1** Classification of spirochaetes

| Genus | Species | Notes |
|---|---|---|
| *Treponema* | *pallidum* | Syphilis (➤89) |
| | *pallidum* subsp. *pertenue, carateum,* *pallidum* subsp. *endemicum* | Non-venereal treponematoses |
| *Borrelia* | *burgdorferi* | Lyme disease (➤323) |
| | *recurrentis* and other spp. | Relapsing fever (➤326) |
| *Leptospira* | *interrogans* | Leptospirosis (➤327) |
| (*Anaerobiospirillum* spp.) | | Isolated from faeces and blood of some immunocompromised patients with diarrhoea |
| (*Mobiluncus* spp.) | | Associated with bacterial vaginosis (➤82) |
| (*Spirillum* | *minus*) | One cause of rat-bite fever (➤306) |

**Table 33.2** Non-venereal treponematoses

| Species | Disease | Environment | Clinical features |
|---|---|---|---|
| *Treponema pallidum* subsp. *pertenue* | Yaws (syn. frambesia tropica) | Humid tropics. Predominantly a disease of childhood. Skin-to-skin transmission | Papular skin lesions which may ulcerate. Periostitis and dactylitis. Approximately 10% develop destructive lesions of skin or bone. CNS, CVS, and congenital disease do not occur |
| *Treponema pallidum* subsp. *endemicum* | Non-venereal endemic syphilis ('bejel', 'njovera') | Arid subtropical or temperate areas. Rural populations where living conditions/hygiene are poor. Mouth-to-mouth transmission via shared utensils | Initial lesion usually mucous patches in the mouth, followed by skin lesions resembling those of secondary venereal syphilis. Gummata of skin, long bones, nasopharynx occur, but CNS and CVS disease are very rare |
| *Treponema carateum* | Pinta ('carate') | Arid tropical Americas. Skin-to-skin transmission | Confined to skin. Maculopapular pigmented rash, healing to leave depigmented scars |

## *Borrelia* spp. (Table 33.1)

### Clinical syndrome

**Lyme disease (LD) (syn. tick-borne borreliosis)**
A multisystem disorder caused by the spirochaete *Borrelia burgdorferi* and transmitted by bite of hard ticks.

**Epidemiology and transmission:** About 40% of UK cases give a history of tick bite. Risk of transmission occurs in areas where ticks are found, especially during late spring and summer where immature, nymphal ticks feed. Ticks, mice, deer, other mammals, and birds act as reservoirs. It is widely distributed in Europe, China, Japan and Australia. In the USA, it is found mainly in the north-east (New England), California, Texas, Wisconsin and Minnesota. It is comparatively rare in the UK ($\Sigma \approx 170$ since 1996) and the rise in incidence in the early 1990s was probably due to increased recognition. Infection occurs across southern England from Kent to Devon (over a quarter of UK cases come from Hampshire, Wiltshire and Dorset, especially associated with the New Forest and Salisbury Plain), in East Anglia, Yorkshire, Cumbria and the Scottish Highlands. It is very unlikely in the absence of a history of travel to an endemic area. Since 1996,

14% UK cases were acquired abroad and only 5% were acquired occupationally (forestry and farm workers). Serosurveys among occupational risk groups suggest that asymptomatic infection is common.

*Borrelia burgdorferi sensu lato* is divided into at least 10 genospecies, of which three are major human pathogens. The commonest European genospecies (*Borrelia garinii* and *afzelii*) are genotypically distinct from those from N. America (*Borrelia burgdorferi sensu stricto*) and have differing pathogenicity. *Borrelia burgdorferi sensu stricto* tends to cause chronic arthritis, *Borrelia garinii* is apparently more neurotropic, and *Borrelia afzelii* is associated with late cutaneous disease. In Europe, the main vector is hard ticks of the *Ixodes ricinus* complex, while in the USA *Ixodes scapularis* or *pacificus* are responsible.

May be co-acquired with ehrlichiosis (➤ 302) and babesiosis (➤ 229) from infected ticks (Table 33.3).

**Pathogenesis:** Several mechanisms of neuronal injury have been proposed, including adhesion to neurones and triggering of local cytokine release.

*(continued...)*

Patients have raised serum and CSF levels of inter-leukin-6. Antibodies to myelin have been demon-strated, and immune complex deposition may occur. In joints, sustained infection induces pro-duction of erosive matrix metalloproteinases.

**Clinical features:** Variable, and may be severe or mild, pathognomonic or non-specific. They have been arbitrarily divided into three stages, but these may overlap.

**Stage 1** (early localized LD): 7 (range 3–32) days after tick bite, a characteristic rash develops at the site of inoculation in 50–75% of cases. This is an expanding, annular, bright red, hot, painless plaque with central clearing, called erythema chronica migrans (ECM). This is often accompanied by local lymphadenopathy and constitutional flu-like symp-toms, headache, meningism and arthralgia.

**Stage 2** (early disseminated LD) occurs weeks to months after the original tick bite. In some patients, secondary ECM lesions occur elsewhere on the body, usually a few days after the primary lesion. More severe constitutional symptoms and general lymphadenopathy occur. Neurological symptoms affect ≈15% of patients, including facial palsy and other cranial nerve lesions, aseptic meningitis, peripheral neuropathy or radiculo-pathy causing pain, sensory loss and weakness in limbs or trunk. Symptoms tend to be migratory and intermittent. Encephalitis, psychosis and focal neurological deficit occur, but are rare in the UK. Cardiac manifestations occur in ≈10% of patients during this stage. A–V block occurs in ≈90% of such cases—it may be complete, but is usually reversible. Pericarditis occurs less often, and con-gestive cardiac failure occurs very rarely. Arthritis may occur during stage 2 or 3 and affects a large proportion of patients (≈50% in the USA). It is usually a recurrent monoarthritis or asymmetrical oligoarthritis affecting large joints, or more rarely a symmetrical seronegative rheumatoid arthritis-like illness. It usually resolves after several years, but in a minority the intermittent pattern gives way to chronic arthritis with erosive changes.

**Stage 3** (late persistent LD) consists of arthritis, which is relatively frequent, and late neurological complications (neuropsychiatric disease, focal neu-rological deficits and intermittent incapacitating fatigue), all of which are rare. Acrodermatitis chronica atrophicans is a doughy, blotchy discol-oration of the skin of the extremities which resem-bles the changes of peripheral vascular disease, and occurs as an unusual late complication, usually in elderly women. Borreliae have been cultured from these lesions up to 10 yrs after onset.

**Infection during pregnancy** has been associated with miscarriage, but there is no firm link with con-genital abnormality.

**Diagnosis:** Clinical, based on the features described above and a history of travel to an endemic area and possible exposure to ticks. Non-specific findings which may be present include raised ESR, abnormal liver function tests, raised IgM, leucocytosis and microscopic haematuria. Culture has a very low yield except very soon after infection. In patients with meningitis, CSF findings are typical of aseptic meningitis (➤97); CSF may be examined for the presence of specific antibodies. Serology is available, but must be interpreted with care, particularly in the absence of definite clinical evidence of LD, and taking a good travel history is essential. Serology is not usually positive until some weeks after the onset of the illness (≈90% by 4 weeks), and prompt antibiotic therapy may ablate an antibody response. Serology should not be performed on patients who present only with a history of a tick bite without compatible clinical signs or symptoms. Patients presenting with classical ECM should be treated for LD regardless of serological results. In contrast, serology is extremely valuable in the investigation of patients presenting with extracutaneous lesions, because results are almost always positive and negative serology suggests an alternative diagnosis. False-positives occur, particularly in rheumatoid disease, infectious mononucleosis and syphilis. A screening ELISA is performed, then Western blotting is used to confirm specificity (≈95% specific at 4 weeks). Individuals from endemic areas commonly have persistently positive serology in the absence of clinical disease, and serology is unhelpful in fol-lowing the response to treatment because titres often remain high for years. PCR is available (✈) and may be applied to serum, CSF and joint fluid. Interpretation of all test results requires close liaison with the reference laboratory (☎).

**Management:** Current antibiotic recommenda-tions are shown in Table 33.4. Over 90% patients with ECM have a satisfactory response to these regimens.

*(continued...)*

Neurological involvement other than Bell's palsy is an indication for parenteral treatment. Some experts would recommend CSF examination for patients with Bell's palsy, and parenteral therapy for those with abnormal CSF. Arthritis often responds to oral therapy, but parenteral therapy should be given if there is concomitant neurological disease, or if arthritis is persistent or recurrent ☎.

**'Chronic Lyme disease':** Some patients continue to suffer symptoms despite treatment for 4 weeks with parenteral antibiotics. It is not known whether this is due to ongoing infection or some other (e.g. autoimmune) process, but controlled trials have established that further antibiotic therapy is no more effective than placebo.

↪ Klempner, N Engl J Med 2001; 345: 85

**Immunity:** After treatment for one episode, patients are probably still at risk of infection.

**Prevention:** Important measures include avoidance of tick bites (➤191) and prompt removal of any ticks attached to skin because transmission requires prolonged attachment of tick (incidence of infection from nymphal female *Ixodes scapularis* estimated 20% when attached for >72 h, but <1% when <72 h). Antibiotic prophylaxis is currently not routinely recommended for individuals with a history of tick bite as the risk of acquiring infection is very low, even in endemic areas, and is outweighed by the risk of adverse drug reactions. Some authorities recommend doxycycline prophylaxis (e.g. single 200 mg oral dose) given within 72 h of removal of a tick that has been attached for at least 24 h to a patient over 12 yrs of age in a hyperendemic area (principally, in limited parts of New England). All patients with a confirmed tick bite in an endemic area should be followed up for development of objective signs, especially skin rash at the site of the bite, and fever >38°C within 30 days of exposure. Recombinant vaccine available for certain high risk groups in the USA.

↪ Steere AC, N Engl J Med 2001; 345: 115; Wormser GP, Guidelines for the treatment of Lyme disease. Clin Infect Dis 2000; 31: S1–14 (also at 🖥 www.journals.uchicago.edu/CID/

**Table 33.3** Diseases spread by ticks

| | | |
|---|---|---|
| Bacteria | *Borrelia burgdorferi* (Lyme disease) | ➤323 |
| | Ehrlichiosis (*Ehrlichia chaffeensis*—human monocytic ehrlichiosis; human granulocytic ehrlichiosis) | ➤302 |
| | *Francisella tularensis* (tularaemia) | ➤307 |
| Viruses | Reovirus (Colorado tick fever etc.) | ➤350 |
| | Flavivirus (encephalitis; Kyansur forest disease, Omsk haemorrhagic fever, etc.) | ➤354 |
| | Bunyavirus (Crimean–Congo haemorrhagic fever etc.) | ➤354 |
| Protozoa | *Babesia* spp. | ➤229 |
| Rickettsias | *Rickettsia rickettsii* (Rocky mountain spotted fever) | ➤329 |
| | *Rickettsia conori* (boutonneuse fever) | |
| | *Rickettsia siberica* (Siberian tick typhus) | |
| | *Rickettsia australis* (Queensland tick typhus) | |

**Table 33.4** Treatment of clinical stages of Lyme disease

| Stage of disease | Regimen | Comments |
| --- | --- | --- |
| Erythema chronica migrans, Bell's palsy, first and second degree heart block, arthritis | Doxycycline 100 mg q12h oral (1st choice) or amoxicillin 500 mg q8h oral (child: 50 mg/kg/day up to adult dose) or cefuroxime axetil 500 mg q12h oral for 21–28 days | Treat Bell's palsy for 30 days |
| Neurological manifestations other than Bell's palsy (e.g. meningitis, encephalopathy, radiculopathy). Third-degree heart-block. Persistent or recurrent arthritis | Ceftriaxone 2 g q24h iv (child 75 mg/kg/day) or benzylpenicillin 2.4 g q4h iv (child 150 mg/kg/day) or cefotaxime 2 g q8h iv (child: 150 mg/kg/day in 3–4 divided doses) for 14–28 days | |

**Table 33.5** Organisms causing relapsing fever

| Species | Transmission | Distribution |
| --- | --- | --- |
| *Borrelia recurrentis* | Louse-borne | Worldwide |
| *Borrelia latychevi* | Tick-borne | Iran |
| *Borrelia persica* | Tick-borne | Asia |
| *Borrelia hispanica* | Tick-borne | Spain |
| *Borrelia parkeri, B. turicatae, B. hermsii* | Tick-borne | N. America |
| *Borrelia venezuelensis* | Tick-borne | S. America |

## Clinical syndrome

### Relapsing fever

Febrile illness transmitted by ticks or lice, characterized by several episodes of clinical relapse. Spirochaetes can usually be seen in the peripheral blood during attacks, but fibrin strands or leptospires may be mistaken for them, hence this investigation should only be performed by experts (✈).

**Risk factors:** Louse-borne relapsing fever is a disease of war and starvation, usually occurring as epidemics wherever people are clothed but impoverished. There is no animal reservoir. Tick-borne relapsing fever is a zoonosis maintained in wild rodents. Endemic foci exist in Asia, Africa, and the Americas, the Middle East and in some Mediterranean areas, particularly Spain (Table 33.5).

**Incubation period:** Eight (3–32) days.

**Clinical features:** Fever, headache, prostration and myalgia. Confusion and cough productive of sputum are common. Myocarditis, meningoencephalitis, hepatosplenomegaly, jaundice and hepatic failure may occur. Thrombocytopenia, DIC and a haemorrhagic rash may complicate severe cases. Mortality 2–10% untreated.

Episodes last 4–7 days and if untreated end by crisis, with a sudden fall in temperature and occasionally hypotension. Remission lasts a similar period, and is followed by relapse and a further febrile episode. This occurs two or three times in louse-borne disease and up to 10 times in tick-borne disease.

**Microbiological investigations:** Parasitaemia, with extracellular spirochaetes, can be demonstrated by examination of thick blood films as for malaria (✈). Animal inoculation and serology are also available.

**Other investigations:** Neutrophilia and mild anaemia are common during episodes.

**Antibiotic management:** Tetracycline 500 mg q6h for 7 days. Erythromycin is also effective. Herxheimer-type reactions to treatment are common, with sudden deterioration in clinical condition.

# Leptospira interrogans

## Clinical syndrome

**Leptospirosis (syn. Weil's disease, canicola fever)**
A spirochaetal infection of variable severity acquired by contact with urine of infected mammals. Probably the most widespread zoonosis in the world. Leptospires are unusual among spirochaetes in possessing a lipopolysaccharide-rich outer membrane.

**Epidemiology and transmission:** Distributed worldwide. Occurs in the UK, although uncommon and has fallen a little in incidence ($\Sigma \approx 60$ in early 1990s, $\approx 40$ currently; $\approx 1$–3 deaths). Tropical fresh water provides the best environment for spirochaete survival, and large outbreaks have followed the flooding caused by recent climate changes in S. America. Most often associated with renal infection in rats and dogs, but any animal may be implicated. Transmission occurs by contact of skin or mucous membranes with urine, tissues or urine-contaminated water. There is usually an exposure history. Risk factors include occupations (e.g. agriculture, sewage and abattoir workers) and recreational exposures (e.g. fishing, canoeing). *Leptospira ictohaemorrhagiae* used to be divided in to over 200 serovars, which were grouped in to serogroups; this has been replaced with a genotypic classification in which a number of species (e.g. *Leptospira interrogans, noguchii, santarosai*) contain the original serogroups. Unfortunately this is confusing clinically, because many serogroups belong to several species, and most reference laboratories report isolates according to the older classification at present. Multiple serovars of *Leptospira interrogans* are responsible for disease, including *icterohaemorrhagiae* (rats), *canicola* (dogs) and *hardjo* (cattle).

**Pathogenesis:** Extensive damage to capillary endothelial cells, and in severe cases widespread visceral haemorrhages, renal failure and hepatocellular failure. A variety of virulence factors have been identified, including hyaluronidase and a glycolipoprotein toxin (important for disruption of endothelial cell junctions).

**Incubation time:** Seven to 12 days (range 2–26 days).

**Clinical features:** Variable severity, but only rarely asymptomatic. Usually a self-limited febrile illness ($\approx 90\%$) with headache, prominent severe myalgia, rigors, arthralgia, neck stiffness and prostration. Generalized abdominal pain, epistaxis, mild haemoptysis and GI upset also occur. On examination, conjunctival suffusion and a transient truncal rash, which may be macular, maculopapular, purpuric or urticarial, hepatomegaly, meningism and mild confusion.

Leptospirosis is classically described as a biphasic illness, although this probably only occurs in a minority of cases. During the initial phase, which lasts 4–7 days, leptospires are present in blood. This is followed by an asymptomatic period lasting 1–5 days, followed by a recurrence of fever lasting 4–30 days, during which organisms are present in urine. Neurological symptoms such an meningism are common during this stage. In a minority of patients the initial phase develops into a severe illness with jaundice, renal failure, widespread haemorrhages, shock and confusion (Weil's disease). Most deaths are due to renal failure, and dialysis may be required, but permanently impaired renal function is rare in patients who recover. Adrenal haemorrhage and severe pulmonary haemorrhage occur rarely. Mortality associated with dyspnoea at presentation, oliguria, high WBC, ECG abnormalities and abnormal CXR.

**Investigations:** Diagnosis is often suspected on epidemiological grounds. Culture is difficult (send blood culture bottles to ⌁ within first 5 days of symptoms), and diagnosis is usually confirmed by serology (IgM antibodies usually produced 7–14 days after onset, usually detected by screening CFT; positives referred for specific IgM EIA and microagglutination tests ⌁). Serogroup-specific responses may be seen later, necessitating repeated testing. Immunofluorescence-based

*(continued...)*

tests may be used with tissue. PCR diagnosis not currently available in the UK. Microscopy of blood or urine is unreliable outside reference laboratories. Anaemia, thrombocytopenia and neutrophilia are common. The WBC is usually 5–15 000 $\times$ $10^9$/L. Proteinuria and microscopic haematuria are common. Uraemia, abnormal liver function tests and disordered coagulation occur in sicker patients. CSF shows a pleocytosis, initially polymorphs, but later mainly mononuclear, with normal glucose and normal or elevated protein. CXR infiltrates are common.

**Management:** Antibiotic therapy shortens duration of illness, particularly if given early. Doxycycline (100 mg q12h for 7 days) and benzylpenicillin are both effective, although no comparative trial has been performed. Supportive therapy for severe complications may be necessary. The renal impairment is usually fully reversible with successful therapy. Penicillin may induce a Jarisch–Herxheimer reaction, which worsens outcome, hence patients should be observed carefully for development of shock during treatment.

**Prevention:** Depends on limiting exposure to infective water and animals. If this cannot be achieved, e.g. for sewer workers or military personnel, chemoprophylaxis with doxycyc-line (200 mg weekly) is effective but rarely indicated. There are anecdotal reports of person-to-person spread in hospitals, therefore patients should be isolated with body fluid precautions during the early stages of treatment. Vaccination against specific serovars for persons at occupational risk has been used in some countries.

# Chapter 34

# Mycoplasmas, chlamydias and rickettsias

## Mycoplasmas (Table 34.1)

The smallest prokaryotic organisms able to grow in cell-free culture media. Multiply by binary fission, often producing branching filaments which fragment to produce single pleomorphic cells. Several species have specialized structures at one or both ends of the cell by which they attach to respiratory or genital mucosa.

**Laboratory diagnosis:** Culture is not routinely performed, but sometimes isolated on blood agar plates or from blood cultures. Serology is available. Patients with atypical pneumonia due to *Mycoplasma pneumoniae* may develop cold agglutinins ($\approx$25%), which were used in the past as surrogate for specific serology. Haemolytic anaemia may occur as a complication.

**Treatment:** Tetracyclines, quinolones or macrolides are used. See individual syndromes.

**Comments:** In patients with hypogammaglobulinaemia, mycoplasmas (particularly *M. hominis* and *U. urealyticum*) may cause suppurative arthritis, subcutaneous abscesses, persistent urethritis and cystitis. Sternal wound infections due to *M. hominis* have occurred in heart and lung transplant patients.

## Chlamydiae (Table 34.2)

Small, non-motile Gram-negative bacteria which are obligate intracellular parasites. Unlike viruses, they contain both DNA and RNA, ribosomes and a cell wall and they divide by binary fission. They do not have peptidoglycan and cannot produce ATP, for which they depend on the host cell (hence 'energy parasites').

Metabolically inert infectious particles ('elementary bodies') are 300–350 nm in diameter. Once inside the host cell the organisms become metabolically active and increase in size to 800–1000 nm diameter ('reticulate bodies').

Serological evidence of previous *Chlamydia pneumoniae* infection in $\approx$50% by adult life; estimated incidence of human infection is 2–4 episodes per life. A number of large outbreaks have been described, mainly in N. Europe.

**Laboratory diagnosis:** Organisms can be cultured in eggs or tissue culture, but this is not routinely performed. Sensitive ELISA or immunofluorescent techniques are used routinely to demonstrate chlamydial antigens in respiratory or genital secretions. Serology is also used (IgG and IgM), although this does not routinely distinguish among species. Tests for chlamydia DNA (PCR or ligase chain reaction — LCR) are now widely available, with high sensitivity and specificity and are now the first line investigation for all specimen types (➤87).

**Treatment:** Quinolones, tetracyclines or macrolides are used. See individual syndromes.

## Rickettsiae (Tables 34.3, 34.4)

Rickettsiae are obligate intracellular Gram-negative parasites. Most are zoonoses spread to humans by arthropods. Rickettsiae replicate within the cytoplasm of endothelial cells and smooth-muscle cells of capillaries, arterioles and small arteries causing necrotizing vasculitis. Rickettsial infections vary greatly in severity, depending on the infecting species. Most are febrile infections with a characteristic rash. An 'eschar', a black ulcerated lesion, may develop at the site of inoculation. Severe, often fatal,

**Table 34.1** Classification of mycoplasmas

| Genus | Species | Notes |
|---|---|---|
| Mycoplasma | pneumoniae | 'Atypical' pneumonia (➤26), clinically indistinguishable from 'typical' pneumococcal pneumonia. 4-yearly peaks of confidence. Commonest in children, but may be severe in the elderly. Rarely associated with acute neurological complications, haemolytic anaemia, pericarditis, Stevens–Johnson syndrome and erythema nodosum. Mortality ≈5%. |
|  | hominis | Non-gonococcal urethritis, salpingitis (➤92). Puerperal infections including bacteraemia. Respiratory infections in neonates (esp. low birth weight) |
| (Acholeplasma spp.) |  | Rare cause of human respiratory tract infection |
| Ureaplasma | urealyticum | Non-gonococcal urethritis. Rare neonatal meningitis |

**Table 34.2** Classification of chlamydias

| Genus | Species | Serovars | Notes |
|---|---|---|---|
| Chlamydia | trachomatis | A, Ba, B, C | Trachoma (➤106) |
|  |  | D–K | Inclusion conjunctivitis (➤106) |
|  |  |  | Ophthalmia neonatorum (➤107) |
|  |  |  | Genital infections (➤87) |
|  |  |  | Respiratory infection in neonates (➤142) |
|  |  | L1–L3 | Lymphogranuloma venereum (➤94) |
|  | psittaci |  | Psittacosis (➤26). Control by bird importation regulations, isolation of newly imported birds etc. highly effective at reducing human cases |
|  | pneumoniae (formerly 'TWAR' agent) |  | Pharyngitis, 'atypical' pneumonia (➤26) with peak incidence during teenage years. Disputed cause of cardiovascular disease |

multisystem involvement occurs with several species.

All rickettsial infections are rare as imported diseases to the UK, with the exception of tick typhus, which occurs occasionally in tourists after rural exposure, e.g. on safari.

*Coxiella burnetii* is currently classified with the rickettsiae, but is biologically distinct. Q fever, the disease caused by systemic infection with *Coxiella burnetii*, occurs in the UK, but is rare (see below).

**Clinical features:** Summarized in Tables 34.3 and 34.4.

**Diagnosis:** Usually clinical, confirmed by serology. Infection with rickettsiae induces antibodies that react with certain strains of the bacterium *Proteus*. This cross-reaction forms the basis of the Well–Felix test, which uses different strains of *Proteus* to differentiate among rickettsial infections. The Well–Felix test is neither sensitive nor specific and has been replaced by specific serology for all important rickettsial infections. Organisms may be seen on biopsy of the skin lesions of Rocky Mountain spotted fever.

Table 34.3 *Rickettsia* I: spotted fever group

| Species | Disease | Distribution | Ecology | Hosts/route | Incubation (days) | Clinical features |
|---|---|---|---|---|---|---|
| *R. rickettsi* | Rocky Mountain spotted fever | USA, Canada, Mexico, S. America | Typically rural, but may occur in urban areas | Ticks, rodents, dogs, foxes/tick bite | 7 (2–14) | Fever, severe headache, myalgia. Eschar in 20%. Widespread maculopapular rash on days 3–5, becoming petechial, purpuric and necrotic. Severe multisystem involvement (pulmonary, renal, GI, neurological, cardiac). Thrombocytopenia, DIC. Mortality 15–20% untreated |
| *R. conori* | African tick typhus ('boutonneuse fever') | Mediterranean, Black Sea, Caspian Sea littorals, Middle East, India, Africa | Usually associated with rural exposure to ticks | Rodents, dogs/tick bite | 5–7 | Eschar with tender local lymphadenopathy. Generalized maculopapular rash and conjunctival injection on days 4–5. Systemic features otherwise mild. Mortality very rare |
| *R. australis* | Queensland tick typhus | Australia | As for African tick typhus | Marsupials/tick bite | 7–10 | As for African tick typhus |
| *R. siberica* | Siberian tick typhus | Central Europe, Central Asia | As for African tick typhus | Rodents/tick bite | 2–7 | As for African tick typhus |
| *R. akari* | Rickettsial pox | N. America, S. Africa, CIS, Korea | Urban over crowding, rodent contact | Rodents/mite bite | 5–10 | As for African tick typhus. Rash is vesicular, resembling chickenpox |

**Table 34.4** *Rickettsia* II: typhus group

| Species | Disease | Distribution | Ecology | Hosts/route | Incubation (days) | Clinical features |
|---|---|---|---|---|---|---|
| *R. prowazeki* | Epidemic louse-borne typhus ('classic typhus') | Worldwide | In colder areas, where people are louse-infected. Typically associated with war and famine | Humans are the reservoir/ transmitted by louse faeces scratched into skin | 12 (7–14) | Fever, headache, severe constitutional symptoms. Early neurological (deafness, delirium) and GI symptoms. Generalized maculopapular rash on day 4–7 of illness. Thrombocytopenia. Severe multisystem involvement. Mortality 20–50% untreated |
| | Brill–Zinsser disease | | Recrudescent infection in latently infected persons | B–Z patients may act as reservoir for epidemic typhus | | Months to years after recovery from typhus, patients develop a similar but milder illness, lasting ≈2 weeks, with no significant mortality |
| *R. typhi* (mooseri) | Murine typhus ('endemic or flea typhus') | Worldwide | Where rats and humans share buildings | Rodents/flea faeces scratched into skin | 12 (7–14) | Clinical features similar to louse-borne typhus, but much milder. Mortality <1% |
| *R. tsutsugamushi* (orientalis) | Scrub typhus ('tsutsugamushi fever, mite typhus') | Asia, India, Australia, Oceania | Circumscribed rural foci ('typhus islands') where rats, mites and rickettsiae coexist | Rodents/mite bite | 12 (6–21) | Eschar is common. Otherwise similar to louse-borne typhus, but usually less severe. Significant mortality occurs |

**Management** *Rickettsia* spp.: doxycycline 100 mg 12-hly or tetracycline 500 mg 6-hly for all rickettsial infections. Chloramphenicol 50 mg/ kg/day (adult max: 4 g/day, child <8 yrs max: 2 g/day) may be used in children under 8 yrs and in pregnancy.

## *Coxiella burnetii* (Q fever, 'Balkan grippe')

*Coxiella burnetii* is biologically distinct from other rickettsiae. It grows in phagosomes rather than in the cytoplasm of infected cells (it grows well in the acidic environment of the phagosome), and its spores survive in the environment for prolonged periods. Alveolar macrophages and liver Kupffer cells are especially prone to infection.

**Epidemiology and transmission:** Zoonosis acquired worldwide by aerosol or direct contact, usually from occupational exposure to cattle or sheep, but may be acquired from almost any mammal or bird. Occasional acquisition from unpasteurized milk or dairy products. Person-to-person spread occurs, but not often enough to merit isolation of cases. Exposure to parturient cats or stillborn kittens is an important risk factor. Frequently found in ticks, but transmission to humans is thought to be very rare via this route. The organism is highly infectious, and is a hazard to staff in the laboratory and post-mortem room ☣. $\Sigma \approx 140$.

In some areas (e.g. Spain and Australia), *Coxiella burnetii* is more common, accounting for a significant proportion of community-acquired atypical pneumonias.

**Clinical features:** After an incubation period of ≈2–5 weeks, sudden onset of fever, rigors, headache (≈80%), myalgia (≈60%), arthralgia, chest pain (≈30%) and dry cough. Q fever may present as a respiratory infection, with signs consistent with 'atypical' pneumonia (➤26), as a systemic febrile illness or as an acute hepatitis (≈50%). Clinically detectable hepatomegaly is common, but jaundice is rare. Rash occurs in about 15% cases, with pink macules or purpuric red papules on the trunk. Rarer presentations are reported, including pleuropericarditis (≈1%), myocarditis (≈1%), haemolytic anaemia, meningo-encephalitis (≈1%), arthritis, glomerulonephritis, thyroiditis and epididymo-orchitis. The peripheral blood leucocyte count is normal in 90%. Infection is almost always self-limited, even without therapy: defervescence normally occurs after 5–14 days, but 60% of patients >40 yrs of age are febrile for longer than 14 days. Mortality is ≈1%, often associated with myocarditis. Q fever in pregnancy is associated with increased risk of miscarriage.

**Organisms:** *Coxiella burnetii.*

**Microbiological investigations:** Culture is difficult and hazardous for laboratory staff. Diagnosis is confirmed by serology. *Coxiella burnetii* undergoes antigenic variation during infection. IgG and IgM antibodies to phase II antigens indicate acute infection. Phase I IgA and IgG antibodies are associated with chronic Q fever. Cross-reactions occur with *Bartonella* infections, leading to diagnostic confusion (➤308, ➤310). Autoantibodies (mitochondria, smooth muscle etc.) are commonly found in infected patients' serum.

**Other investigations:** Abnormal liver function is common. CXR often shows diffuse infiltration and rounded opacities, even if auscultation is normal.

**Antibiotic management:** Treatment is indicated for all cases to reduce risk of developing chronic Q fever. Doxycycline (drug of choice), tetracycline or chloramphenicol for 2–3 weeks. Ciprofloxacin is active *in vitro*, but has not been subjected to clinical trial, and the newer macrolides may also be effective.

**Comments:** Chronic Q fever is very rare (➤50) and some cases diagnosed in the past may have been *Bartonella* infections with serological cross-reaction. It presents usually as a culture-negative endocarditis (≈65%), most commonly affecting the aortic valve, and may be accompanied by a protean and clinically confusing range of clinical manifestations (e.g. acute renal failure, stroke, chronic hepato- or splenomegaly and postoperative fever). Other cases have presented with vascular infection (aneurysm, vascular graft), interstitial pulmonary fibrosis, placentitis and osteomyelitis. Most patients are over the age of 40 and have pre-existing rheumatic heart disease, but very few have been diagnosed in the past with acute Q fever. Immunocompromised and pregnant hosts may be at higher risk, but ≈75% cases are in males overall. Prolonged (≈1 yr), even lifelong, treatment with tetracycline and rifampicin or co-trimoxazole is required; doxycycline plus chloroquine has been recommended recently. Valve replacement is often necessary.

# Chapter 35

# Virology

## Classification of viruses (Table 35.1)

Viruses are obligate intracellular parasites which require host cells to replicate. They contain either DNA or RNA, but not both, and this forms the basis of the fundamental classification into DNA and RNA viruses. Viruses are then grouped into families on the basis of shared biological and structural properties, but members of the same family can cause very different diseases. Similarly, almost identical illnesses may be caused by viruses which are structurally entirely different.

Virus infections are largely species-specific, but many viruses that primarily cause disease in animals are important human zoonoses.

## Adenoviruses

A family of DNA viruses divided into 49 serotypes, causing a broad range of clinical syndromes, in particular respiratory tract infection and conjunctivitis. Many serotypes have not been associated with human disease. Some adenoviruses cause tumours in animals. Common worldwide.

**Key biological features:** Virus replication occurs in epithelial cells. Latent infection of lymphoid tissue may occur.

**Reservoir:** No animal reservoir for serotypes causing human disease.

**Transmission:** Respiratory, direct contact or orofaecal, depending on serotype.

**Incubation period:** Typically 4–5 days; 4–28 days for epidemic keratoconjunctivitis.

**Immunization:** Not available.

**Diagnosis:** Serology, viral culture.

**Major clinical associations:** Table 35.2.

**Antiviral therapy:** None.

**Comments:** Immunosuppressed patients and neonates may develop severe disseminated adenovirus infection, which may be fatal.

## Herpesviruses

Common worldwide. Over 150 herpesviruses have been described in many species (vertebrate and invertebrate), of which nine have been shown to cause disease in humans (Table 35.3). No animal reservoir for viruses causing human disease.

**Key biological features:** Herpesvirus infections are characterized by primary infection that can be mild or asymptomatic, followed by the establishment of latent infection. Reactivation of the virus occurs months to years later, and may cause asymptomatic shedding of virus or clinical disease, such as cold sores due to HSV or herpes zoster due to VZV, in patients who are immunocompetent. Primary or recurrent infection may be severe in the immunocompromised. EBV has the ability to immortalize B cells *in vitro* and has been associated with malignancies (lymphoma and nasopharyngeal carcinoma). Like most viruses with a lipid envelope, they are relatively fragile and most easily transmit on contact with warm moist mucosae, typically by oral secretions or genital contact.

### Herpes simplex virus (syn. HHV-1, HHV-2)

HSV-1 and HSV-2 cause a wide range of clinical syndromes. Clinical features depend on the

**Table 35.1** Medically important viruses

| Group | Most important members | Size (nm) | Morphology | Envelope | Genome type | Genome size (kb) | |
|-------|------------------------|-----------|------------|----------|-------------|------------------|---|
| **DNA viruses** | | | | | | | |
| Adenoviridae | Adenoviruses | 70–90 | Icosahedral | No | Linear dsDNA | 36–38 | ➤334 |
| Herpesviridae | Herpes simplex types 1 & 2, Epstein–Barr virus, varicella-zoster virus, cytomegalovirus, human herpes virus type 6 and 7, Kaposi's sarcoma-associated herpesvirus (HHV-8) | 120–200 | Icosahedral capsid 100–110 nm | Yes | Linear dsDNA | 120–240 | ➤334 |
| Poxviridae | Molluscum contagiosum, orf | 300 × 240 × 100 | Brick-shaped | Yes | Linear dsDNA | 130–380 | ➤341 |
| Parvoviridae | Parvovirus B19 | 20 | Icosahedral | No | ssDNA | 5 | ➤341 |
| Papovaviridae | Human papillomaviruses, polyomaviruses | ≈50 | Icosahedral | No | Circular dsDNA | 5–8 | ➤342 |
| Hepadnaviridae | Hepatitis B virus | 42 | Spherical | Yes | Partially ss/partially ds DNA | 3.2 | ➤344 |
| **RNA viruses** | | | | | | | |
| Orthomyxoviridae | Influenza types A, B & C | 80–120 | Spherical | Yes | ss(−)RNA | 10–14 | ➤344 |
| Paramyxoviridae | Parainfluenza, mumps, measles, RSV | 150–300 | Spherical | Yes | ss(−)RNA | 16–20 | ➤346 |
| Coronaviridae | Coronavirus | 60–220 | Spherical | Yes | ss(+)RNA | 20–30 | ➤347 |
| Picornaviridae | Poliovirus, coxsackievirus, echovirus, other enteroviruses, hepatitis A virus, rhinovirus | 25–30 | Icosahedral | No | ss(+)RNA | 7.2–8.4 | ➤347 |

*(Continued)*

**Table 35.1** (*Continued*)

| Group | Most important members | Size (nm) | Morphology | Envelope | Genome type | Genome size (kb) | |
|---|---|---|---|---|---|---|---|
| Reoviridae | Rotavirus, reovirus | 60–80 | Icosahedral | No | dsRNA | 16–27 | ➤350 |
| Retroviridae | HTLV-I, HTLV-II, HIV types 1 & 2 | 100 | Spherical | Yes | Diploid ss(+)RNA | 7–11 | ➤351 |
| Togaviridae | Rubella. Arboviruses causing encephalitis | 60–70 | Spherical | Yes | ss(+)RNA | 10–12 | ➤352 |
| Flaviviridae | Yellow fever, dengue, hepatitis C virus. Arboviruses causing encephalitis | 40–50 | Spherical | Yes | ss(+)RNA | 9.5–13 | ➤352 |
| Bunyaviridae | Hantaan. Arboviruses causing encephalitis. Crimean–Congo haemorrhagic fever | 90–100 | Spherical | Yes | ss(ambisense)RNA | 11–21 | ➤354 |
| Arenaviridae | Lassa | 50–300 | Spherical | Yes | ss(ambisense)RNA | 10–14 | ➤356 |
| Filoviridae | Marburg, Ebola | ≈800 × 80 | Filamentous with helical nucleocapsid | Yes | ss(−)RNA | 19 | ➤357 |
| Rhabdoviridae | Rabies | 180 × 75 | Bullet-shaped | Yes | ss(−)RNA | 13–16 | ➤357 |
| Astroviridae | Astrovirus | 27–32 | Spherical | No | ss(+)RNA | 7.2–7.9 | ➤350 |
| Caliciviridae | Calicivirus | 27–38 | Spherical | No | ss(+)RNA | 7.4–7.7 | ➤350 |
| Hepatitis E | Currently unclassified | 32 | Icosahedral | No | ss(+)RNA | 7.5 | ➤75 |

Genome type: (+) message sense, (−) complementary to message. ss, single stranded; ds, double stranded.

**Table 35.2** Clinical associations of adenovirus infection

| Clinical syndrome | Serotypes | Comments | |
|---|---|---|---|
| Upper respiratory tract infection | 1, 2, 4, 5, 6 | Primarily in children under 5 yrs | ➤19 |
| Lower respiratory tract infection | 3, 4, 7 | Primarily young adults | ➤23 |
| Pharyngoconjunctival fever | 3, 7 | 'Swimming-pool conjunctivitis' — primarily in children under 10 yrs | ➤106 |
| Epidemic keratoconjunctivitis | 8, 19, 37 | 'Shipyard worker's eye' | ➤106 |
| Meningoencephalitis | 2, 6, 7, 12 | Primarily in children under 10 yrs | ➤100 |
| Haemorrhagic cystitis | 7, 11, 21 | | |
| Intussusception | 1, 2, 4, 5 | Primarily in children under 5 yrs | |
| Diarrhoea | 2, 3, 5, 40, 41 | | ➤58 |
| Encephalitis | 7, 12, 32 | In AIDS and other immunocompromised patients | ➤162 |
| Pneumonia, urinary tract infection, disseminated infection | 5, 31, 34, 35, 39 | | |
| Fatal disseminated infection in neonates | 3, 7, 21, 30 | | |

**Table 35.3** Herpesviruses causing disease in humans

| Subfamily | Important human viruses | |
|---|---|---|
| Alphaherpesviruses | Herpes simplex types 1 & 2 | HHV-1, HHV-2 |
| | Varicella-zoster virus | HHV-3 |
| Betaherpesviruses | Cytomegalovirus | HHV-5 |
| | Human herpes virus types 6 and 7 | HHV-6, HHV-7 |
| | Simian herpes B | |
| Gammaherpesviruses | Epstein–Barr virus | HHV-4 |
| | Kaposi's sarcoma-associated herpesvirus | HHV-8 |

route of infection (e.g. oral, genital, cutaneous) and host factors, particularly previous exposure to HSV, generalized immunodeficiency, intercurrent illness (e.g. eczema). After primary infection, latent infection is established in sensory ganglia (principally the trigeminal ganglion and the dorsal root ganglia of the spinal cord).

**Epidemiology:** Endemic infection is maintained by asymptomatic shedding of virus from latently infected individuals. In developing countries, childhood infection is very common, with seroprevalence typically 90% by age 10 yrs. In developed countries, infection tends to occur later, in adolescence or early adulthood.

**Immunization:** Not available, although vaccines against HSV-2 are in development. Prior exposure to either HSV-1 or HSV-2 gives **partial** immunity to infection by the other virus.

**Incubation period:** 2–12 (mean 4) days for symptomatic primary infection. Many primary infections are asymptomatic.

**Transmission:** HSV-1 is transmitted non-sexually, primarily via saliva, and frequently from asymptomatic shedders. Both HSV-1 and HSV-2 may be transmitted sexually in genital secretions. Approximately 30% of first episodes of genital herpes are due to HSV-1, but the recurrence rate is much higher for HSV-2.

**Clinical features:** Table 35.4.

**Management:** Systemic aciclovir (ACV) shortens the duration of primary attacks of cutaneous, oral and genital herpes, but is less effective against recurrent disease, even when started at the onset of prodromal symptoms. For this reason, it is generally not indicated for cold sores or recurrent genital herpes, unless particularly frequent or severe. In patients with frequent recurrences and in the immuno-compromised, prophylactic therapy may be given with ACV 400 mg 12hly to reduce the frequency and severity of attacks ($\succ$158). Disseminated or severe HSV infection (e.g. encephalitis) should be treated with intravenous ACV. Ophthalmic HSV infections may be treated topically.

**Famciclovir** and **valaciclovir** offer reduced dosing frequency at higher cost.

**Complications:** Severe **disseminated visceral infection**, which may be fatal, occurs extremely infrequently, most often in women during the third trimester of pregnancy. **Eczema herpeticum** (syn. Kaposi's varicelliform eruption) is due to disseminated cutaneous infection in patients with pre-existing atopic dermatitis. It can be widespread and severe, and is an indication for systemic antiviral therapy. **Erythema multiforme** (Stevens–Johnson syndrome) is an allergic manifestation, causing target lesions on the skin and mucosal ulceration. Differentia-

**Table 35.4** Clinical features of herpesvirus infection in humans

| Clinical syndrome | | Relative frequency of HSV-1 and HSV-2 | Recommendations for aciclovir (ACV) use |
|---|---|---|---|
| **Primary infection** | | | |
| Acute stomatitis | $\succ$129 | Usually HSV-1 | Systemic ACV may shorten attack |
| Acute keratoconjunctivitis | $\succ$107 | Usually HSV-1. HSV-2 in neonates | Topical ACV |
| Neonatal infection | $\succ$129 | HSV-2 in two-thirds of cases | Intravenous ACV (10 mg/kg 8 hly) |
| **Recurrent infection** | | | |
| Herpes labialis | $\succ$118 | HSV-1 | Topical or oral ACV may shorten attack if started promptly |
| Herpes keratitis | $\succ$107 | HSV-1 | Topical ACV |
| **Primary or recurrent infection** | | | |
| Cutaneous herpes | $\succ$118 | HSV-1 | Oral ACV (200–400 mg p.o. 5 times daily) shortens primary attack. Less effective in recurrent disease. Topical ACV is not recommended |
| Paronychia ('herpetic whitlow') | $\succ$118 | HSV-1 in children, health workers. HSV-2 in adults | |
| Genital herpes | $\succ$88 | 60–70% HSV-2 | |
| Eczema herpeticum | $\succ$338 | Usually HSV-1 | Intravenous ACV (10 mg/kg 8 hly) |
| Encephalitis | $\succ$101 | Nearly always HSV-1 | |
| Meningitis | $\succ$100 | Usually HSV-2 | |
| Disseminated disease in immunodeficient | $\succ$338 | HSV-1 or HSV-2 | |

tion from HSV infection itself can be difficult, but the vesicular lesions of erythema multiforme have thicker, longer-lived roofs than the vesicles of HSV infection, and virus cannot be isolated from them.

## Varicella zoster virus (VZV, HHV-3) ①
Clinical associations:
Varicella ➤130.
Congenital infection ➤131.
Severe infection in neonates ➤131.
Herpes zoster ➤132.

## Epstein–Barr virus (EBV, HHV-4)
EBV infects B lymphocytes and epithelial cells. Latent infection is established in B cells. *In vitro* infection of B cells renders them immortal, capable of indefinite *in vitro* propagation ('transformation'). This property of transformation is reflected in the ability of EBV to induce human lymphoma under certain circumstances.

**Epidemiology:** Adult seroprevalence rates are typically >90% worldwide. Age at primary infection is lower in developing countries, where infection is typically acquired in childhood.

**Transmission:** Via oropharyngeal secretions. Asymptomatic shedding of virus is very common.

**Clinical associations:** Primary infection is often asymptomatic.
**Infectious mononucleosis** ➤133.
**Fatal acute mononucleosis** in carriers of XLP gene ➤134.
**Lymphoma: Burkitt's lymphoma** is seen in equatorial Africa and New Guinea. It is associated with a low age of EBV infection and hyperendemic malaria. It presents as a rapidly-growing tumour of children, usually affecting the jaw or abdominal organs. EBV is present in the majority of AIDS-associated lymphomas. **Polyclonal B-cell lymphoproliferation** occurs in immunodeficient patients (e.g. post-transplant or HIV seropositive).
**Nasopharyngeal carcinoma:** EBV is strongly associated with undifferentiated carcinoma of the nasopharyngeal epithelium, seen primarily in Chinese, Eskimos and Greenlanders. A chemical cofactor may be involved.
**Oral hairy leukoplakia** ➤160.

Severe **persistent illness** associated with EBV is extremely rare, but a few patients have been described with immunodeficiency and disseminated viral infection, including hepatitis, pneumonitis, splenomegaly and pancytopenia. Such individuals have an unusual serological profile, with high titres of anti-VCA IgG and anti-EA, and low titres of anti-EBNA antibodies.

**Diagnosis:** ➤133.

# Chronic fatigue syndrome

Chronic fatigue syndrome (CFS, syn. 'post-viral syndrome' and 'myalgic encephalomyelitis') is characterized by intermittent feverishness, fatigue, myalgia and cognitive disturbances, including poor concentration. Patients in whom CFS is diagnosed represent a heterogeneous group in whom both physical and psychological features are important. Extensive studies have failed to demonstrate any link between EBV infection and CFS. Patients with CFS rarely have a diagnosable underlying infectious illness, and viral serology plays no part in the management of CFS.

🖳 www.doh.gov.uk/cmo/cfsmereport

# Cytomegalovirus (CMV, HHV-5)

CMV causes only mild disease in the immunocompetent, but can be serious in the immunosuppressed or when infection occurs in pregnancy. Like other herpesviruses, acute primary infection is followed by the establishment of latency. Reactivation and clinical disease may occur if the patient becomes immunodeficient, e.g. post-transplantation.

**Epidemiology:** Infection occurs worldwide. In developed countries, peaks of seroconversion occur during early childhood, and then during the second and third decades of life, when patients become sexually active. Seroprevalence increases throughout life and is >80% at age 60 yrs.

**Transmission:** Mainly via oropharyngeal secretions or urine, particularly from children. Asymptomatic shedding of virus and sexual transmission are common. Transmission by blood products or solid organ transplant are important, particularly as transplant recipients will be immunosuppressed.

**Incubation period:** Variable. Typically 3–8 weeks when the time of transmission is known (e.g. following infection by blood transfusion).

**Immunization:** Not available.

**Diagnosis:** Seroconversion or a rise in antibody titre suggests active CMV infection. Culture of CMV does not always indicate active infection, as healthy seropositive individuals continue to shed virus intermittently in saliva and urine. **CMV viraemia** detected by isolation of virus from buffy coats correlates well with active infection. Conventional culture is slow, and a number of methods have been developed in which CMV is demonstrated early in culture by immunofluorescent detection of viral antigens. **PCR** is now routinely available and correlates well with the results of culture. **Biopsy** of infected tissue may be diagnostic; CMV causes characteristic histological changes, including 'owl's eye' inclusion bodies.

### Clinical associations

**Acute mononucleosis:** Acute primary CMV infection in immunocompetent patients causes a mononucleosis-like illness with fever, malaise and hepatosplenomegaly. Pharyngitis and lymphadenopathy occur in only ≈30% of patients, in contrast to EBV-associated mononucleosis. Abnormal liver function tests and atypical mononucleosis are normally seen. Heterophile antibodies do not occur (➤134). Guillain–Barré syndrome and Bell's palsy have been reported as complications.

**Congenital infection:** Primary maternal infection during pregnancy results in foetal infection in 50% of cases. Congenital infection and structural defects are seen in approximately 10% of these. Infants with cytomegalic inclusion disease present within a few days of birth with hepatosplenomegaly, thrombocytopenia and petechial rash. Intrauterine growth retar-

dation and failure to thrive are common. Encephalitis, microcephaly and intracranial calcification may occur. Mental and physical retardation affect the majority of patients. Infected infants without these severe features have a significant risk of sensorineural deafness (➤141).

**Neonatal infection:** Premature infants who acquire CMV (e.g. by transfusion) may develop 'grey baby' syndrome, with pallor, hypotension and respiratory distress.

**Infection in the immunocompromised:** CMV infection of variable severity may occur after transplantation of solid organs, causing fever, hepatitis, leucopenia, pneumonitis and graft rejection (➤176). In bone-marrow transplant patients, a severe, frequently fatal interstitial pneumonitis occurs after CMV infection or reactivation (➤177). Infection in HIV patients causes a number of clinical syndromes, including chorioretinitis and colitis (➤166).

**Antiviral therapy:** Infection in immunocompetent patients does not require treatment. In the immunocompromised host, ganciclovir, cidofovir and foscarnet (➤166) are effective. Interstitial pneumonitis in bone marrow transplant patients responds poorly to GCV, but may respond to GCV given with CMV hyperimmune globulin. Aciclovir is not effective as therapy for established CMV infections, but is useful as prophylaxis in transplant patients (Table 35.5). Valganciclovir is an oral pro-drug of ganciclovir which will probably replace ganciclovir for most indications.

**Table 35.5** Activity of antiherpes agents

| Agent | HSV1/2 | VZV | CMV | |
|---|---|---|---|---|
| Aciclovir, famciclovir, valaciclovir | +++ | ++ | − | ➤362 |
| Ganciclovir | + | + | +++ | ➤166 |
| Foscarnet | ++ | + | ++ | ➤166 |
| Cidofovir | + | ++ | +++ | ➤166 |

## Human herpes viruses 6 & 7 (HHV-6, HHV-7)

### Clinical associations

**Exanthema subitum** (syn. roseola infantum) ➤ 134.

HHV-6 has been associated with a mononucleosis-like illness in adolescents and adults, and with interstitial pneumonia, hepatitis, myelosuppression and encephalitis in transplant recipients. A putative link to multiple sclerosis has been suggested.

**Antiviral therapy:** HHV-6 is sensitive *in vitro* to ganciclovir and foscarnet, but there are no published studies of clinical utility.

**HHV-7** is similar to HHV-6 and probably causes some cases of exanthema subitum. Adult seroprevalence in developed countries >85%.

## Human herpes virus 8 (HHV-8, Kaposi's sarcoma-associated herpes virus, KSHV)

No clinical disease has been associated with acute infection by HHV-8. Adult seroprevalence varies between <1% for the UK and ≈10–25% in some Mediterranean areas. Seroprevalence is higher among homosexual men, suggesting sexual transmission. HHV-8 is a cofactor in the development of Kaposi's sarcoma both in patients co-infected with HIV (➤ 168) and in non-HIV-associated endemic KS. It is also associated with primary effusion lymphoma in immunosuppressed patients.

**Simian herpes B** causes benign latent infection in macaques, and may rarely be transmitted to man by monkey bites. After an incubation period of 3 days to 3 weeks, pain, redness and a vesicular rash develop at the site of the bite. There may be local neurological signs or encephalitis, which may be fatal. Prompt parenteral aciclovir therapy is essential, and is given prophylactically to animal handlers bitten by monkeys whose B virus status is unknown.

## Poxviruses

A large family of DNA viruses, members of which infect invertebrate and vertebrate hosts, including man (Table 35.6).

**Reservoir:** There is no animal reservoir for molluscum contagiosum and smallpox (a fact which was essential in the eradication of smallpox by vaccination). Other poxviruses are acquired as zoonoses from a variety of animals and, with the exception of monkeypox, only cause superficial skin infection in man.

**Transmission:** Direct contact with an infected person or animal. Orf is the only zoonotic poxvirus common in the UK. Patients always have an occupational exposure to sheep or goats, and often the animals are known to have orf.

**Antiviral therapy:** None.

## Parvoviruses ①

Parvovirus B19 is the only member of this group pathogenic in man. The only known host cell for human parvovirus is the erythrocyte precursor; this site of infection explains the ability of the virus to cause aplastic crises in patients with pre-existing haemolytic anaemia (e.g. sickle-cell disease).

**Reservoir:** Man.

**Epidemiology:** Worldwide. Common in children. Typically occurring in epidemics, usually 4–5 yrs apart. Infection is commonest between 5 and 14 yrs. Seroprevalence typically 20% at 10 yrs, 50% at 50 yrs.

**Transmission:** Highly contagious, probably via respiratory route.

**Incubation period:** 4–20 days.

**Diagnosis:** By detection of specific IgM or a rise in IgG. Molecular techniques such as nucleic acid hybridization can be used to demonstrate parvovirus antigens in serum.

### Clinical associations

**Erythema infectiosum ('fifth disease') in children** ➤ 135.

**Arthritis** is a common complication in adults. Arthralgia occurs in ≈75% of cases in

**Table 35.6** Human poxvirus infections

| Virus | Group | Major hosts | Disease |
|---|---|---|---|
| **Poxviruses restricted to humans** | | | |
| Variola | Orthopoxvirus | None | Smallpox ⊠ (eradicated) |
| Molluscum contagiosum | Molluscipoxvirus | None | Molluscum contagiosum (➤119) |
| **Common zoonotic poxviruses** | | | |
| Orf | Parapoxvirus | Sheep, goats | Orf (➤119) |
| Vaccinia | Orthopoxvirus | Laboratory virus | Used as smallpox vaccine |
| Paravaccinia | Parapoxvirus | European cattle | 'Milker's nodules': small indolent papules on hands |
| **Rarer zoonotic poxviruses** | | | |
| Bovine papular stomatitis | Parapoxvirus | European cattle | Localized skin infection, similar to orf |
| Monkeypox | Orthopoxvirus | Monkeys, squirrels | Smallpox-like systemic illness. Restricted to tropical rainforests of W. and central Africa, esp. Zaire |
| Cowpox | Orthopoxvirus | Cows | Localized skin lesions with lymphadenopathy, fever and systemic upset |
| Tanapox | Yabapoxvirus | Monkeys | Localized skin infection |
| Yabapox | Yabapoxvirus | Monkeys | Localized skin infection |

patients over 20 yrs; 60% have joint swelling, which superficially resembles the acute onset of rheumatoid disease. The vast majority recover with no residual joint damage. In children, arthritis is much less common; under 9 yrs of age, only 5% have arthralgia and 3% have joint swelling.

**Infection in patients with haemolytic anaemias**, such as sickle-cell disease, thalassaemia or hereditary spherocytosis may cause **transient aplastic crises**. Infection in the **immunocompromised** (HIV, immunosuppressive drugs, haematological malignancy) can cause persistent infection with chronic anaemia. **Intrauterine infection** infrequently ($\approx$2–10% of maternal infections) causes fetal anaemia, hydrops fetalis (treated by intrauterine blood transfusion) and fetal death. Risk is highest in the first trimester.

**Specific management:** Erythema infectiosum is self-limiting. Chronic anaemia usually responds to iv immunoglobulin.

🖥www.phls.co.uk/topics_az/parvovirus/
gen_info.htm

## Papovaviruses

The papovavirus family contains two subfamilies: papillomaviruses, which cause warts and cervical cancer, and polyomaviruses, which cause disease in the immunocompromised host.

### Papillomaviruses

Very many papillomaviruses have been described. They are each strictly restricted to one species. Over 80 human papillomaviruses (HPV) have been isolated.

**Key biological features:** HPVs grow only in epithelial cells, where they cause benign proliferation of the epithelium. HPVs associated with mucosal infection do not infect skin and vice versa. Certain types of HPV are strongly associated with cervical cancer. Others may cause skin cancers in immunosuppressed individuals and in patients with the rare inherited disorder epidermodysplasia verruciformis.

**Transmission:** By direct contact with an infected person or contaminated object. Swimming-pool transmission occurs. Older children and young adults are most affected; ≈10% of the adult population have warts. Genital warts are spread by sexual contact. Infection may be clinically silent.

**Incubation period:** Warts develop between 1 and 20 months after infection.

**Immunization:** None.

**Diagnosis:** Diagnosis is clinical. Viral culture is not available. A variety of molecular techniques, including PCR and nucleic acid hybridization, are often used in epidemiological research.

**Clinical associations:** Table 35.7.
**Juvenile-onset respiratory papillomata** are due to infection with HPVs causing mucosal warts, probably acquired intrapartum from the maternal genital tract.

**Antiviral therapy:** Specific antiviral therapy is not available. For cutaneous warts, topical preparations of salicylic acid are available. For genital warts, local caustic agents such as podophyllin or trichloracetic acid may be used. Podophyllin is very irritant and excess topical application can lead rarely to systemic toxicity with nausea, vomiting, lethargy and neuropathy. It is anti-mitotic and is therefore contraindicated in pregnancy and infancy. Cryotherapy and surgery may be necessary in some cases.

## Polyomaviruses
Two viruses in this group cause disease in humans. Both JC virus (JCV) and BK virus

**Table 35.7** Clinical associations of human papilomaviruses

| Clinical manifestation | Type |
| --- | --- |
| **Cutaneous warts** | |
| Plantar warts | 1, 2 |
| Common warts | 2, 1, 4 |
| Flat warts | 3, 10, 28, 41 |
| **Mucosal (primarily genital) warts (>91)** | |
| Condylomata acuminata | 6, 11 |
| Flat condylomata | 6, 11, 16, 18, 31 and others |
| Cervical cancer | |
| Strong association | 16, 18 |
| Moderate association | 31, 33, 35, 45, 51, 52, 56 |
| Weak or no association | 6, 11, 42, 43, 44 |
| Association with vulval cancer | 16 |
| Respiratory papillomata | 6, 11 |
| Conjunctival papillomata | 6, 11 |
| Oral mucosal warts | 6, 11, 13, 16, 32 |
| Warts on lips | 2 |

(BKV) are usually only clinically significant in immunosuppressed patients. In both cases, clinical disease is usually due to reactivation of latent viral infection.

**Transmission:** Probably via the respiratory route. Seroprevalence among children in the developed world is 50% at 3 yrs for BKV, and 10–14 yrs for JCV.

**Immunization:** Not available.

**Diagnosis:** Serology is not helpful, as latent infection is very common. Detection of virus by electron microscopy of urine or tissue, or demonstration of viral antigens or DNA by ELISA or PCR are required to confirm active viral replication. PCR on plasma has been used in renal transplant recipients.

**Major clinical associations:**
JCV causes **progressive multifocal leuco-encephalopathy** (>163) in patients with AIDS.

BKV causes **haemorrhagic cystitis** in immunosuppressed patients, particularly bone-marrow transplant recipients. Viruria is common post-renal transplant, but does not always indicate significant disease. BKV infection has been implicated in the development of post-transplant ureteric stenosis. BKV has recently been implicated as a cause of **interstitial nephritis** in renal transplant recipients, affecting up to 5% of transplants and resulting in graft failure in ≈50% of those affected. Differentiation from graft rejection is difficult.

## Hepadnaviruses

This family includes hepatitis B and a variety of related viruses causing hepatitis in animals (e.g. ground squirrel hepatitis virus, duck hepatitis B virus).

**Key biological features:** As well as causing acute hepatitis, HBV establishes latent infection in a small percentage of patients, causing chronic active hepatitis, cirrhosis and hepatocellular carcinoma. **Hepatitis D virus** is a defective RNA virus (36 nm virion, ssRNA 1.7 kb genome) that depends on HBV for replication, and is coated in HBV surface antigen. Infection is therefore restricted to those who are previously or simultaneously infected with HBV.

**Reservoir:** Man.

**Transmission:** By blood and blood products, by sexual transmission and vertically before, during and after delivery. Infectivity varies, depending on carrier status (➤70, 73).

**Diagnosis:** By serology (➤71).

**Immunization:** ➤72.

**Major clinical associations:**
Hepatitis B ➤70.
Hepatitis D ➤73.
Chronic active hepatitis, cirrhosis, hepatocellular carcinoma ➤71.

## Orthomyxoviruses: influenza virus types A, B & C

Influenza viruses primarily cause upper respiratory tract infection. Their importance lies in their ability to cause epidemic disease. Most clinical infections are due to types A and B.

**Key biological features:** Classified serologically into types A, B and C. The antigens that differentiate the three types are internal matrix and nucleoproteins, which are relatively stable and are not accessible to host antibodies. The virus also carries two major surface antigens, haemagglutinin (HA) and neuraminidase (NA), which are variable and are important targets for host antibodies. All three types of virus may alter both HA and NA gradually by mutation, a process known as **antigenic drift**. In addition, for influenza type A (but not types B or C), there are at least 13 subtypes of HA and at least nine subtypes of NA. The emergence of strains expressing different combinations of surface antigens is called **antigenic shift**. So far only $H_{1-3}$ and $N_{1-2}$ have been found in human influenza viruses. These two processes allow the virus to escape host immune responses. Rapid killing of ciliated respiratory epithelium, with impaired respiratory defences for ≈3 weeks.

**Epidemiology:** Infection occurs worldwide. Endemic cases occur continuously in most communities. Focal epidemics associated with antigenic drift occur every few years. Pandemics due to antigenic shift occur every 10–20 yrs. For example, the severe pandemic of 1918 followed the replacement of $H_3N_8$ by $H_1N_1$ as the predominant strain. Since 1977, $H_1N_1$ and $H_3N_2$ subtypes have frequently circulated at the same time. Influenza viruses have a segmented genome, which can result in high rates of reassortment among viruses which coinfect the same cell. It has been suggested that pandemic strains may arise by reassortment of genes between human and animal influenza viruses which simultaneously infect a human host. There was concern that such a reassortment might have occurred when influenza $H_5N_1$ infections were detected in humans, including several fatalities, in Hong Kong in March 1997 at the time of an extensive outbreak of avian influenza $H_5N_1$ in poultry. However, this outbreak of influenza A remained localized to a relatively few cases in humans, for reasons that are not well understood.

**Transmission:** Droplet spread by the respiratory route.

**Incubation period:** 1–5 days.

**Infectious period:** For 1 week after the development of symptoms.

**Immunization:** Vaccine is prepared on an annual basis from recently isolated viruses to take account of antigenic drift. It is usually trivalent, containing 2 type A strains and 1 type B strain and typically gives ≈70% protection for about 1 yr. It is usually given as a single dose in late October/early November. (Children aged 6–35 months: dose is repeated after 4–6 weeks if receiving vaccine for the first time.) It is recommended for patients with cardiac, renal and pulmonary disease (including asthma), for patients with diabetes mellitus and other endocrine disorders, for the immunocompromised, and people >65 yrs. Influenza vaccination is also advocated for patients on long-term aspirin treatment, in an attempt to reduce the risk of Reye syndrome, and is offered to healthcare workers to protect patients, and to prevent disruption of services.

⌨ www.doh.gov.uk/flu/

**Diagnosis:** Most cases occur in the context of local epidemics. Diagnosis may be confirmed by serology, culture or (best) demonstration of viral antigens in respiratory secretions by immunofluorescence (nasopharyngeal aspirate or throat swab).

**Clinical features:** Infection is commonest in children but more severe in the elderly, in whom secondary bacterial pneumonia is more common. Acute onset of fever, rigors, cough and constitutional symptoms including headache, malaise and myalgia. Coryza and sore throat are common but less pronounced than with other viral causes of URTI. Fever and constitutional symptoms usually last 3–4 days. Cough and malaise usually resolve by 1 week. Nausea, vomiting and diarrhoea may occur, particularly in children.

**Complications:** Secondary bacterial pneumonia is common in the elderly and is frequently severe. Infection by *Staphylococcus aureus* is commoner post influenza than under other circumstances and cases of toxic shock syndrome have followed flu (➤84). Other secondary bacterial invaders include *Streptococcus pneumoniae* and *Haemophilus influenzae*. Primary viral pneumonia is uncommon but frequently severe (➤23). It occurs most often in patients with previous cardiac disease, such as mitral stenosis, and during the third trimester of pregnancy. Myocarditis, polymyositis and neurological sequelae including encephalopathy and Guillain–Barré syndrome occur very rarely. Reye syndrome occurs very rarely, usually in association with aspirin use and influenza B. Mean of 10 000 cases of excess mortality attributable to influenza in England and Wales p.a. since 1980.

**Antiviral therapy: Amantadine** is effective for treatment, within 48 h of onset, and prophylaxis of influenza A, but not B or C. Side effects, which occur in 1–5% of patients, include insomnia and agitation. It is very rarely used.

**Zanamivir** (Ralenza™) is an inhaled neuraminidase inhibitor which has been demonstrated to be effective in the prophylaxis and therapy of influenza A and B infections in humans. Most available evidence relates to use in younger persons not at high risk of complications. Current UK guidelines state that zanamivir should only be used for treatment of patients at high risk of complications (defined above for immunization) when flu is circulating (defined as >50 cases per 100 000 population). There is no evidence to guide the use of zanamivir in patients with severe manifestations of influenza.

⌨ www.nice.org.uk
⌨ www.doh.gov.uk/zanamivirguidance

| Genus | Important human viruses | Comments |
|---|---|---|
| Paramyxovirus | Parainfluenza types 1–4 | ➢346 |
| | Mumps | ➢128 |
| | Nipah | ➢346 |
| | Hendra | ➢347 |
| Morbillivirus | Measles | ➢126 |
| Pneumovirus | Respiratory syncytial virus (RSV) | ➢346 |

**Table 35.8** Paramyxoviruses causing disease in humans

## Paramyxoviruses (Table 35.8)

### Parainfluenza virus

**Reservoir:** Man.

**Transmission:** Droplet spread by the respiratory route.

**Epidemiology:** Infection occurs worldwide. Children under 5 yrs are most often affected. Parainfluenza has four serotypes, but does not have the capacity for antigenic shift and drift, and does not therefore cause epidemic disease.

**Incubation period:** 2–6 days.

**Immunization:** Not available.

**Diagnosis:** Viral culture, immunofluorescent antigen detection. Serology is unhelpful, because infection is widespread, and differentiation between types 1–4 is difficult.

#### Major clinical associations

**Upper respiratory tract infection** in children under 5 yrs (➢19). **Lower respiratory tract infection**, which may be severe, is seen in infants under 6 months. Parainfluenza type 3 is particularly associated with bronchiolitis in this age group (➢23).

**Antiviral therapy:** None.

### Respiratory syncytial virus

**Transmission:** Self-inoculation of mucous membranes after contact with infected secretions or contaminated objects.

**Epidemiology:** Demonstrated in 40–50% of children with bronchiolitis and 25% with pneumonia admitted to hospital. In temperate parts of the world, RSV infection has a striking seasonal incidence with peaks occurring in the winter months. These do not occur in tropical areas, and are thought to be due to crowding rather than any climatic effect. Increasingly recognized in adults and the elderly.

**Incubation period:** 2–6 days.

**Immunization:** Active immunization is not available. **Palivizumab** is a monoclonal antibody that reduces morbidity in infants at risk of severe RSV (e.g. ex-premature, or with chronic lung disease). It is very expensive and UK prescribing is tightly controlled ☎.

**Diagnosis:** Serology is unhelpful. Viral culture and rapid diagnostic tests for viral antigens (including ELISA and direct immunofluorescence) in material obtained by nasopharyngeal aspiration are widely used.

**Major clinical associations:**
URTI ➢17.
Croup ➢20.
Otitis media ➢17.
Bronchiolitis in infancy ➢23.
Viral pneumonia ➢23. Causes severe disease in children with immunodeficiency or congenital heart and lung disease.

**Antiviral therapy:** Ribavarin has been used, but its efficacy has not been firmly established ☎.

**Nipah virus** is a newly described paramyxovirus which caused an outbreak of encephalitis in more than 200 patients in Malaysia in 1998–99.

**Transmission:** Presumed to be by direct contact with respiratory secretions and urine of pigs. No cases of human-to-human transmission have thus far been documented.

**Epidemiology:** Patients were predominantly involved in pig farming.

**Incubation period:** 7–40 days.

**Clinical features:** Causes severe illness in pigs, and infection in humans is associated with a mortality rate of approximately 30–40%. Initial presentation is non-specific, characterized by the sudden onset of fever, headache, myalgia, nausea and vomiting. In ≈60%, the disease rapidly progresses, with a deterioration in the state of consciousness, leading to coma, seizures and diverse neurological signs including brainstem involvement within 5–7 days.

MRI shows multiple, small, asymmetrical focal lesions in the subcortical and deep white matter without surrounding oedema probably representing areas of microinfarction that have also been observed on histopathology. CT scans are often normal. CSF and EEG are abnormal.

**Hendra virus** is a paramyxovirus that caused an outbreak of severe respiratory illness in horses in Australia in 1994. Two humans with close contacts to sick horses were affected, and one died. There has been one further fatal human case, in which a farmer died from meningoencephalitis 13 months after close contact with two horses affected by the same disease. The natural host for Hendra virus is believed to be fruit bats, but all human cases of Hendra infection appear to have been acquired through exposure to infected horses.

Ribavirin has *in vitro* activity against Hendra and Nipah virus, and preliminary studies suggest it is effective in human infection.

## Coronaviruses

Two coronaviruses (strains 229E and OC43) cause disease in humans.

**Reservoir:** Man.

**Transmission:** Respiratory droplet spread.

**Epidemiology:** Infection occurs worldwide, primarily in children. Seroprevalence is 90–100% in adults in most communities.

**Incubation period:** 2–5 days.

**Immunization:** Not available.

**Diagnosis:** Viral culture is difficult. Serology is not routinely available.

### Clinical features
**Upper respiratory tract infection** resembling the common cold, with fever, cough coryza and sore throat. Lower respiratory involvement is extremely rare.

**Antiviral therapy:** Not available.

**Comments:** Coronavirus-like particles have been seen by electron microscopy in the stools of some patients with diarrhoea, but these viruses have not been isolated in culture and their identity has yet to be established.

## Picornaviruses

The family *Picornaviridae* contains two large genera of medical importance: *Enteroviridae* and *Rhinoviridae*. The enteroviruses include the polioviruses, echoviruses, coxsackieviruses and numbered enteroviruses. They were all originally isolated from stools, often as part of efforts to control poliomyelitis. The original classification of non-polio enteroviruses into Coxsackie A and B, and echoviruses was made on the basis of their pathogenicity for suckling mice (Coxsackie A viruses are those that cause flaccid paralysis in mice and type B viruses cause spastic paralysis), and does not reflect the clinical features of infection in man. Echovirus (**e**nteric **c**ytopathic **h**uman **o**rphan viruses) are those enteroviruses which do not cause disease in mice. Since 1967, this system of classification has been abandoned and newly discovered enterovirus serotypes are now assigned to the group enterovirus and numbered sequentially (e.g. enterovirus 70).

Hepatitis A virus (➤70) has recently been reclassified as hepatovirus, the only member of the genus Heparnavirus, within the family *Picornaviridae.*

## Polioviruses ✉ ①

**Key biological features:** Poliovirus types 1, 2 and 3 are distinguished serologically, but cause similar disease. The primary site of infection is the epithelium of the intestine and respiratory tract. Neurological involvement with destruction of anterior horn cells and development of paralysis is relatively infrequent.

**Reservoir:** Man.

**Transmission:** Mainly oro–faecal. Spread via the respiratory route occurs and is more important in the developed world where standards of sanitation are higher.

**Epidemiology:** Infection occurs worldwide, but is now very rare in the developed world as a result of successful mass immunization. Polio, like smallpox, is a realistic target for global eradication, as there is no animal reservoir and the vaccine gives good protection. Most cases occurring in the developed world are now associated with vaccine strains (see below).

**Incubation period:** 7–14 days (range 3–35).

**Infectious period:** From 36 h after *exposure.* Virus continues to be excreted in the stools for many weeks (typically 2–4 but often longer).

**Immunization:** Inactivated (Salk) polio vaccine (IPV) was introduced in 1956 and replaced by live attenuated oral polio vaccine (OPV, the Sabin vaccine) in 1962. Persons born before 1958 may therefore not have been immunized. OPV contains live attenuated strains of all three polio types, and provides good mucosal immunity. Vaccine strain virus may be excreted in the stools for many weeks after administration. Because of the very small risk of OPV-associated polio, recently immunized patients and parents of immunized infants should observe careful personal hygiene (particularly washing hands after changing nappies). Paralytic polio following OPV has been estimated to occur in ≈1 in 1 200 000 recipients and 1 in 5 000 000 contacts.

OPV is currently recommended for the immunization of infants from the age of 2 months. Three doses at monthly intervals should be given at the same time as diphtheria/tetanus/pertussis and Hib vaccine (➤417). Non-immunized adults should also receive three doses at monthly intervals. Travellers to polio-endemic or epidemic areas and healthcare workers exposed to cases of polio should receive a booster dose. OPV is safe for use in HIV patients, but is contraindicated in other immunosuppressed patients, for whom IPV is available.

**Diagnosis:** Culture of virus from stool, throat swab or CSF is required to confirm the diagnosis. Two stool samples 24–48 h apart should be obtained as soon as possible after the onset of paralysis in suspected cases. Molecular methods exist but are not routinely available.

**Clinical features:** Fever, headache, malaise and mild gastrointestinal symptoms constitute the only signs of illness in the majority of cases. A small number of patients develop neurological involvement with meningism, usually occurring 3–10 days after the onset of illness. In ≈1 in 1000 cases in children (one in 75 in adults), paralytic polio follows with rapid onset of asymmetrical paralysis, usually affecting the legs. The tendon reflexes are reduced or absent, and there is no sensory deficit. Muscle pain is common. Bulbar paralysis or involvement of the muscles of respiration may also occur. Some functional recovery (occasionally complete) may occur. Denervation is followed by atrophy of affected muscle groups. Neuromuscular symptoms may in some cases continue to progress for many years after acute poliomyelitis.

CSF protein and glucose are usually normal. There is a CSF pleocytosis consistent with viral meningitis (➤97). Differentiation from Guillain–Barré syndrome (GBS) is important, since in that condition the prognosis is better. In GBS, paralysis and sensory deficit are usually symmetrical and ascending, fever is usually absent, the CSF protein is grossly elevated, and pleocytosis is usually mild or absent.

**Antiviral therapy:** There is no specific antiviral therapy. Physical exercise may exacerbate paralysis, and bed rest is indicated during the acute attack. Supportive therapy, including mechanical ventilation, may be required if the respiratory muscles are involved.

**Post-polio syndrome:** A small percentage of polio patients experience a recrudescence of paralysis and muscle atrophy decades after paralytic polio. This is poorly understood; it is not currently thought to be due to active viral infection and has been attributed to the additive effects of physiological aging and long-standing neuromuscular disease.

## Coxsackieviruses, echoviruses, enteroviruses 68–71

**Key biological features:** Like poliovirus, these viruses multiply in the epithelium of the respiratory and gastrointestinal tracts. Virus may be isolated from the stools for many weeks after infection.

**Reservoir:** Man.

**Transmission:** Oro–faecal. Person-to-person, via respiratory or conjunctival secretions.

**Incubation period:** Typically 2–5 days.

**Infectious period:** From the onset of symptoms for several weeks as virus persists in stools.

**Epidemiology:** Infection occurs worldwide. Epidemics due to one serotype occur on the background of endemic cases.

**Immunization:** Not available.

**Diagnosis:** By viral culture from stools, respiratory secretions or CSF. Positive enterovirus IgM indicates recent infection.

**Major clinical associations:** Infection is often asymptomatic or associated with a mild febrile 'flu-like' illness. Most clinical syndromes are associated with a number of different serotypes. With few exceptions, clinical features are not sufficiently distinctive to allow clinical diagnosis of the serotype involved.

Viral meningitis (➤100).

Rarely **viral encephalitis** (➤102) or a paralytic illness resembling polio but not as severe.

**Upper respiratory tract infection** (➤19), **herpangina** (➤135), **hand, foot and mouth disease** (➤135).

Myocarditis (➤55), pericarditis (➤53).

**Acute haemorrhagic conjunctivitis** (➤106), usually due to enterovirus 70 or Coxsackie A24.

**Disseminated neonatal infection** (➤139).

**Bornholm's disease** (syn. 'Devil's grip'): Sudden onset of severe unilateral pain in the intercostal muscles of the chest, worse on breathing. There may be pain in the muscles of the trunk, neck and limbs. Pleurisy and pericarditis may occur. Resolution takes place over 2–3 weeks.

**Antiviral therapy:** Not available.

## Rhinoviruses

**Reservoir:** Man.

**Transmission:** Via respiratory secretions, by direct contact, droplet spread or fomites.

**Incubation period:** 1–4 days.

**Infectious period:** Usually for ≈7 days after the onset of symptoms. Viral shedding may occasionally continue for several weeks.

**Immunization:** Not available.

### Clinical features

**Common cold:** Fever, malaise, sneezing and coryza lasting 3–7 days. Infection may be asymptomatic (➤19).

**Complications:** Sinusitis (➤17), exacerbation of chronic obstructive airways disease (➤24) and secondary pneumonia (➤25). Viral pneumonia does not occur.

**Table 35.9** Reoviruses

| Genus | Important human viruses | Comments |
|---|---|---|
| Reoviruses | | Probably causes some mild URTI and gastrointestinal infections |
| Rotaviruses | Rotavirus group A and B | An important cause of viral diarrhoea (➤350) |
| Orbiviruses | Colorado tick fever virus | |

## Reoviruses (Table 35.9)

### Colorado tick fever

**Reservoir:** Rodents, deer.

**Transmission:** By tick vector—*Dermacentor andersoni*.

**Epidemiology:** Infection is restricted by the geographical distribution of the tick vector to western USA and Canada. Infection is always associated with an occupational or recreational history of tick exposure.

**Incubation period:** 3–6 days.

**Immunization:** Not available.

**Diagnosis:** Serology, detection of viral antigens in serum by immunofluorescence. Not routinely available.

**Clinical features:** Fever, rigors, headache, malaise. Recovery is usually complete by 7–10 days. ≈10% complicated by meningoencephalitis, particularly children. Very rare haemorrhagic manifestations.

**Antiviral therapy:** Not available.

**Comments:** In addition to Colorado tick fever, the genus *Orbivirus* contains many important animal pathogens, all of which are vector-borne (tick, mosquito, midge). Some occasionally cause human disease, e.g. Kemerovo (Russia) and Lipovnik (Czech Republic).

### Rotaviruses and other agents causing viral gastroenteritis

Diarrhoea and vomiting are particularly associated with infection by rotavirus, adenovirus (➤334), astrovirus, calicivirus and Norwalk and Norwalk-like viruses (small round structured viruses, *Norovirus*).

**Epidemiology:** Infection occurs worldwide. In the developed world, rotavirus is responsible for ≥50% of diarrhoeal illness in children requiring hospitalization. In the developing world, viral diarrhoea and dehydration account for several million childhood deaths per annum. Rotavirus infections have a seasonal incidence in temperate regions, peaking in winter months. Rotavirus, astrovirus and calicivirus are typically infections of infants and children. Norwalk is more often associated with epidemics or family outbreaks and affects individuals of all ages.

**Key biological features:** Replication occurs in the small intestine, causing malabsorption and osmotic diarrhoea. Colitis is not a feature and faecal pus cells are not seen.

**Reservoir:** Man.

**Transmission:** Oro–faecal, by direct contact, contaminated water or food, particularly cold foods requiring handling, such as salads and sandwiches. Inhalation of aerosol from vomit or faeces. The infectious dose of rotavirus is tiny ($\approx$10–100 virions), and during acute infection faeces may contain $10^{11}$ virions/g. Minor contamination of the environment may therefore be highly significant, particularly in nosocomial infection.

**Incubation period:** 1–2 days.

**Immunization:** Not available.

**Table 35.10** Retroviruses

| Genus | Important human viruses | Comments |
|---|---|---|
| Oncoviruses | Human T-cell lymphotrophic virus (HTLV) I and II | Genus includes many oncogenic animal viruses |
| Lentiviruses | Human immunodeficiency virus (HIV) 1 and 2 ($\blacktriangleright$143) | Animal viruses include slow viruses (e.g. visna) and immunodeficiency viruses (e.g. simian immunodeficiency virus, SIV) |
| Spumaviruses | No human pathogens | |

**Diagnosis:** Electron microscopy of stools. This can be made more sensitive by using specific antisera to concentrate viruses (immuno-electron microscopy). For rotavirus rapid diagnostic methods based on specific monoclonal antibodies, such as latex agglutination or ELISA, or detection of rotavirus genome by electrophoresis (PAGE) are in widespread routine use, but are less sensitive and specific. Caliciviruses and astroviruses have characteristic appearances on electron microscopy, but detailed knowledge of their structure is lacking.

**Clinical features:** Vomiting, diarrhoea, abdominal cramps, dehydration. Fever and constitutional symptoms such as headache and myalgia are common. Recovery normally occurs in 2–4 days. Infection may be severe or prolonged in immunodeficient or malnourished patients. Asymptomatic infection and faecal shedding are common ($\blacktriangleright$10). Outbreaks among staff and patients on wards for the elderly can be disruptive and difficult to control ☎. Clean spillages with hot water and detergent. Close wards to new admissions. Isolate patients and keep affected staff off work for 48 h after last episode of diarrhoea or vomiting.

**Antiviral therapy:** No specific antiviral therapy. Supportive treatment, in particular correction of dehydration, is paramount. Rotavirus vaccines are in development.

# Retroviruses (Table 35.10)

**Key biological features:** Retroviruses have a reverse transcriptase enzyme that transcribes their RNA genome into DNA, which then integrates into the host genome. The biology of HIV infection is discussed elsewhere ($\blacktriangleright$143).

## HTLV-I

**Reservoir:** Man.

**Transmission:** Sexual transmission. By blood products (therapeutic or as a result of IVDU). Vertical transmission, particularly by breast feeding.

**Epidemiology:** Infection common in certain countries, particularly Japan, the Caribbean islands and South America. Unusual in UK residents.

**Immunization:** Not available.

**Diagnosis:** Serology indicates infection, but disease affects only a small percentage of infected individuals.

**Major clinical associations:** No acute clinical illness has been associated with acquisition of HTLV-I.

    **Adult T-cell leukaemia/lymphoma** (ATL) affects $\approx$1% of infected individuals. It presents at a mean age of 50 yrs and the latent period between infection and development of disease is $\geq$20 yrs. It presents as an aggressive leukaemia or lymphoma due to clonal expansion of lymphocytes (shown to contain the virus).

    **Tropical spastic paraparesis** is a progressive spastic myelopathy with pyramidal, sensory and sphincteric disturbance. It occurs after a variable latent period, which has been as short

**Table 35.11** Togaviruses

| Genus | Important human viruses | Comments |
|---|---|---|
| Rubiviridae | Rubella | ➤127 |
| Alphaviridae | Eastern and Western equine encephalitis viruses, Venezuelan equine encephalitis virus | Arthropod-borne viruses causing encephalitis (➤102) |
| | Chikungunya (SE Asia, Africa) O'nyong-nyong (Africa) Ross River virus (Australia, S. Pacific) Sindbis (Africa, Asia, Russia, Australia, Europe) Mayaro (Caribbean, S. America) | Arthropod-borne viruses causing febrile illness similar to dengue, often with prominent arthralgia (➤123) |

**Table 35.12** Commoner human flavivirus infections

| Virus | Comments |
|---|---|
| Yellow fever virus | ➤352 |
| Dengue virus serotypes 1–4 | ➤353 |
| Kyansur Forest disease/Omsk haemorrhagic fever | ➤354 |
| **Arthropod-borne viruses causing encephalitis (➤102)** | |
| Japanese B encephalitis | ➤354 |
| Tick-borne encephalitis | ➤354 |
| Powassan | Rare tick-borne zoonotic encephalitis of N. America |
| St Louis encephalitis, Murray Valley encephalitis | |
| **Arthropod-borne virus causing febrile illness similar to dengue** | |
| West Nile virus (India and E. Africa) | ➤102, 354 |

as a few months in patients infected by blood transfusion, but is usually many years; 20–40% of patients are seronegative for HTLV-I suggesting that this is a heterogeneous syndrome. Most patients have high-titre antibodies and infectious virus in their CSF.

HTLV-I is also associated with a **chronic inflammatory arthropathy**, which can also occur in patients with ATL.

### HTLV-II

This virus appears to be transmitted by blood products, as there is a high prevalence among IVDUs. It has been associated with hairy T-lymphocytic leukaemia, and chronic lymphocytic leukaemia.

## Togaviruses (Table 35.11)

Rubella ➤127.

## Flaviviruses

Apart from the important human pathogens listed in Table 35.12, there are many named vector-transmitted flavivirus infections that cause disease in geographically restricted areas, e.g. Edge Hill (Australia), Negishi (Japan, China, Russia).

### Yellow fever (YF) ✉

**Epidemiology:** Found in tropical South America and sub-Saharan Africa, between 15° N and 15°

S. In urban YF, which currently occurs only in Africa, human-to-human transmission occurs via mosquito bite (*Aedes aegypti*). In jungle YF, infection is maintained by enzootic infection of monkeys, transmitted by *Hemagogus* and *Aedes* spp. mosquitoes. In this situation, human infection follows jungle exposure.

**Incubation period:** 3–6 days.

**Infectious period:** Blood is infective for mosquitoes for the first 3–5 days of illness. YF is not transmissible by contact.

**Clinical features:** Typically a biphasic illness. Abrupt onset of fever, rigors, headache, backache, myalgia, nausea and vomiting. After 3–4 days, symptoms and fever remit for 1–2 days and then recur. Jaundice, hepatic and renal failure, which may progress to acute tubular necrosis, disseminated intravascular coagulopathy, mucosal bleeding, GI haemorrhage and myocarditis may occur. Case fatality rate depends on the quality of supportive management, but may be as high as 40%.

**Investigations:** Leucopenia, thrombocytopenia, abnormal liver function tests and disordered clotting. Diagnosis is confirmed by serology, by the identification of viral antigens in serum by a number of rapid diagnostic methods, or by culture of the virus.

**Antiviral therapy:** None.

**Supportive management:** Attention to fluid balance, specific treatment for coagulopathy, and management of renal and hepatic failure may all be required. Secondary bacterial sepsis may occur.

**Immunization:** Recovery from YF gives complete lifelong protection against further attacks. A live attenuated vaccine is available. Immunization (➤193), confirmed by a valid certificate, is required for entry to many countries. A single dose of vaccine gives ≥99% protection. Revaccination is required after 10 yrs, although protection probably lasts for life. Vaccination is currently recommended in the UK for laboratory workers handling infected material, travellers over the age of 9 months intending to visit infected areas, and persons requiring a valid certificate of immunization for entry into particular countries. Vaccination is not recommended under the age of 9 months, unless exposure is unavoidable.

## Dengue

**Epidemiology:** Four serotypes, widely distributed in Asia, Africa, Northern Australia, Central and South America, including the Caribbean. Animal reservoirs, e.g. monkeys, exist in some regions. Transmission occurs by the bite of an infected mosquito, usually *Aedes aegypti*.

**Incubation period:** 3–14 days (usually 7–10).

**Infectious period:** Blood is infective for mosquitoes for the first 5 days of illness. Person-to-person spread does not occur.

**Clinical features:** Abrupt onset of fever, rigors, severe headache and backache, myalgia, arthralgia, nausea and vomiting. Generalized maculopapular rash and lymphadenopathy develop, usually as fever wanes after 3–5 days. A second lower peak of fever is often seen. Leucopenia, thrombocytopenia and abnormal liver function tests are usual.

**Antiviral therapy:** None.

**Complications: Dengue haemorrhagic fever** (DHF). This syndrome typically presents with rapid clinical deterioration and shock after 2–5 days of milder febrile illness. DHF is thought to be caused by second infections with a different dengue serotype in individuals with protective immunity against one serotype, a phenomenon known as antibody-dependent enhancement. It is commoner in children and may occur in epidemics following the introduction of a new dengue serotype to susceptible populations. DHF is characterized by abnormal vascular permeability, hypovolaemia and abnormal clotting. Classical clinical signs include hypotension and tachycardia, restlessness and sweating, facial pallor with circumoral cyanosis and hepatomegaly. Spontaneous bruising and GI haemorrhage may occur. Mortality rates may be as high as 40%. Fluid replacement and treatment of coagulopathy are required. After 24–36 h of crisis, recovery is fairly rapid in those that survive.

## Japanese B encephalitis

**Epidemiology:** Endemic in Indian sub-continent, SE Asia, NE Asia, including Japan. A zoonosis, primarily acquired from pigs, that infects humans as an incidental host. It is a major public health problem in Asia where an estimated 50 000 cases occur annually.

**Transmission:** By *Culex* mosquitoes.

**Incubation period:** 5–15 days.

**Infectious period:** Person-to-person spread does not occur.

**Clinical features:** Most infections are subclinical. Can cause severe encephalitis, indistinguishable from other viral encephalitides (➤102). Case fatality rate is 10–30%; long-term disability is seen in 30% of survivors.

**Immunization:** (➤193).

## Tick-borne encephalitis

**Epidemiology:** Endemic in Scandinavia, Central and Northern Europe. Occurs rarely in Scotland. Also Siberia, where it tends to be more severe.

**Transmission:** By the tick *Ixodes ricinus* in Europe.

**Incubation period:** 7–14 days.

**Clinical features:** European forms cause mild biphasic meningoencephalitis. Siberian form more severe (polio-encephalomyelitis) with significant mortality.

**Immunization:** (➤194).

## West Nile virus

Mosquito-borne avian zoonosis causing an illness similar to dengue. Previously restricted to Africa, Eastern Europe and Asia, cases were reported in New York in 1999 and Israel in 2000.

Currently spreading west across the USA. Serosurveys suggest 20% of infected persons developed febrile illness, <1% had encephalitis, among whom mortality was ≈5%, commoner in the elderly. These epidemics were associated with high death rate among birds (particularly crows in New York). Control by mosquito vector avoidance and control. Subunit vaccines in development.

## Kyansur Forest disease/Omsk haemorrhagic fever ✉

These two closely related viruses are geographically restricted to the Kyansur Forest in India and the steppes of Siberia, respectively.

**Transmission:** By tick bite. Person-to-person spread does not occur.

**Incubation period:** 3–8 days.

**Clinical features:** Febrile illness with myalgia, GI disturbance and conjunctivitis. There may be a papulovesicular eruption on the soft palate and cervical lymphadenopathy. Encephalitis and haemorrhage may occur. Case fatality rate is estimated at 1–10%.

## Hepacivirus

Hepatitis C virus has recently been reclassified as the only member of the new genus hepacivirus, in the family *Flaviviridae* (➤73).

# Bunyaviruses

Over 200 bunyaviruses have been described. They are nearly all arthropod-borne infections causing fever and occasionally encephalitis. They are restricted geographically and are often named after the region in which they occur (Table 35.13).

## Crimean–Congo haemorrhagic fever (CCHF) ✉④

**Epidemiology:** Widely distributed throughout tropical Africa, the Middle East, Southern USSR and the Balkans.

**Reservoir/Transmission:** Hares, birds and *Hyalomma* spp. ticks, which are also the vector

**Table 35.13** Human bunyavirus infections

| Serogroup | Important human viruses | Comments |
|---|---|---|
| California | California<br>La Crosse<br>Jamestown Canyon | Arthropod-borne viruses causing encephalitis (➤102) |
| Phlebovirus | Rift Valley fever<br>Sandfly fever<br>Toscana virus | Mosquito vector. E. Africa<br>Sandfly vector. Mediterranean area and Middle East<br>Sandfly vector. Italy |
| Nairovirus | Crimean–Congo haemorrhagic fever virus | (➤354) |
| Hantavirus | Hantaan virus | Haemorrhagic fever with renal syndrome (Old World) (➤355) |
| | Sin Nombre (Four Corners) virus | Hantavirus pulmonary syndrome (USA) (➤356) |

for human infection. Nosocomial person-to-person spread has occurred.

**Incubation period:** 3–12 days.

**Clinical features:** Fever, malaise, headache, severe myalgia. Facial flush and conjunctival injection. Palatal petechiae and petechial rash on trunk. GI haemorrhage and haematuria may develop in association with severe hepatitis. Leucopenia, thrombocytopenia, disordered liver function tests and abnormal renal function are common. Reported case fatality rates vary from 5% to 50%.

**Diagnosis:** By serology or by isolation of virus from blood.

**Antiviral therapy:** CCHF is sensitive to ribavarin, and there are limited clinical data suggesting useful efficacy.

**Immunization:** Killed vaccine is available in E. Europe and China—no published trials.

### Hantavirus infections

Hantaviruses have been associated with two distinct human infections. Hantaan virus causes **haemorrhagic fever with renal syndrome** in the Old World, esp. Asia. Sin Nombre virus causes **hantavirus pulmonary syndrome** in the New World.

### Haemorrhagic fever with renal syndrome ⊠

**Epidemiology:** Common throughout Japan, Korea, China. Rarer in Europe, although serological evidence suggests subclinical infection, including in the UK.

**Reservoir:** Rodents.

**Transmission:** By direct contact with rodent urine, or fomites contaminated with rodent urine. Person-to-person spread does not occur.

**Incubation period:** Usually 12–21 days (range 5–42 days).

**Immunization:** Not available.

**Clinical features:** Mild non-specific prodrome followed by abrupt onset of fever, headache, myalgia and GI disturbance. Haemorrhage (petechiae and GI) may develop, with severe hypovolaemic shock and acute renal failure. Leucocytosis, thrombocytopenia, abnormal renal function and prolonged bleeding time are commonly seen.

**Antiviral therapy:** Ribavarin has been shown to be effective in China; further trials are ongoing.

## Hantavirus pulmonary syndrome

First recognized in 1993 in the Four Corners region of SW USA, and now known to be caused by the newly characterized Sin Nombre virus (also known as Four Corners virus). By 1997, cases had been reported in 26 US states, Canada and S. America. Cases due to other hantaviruses (Bayou virus, Black Creek Canal virus, New York virus) have been described.

**Reservoir:** Rodents.

**Transmission:** By inhalation of aerosolized rodent excreta.

**Incubation period:** ≈3 weeks.

**Clinical features:** After a non-specific prodrome, non-cardiogenic pulmonary oedema, shock and thrombocytopenia develop. Case fatality rates of ≈50% have been reported.

**Antiviral therapy:** Ribavarin is effective *in vitro*, but a limited clinical trial showed no benefit in human infection.

## Viral haemorrhagic fever (VHF) ✉④☧

Viruses from several families cause febrile infections associated with severe haemorrhage and shock, including bunyaviruses, arenaviruses and filoviruses.

> Special isolation procedures are required to prevent cross-infection of patients, staff and laboratory workers (➤206).

## Arenaviruses ✉④

**Epidemiology:** Geographically restricted, as indicated in Table 35.14. Primarily rural disease of developing countries. Infection is associated with rodent exposure, occupational or domestic. Lassa fever (LF) is hyperendemic in two distinct areas of W. Africa (Nigeria; Sierra Leone, Guinea and Liberia), where there are an estimated 400 000 cases p.a., with an overall mortality of ≈2%.

**Reservoir:** Rodents. For LF, the multimammate mouse *Mastomys natalensis*.

**Transmission:** From rodent to human by contact with urine. Person-to-person transmission has been recorded, but it is not common, especially in hospitals in the developed world. Isolation is essential (➤206).

**Incubation period:** Usually 6–21 days.

**Infectious period:** Virus may be isolated from the urine of patients with LF for 3–9 weeks post infection.

**Immunization:** Not available.

**Diagnosis:** Serology, viral culture.

**Table 35.14** Arenavirus infections

| Virus | Distribution | Comments |
| --- | --- | --- |
| Lymphocytic choriomeningitis virus (LCV) | Worldwide | A pathogen of mice. Human cases are rare. May cause severe meningoencephalitis |
| Lassa fever (LF) | W. Africa | ➤356 |
| Argentine HF (AHF, Junin) | Argentina | Vaccine available |
| Bolivian HF (BHF, Machupo) | Bolivia | |
| Venezuelan HF (Guanarito) | Venezuela | |
| Brazilian HF (Sabia) | Brazil | Very rare |

Clinical features: Gradual onset of fever, headache, myalgia, vomiting and diarrhoea. Pharyngitis with exudate is common in LF but unusual in AHF and BHF. Bleeding from mucosal surfaces and into skin may occur (15–20% of LF, >50% in AHF and BHF). Petechiae and jaundice are not seen in LF, but a petechial rash is common in AHF and BHF. Death is associated with haemorrhage, shock and non-cardiogenic pulmonary oedema. Fatality rates of 15–30% are reported for hospital cases, but serology indicates that subclinical infection is common.

Antiviral therapy: Ribavarin (➤361) improves prognosis significantly in LF and may be of benefit in other arenavirus infections. Convalescent serum has also been used.

## Filoviruses ④☒

Two filoviruses, Marburg and Ebola, cause similar severe, often fatal haemorrhagic illnesses in monkeys and humans. Unlike Lassa, filoviruses are not endemic in humans, and occur in small epidemics with high attack rate and mortality.

Marburg ('Green Monkey disease') was first recognized after an outbreak in 1967 in German lab workers handling infected African Green monkeys imported from Uganda. Since then, sporadic cases have been reported from Kenya and Southern Africa. In 1999–2000 there was an outbreak in Congo (formerly Zaire) involving up to 100 cases with high mortality.

Ebola was first described in 1976 in S. Sudan and W. Zaire (>600 cases, mortality 72%). Subsequent major outbreaks have occurred in Kikwit, Zaire in 1995 (315 cases, mortality 81%), in Gabon in 1994–6 (≈130 cases, mortality 63%) and in Uganda in 2000 (425 cases, mortality 53%). At the time of writing (early 2002), there is an ongoing epidemic in Gabon, with ≈50 cases and ≈40 deaths.

Reservoir: Probably monkeys, possibly bats.

Transmission: Person-to-person transmission occurs by direct contact. Isolation is essential (➤206).

Immunization: Not available.

Diagnosis: Serology, viral culture.

Clinical features: Abrupt onset of fever, headache, myalgia, malaise, followed by GI and then generalized haemorrhage. Maculopapular rash develops 7–10 days after onset. Lab findings include neutrophilia, thrombocytopenia and raised ALT.

Antiviral therapy: Not available.

🖳www.who.int/emc
🖳www.cdc.gov/ncidod

# Rhabdoviruses

## Rabies ☒ ④

Key biological features: Rabies virus (genus Lyssavirus) causes encephalitis and neuronal degeneration. Post-mortem histology of brain shows changes similar to other viral encephalitides. Negri bodies are pathognomic cytoplasmic inclusion bodies, present in 70–90% of cases. Virus may also be found extracranially, e.g. in salivary glands, corneal epithelium and cutaneous nerves.

Epidemiology: Rabies is now rare in all developed countries, but remains common elsewhere. Rabies-free areas include United Kingdom, most West Indian islands, Finland, Iceland, Sweden, Japan, Taiwan, New Zealand.

Reservoir: Many different mammalian species, particularly canines, cats, bats. Since 1903, all UK cases have been imported, nearly all after dog bites. In 2002 a patient in Scotland died after acquiring rabies from a bat.

Transmission: Infection occurs by inoculation of virus into peripheral tissues usually by the bite of an infected animal. Virus ascends along peripheral nerves to the CNS and then descends to skin, cornea and salivary glands. Virus does not penetrate intact skin. Human-to-human transmission via saliva is theoretically possible, but has only been recorded after corneal grafting. Isolation procedures are indicated. Infection has occurred by inhalation and inoculation onto mucous membranes.

**Incubation period:** Usually 3–78 days; >90 days in 15%. Range 9 days to several years. Heavy contamination and cephalic location of bite are associated with short incubation.

**Immunization:** Two safe modern vaccines are available (HDCV, PCEC ➢194). Older vaccines, such as duck embryo vaccine (DEV), are cheaper but are associated with a high incidence of minor local and systemic adverse effects, and very infrequently with encephalitis. DEV is still widely used in developing countries. Rabies specific immunoglobulin (RIG) is now prepared from serum of hyperimmunized individuals. See below under 'Prevention' for recommendations on vaccine use.

**Diagnosis:** Serology, viral culture, antigen detection in tissue and histology.

**Major clinical associations:** Infection is not inevitable after exposure. Risk depends on degree of contamination, post-exposure treatment and vaccination status. Once infection is established, death is inevitable. (Three cases of recovery have been reported.) Following incubation, there is a 2–10 day prodrome of fever, headache, GI symptoms, anorexia and fatigue. Mental changes may be present at this stage. Pain and paraesthesiae at the site of the bite may occur. The prodrome is followed by the neurological phase, which lasts 2–7 days. This may be 'furious', with disorientation, hallucinations and hyperactivity. Pharyngeal and laryngeal spasms causing choking or vomiting may be triggered by attempts to eat or drink, causing the classical symptom of hydrophobia. Other stimuli, such as cold air, loud noises or bright lights may also trigger spasms, which may progress to generalized convulsions. Some 20% develop 'dumb' rabies, with paralysis, either ascending and symmetrical, or more pronounced on the side of the bite. The neurological phase is followed by coma (usual duration 3–13 days) and death.

**Antiviral therapy:** No treatment is effective once infection has developed. Full supportive therapy is given, but the chance of survival is very slight.

**Prevention:** Prevention depends on avoiding contact with infected animals, pre-exposure vaccination of those at risk of contact, and post-exposure vaccination of patients who present after being bitten. Fox rabies has been well controlled in Europe by the use of oral vaccine distributed on bait.

**Pre-exposure vaccination** (➢194) is currently recommended in the UK for laboratory workers handling virus, those likely to have occupational exposure to imported animals (e.g. zoo workers, bat handlers, Customs officials), workers in enzootic areas whose occupation puts them at risk of exposure, and travellers to enzootic areas who are at risk of being infected and who are undertaking long journeys where medical aid may not be immediately available. Three doses of HDCV are given on days 0, 7, 28.

**Post-exposure management:** Bite wounds should be scrubbed with soap and water for 5 min under a running tap as soon as possible. The animal should be captured and observed for 10 days if possible. Local advice should be sought about the risk of rabies associated with the species of animal involved. If preventive treatment is considered necessary, vaccine (six doses on days 0, 3, 7, 14, 30, 90) should be started immediately. Rabies-specific immunoglobulin (20 IU/kg) should be given; half infiltrated around the bite and half given im. Previously immunized individuals should receive two doses of HDCV; RIG is not required.

In the UK, rabies concerns always involve patients returning from enzootic areas. Advice may be sought the Communicable Diseases Branch of the Department of Health (020 7972 4481, or out of hours 020 7210 3000), from the Virus Reference Laboratory, Central Public Health Laboratory (020 8200 4400) and from the Scottish Centre for Infection and Environmental Health (0141 946 7120).

⬛www.doh.gov.uk/memorandumonrabies/

**Vesicular stomatitis virus** (genus *Vesiculovirus*) is an infrequent cause of fever, with oral mucosal vesicles, spread by sandflies, usually in animal handlers. Widespread distribution in tropical and subtropical regions of N. and S. America.

**Table 35.15** Slow virus infections of the CNS

| Family | Virus | Disease | Comments |
|---|---|---|---|
| Polyoma | JC virus | Progressive multifocal leucoencephalopathy | ➤163, 343 |
| Paramyxovirus | Measles | Subacute sclerosing panencephalitis | ➤127 |
| Togavirus | Rubella | Rubella panencephalitis | Very rare complication of congenital or early childhood rubella. Presents in teens with intellectual impairment, seizures, myoclonus, spasticity and ataxia |

# Slow virus infections of the CNS

Several conventional viruses cause CNS infections that develop over months or years (Table 35.15).

# Diseases caused by prions ☷

Prion diseases (Table 35.16) are neurodegenerative conditions with a long incubation period and inexorable progression to death once symptoms appear. They share the following neuropathological features: neuronal loss, glial proliferation, absence of an inflammatory response and vacuolation leading to a spongiform appearance.

Prions are now believed to be infectious proteins with no nucleic acid. Prion proteins have the same amino-acid sequence as a cellular protein, but a different three-dimensional conformation—i.e. they are folded differently. Prions 'reproduce' by stimulating the cellular protein to adopt the abnormal conformation of the prion protein, typically changing from a structure rich in α-helices to one rich in β-sheets. These changes are associated with loss of function and resistance to degradation. Animal models suggest that prion proteins accumulate first in follicular dendritic cells in the peripheral lymphoid system, and are then transported to the CNS by axonal transport. Disease results from accumulation of abnormal protein in the CNS. This process can also occur as a consequence of an inherited or sporadic genetic mutation leading to an abnormal cellular protein. Inherited mutations in the cellular protein are also involved in susceptibility to exogenous prion proteins and the pattern of disease that results.

**Five human prion diseases** have been described (Table 35.16). Closely related diseases in animals include scrapie in sheep and bovine spongiform encephalopathy (BSE, 'mad cow disease').

The epidemic of BSE in the UK in the 1980s has been attributed to feeding cattle prion-contaminated meat and bone meal, following changes in rendering practices. Subsequently, a new form of Creutzfeld–Jakob disease (CJD) known as **new variant CJD** (vCJD) has been identified in humans. vCJD is different from previous forms of CJD in the following ways: younger age (mean 29 vs. 65 yrs); less rapid progression (mean 14 vs 4 months from onset to death); different presenting symptoms, with prominent sensory and psychiatric symptoms at onset. Most cases of vCJD have initially been diagnosed as depression. There is increasing evidence that vCJD represents bovine-to-human transmission of BSE, and suggestions that BSE is derived from scrapie.

New regulations on animal feeding and husbandry have led to a dramatic decline in cases of BSE, but the extent of the human epidemic of vCJD remains to be seen. By the end of 2002 there had been ≈120 deaths from confirmed or probable vCJD, with a further 10 probable cases still alive.

**Table 35.16** Human prion diseases

| Disease | Mechanism | Clinical features |
|---|---|---|
| Kuru | Restricted to the Fore people of Papua New Guinea. Disease is disappearing with the discontinuation of cannibalism | Ataxia, dysarthria and tremor, progressing to chorea, flaccid paralysis and death 3–9 months after onset |
| Creutzfeld–Jakob disease Iatrogenic (iCJD) | Infection via human growth hormone, dura mater grafts, etc. | Memory loss, abnormal behaviour and personality change followed by myoclonus, ataxia and extrapyramidal rigidity. Progression to death over 4–7 months |
| Familial (fCJD) | Inherited mutation in prion protein gene | |
| Sporadic (sCJD) | ?Somatic mutation in prion protein gene | |
| New variant Creutzfeld–Jakob disease (vCJD) | ?Infection by bovine prions. Almost all cases reported in UK | Mean age at onset 29 yrs. Sensory and psychiatric abnormalities prominent at outset. Dementia and motor signs follow. Mean duration to death 14 months |
| Gerstmann–Sträussler–Scheinker syndrome (GSS) | Autosomal-dominant mutation in prion protein gene | Extensive spinocerebellar involvement, causing severe gait disturbance, incoordination and dysarthria in addition to dementia |
| Fatal familial insomnia (FFI) | Inherited mutation in prion protein gene. First reported in Italian families, but kindreds now identified worldwide | Rapidly fatal (mean duration 13 months) occurring in midlife. Progressive insomnia, behavioural changes and eventually motor symptoms. Endocrine disturbance (hyperhidrosis, hyperthermia, tachycardia, hypertension) |

Prions are resistant to treatments that inactivate conventional viruses, such as boiling, irradiation and disinfectants including alcohol, aldehydes and β-propriolactone. They are an infection hazard to staff handling neurological material post mortem. Transmission of CJD has occurred after corneal and dura mater transplantation, by purified human growth hormone and by contaminated stereotactic electrodes. Based on experimental work with scrapie, these agents might be destroyed by autoclaving at 132°C for 1 h or by immersion in 1 N sodium hydroxide.

Measures are in place to reduce risk of transmission by blood products and reusable surgical instruments, particularly those used in procedures which involve extensive handling of lymphoid tissue, e.g. tonsillectomy ☎. Adequate washing and cleaning of reusable instruments and selective use of disposable equipment are mainstays of risk management.

↪ Collinge J, Lancet 1999; 354: 317
↪ Prusiner SB, New Engl J Med 2001; 344: 1516
💻 www.bse.org.uk
💻 www.doh.gov.uk/cjd/index.hm
💻 www.defra.gov.uk/animalh/bse/index.html

**Table 35.17** Summary of antiviral therapy*

| Agent | Indications, comments | Adverse effects |
|-------|----------------------|-----------------|
| Aciclovir | Herpes simplex (➤129, ➤334) and herpes zoster virus infections (➤130, ➤339) | Rare. Rash, GI upset, CNS toxicity. Renal toxicity due to crystalluria |
| Valaciclovir | Pro-drug of aciclovir. Similar range of activity and adverse effects. Achieves high intracellular levels with simpler dosage schedule | |
| Famciclovir | Pro-drug of penciclovir. Similar range of activity and adverse effects. Achieves high intracellular levels with simpler dosage schedule | |
| Ganciclovir | Life- or sight-threatening CMV infection in immunocompromised patients. For use in HIV infection ➤166. For use in renal failure see data sheet. Oral preparation is poorly absorbed, and used mainly in maintenance therapy | Common. Severe myelotoxicity. Contraindicated in pregnancy and lactation. Fever, rash, abnormal liver function. |
| Valganciclovir | Recently licensed oral pro-drug of ganciclovir that will probably replace ganciclovir for most indications (➤166) | |
| Foscarnet | Alternative to ganciclovir for CMV retinitis in AIDS (➤166) | Nephrotoxicity, hypo- or hypercalcaemia, hyperphosphataemia, anaemia, hepatotoxicity, nausea. Maintain hydration and reduce dose in renal impairment 🗎 |
| Amantadine | Prophylaxis of influenza A (➤345) | Nausea, insomnia, fits |
| Zanamivir | Prophylaxis and treatment of influenza (➤345) | |
| Ribavarin Inhaled | Severe RSV bronchiolitis in infants (➤23). | No significant adverse effects, but administration to ventilated children is difficult |
| Oral | In combination with interferon for treatment of HCV (➤74). Experimental use in Lassa fever (➤357), haemorrhagic fever with renal syndrome (➤355) and Congo–Crimea HF (➤354) | Haemolytic anaemia, nausea, stomatitis 🗎 |

* For anti-HIV drugs ➤148.

**Investigations:** CSF is normal. EEG is abnormal, but the changes are not diagnostic. Diagnosis is usually made clinically and confirmed by post-mortem neuropathology. Tests to measure prion protein in blood and other accessible tissues are in development.

# Summary of antiviral therapy

The availability of antiviral drugs has improved considerably over the past decade. Table 35.17 summarizes the characteristics of currently available drugs. Anti-HIV therapy is discussed elsewhere (➤148). Dosing of aciclovir in renal failure is shown in Table 35.18.

**Table 35.18** Aciclovir dosing in renal failure (doses in parentheses for serious infection)

| | | Serum creatinine ($\mu$mol/L) | | |
|---|---|---|---|---|
| | Normal dose | 150–300 | 300–700 | >700; dialysis |
| Oral | For HSV treatment: 200 mg (400 mg) 5 times daily<br>Prophylaxis: 200 mg (400 mg) q6h<br>Varicella and zoster: 800 mg 5 times daily | For HSV, see left. | For HSV, see left.<br><br>For varicella and zoster: 800 mg q8h (q6h) | For HSV treatment: 200 mg q12h<br>Varicella and zoster: 800 mg q12h |
| IV | 5 (10) mg/kg q8h | 5 (10) mg/kg q12h | 5 (10) mg/kg q24h | 2.5 (5) mg/kg q24h |

Effect of dialysis: HD: >50%. PD: 5–20%. Give dose after HD.

# Chapter 36

# Fungi

Primitive eukaryotes, the vast majority of which are saprophytic and do not cause disease in humans. Many of the remainder are frequent human commensals. Disease may be caused by tissue invasion, by release of toxins (e.g. aflatoxins), and/or by immunological stimulation (e.g. asthma). Most pathogenic fungi are dimorphic (capable of existing in two forms, depending upon environmental conditions). Each pathogenic fungus causes infection within the human body in one or other of these two forms:

• Hyphal or mould-like (e.g. *Aspergillus* spp.): branching filaments, interweaving to form a mycelium, often (outside the body) forming specialized reproductive bodies carrying asexual or sexual spores (Table 36.1).

• Yeast-like (e.g. *Candida* spp.): single spherical or oval cells, reproducing by asexual budding. Yeast forms often produce unbranched chains of elongated cells, known as a pseudomycelium (Table 36.2).

Provisional identification of fungi is performed in most diagnostic laboratories by a combination of microscopical and colonial morphology, and some biochemical tests. All stain Gram-positive. Commercial identification kits now quite reliable for yeasts, and indicator media useful for preliminary identification (e.g. ChromAgar). Atypical or unfamiliar isolates ✈. Antimicrobial sensitivity testing of fungi not performed by most laboratories (✈), but new commercial kits are reliable with experience.

Population-based studies in the USA have revealed that fungal infection is the seventh most common cause of infectious disease-related death, and that the commonest causative agents of infection in order of frequency are *Candida* spp. (72.8 million cases p.a.), *Cryptococcus* spp., *Coccidioides* spp., *Aspergillus* spp., and *Histoplasma* spp. (7.1 million). HIV infection is the commonest predisposing factor, in 47%.

Definitive or adjunctive surgical management of serious fungal infection should be considered especially with: fungal endocarditis; endophthalmitis; osteomyelitis and fungal septic arthritis; early bleeding from primary aspergilloma; invasive fungal sinusitis; and primary invasive fungal infection of the gastrointestinal tract. Other adjunctive treatments that may be appropriate under particular clinical conditions include: white cell transfusion; colony-stimulating factors (e.g. GCSF) and gamma interferon; hyperbaric oxygen.

## *Aspergillus fumigatus*

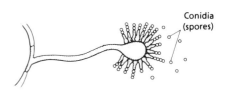

Conidia (spores)

Conidiophore ('fruiting body')

**Pathogenesis:** Virulence factors largely unknown, but a variety of adhesins, pigments, toxins and enzymes have been proposed: no single factor is believed to be crucial. Alveolar macrophages kill spores ('conidia'), and principally neutrophils kill hyphae.

**Epidemiology:** Air-borne spores ubiquitous from decaying vegetation. Inhalational route, spores germinate within airways; *Aspergillus* spp. can be isolated from nose swabs of ≈1% normal individuals (usually transient colonization), but nasal colonization does not always precede invasive lung disease. Also found in some foods (e.g. pepper) and water. Risk of

Table 36.1 Moulds

| Genus | Species | Notes |
|---|---|---|
| **Aspergillus** | **fumigatus**, **flavus**, niger, terreus, nidulans, etc. | Cause allergic, localized and invasive aspergillosis (➤363) |
| Mucor spp., Rhizopus spp., Absidia spp. etc.: 'zygomycetes' | | Rare, invasive infections in the immunocompromised and diabetic host, especially of the paranasal sinuses: 'zygomycosis', 'mucormycosis', or 'phycomycosis' (➤369) |
| Pseudallescheria | boydii | Miscellaneous group of filamentous fungi, occasionally causing invasive infections in the immunocompromised host (➤370). Many other fungi more rarely may cause of this type infection |
| Fusarium | spp. | |
| Penicillium | marneffei and others | |
| Scedosporium | spp. | |
| Paecilomyces | lilacinus | |
| **Ringworm fungi:** | | Infecting stratum corneum of skin, hair and nails (➤117) |
| **Epidermophyton** | spp. | |
| **Microsporum** | spp. | |
| **Trichophyton** | spp. | |
| Mycetoma and chromoblastomycosis fungi: (Madurella, Acremonium, Actinomadura, Exophiala, Fonsecaea, Phialophora, Cladosporium spp., etc.) | | Causes of mycetoma (eumycetoma—involving fungi) and chromoblastomycosis, superficial skin infections in the tropics |
| (Rhinosporidium) | (seeberi) | Causes rhinosporidiosis, a granulomatous disease of nasal and conjunctival mucosae, especially in India |
| **Pneumocystis** | **carinii** (renamed P. jiroveci) | Previously classified as a protozoon: re-designated based on DNA homology and membrane sterol content (➤156) |

invasive disease up to 40% in patients after BMT with neutropenia ($<0.5 \times 10^9$/L) for >20 days. Rising incidence of cases in past 20 yrs due to improved recognition and diagnosis, and increased numbers of susceptible individuals. $\Sigma$ risen from ≈25 invasive infections in 1990 to ≈100 in 1999.

Higher rate of recurrence in subsequent episodes of chemotherapy in those with previous Aspergillus infection (➤176). Occasional outbreaks of invasive disease in the immunocompromised associated with disturbance of fungal growth in hospital buildings (e.g. damp organic insulation material) in construction work, ventilation systems. Strain typing is in its infancy.

After **allogeneic** bone-marrow transplants, Aspergillus infection is seen in about 7% related and 10% unrelated grafts, and is commoner after engraftment. Within 40 days of transplant it is associated with season of the year (spore counts in air are highest in late summer) and nursing out of HEPA-filtered air. After that time risk factors include graft-versus-host disease, neutropenic episodes and corticosteroid use. After **autologous** grafts it occurs in only 2.6% of cases and is commoner earlier (before engraftment, around 2 weeks after

**Table 36.2** Yeasts

| Genus | Species | Notes |
|---|---|---|
| *Candida* | *albicans*, *tropicalis*, *parapsilosis*, *lusitaniae*, *glabrata*, *guilliermondii*, *krusei*, *dubliniensis*, *pseudotropicalis*, *rugosa*, *stellatoidea* | *Candida glabrata* is also known as *Torulopsis glabrata* (➤367) |
| *Cryptococcus* | *neoformans* | Capsulate yeast (➤368) |
| (*Trichosporon* (*Rhodotorula* | *beigelii*) spp.) | Disseminated infections in immunocompromised patients |
| *Histoplasma* | *capsulatum* (*duboisii*) | Widespread environmental distribution, especially in eastern USA and tropics (➤369) |
| (*Coccidioides immitis, Blastomyces dermatididis, Paracoccidioides brasiliensis*) | | Restricted environmental distribution, especially in the Americas (➤369, 370) |
| (*Sporothrix* | *schenkii*) | Skin sepsis, satellite lesions and lymphangitis following local trauma associated with moist vegetation; rare pulmonary and systemic infection in the immunocompromised |
| *Malassezia* | *furfur* | Lipophilic. Causes pityriasis versicolor, and iv catheter infection and fungaemia in infants receiving parenteral lipid therapy. Also called *Pityriasis versicolor* and *ovale* |

transplantation) and is associated only with episodes of neutropenia. Other groups at highest risk include chronic granulomatous disease, lung transplant recipients, and acute myeloid leukaemia if nursed out of HEPA filtered air.

**Spectrum of disease: Allergic aspergillosis** includes: (i) allergy to inhaled aspergillus antigens, common in atopic patients (raised IgE levels); (ii) colonization of airways causing asthma, eosinophilia, plugging of airways; and (iii) inhalation of high spore concentrations ⇨ fever, breathlessness (allergic alveolitis) ⇨ progressive lung damage if repeated (e.g. maltster's lung from *Aspergillus clavatus*). **Local infection** (**aspergilloma**)—colonization of pre-existing pulmonary cavities (esp. post-tuberculous) usually asymptomatic, with no local invasion (eventual erosion of pulmonary arteriole ⇨ haemorrhage in up to 50%, but usually minor). Ulcerative tracheobronchitis in lung transplant

recipients. **Invasive aspergillosis** (IA)—in immunocompromised patients only (➤173). Usual site of invasion is lung, later spread haematogenously to many organs ⇨ arterial thrombosis or infarction with local invasion. Fever, unresponsive to antibiotics, is usual. Pulmonary infection presents with cough (≈90%), chest pain (≈75%) and haemoptysis (≈50%). Occasional primary infection of nasal sinuses ⇨ local invasion of orbit and brain; and iv catheter infection. Cerebral involvement carries grave prognosis. Rare endocarditis (most commonly PVE, acquired at time of valve insertion) with large, friable vegetations. IA in liver transplantation associated with prior poor graft function, CMV infection and renal failure. IA plus respiratory failure requiring ICU management has a 92% mortality rate.

**Laboratory diagnosis and other methods: Allergic aspergillosis**—plugs of mycelium visible in sputum, serum precipitins positive.

**Aspergilloma** best visualized radiologically; sputum usually microscopy- and culture-negative. Hyphae in **IA** best seen in biopsies; various serological and DNA-based assays under assessment, but none currently proven sufficiently sensitive and specific to be generally recommended. Isolation from any colonization site in bone-marrow and liver transplant recipients is predictive of infection, but this is not predictive in other patients. Early CT scanning of chest is especially helpful, with distinctive 'halo' (day 3–5, often disappeared by day 7) and 'air crescent' (around day 14, often associated with rising granulocyte count) representing haemorrhage and consolidation around pulmonary infarcts.

Growth on Sabouraud's agar visible in 1–7 days (occasionally up to 10 days). Will grow on blood agar, and frequently contaminates plates incubated for long periods. Quantitation and repeated isolation helpful to assess significance. Growth frequently scanty from biopsies in IA, and blood cultures rarely positive even in IE. IA still often diagnosed post mortem, especially in allogeneic bone-marrow transplants, but recently introduced diagnostic tests allowing early confirmation, and use of modern therapeutic regimens, appear to have reduced direct IA mortality from 50–90% to about 25%—confirmatory studies are required.

**Treatment:** Corticosteroid-dependent **allergic aspergillosis** may be improved by addition of oral itraconazole. Symptomatic **aspergilloma** usually requires surgical excision; possible role for local instillation of amphotericin B. For **IA**, seek urgent specialist advice and follow local protocols ☎. Amphotericin B (especially lipid preparations) remains first-line therapy in most units. Itraconazole is under assessment, particularly since availability of parenteral preparation, but will probably be used mainly for continuation treatment after initial control with amphotericin. Combined amphotericin and itraconazole therapy generally should be avoided but has been recommended in cerebral aspergillosis (☎). A recent RCT comparing the new azole voriconazole (➤375) with conventional amphotericin in confirmed or probable IA showed superior efficacy with significantly

improved survival and fewer adverse effects for voriconazole. This new agent is likely to replace amphotericin B as first-line therapy in many units. The candins (➤376) also offer promising activity against *Aspergillus* spp. Caspofungin (➤376) has shown useful efficacy in several trials of patients with IA who were failing or intolerant of conventional therapy. These agents will undoubtedly be important in the future therapy of IA, although their precise roles have yet to be determined.

Therapy should begin as soon as diagnosis of invasive aspergillosis seriously entertained—failure is associated with treatment delay. Surgical resection of lesions may be useful in selected cases. Recovery of granulocyte count improves outlook, but may acutely worsen CXR appearances and clinical state.

➥ Stevens D, Practice guidelines for diseases caused by *Aspergillus*, Clin Inf Dis 2000; 30: 696

➥ Herbrecht R, New Engl J Med 2002; 347: 408

**Prevention:** Dust screening of hospital building works. HEPA filtration of air supply to bone-marrow transplant units and ICUs caring for many immunocompromised patients (although many episodes undoubtedly acquired out of hospital, hence effectiveness of this expensive measure is not certain). Some have recommended patients should wear dust-mist respirator masks when leaving HEPA-filtered accommodation for investigations in other hospital departments. Antifungal prophylaxis of immunosuppression episodes is under assessment, but nebulized and iv amphotericin B and oral itraconazole have been used with some reported success in the highest risk groups (i.e. allogeneic stem cell, liver and lung transplants, and all undergoing transplantation who have had prior episodes of IA).

*Aspergillus flavus* causes similar infections to *A. fumigatus*, but is less commonly isolated from invasive disease. *Aspergillus niger* forms black colonies on solid media, and is most frequently isolated from chronic otitis externa. Occasionally isolated from invasive disease.

Many other moulds (e.g. *Penicillium* spp., *Thermoactinomyces* spp.) are associated with extrinsic allergic alveolitis.

# Candida albicans

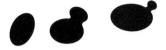

Responsible for ≈90% *Candida* spp. infections and 40–50% cases of fungaemia.

**Pathogenesis:** Adhesion to epithelia, phospholipase and proteinase production, and formation of hyphae are major virulence factors.

**Epidemiology:** Usually causes endogenous infections: *Candida albicans* is a normal oropharyngeal, vaginal and gut commensal. Overgrowth on mucosae follows destruction of normal bacterial flora (yeast takes over epithelial binding sites)—commonly with antibiotic therapy, diabetes, persistently moist skin. Other factors include pregnancy, infancy, old age, steroids, neutropenia, organ transplants, iron deficiency. Bladder catheter ⇨ colonization, may ⇨ infection. Systemic candidiasis may follow contamination of lemon juice used to dissolve heroin by IVDUs (➤162). Epidemiology often difficult to elucidate, because recurrent episodes in single patients may involve strains with variation in typing markers. Nosocomial outbreaks occasionally proven.

Incidence of invasive infection in hospitals has risen 10-fold in past 10 yrs: *Candida* spp. are now the commonest significant nosocomial blood culture isolate in ICUs in the USA, and the third or fourth commonest over all units. Risk factors for *Candida* infection in ICU include abdominal surgery (especially re-operation for anastomotic leak or abscess, pancreatitis), burns, central venous catheters and TPN, prolonged antibiotic therapy, organ transplantation. Σ ≈750 invasive infections.

**Spectrum of disease:** Thrush—superficial infection of mucous membranes (➤160); may progress to local invasion (e.g. oesophagitis in AIDS ➤160). Moist skin areas, nappy rash, paronychia, onychomycosis, otitis externa (➤17). Development of **invasive candidiasis** usually requires several predisposing factors, and haematogenous spread is uncommon without iv access (iv catheter infection, IVDUs). **Intraperitoneal infection** common following treatment of serious peritoneal bacterial sepsis—especially after pancreatitis. **Endophthalmitis** has been reported in up to 60% cases of candidaemia—hence perform ophthalmoscopy and ask patient about blurred vision. **Endocarditis** (from candidaemic infection of previously abnormal valves) and PVE (usually acquired at time of implantation). **Hepatosplenic candidiasis** becomes clinically apparent with granulocyte recovery during cycles of chemotherapy and after bone marrow transplantation. **Neonatal candidaemia** and meningitis encouraged by iv and umbilical catheters and prolonged antibiotics. **Chronic mucocutaneous candidiasis** is associated with granulocyte disorders (➤172).

**Laboratory diagnosis:** Round or oval budding yeasts; pseudomycelium and mycelium commonly seen in superficial and invasive disease. Strict aerobes, growing on many solid media in 24–72 h ⇨ alcoholic-smelling, heaped colonies. Modern blood culture systems usually positive in most bottles in 48–96 h in cases of candidaemia. Although speciation is slow (ChromAgar, commercial biochemical kits or ✈), formation of 'germ tubes' on incubation in serum (3 h) is virtually diagnostic of *C. albicans*, hence implies isolate is likely to be sensitive to azoles. Positive cultures from normal carriage sites need careful clinical interpretation, and quantitation may be helpful. *Candida* may be a contaminant of blood cultures, but differentiation from true infection is impossible prospectively, hence treatment usually mandatory. Superficial infections often diagnosed clinically. Consider possibility of invasive disease in ICU patients with superficial and urinary candidiasis, iv catheters and fever: systemic candidiasis is very rare without superficial colonization. Serology rarely useful diagnostically; rapid antigen and cell component detection systems under development—(e.g. ELISA for cell-wall mannans or enolase, and PCR) but of unproven diagnostic value at present.

**Treatment:** Topical therapy used for superficial infections (➤374). Virtually all strains sensitive to amphotericin B, which many still consider drug of choice for invasive disease. Combination with flucytosine possibly of value in systemic neonatal infection, but routinely avoid because of risk of toxicity. Oral azole therapy usually successful in AIDS oesophagitis (➤160). *C. albicans* rarely resistant to azoles (except after prolonged prophylactic use in, for example, AIDS), which are useful continuation therapy after initial control with amphotericin. Most non-*albicans* species are less reliably susceptible. Azoles increasingly now used as first choice for moderately serious *Candida* infections (e.g. 400–800 mg/day fluconazole). Outcome of invasive and fungaemic infections improved if at least 3 weeks' therapy at high dose is given but, in a non-compromised patient who responds promptly, 10–14 days is probably sufficient. IV catheter infections require line removal and IE usually requires valve replacement for control of infection. Changing urethral catheter may resolve urinary colonization.

> Rex JH, Practice guidelines for the treatment of candidiasis. Clin Infect Dis 2000; 30: 662

**Prevention:** Multiple recurrent superficial episodes may respond to intermittent antifungal prophylaxis, at the risk of encouraging resistance. Diabetic control. Oral azole prophylaxis in HIV patients is no longer recommended because of the inevitable occurrence of resistance. Fluconazole (100 mg/day) and non-absorbed antifungals reduce incidence of clinical candidiasis during immunosuppressive episodes. Hand hygiene with alcoholic antiseptics between each patient contact.

*Candida parapsilosis* and *tropicalis* are skin commensals isolated from a higher proportion of iv catheter infections and endocarditis than *C. albicans*; each now isolated from 10–20% candidaemias overall. *Candida parapsilosis* multiplies rapidly in glucose-containing solutions and has a propensity to adhere to synthetic materials. *Candida glabrata* (syn. *Torulopsis glabrata*) is frequently fluconazole- and itraconazole-resistant, and its infections on ICUs are associated with a low survival rate — 50% compared with 60% for *tropicalis*, 90% for *albicans* and 95% for *parapsilosis*. *Candida tropicalis* and *glabrata* infections have risen steadily in prevalence compared with those caused by *Candida albicans* during the past 15 yrs.

**Candida krusei** forms elongated yeast cells looking like grains of rice, and is resistant to fluconazole. It is occasionally found in a variety of environmental sites, but only rarely from human mucosae. It is increasingly seen colonizing patients receiving fluconazole prophylaxis, and may cause significant infection in this group. It appears to be less virulent than *Candida albicans*.

**Candida dubliniensis** has been recently associated with oropharyngeal and occasional systemic infections in patients with AIDS. It is commonly fluconazole-resistant (or resistance emerges early during therapy), and is readily confused with *Candida albicans* in commonly used identification schemes.

Agents useful against non-*albicans* species include amphotericin B, the new azoles voriconazole, ravuconazole and posaconazole, and the candins, including the newly-released caspofungin ☎. It is likely that several more of these antifungals will reach the market in the next few years.

## Cryptococcus neoformans

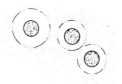

India ink preparation of CSF, showing capsules

Capsulate, spherical yeast.

**Pathogenesis:** Antiphagocytic mucopolysaccharide capsule; capsule production increased by host immune response.

**Epidemiology:** Present worldwide in bird droppings and elsewhere in environment. Frequently inhaled to cause asymptomatic or mild infection (lung granuloma), which resolves with intact CMI. Rare chronic cryptococcoma formation, with surrounding fibrosis. Progression (recrudescence or reinfection), especially in AIDS and others with CMI deficits. Typing available (✈). Σ ≈ 30.

**Spectrum of disease:** Commonest cause of fungal meningitis; occasionally also chronic skin and pulmonary sepsis, osteomyelitis. Recurrent infections, particularly meningitis, in HIV (➤164).

**Laboratory diagnosis:** Seen in CSF wet preparation and Gram stain in up to 50% of cases—differentiated from host lymphocytes by demonstration of capsule by India ink-negative stain. Sometimes little capsule seen, especially in AIDS. Budding visible, but forms no mycelium or pseudomycelium. Demonstrated by tissue fungal stains in biopsy material. Most rapid, sensitive and specific diagnostic method is capsule detection by latex agglutination or ELISA (many laboratories send to ✈) in CSF and serum. CSF and serum are positive by antigen tests in >90% of cases of meningitis. Repeat if initially negative and diagnosis strongly suspected clinically. Usually readily cultured from CSF, blood, urine and sputum on Sabouraud's agar (≈90% cases; also grows on blood agar) to cream, opaque, waxy colonies in 48–96 h, but can take up to 3 weeks (confirm identity in ✈). Grows best at 30–32°C.

**Treatment:** Amphotericin B ± flucytosine until stable, then fluconazole (➤165). Fluconazole + flucytosine has also been used. Antigen detection and serology useful to follow progress of treatment, but proof of correlation between clinical response and titres is lacking.

## Histoplasma capsulatum

Found as a saprophyte in soil contaminated with bat and bird droppings, especially in eastern USA, but is also widespread in tropical and some temperate areas. It normally causes subclinical or self-limited lung infection, but occasionally causes chronic or acutely progressive pneumonia and disseminated infection in the immunocompromised (including AIDS).

Acute symptomatic pulmonary histoplasmosis occasionally seen in normal hosts 7–21 days after inhalation of infective spores (conidia). Diagnosed by microscopy of sputum, pus, tissue biopsies for yeast cells within macrophages. Can be cultured on Sabouraud's agar at low temperature for up to 6 weeks (☣). Serology and antigen detection available (✈). Amphotericin B and azoles have been used in treatment (discuss with ✈). Culture is a reliable test of cure, but antigen assays give variable results even in successfully treated patients.

*Histoplasma duboisii* mainly causes skin and subcutaneous histoplasmosis in Africa.

## Coccidioides immitis

A soil saprophyte, found only in dry regions of the south-western USA and north Mexico. Infection associated with inhalation of arthroconidia, especially from soil disturbance, e.g. dust storms, construction work and archaeological excavations. Serological evidence of exposure is common in the indigenous population (over 90% in some areas) following self-limited lung infections. Sixty per cent are subclinical, but about 30% present as 'influenza' and the remainder as progressive pulmonary disease (associated with diabetes, smoking and old age) and disseminated infection (associated with immunosuppression, pregnancy, and black or Asian race). Long-lived immunity results in the immunocompetent. Diagnosed by seeing 'spherules' in sputum, pus and tissue biopsies. Grows within 3 weeks on Sabouraud's agar (☣). Serology available (✈). Amphotericin B and azoles have been used in treatment (discuss with ✈).

## Zygomycosis ('mucormycosis')

Commonest isolates belong to *Mucor*, *Rhizopus*, *Absidia*, *Rhizomucor* and *Cunninghamella* genera; often referred to as 'mucormycosis'. Widespread saprophytes of rotting vegetation, acquired mainly by inhalation of spores; occasionally inoculated directly to skin or ingested. Clinical manifestations include rhinocerebral, pulmonary, cutaneous, gastrointestinal and disseminated infections.

**Risk factors:** Diabetes, particularly with ketoacidosis, lymphoma, leukaemia, neutropenia, long-term steroid or other immunosuppressive therapy, granulocyte function disorders, and desferrioxamine therapy of dialysis patients with aluminium or iron overload. Skin trauma, burns, IVDU, iv catheters may lead to local infections in the immunocompetent host (e.g. from contaminated wooden tongue depressors used as splints for iv catheters in neonates). Steadily rising incidence since mid-1980s. Very rare reports of rhinocerebral zygomycosis in the absence of apparent risk factors.

**Clinical features:** Vascular invasion by hyphae causes infarction and necrosis of host tissues. Deterioration usually very fast; rare descriptions of indolent course. Commonest presentation is **rhinocerebral infection**, presumed to start with inhalation of spores into the paranasal sinuses. Presents as an acute severe pansinusitis, rapidly spreading to contiguous structures including palate, orbit and brain with tissue necrosis of the palate, destruction of the turbinates, perinasal swelling, and erythema and cyanosis of the overlying facial skin. **Pulmonary zygomycosis** presents as a rapidly progressive diffuse pneumonia, which can spread to contiguous structures such as the mediastinum and heart. Most patients have fever with hemoptysis. Local inoculation of spores into the dermis may cause **cutaneous infection**, usually manifesting as a single, painful, indurated area of cellulitis. Renal, gastrointestinal and CNS infection have also been reported.

**Diagnosis:** Readily cultured on most media and identified by morphology of hyphae and sporangiospores (confirm by ✦). Clinically, the diagnosis depends on the clinician suspecting zygomycosis and pursuing invasive investigations to obtain tissue, for example by sinus endoscopy or bronchoscopy. CT and MRI scans may be used to evaluate involvement of contiguous structures.

**Treatment:** Radical, often disfiguring, surgical resection is essential: response to antifungal agents is variable, but high-dose lipid formulations of amphotericin B (e.g. liposomal amphotericin B 5–15 mg/kg/day) have been used with success (discuss therapy with ✦). Granulocyte colony-stimulating factors may be helpful. Overall mortality for rhinocerebral disease is up to 50%, depending on site and speed of diagnosis, and >80% for pulmonary zygomycosis.

## Other fungi

***Trichosporon beigelii*** is widely distributed in decaying vegetation, soil and the air. It causes occasional disseminated infections in immunocompromised patients, especially those with acute leukaemia; blood cultures are often positive. $\Sigma$ 1–2 invasive infections. It may cross-react in *Cryptococcus* antigen assays. Most experience has been gained with amphotericin B, although itraconazole may be effective. Recovery from neutropenia is important for eradication.

***Blastomyces dermatididis*** ♟ causes chronic pulmonary, skin and bone infections in patients from parts of the USA and Canada. ***Paracoccidioides brasiliensis*** ♟ causes chronic pulmonary, skin and mucosal infections in patients from tropical forest regions of South and Central America. Both usually diagnosed by microscopy of sputum, pus or tissue biopsies, and grow slowly on Sabouraud's agar. Serology is useful for paracoccidioidomycosis (✦). Amphotericin B and azoles have been used in treatment of both (discuss with ✦).

***Penicillium marneffei*** ♟ is a dimorphic fungus that causes invasive infections in immunocompromised patients in SE Asia (including short-term visitors), especially those infected with HIV (➤143). About 20% cases lack predisposing factors. Infection occurs mainly during the rainy season, and may be derived from colonized bamboo rats or a soil reservoir. Usually presents with fever, weight loss, lymphadenopathy, cough, skin lesions and anaemia (differential diagnosis of tuberculosis (➤38), cryptococcosis and histoplasmosis). Hepatosplenomegaly is common in children. A generalized papular rash is seen frequently, sometimes resembling molluscum contagiosum. Granulomatous lesions in reticuloendothelial system and abscesses in various organs are characteristic, although granulomas are not seen in immunocompromised hosts. Readily grown from skin, pus, blood, sputum and bone marrow on Sabouraud's agar in 48 h at 25°C to yield red colonies surrounded by red diffusable pigment (other *Penicillium* spp. may produce red pigment; send for identification ✈). Significant risk of laboratory-acquired infection. Generally responds to amphotericin B or itraconazole (75% response rate after 8 weeks' therapy). Long-term maintenance therapy is necessary in patients with AIDS to prevent recurrence.

*Fusarium* spp. are widely distributed plant pathogens, and cause keratitis in the immunocompetent host (especially associated with travel in dusty environments ➤107), and sinusitis, skin ulcers, pneumonia and other invasive infections in the immunocompromised, diabetics, etc. (➤174). Blood cultures are much more commonly positive than with *Aspergillus* infections, but *Fusarium* has a similar propensity for causing infarcts, especially in the skin.

*Scedosporium* spp. cause similar pulmonary infections to *Fusarium*, but with an especially poor prognosis (survival >1 month of diagnosis is rare).

Both *Fusarium* and *Scedosporium* may respond to amphotericin or itraconazole, but *in vitro* susceptibility is seen in only c. 15%, and some of the new azoles (voriconazole and posaconazole) may prove more effective.

*Pseudallescheria boydii* (recently renamed as a *Scedosporium* sp.) is frequently found in polluted waters and manure. It causes pneumonia, meningitis and systemic abscesses after near-drownings, and pneumonia in the immunocompromised. It is usually resistant to amphotericin B and flucytosine, and treatment requires surgical drainage. Itraconazole has been used successfully.

*Sporothrix schenkii*, usually associated with local sepsis and lymphangitic lesions after traumatic inoculation of moist vegetable matter,

occasionally causes pulmonary infection in COPD and disseminated infections in patients with AIDS. Itraconazole or amphotericin B have been used.

Many other fungi of diverse genera may rarely cause human infections, especially of immunocompromised patients, e.g. *Malassezia* spp. Σ 1–2, *Rhodotorula* spp. Σ 2–3, *Saccharomyces* spp. Σ 2 invasive infections. Referral to a reference laboratory is important for any isolate considered clinically relevant, because correct identification often has epidemiological and prognostic significance, and antifungal susceptibility testing is important.

## Antifungal agents

Susceptibility testing of fungi has generally been considered technically demanding and poorly predictive of clinical response, but recent technical developments (especially the introduction of the E-test methodology for many agents and international standardization of methodologies) appear to produce useful correlation of laboratory and clinical results. Many laboratories currently still refer fungi to reference laboratories for susceptibility testing. Susceptibility tests should be performed in the light of an isolate's identity and the clinical situation from which it came. In general, they should be performed on yeasts from serious or recurrent infections, and from all moulds causing invasive infection.

Adjuvant therapy of fungal infections with immune-stimulating factors (e.g. granulocyte colony-stimulating factor and interferon) has shown promise, especially in patients with deficits in neutrophil function, and in neutropenic patients in whom restoration of neutrophil numbers may be expected reasonably quickly. Some benefit has also been demonstrated for neutrophil transfusions in patients with invasive *Candida* infections.

Antifungal agents have no cross-activity against bacteria, and are frequently prescribed to treat *Candida* spp. superinfections resulting from antibacterial use. Cessation of antibacterial therapy is often an important factor in successful management of thrush. Only five different classes of antifungal agent are currently licensed, but a number of examples of novel groups are about to be released to the market. Many can be used topically (including oral usage of non-absorbable antifungals) or systemically.

## Polyenes: Amphotericin B

Bind to ergosterol present in fungal (but not mammalian) cell membranes. The resulting deformity of the membrane allows leakage of intracellular ions and enzymes, causing cell death. Fungicidal at higher concentrations. May possess immune stimulating properties.

**Uses:** Active against most yeasts and systemically infecting fungi (including *Aspergillus* spp. and the dimorphic fungi), and the amoebae *Naegleria* spp. and *Hartmanella* spp. Also used in leishmaniasis (➤221). Dermatophytes, *Pseudallescheria boydii*, *Aspergillus flavus* and *terreus*, *Scedosporium* spp. and *Fusarium* spp. are more likely to be resistant or less susceptible (hence susceptibility testing is important ➤). Occasional acquired resistance in *Candida* spp. (*tropicalis*, *krusei*, *guilliermondii* and *lusitaniae*; very rare in the clinically commoner *Candida albicans*, *parapsilosis* and *glabrata*). Despite toxicity, still considered by many to be **agent of choice** for many serious fungal infections, including systemic candidiasis, aspergillosis and cryptococcosis. Oral prophylaxis and treatment of GI tract yeast infection. Combination with flucytosine allows lower doses of both in cryptococcal meningitis, but little evidence of benefit for combinations with azoles (theoretical risk of antagonism).

**Administration:** There are iv and oral preparations; occasionally instilled into bladder, abscesses, joints, CSF; not absorbed from gut. CSF ✗ (but effective in combination for cryptococcal meningitis), urine ✓. Slow build-up to full dosage reduces unwanted effects, but may risk inadequate early therapy in immunocompromised patients (hence 'accelerated regimen' used). Monitor renal function. Serum levels do not correlate with side effects, so assay not helpful. Many centres administer by infusion over 4–12 h 0.8–1 mg/kg/day for *Candida*

infection, 1 mg/kg/day (occasionally up to 1.5 mg/kg/day) for filamentous fungal infection. Preliminary evidence suggests slow infusion over 24 h may reduce adverse effects to same rate as is seen with lipid-associated preparations; confirmation, and proof of efficacy are awaited (Table 36.3).

Amphotericin B is generally administered until neutrophil recovery, clinical and radiological response, and a cumulative dose of at least 2 g has been given, but there is currently little high-quality evidence to guide course lengths.

**Adverse effects:** Fever ($\approx$50%), rigors ($\approx$50%), vomiting, thrombophlebitis after iv administration (minimized by analgesics, antihistamines, iv pethidine, iv hydrocortisone). Amphotericin B increases membrane permeability, hence hypokalaemia, hypomagnesaemia, nephrotoxicity ($\approx$30%) and cardiac arrythmias may be seen. Also hepatic dysfunction, cerebral irritation, peripheral neuropathy. Amphotericin-associated renal failure in patients treated for aspergillosis after bone-marrow transplantation is not always reversible, and proven to increase mortality, length of hospital stay and treatment costs. Much lower risk of such adverse events after solid organ transplantation.

Three '**lipid-associated formulations of amphotericin B**' (LAFsAB) are available, each with different lipid constituents, amphotericin content, and pharmacokinetic properties. All are less nephrotoxic than amphotericin B (but are **not** free from risk of side effects, which include all those listed above for the native compound), may be given in higher doses and are significantly more expensive. Reduced toxicity may be due to slow, sustained release of active drug; also tend to concentrate amphotericin in reticuloendothelial tissues. In some hospitals caring for large numbers of immunocompromised patients, more is now spent on LAFsAB than on any other antimicrobial agent. More comparative data are currently required to prove any LAFAB to be more effective for some or all applications. Animal models generally suggest greater efficacy because a greater daily dose may be given; however, weight-for-weight of amphotericin the new preparations some-

**Table 36.3** Antifungal doses (doses for severe infection in parentheses)

| Drug (cautions, interactions) For codes, see footnote | Dose if serum creatinine (µmol/L) | | | | Effect of dialysis |
|---|---|---|---|---|---|
| | Normal dose | 150–300 | 300–700 | >700 | |
| Amphotericin B £(6) | iv: 0.6 mg/kg (1–1.5 mg/kg) q24h. Consider lipid-associated formulations for patients with impaired renal function. Manufacturer recommends discontinuation or dosage reduction if creatinine exceeds 260 µmol/L | | | Doses as column to left, but given 36hly | HD: <5%. Usual regimen |
| | Gradual work-up to full dosage in less severely ill, non-compromised patient: 1 mg in 50 mL infused over 2 h; if tolerated, give 9 mg over next 6 h; if tolerated, increase by 10 mg/day given over 6 h. Accelerated regimen for severely ill, compromised patient: first 1 mg of half full dose over 1–2 h; if tolerated, give remainder of infusion over 12 h, then give full dose from second day over 6 h | | | | |
| Liposomal amphotericin B (AmBisome) (PL 6) ££££ | iv: 1 mg/kg (3 mg/kg) q24h over 60 min | | | | Administration should commence only after HD has finished |
| Amphotericin B lipid complex (Abelcet) (PL 6) ££££ | iv: 5 mg/kg q24h over 120 min | | | | |
| Amphotericin B colloidal dispersion (Amphocil) (PL 6) ££££ | iv: 1 mg/kg (4 mg/kg) q24h over 60–90 min | | | | |
| Fluconazole £££ (PL 2346890 ⊗(1 yr)) Vaginal/penile candidiasis: | Oral: 150 mg single dose | | | | HD: 50%. One dose after each HD; no doses between HD |
| Non-genital mucosal candidiasis: | Oral: 50 mg (100 mg) q24h | | Oral: 50 mg q24h | | |
| Invasive infection: | iv/Oral: 400–800 mg initial dose, then 200 mg (400–800 mg) q24h | | iv/Oral: 400 mg initial dose, then 100 mg (200–400 mg) q24h | | |
| Itraconazole £££ (PLH ⊗ 1246780 △) | Oral: 100 mg (200 mg) q24h iv: 200 mg q12h for 2 days, then 200 mg q24h (maximum 12 days) | | Avoid iv preparation if creatinine clearance <30 mL/min (➤403) | | HD: <5% |
| Ketoconazole £ (PLHO 124680) | Oral: 200 mg (400 mg) q24h | | | | |
| Flucytosine ££ (HPL△) | iv: 37.5 mg/kg (50 mg/kg) q6h | iv: 37.5 mg/kg (50 mg/kg) q12h | iv: 37.5 mg/kg (50 mg/kg) q24h | iv: 50 mg/kg initial dose, then assay | HD: >50% |

**Cautions/contraindications:** P, pregnancy; L, lactation; H, hepatic failure; O, porphyrias (see BNF for details); △, assay needed; ⊗ contraindicated or use not established in children below age stated in parentheses. (➤391). **Interactions:** (➤391): 1, Absorption/metabolism altered by ulcer healing drugs, antacids, calcium/magnesium/zinc/iron salts; 2, anticoagulants; 3, antidiabetics; 4, anti-epileptics; 6, ciclosporin; 7, digoxin; 8, rifampicin; 9, theophylline; 0, terfenadine. £, ££, £££: ➤391.

times appear less effective in these models. Infusion-related toxicity (fever, chills, hypotension, nausea, vomiting) may also be reduced in incidence. Overall incidence of side effects reduced by 30–90% compared with amphotericin B.

LAFsAB are generally now considered the initial agent of choice in patients with renal impairment *ab initio* (e.g. serum creatinine >180 μmol/L), in hepatosplenic candidiasis (➤367) and rhinocerebral zygomycosis (➤369), and they should be substituted for amphotericin B in patients who develop renal impairment during therapy. Administered as a bolus, they are sometimes valuable to reduce the pressure on 'line-time' in patients being treated for haematological malignancies.

**Liposomal amphotericin B** (AmBisome): first LAFAB to be released to the market, and the only liposomal product. Generally given at 1 mg/kg/day for unproven filamentous fungal infection (e.g. febrile episodes in neutropenia that have not responded to 3–5 days antibacterial agents ➤174) or for *Candida* infection. Higher doses, 3–7(–15) mg/kg/day generally given for proven filamentous fungal infection. Dose recommendations not currently based on good evidence, but animal studies suggest higher doses may improve efficacy because of increased penetration to ischaemic lesions of invasive aspergillosis. Limited evidence base for efficacy in candidaemia (Table 36.3).

**Amphotericin B lipid complex** (Abelcet): may have higher rate of infusion related and toxic side effects than liposomal amphotericin B (Table 36.3).

**Amphotericin B colloidal dispersion** (Amphotec or Amphocil): associated with greater administration toxicity than the other LAFsAB (Table 36.3).

'In-house' manufactured mixtures of amphotericin with parenteral fat emulsions have been produced in some hospital pharmacies to avoid the high cost of commercial preparations. These are not recommended, because their properties are entirely uncontrolled, and some studies have shown reduced efficacy and greater nephrotoxicity than the native compound.

## Nystatin

Too toxic for systemic use. Oral and topical treatment of mucosal candidiasis; oropharyngeal and gastrointestinal prophylaxis. Resistance rare, but no systemic absorption, so use as treatment only for minor infections. Inactive against other fungi. Work is underway to develop a liposome-associated formulation which may be usable systemically.

## Azoles

Disrupt ergosterol synthesis (inhibit P-450-dependent 14a demethylation of lanosterol), resulting in formation of abnormal fungal cell membranes and accumulation of toxic sterol intermediates. Fungistatic (although voriconazole and posaconazole may be cidal). All lack activity against the zygomycetes. For itraconazole, fluconazole, miconazole and ketoconazole *in vitro* and *in vivo* cross-resistance is uncommon overall, but well recognized in some *Candida albicans* strains. Use in combination with amphotericin B is controversial (theoretical antagonism). Adverse effects of all include rash, hepatotoxicity (monitor liver function, especially of patients receiving long-term treatment) and interactions with other drugs metabolized via the cytochrome P-450 system.

## Clotrimazole, econazole

Topical treatment of mucosal candidiasis and dermatophyte infection. Recurrence common, especially of vaginal candidiasis, and re-treatment of patient and treatment of sexual partner often effective: azole resistance in recurrent infections is uncommon.

## Fluconazole

**Uses:** Broad spectrum including yeasts (some non-*albicans Candida* spp. show acquired or primary resistance, especially *Candida krusei*) and some dermatophytes. Used single-dose for vaginal candidiasis and now available 'over the counter' in the UK for this indication; prophylaxis, prevention of relapse, and treatment of yeast infections in immunocompromised patients, especially *Cryptococcus neoformans* meningitis in AIDS (➤164). Ineffective in aspergillosis. Shown to be a less toxic alternative to amphotericin B for candidaemia in non-neutropenic patients at 400 mg/day, but optimal dosing not yet determined. Marginally more mycological failures in therapy of non-*albicans* candidaemias.

> ↪ Kontoyiannis D, Fluconazole vs. amphotericin B for the management of candidaemia in adults: a meta-analysis. Mycoses 2001; 44: 125

**Administration:** There are iv and (well-absorbed) oral preparations; CSF✓ (especially with meningitis), urine✓ (Table 36.3).

**Adverse effects:** Less common than with the other systemically available azoles. Nausea, abdominal pain, headache, dizziness, rashes, pruritus.

## Itraconazole

**Uses:** Broadly active against many yeasts, dimorphic fungi and *Aspergillus* spp. Often used as oral follow-on after initial amphotericin B therapy of invasive pulmonary aspergillosis. 'Pulse' therapy of onychomycosis (➤117).

**Administration:** Oral and new iv formulations; oral absorption unpredictable especially in AIDS, but much improved with new liquid formulation solubilized in cyclodextrin oligosaccharides. This new formulation should not be taken with food, and absorption may be reduced by drugs that reduce gastric acidity (e.g. antacids, omeprazole, $H_2$-receptor blockers). CSF✗ (but appears effective in cryptococcal meningitis, perhaps due to intracellular accumulation within host tissues), urine✗. ⚠Serum assay recommended to ensure adequate oral therapy of documented infections (peak 1–2.5 mg/L. Assay after 7 days' therapy, or 7 days after change in dose; sample 2 h after dose) (Table 36.3).

**Adverse effects:** Nausea, abdominal pain, headache, dizziness, rashes, pruritus; occasional hepatotoxicity, Stevens–Johnson syndrome.

Cyclodextrin is excreted renally, so caution is needed in patients with impaired renal function.

## Ketoconazole

**Uses:** Broad spectrum, including systemic mycoses (not *Aspergillus* spp.), candidosis and dermatophytosis. Superseded by fluconazole and itraconazole for many indications largely on grounds of improved pharmacokinetics, unwanted effect profile and efficacy.

**Administration:** Oral, topical formulations; minimal CSF and urinary penetration, improved with very large doses.

**Adverse effects:** Gastrointestinal disturbance (commoner with higher doses), pruritus, rashes; rare hepatotoxicity; occasional painful gynaecomastia, loss of libido (interference with testosterone synthesis).

## Miconazole

**Uses:** Largely superseded by newer azoles; broad spectrum *in vitro*, including *Aspergillus* spp., yeasts and dermatophytes, but clinical response in serious infection often poor.

**Administration:** Oral (little systemic absorption), iv preparations; little CSF or urinary penetration. Can be given intrathecally. Topical preparation widely used for seborrhoeic dermatitis (➤117).

**Adverse effects:** Phlebitis, pruritus, rashes, fever; nausea, vomiting; cardiac dysrhythmia.

## Voriconazole

A recently-licensed derivative of fluconazole with greater *in vitro* activity against many *Candida* spp., including *Candida krusei*, but cross-resistance with itraconazole is usual. Clinically useful activity against *Aspergillus* spp., *Scedosporium* spp., *Fusarium* spp. and some other filamentous fungi, and the dimorphic fungi. Recent trial shows superiority vs. conventional amphotericin in invasive aspergillosis ($\blacktriangleright$365); voriconazole is now licensed in UK for treatment of *Aspergillus* spp., *Scedosporium* spp., *Fusarium* spp. and serious fluconazole-resistant *Candida* infections. Trials have also shown equivalent efficacy to amphotericin B in empirical therapy of febrile neutropenic patients, but it is not yet licensed for that indication. In addition to established efficacy, voriconazole offers considerable advantages over amphotericin in terms of ease of administration and adverse effects, and it is likely to play a major role in the management of serious fungal infections.

**Administration:** May be given iv or orally 🖹. iv: 6 mg/kg q12h for 24 h, then 4 mg/kg q12h. Oral: 400 mg (reduced to 200 mg if body weight <40 kg) q12h for 24 h, then 200 mg (reduced to 100 mg if body weight <40 kg) q12h. Not significantly removed by HD. No dose adjustment required in renal impairment for oral formulation, but the iv preparation is relatively contraindicated in moderate to severe renal failure (creatinine clearance <50 mL/min) because of accumulation of the iv vehicle 🖹. CSF ✓ urine ✓. Many significant drug interactions occur, notably with warfarin, rifamycins and phenytoin 🖹.

**Adverse effects:** Transient, infusion-associated altered perception of light and dark ($\approx$20%), visual hallucinations ($\approx$4%) both commoner during the first week of therapy. Nausea, diarrhoea, headache, dizziness, rashes. Abnormal liver function.

**Ravuconazole** and **posaconazole** are similar, but appear to have enhanced antifungal activity.

## Candins

A novel group of peptides that inhibit fungal cell wall synthesis ((1,3)-beta-D-glucan synthetase is the target). A number of agents are in advanced clinical trials (mainly in patients refractory or intolerant to other antifungal therapy); candins have demonstrated fungicidal activity against all *Candida* spp., a number of filamentous fungi and *Pneumocystis carinii*, but not *Cryptococcus neoformans*. Technical problems currently limit testing of *in vitro* susceptibility of filamentous fungi. Cross-resistance with established agents appears not to be a problem. Available by once-daily iv injection only (because high molecular weight prevents oral absorption). Probably CSF ✗, urine ✗, although responses have been reported in cerebral aspergillosis. No interactions with cytochrome P-450 system, and side effect profiles appear similar to that of fluconazole with somewhat more frequent incidence of hepatotoxicity.

## Caspofungin

The first candin. Recently licensed in the USA and Europe for invasive aspergillosis in patients who are intolerant of or refractory to conventional anti-fungal therapy ☎.

**Administration:** IV infusion over an hour.

**Dose:** Loading dose 70 mg. Subsequently 70 mg q24h for body weight >80 kg, 50 mg daily if <80 kg. Reduce dose to 35 mg q24h in moderate liver damage; 50 mg with mild hepatic impairment. No reduction is required in renal impairment.

**Adverse effects:** Fever, headache, abdominal pain, nausea, diarrhoea, vomiting, rash and pruritus. Phlebitis. Altered liver enzymes.

**Cautions:** PL ☹ ($\blacktriangleright$391).

## Flucytosine

Metabolized in the fungal cell to 5-fluorouracil which inhibits nucleic acid synthesis.

**Uses:** Combined with amphotericin B in cryptococcosis and severe *Candida* spp. infection (including hepatosplenic candidiasis, endocarditis, meningitis and peritonitis). May enable lower dosing of amphotericin. Primary resistance $\approx$10%. Acquired resistance common if flucytosine used alone (except short courses for lower UTI).

**Administration:** Well absorbed orally (iv available); CSF ✓, urine ✓ 🜄 (peak 25–50 mg/L; max. safe level 80 mg/L) (Table 36.3).

**Adverse effects:** Marrow aplasia and mucositis (especially with serum level >100 mg/L; often a result of renal failure secondary to amphotericin B toxicity); nausea, vomiting, diarrhoea, rashes, CNS effects; rare hepatotoxicity. Some authorities advocate keeping peak serum levels <60 mg/L, and descriptive published studies of such regimens in combination with amphotericin B show side effects to be very uncommon.

## Griseofulvin and terbinafine

**Griseofulvin** is used for the oral treatment of dermatophyte infections but has largely been superseded by terbinafine.

**Terbinafine** is an allylamine that inhibits squalene epoxidase, leading to inhibition of ergosterol synthesis and accumulation of toxic squalene. It is more effective than griseofulvin in nail infections, and shorter courses are required. Occasional gastrointestinal disturbance, rashes. Rare hepatotoxicity, toxic epidermal necrolysis and erythema multiforme. Metabolized via cytochrome P-450 system, but has only moderate affinity for the enzymes so few problem interactions are seen.

**Dose:** 250 mg q24h; 2–6 weeks in skin infection, 6–12 weeks or longer in nail infection. Reduce dose by 50% if creatinine clearance <40 mL/min (➤403).

Drugs active against a number of other fungal targets (e.g. chitin synthetase, cell wall mannoproteins, elongation factors) are under active development, and several of these will undoubtedly reach the market in the next few years.

# Antibiotic Therapy

# Chapter 37

# Antibiotics: theory, usage and abuse

In any community, the results of widespread antibiotic usage are reflected in the prevalence and distribution of antibiotic resistance in common pathogens. **Antibiotic usage is the only form of medical treatment where the choice of therapy for one patient can affect diseases suffered in the future by another, by selection of resistant organisms followed by cross-infection to the new host.**

## Mechanisms of antibiotic action

Rely upon **selective toxicity** versus microbial rather than human structures and metabolism (Table 37.1).

## Antibiotic sensitivity, resistance and 'activity'

### Susceptibility testing

Results of susceptibility testing of bacteria are reported by most laboratories as 'sensitive' or 'resistant', with some using an 'intermediate' category. These results are based upon *in vitro* tests, which may include:

**Disk diffusion**: Zone of inhibition around antibiotic-containing disk after overnight incubation of bacterial lawn on solid agar. If zone diameter of test organism is ≥3 mm less than that of control sensitive organism, result is 'resistant'. A variety of nationally and internationally accepted testing methodologies are used. The aim is to increase standardization, hence comparability of results for surveillance purposes.

**Breakpoint test**: Growth of a spot inoculum of bacteria on solid medium containing a known concentration of antibiotic, the 'breakpoint concentration', chosen to allow the growth of 'sensitive' micro-organisms and inhibit the growth of 'resistant' ones.

**Direct detection of resistance mechanism:** e.g. extracellular β-lactamase activity of *Neisseria gonorrhoeae* by rubbing a colony on a paper strip containing chromogenic cephalosporin—colour change = β-lactamase positive. **PCR** is now used for the rapid detection of the presence of some resistance genes, e.g. rifampicin resistance in mycobacteria.

More detailed tests, which attempt to quantify the specific 'activity' of antibiotics, include:

**Minimum inhibitory concentration (MIC):** lowest concentration of an antibiotic to inhibit multiplication of an organism in broth culture or on solid agar. Now much more simply, economically and reliably performed by use of 'E-test' strips, which contain a gradient of antibiotics which diffuse into solid medium. MIC read at intersection of zone of growth with edge of strip at 24 h.

**Minimum bactericidal concentration (MBC):** lowest concentration of an antibiotic to kill an organism—usually shown by subculture of MIC broth to antibiotic-free medium to demonstrate death or viability of bacteria within it.

Laboratory reports of sensitivity or resistance are educated guesses about what may happen in a real patient: disk contents, zone diameters and breakpoint concentrations are chosen based upon past experience, and on likely concentrations of antibiotic achieved at the site of infection. Many factors will modify activity *in vivo*, including protein binding, penetration to abscesses and privileged sites (CSF, eye, inside cells), immune and phagocytic activity, and presence of foreign bodies. Some antibiotics (e.g. β-lactams) reach high concentrations in the urine, so greater zone diameters and breakpoints are used for these agents to denote resistance in urine isolates.

To limit antibiotics tested to practicable

**Table 37.1** Mechanisms of antibiotic action

| Target | Antibiotic class |
|---|---|
| Cell wall synthesis | Penicillins, cephalosporins, glycopeptides |
| Protein synthesis | Chloramphenicol, macrolides, fusidate, tetracyclines, aminoglycosides, lincosamides, oxazolidinones (linezolid), streptogramins (quinupristin–dalfopristin) |
| DNA/RNA synthesis | Quinolones, rifampicin, 5-nitroimidazoles (metronidazole), nitrofurans |
| Intermediary metabolism | Sulphonamides, diaminopyrimidines |

numbers, laboratories usually test one example of a particular group and assume results for other members of the group—e.g. methicillin for *Staphylococcus aureus* (assume results for all β-lactams), cephalexin for *Escherichia coli* (assume results for all oral cephalosporins).

Some antibiotics kill organisms *in vitro* (**bactericidal**), others only inhibit their multiplication (**bacteriostatic**); clinical relevance of this is dubious.

## Antibiotic resistance

Common resistance mechanisms include: **inactivation** by bacterial enzymes (β-lactamases, aminoglycoside modifying enzymes); **alteration of target molecules** (penicillin-binding proteins); **restriction of entry** to the cell (imipenem in *E. coli*); **bypassing of metabolic pathway** (trimethoprim in enterococci).

Use of virtually any antibiotic results in an increased prevalence of resistance in the bacterial flora of an individual patient, and in the population of which he or she is a member—by **selection** and overgrowth of resistant mutants (e.g. rifampicin resistance in *Neisseria meningitidis*), or by **induction** of innate resistance mechanisms latent within initially apparently sensitive subpopulations (e.g. cefotaxime resistance in *Enterobacter cloacae*). Multiple determinants of resistance may be linked on plasmids or other mobile genetic elements, so exposure to one antimicrobial agent may increase the prevalence of all linked resistances in the population.

Selection and induction during antibiotic treatment is most likely with undrained 'sumps' of infected material (e.g. empyema, abdominal abscess). Resistant bacteria may also appear *de novo* at an infected site by **cross-infection** and **superinfection**—most likely with infections that communicate with the mucous membranes or skin (e.g. abdominal abscess treated with open drainage).

**Current important examples of resistance:** four bacteria are causing particular resistance problems in the UK and USA at the moment: methicillin-resistant *Staphylococcus aureus* (MRSA) (➤251); high-level gentamicin-resistant (HLGR) and vancomycin-resistant enterococci (➤261); cefotaxime/ceftazidime-resistant *Klebsiella* spp. (➤279); and multiply-resistant *Mycobacterium tuberculosis* (➤39).

Other worrying developments include the emergence of glycopeptide intermediate-resistant *Staphylococcus aureus* (GISA ➤252) in several countries, fully vancomycin-resistant MRSA in the USA (➤253), highly resistant *Acinetobacter baunanii* in ICUs in southern Europe and SE Asia (➤294), and the inexorable rise worldwide in resistance to all first-line antibiotics in common pathogens.

⌨ The Path of Least Resistance: www.doh.gov.uk/smacsyn.htm

### Counting the costs

At any one time, about 25% of hospital in-patients are receiving antibiotics, and about 15% of a large hospital's drug budget is spent on antibiotics. When audited, about 15% of this

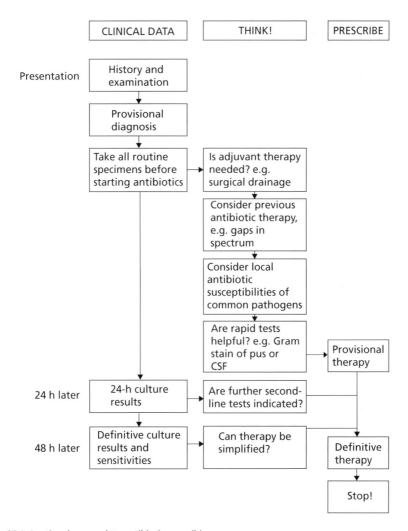

**Figure 37.1** A rational approach to antibiotic prescribing.

usage is inappropriate. Antibiotic expenditure rises annually above inflation in all units, with the largest proportional increases seen recently in antiviral and antifungal agents. Considerable savings can be made by agreement of an **antibiotic policy** allowing bulk purchase of few agents, reduced chance of confusion, and offering treatment guidelines based on local resistance patterns, at the expense of restricted clinical freedom.

The best methods of ensuring cost-effective antibiotic therapy involve:

1 **Agreement of treatment guidelines** between microbiologists and clinicians.
2 **Selective sensitivity reporting** by laboratories.
3 **Regular feedback of usage** to prescribers.
4 **Budgetary inducements** to reduce expenditure.

## Principles of antibiotic usage

Figure 37.1 illustrates a rational approach to antibiotic prescribing.

**Table 37.2** Factors influencing antibiotic choices

| Factor | Notes |
|---|---|
| Antibiotic activity | *In vitro* and *in vivo* vs. likely or known pathogens |
| Concentrations achieved at site of infection | Predictably poor for many in CSF, eye, intracellularly and in abscesses. Some have poor urinary penetration (e.g. macrolides) |
| Bacterial resistance | Local knowledge of resistance patterns; previous antibiotic therapy; likelihood of inducing resistance in the infecting flora |
| Pharmacokinetics | Absorption, excretion, metabolism, penetration. Some give poor tissue levels (e.g. nalidixic acid) |
| Side effects | Adverse drug reactions and interactions; some patients predisposed (e.g. age, renal or hepatic failure). Toxicity (aminoglycosides and VIII nerve), allergy (ampicillin rash), superinfection (thrush, *Clostridium difficile*), administration problems (iv line infection) |
| Cost | Of drug, administration, and monitoring |

**Take specimens for culture before starting antibiotics:** Specimens taken after antibiotics have been given (even only a few hours after) may be grossly misleading.

**Antibiotic choice:** Once it has been decided to treat a patient with antibiotics, there are usually numerous agents that could be **rational therapy**. Few clinical syndromes are so characteristic, and their causative organisms reliably antibiotic sensitive, that a single antimicrobial agent of first choice is always indicated. Rapid tests can sometimes confirm a microbial cause and allow definitive therapy to be started immediately — e.g. Gram stain of CSF confirming *Neisseria meningitidis*, allowing benzylpenicillin monotherapy. Alternatives are always necessary to cater for hypersensitivity in the patient and unusual resistance in the pathogen. Most hospital or practice antibiotic policies give guidelines for antibiotic choice in different clinical situations. Local contemporary knowledge of susceptibility rates of common pathogens to a range of antimicrobial agents is essential, and regular updates should be produced by microbiology laboratories.

**Factors to be considered** when choosing which to use are listed in Table 37.2.

**Route of administration: Intravenous** recommended for severe infection. Bolus doses better than continuous infusion for most indications, but risks of iv access and high costs of administration. **Intramuscular** allows use of depot preparations, but painful (some agents locally toxic), ineffective if patient shocked, and contraindicated with haemorrhagic diathesis. **Oral** best for minor infections and follow-on after initial iv therapy; requires a conscious patient without diarrhoea or vomiting; administration costs low; possibly greater effects on commensal flora of colon. Some antibiotics especially well absorbed orally (e.g. ciprofloxacin, fusidic acid). **Rectal** cheap and often convenient, but not with diarrhoea, and only limited range of agents available for this route (e.g. metronidazole). **Topical** cheap, but hypersensitivity reactions and encouragement of bacterial resistance are problems. Mupirocin (➤414) and antiseptics are preferred.

**Combinations of antibiotics** are most commonly chosen to **broaden spectrum**, although there are a few specific indications for **synergistic action** (penicillin/gentamicin for streptococcal infective endocarditis) **to retard development of resistance** (e.g. isoniazid,

**Table 37.3** Examples of common antibiotic combinations for empirical use

| Antibiotic combination | Suspected source is | Strengths | Weaknesses |
|---|---|---|---|
| Ampicillin, gentamicin, metronidazole | Abdominal, urinary | Broad activity against faecal and urinary pathogens | Nephrotoxicity of gentamicin, not active vs. *Legionella*, *Staph. aureus* |
| Benzylpenicillin, flucloxacillin | Soft tissue | | No Gram-negative or 'atypical' cover |
| Co-amoxiclav | Abdominal, urinary, soft tissue | Single agent, low toxicity | Inadequate vs. 'hard' coliforms and *Pseudomonas* to use alone in severe sepsis. Not active vs. *Legionella* |
| Cefotaxime or ceftriaxone plus metronidazole | Abdominal, urinary, respiratory | Low toxicity | Inadequate vs. 'hard' coliforms and *Pseudomonas* in severe sepsis. Not active vs. *Legionella*, enterococci, *Listeria*. Risk of *Clostridium difficile* diarrhoea |
| Cefotaxime or ceftriaxone plus macrolide | Respiratory | Low toxicity | Not active vs. anaerobes in the event that diagnosis is incorrect. Risk of *Clostridium difficile* diarrhoea |
| Piperacillin/ tazobactam (Tazocin) | Abdominal | Often used as single agent in surgical units | Not effective against most 'hard' coliforms. |

rifampicin, pyrazinamide + ethambutol for *Mycobacterium tuberculosis*) and to **overcome resistance** (e.g. amoxicillin + clavulanate (co-amoxiclav) for many β-lactamase-producing bacteria); rarely enables use of **lower doses of toxic agents** (e.g. amphotericin + flucytosine in cryptococcal meningitis).

Certain cocktails are widely used for empirical therapy, and it is helpful to understand the strengths and weaknesses of each (Table 37.3). These comments need to be modified in the light of the local prevalence of resistant organisms: MRSA, penicillin-resistant pneumococci, high-level gentamicin-resistant enterococci, VRE, multiply-resistant *Acinetobacter* spp.

**Guidelines for stopping:** 'measures of response' to antibiotic treatment include: fever, pulse, respiratory rate, CRP, ESR, WBC, culture results. Antibiotic course-lengths have been defined by clinical trial for only a few infectious syndromes (including tuberculosis ➤38 and gonorrhoea ➤86). Inferences can be made for others, including lower urinary tract infection (➤77), streptococcal infective endocarditis (➤49), *Staphylococcus aureus* bacteraemia (➤249), meningitis (➤96), but length of treatment needed for many common infections including pneumonias, wound infections, abdominal abscess, osteomyelitis and most severe systemic sepsis is based upon scant evidence, and antibiotics are probably often given for too long. When individual guidelines not available, patients best treated iv until a clear clinical response is seen, then orally until signs and symptoms have resolved and for severe, chronic infections such as osteomyelitis, abdominal abscess, 'measures of response' have returned to normal range.

**Reaction to apparent treatment failure:**
• Ask for microbiology or infectious diseases opinion ☎.

- Review diagnosis, results of culture, and therapy:
  - Is the provisional diagnosis of infection still likely?
  - Was the original culture representative?
  - Are further, second-line investigations now indicated?
  - Is more time needed for response? (Serious infections often take 48–72 h to respond clinically.)
- Then consider the following:
  - Is drainage or foreign-body removal indicated?
  - Stop antibiotics and reculture?
  - Is this a drug (antibiotic) allergy?
  - Is there a superinfection or additional pathogen (original site, or different—e.g. iv catheter sepsis)?
  - Has the original pathogen developed resistance?
  - Is there an intracellular-persisting pathogen?

## Prophylactic antibiotics

Antibiotics given just before, during and just after the period of exposure to an infectious agent to reduce the risks of establishment of infection. Audit shows that prophylaxis comprises ≈25% antibiotic usage in hospitals, and up to 50% of these courses are given for too long.

**Principles of use:** consider **incidence** of infection to be prevented, **likely organisms**, their **probable sensitivities** and **period of risk**. Infections deserving prophylaxis should be **common** (e.g. all large-bowel surgery), and/or **catastrophic** (e.g. prosthetic heart valve insertion), and/or proven to be reduced by prophylaxis.

**Disadvantages of prophylaxis** to be weighed against potential advantages: antibiotic costs; encouragement of antibiotic resistance in individual and community; hypersensitivity and adverse drug reactions; false sense of security (prophylaxis is never a substitute for good surgical, aseptic and antiseptic techniques); sometimes delayed presentation rather than prevention of infections.

**Choice of prophylactic regimen:** use high doses of antibiotics that reach high levels at the risk site (e.g. rifampicin rather than penicillin to clear nasopharyngeal meningococci); maintain effective levels throughout risk period (e.g. consider repeating doses during long operations).

**Principles of use:** There are important differences between medical and surgical indications (Table 37.4).

### Surgical prophylaxis (Table 37.5)

First dose given at time of induction of anaesthesia to ensure adequate tissue levels peri-

Table 37.4 Differences between medical and surgical antibiotic prophylaxis

|  | Medical indications | Surgical indications |
|---|---|---|
| Risk period | Often long and ill-defined | Usually short |
| Magnitude of risks | Often low with many confounding variables (hence value of prophylaxis hard to prove) | Often high, or many patients at risk under standardized conditions (hence easier to prove) |
| Routes of antibiotics | Oral usually essential | Parenteral regimen assures high, timely concentrations at sites of risk |
| Infecting organisms | Often a single organism | More usually a range of possibilities |
| Repeated risk? | Often yes | Usually single event only |

**Table 37.5** Surgical prophylaxis

| Operation | Normal regimen | Minor* penicillin allergy | Major† penicillin allergy |
|---|---|---|---|
| **Orthopaedics** | | | |
| Primary insertion of prosthesis | Flucoxacillin 1 g q6h × 3 doses | Cefotaxime 2 g q8h × 2 doses | Vancomycin 1 g × 1 dose‡ |
| Urinary catheter insertion during post-op. period§ | Benzylpenicillin 1.2 g + gentamicin 120 mg × 1 dose | Gentamicin 120 mg × 1 dose | Gentamicin 120 mg × 1 dose |
| **Neurosurgery** | | | |
| Clean craniotomy, shunts, flaps and external drains | Flucoxacillin 1 g, repeated if op. time > 4 h | Cefotaxime 1 g, repeated if op. time > 6 h | Vancomycin 500 mg‡, repeated if op. time > 6 h |
| Acoustic neuroma and transmucosal operations | Cefotaxime 1 g q8h for 24 h | Cefotaxime 1 g q8h for 24 h | Chloramphenicol or vancomycin single dose |
| **Abdominal surgery** | | | |
| Uncomplicated biliary surgery or oesophagectomy | Cefotaxime 1 g, repeated if op. time > 6 h | Cefotaxime 1 g, repeated if op. time > 6 h | Ciprofloxacin 200 mg |
| Complicated biliary surgery (e.g. acute infection) | Cefotaxime 1 g q8h for 48 h | Cefotaxime 1 g q8h for 48 h | Ciprofloxacin 200 mg q12h for 48 h |
| Complicated oesophagectomy (e.g. perforation, spillage) | Cefotaxime 2 g + metronidazole 500 mg q8h for 48 h | Cefotaxime 2 g + metronidazole 500 mg q8h for 48 h | Ciprofloxacin 200 mg q12h + metronidazole 500 mg q8h for 48 h |
| Uncomplicated gastrectomy or colonic surgery | Benzylpenicillin 1.2 g + gentamicin 120 mg + metronidazole 500 mg × 1 dose | Cefotaxime 1 g + metronidazole 500 mg × 1 dose | Ciprofloxacin 200 mg + metronidazole 500 mg × 1 dose |
| Complicated gastrectomy (e.g. gastric stasis, spillage at operation) or complicated colonic surgery¶ (e.g. AP resection, spillage of gut contents) | Benzylpenicillin 1.2 g q6h + gentamicin 120 mg q12h + metronidazole 500 mg q8h for 48 h | Cefotaxime 1 g + metronidazole 500 mg q8h for 48 h | Ciprofloxacin 200 mg q12h + metronidazole 500 mg q8h for 48 h |
| Appendicectomy (uncomplicated) | Metronidazole 500 mg p.r. — 2 doses | | |
| Complicated appendicectomy | As for complicated colonic surgery above | | |
| Aortic/lower limb vascular graft surgery (uncomplicated) | Flucloxacillin 500 mg + gentamicin 120 mg × 2 doses 8 h apart | Cefotaxime 1 g × 2 doses 8 h apart | Vancomycin 1 g single dose‡ |
| Aortic and lower limb vascular graft surgery — bowel ischaemia suspected | Flucloxacillin 500 mg q6h + gentamicin 120 mg q12h + metronidazole 500 mg q8h for 48 h | Cefotaxime 1 g + metronidazole 500 mg q8h for 48 h | Ciprofloxacin 200 mg q12h + metronidazole 500 mg q8h for 48 h |

* Skin rash only. † Anaphylaxis, immediate urticaria or angioneurotic oedema. ‡ Vancomycin infusion is given over 1.5 h, so best started with pre-med. § Give 1 h before catheterization. ¶ ☐ If therapy is prolonged beyond 48 h, gentamicin assays should be performed.
For all indications consider adding/substituting vancomycin or teicoplanin in patients known to be carriers of MRSA, or if MRSA prevalent on unit.
☐ Scottish Inter-Collegiate Guidelines Network, 'Antibiotic prophylaxis in surgery' (Guideline no. 45) at www.sign.ac.uk/guidelines/published/index.html

operatively. 'Cover' for >48 h **never** shown superior to shorter periods, and **single-dose** prophylaxis increasingly proven to be as effective. Prophylaxis proven ineffective for indwelling urinary catheters, CSF leaks, insertion of iv and Tenckoff catheters.

Protocols are usually decided at individual hospitals, based on local antibiotic resistance patterns and purchasing arrangements. The regimens in Table 37.5 are suitable if local protocols are unavailable.

### Medical prophylaxis (Table 37.6)

## Antibiotic assays ⚠

Serum assay is needed when an antibiotic has a narrow 'therapeutic index' (range of serum concentrations between adequate therapy and toxicity), or when absorption, excretion or metabolism is highly variable. Timing of assay samples in relation to administration of doses is important for interpretation; write both times on the request card. Perform assays around doses given early in the day to avoid delays or the need to do tests 'on call'. Many laboratories have standardized on samples taken immediately before a dose ('pre-sample' or 'trough' level) and 60 min after the same dose ('post-sample' or 'peak' level) although single, timed samples are increasingly used for single daily dose aminoglycoside therapy (➤403) and—less commonly at the moment—glycopeptide therapy. Take the first assay sample of a course around the third or fourth dose. Targets for peak and trough levels are shown where relevant in antibiotic dosing charts (➤391).

## Antibiotics in pregnancy

Choice of antibiotics influenced by:
- **Risks to fetus** (teratogenesis greater in first trimester).
- **Effects of the pregnancy on maternal infections** (asymptomatic bacteriuria ➤78, vaginal colonization and premature labour ➤140).
- **Pharmacokinetics** (serum concentrations lower for most antibiotics in pregnancy).

In general, **full doses should be used, but course lengths kept to a minimum.** Important to **send cultures** from pregnant women to guide optimal therapy.

Table 37.7 lists appropriate choices for common clinical scenarios.

## Antibiotic therapy during lactation

Very few antibiotics will be taken in sufficient dosage by a suckling infant to cause harm, but information is lacking on many, and mothers may prefer to interrupt breastfeeding to avoid any possibility of risk. Alteration of the infant's gut flora, and sensitization, may occur. No antibiotic is known to inhibit lactation or the suckling reflex.

Agents **safe** because of the extremely small dosage ingested include clavulanate, cycloserine, ethambutol, penicillins (but risk of sensitization), pyrazinamide and rifampicin.

**Table 37.6** Medical antibiotic prophylaxis

| | |
|---|---|
| **Short-term risks** | |
| Infective endocarditis | (➤53) |
| Contacts of invasive meningococcal and *Haemophilus influenzae* infection | (➤100) |
| Syphilis | (➤91) |
| Gonorrhoea | (➤87) |
| Diphtheria | (➤268) |
| Neonatal Lancefield group B streptococcal infection | (➤140) |
| **Medium-term risks** | |
| Neutropenia | (➤174) |
| Patients in ITU (selective gut decontamination) | (➤34) |
| Travellers' diarrhoea | (➤64) |
| Leptospirosis | (➤327) |
| Lyme disease | (➤323) |
| Malaria | (➤211) |
| Tuberculosis contacts | (➤45) |
| **Long-term risks** | |
| *Pneumocystis carinii* in AIDS, transplantation, etc. | (➤155) |
| Asplenia | (➤170) |
| Sickle-cell disease: penicillin V 250 mg q12h, and see asplenia | |
| Rheumatic fever | (➤257) |
| Recurrent UTI | (➤77) |

**Table 37.7** Antibiotic prescribing in pregnancy

| Infection | Safe first choices for which there is extensive experience for common infections: (possible alternatives in parentheses: ☎) |
|---|---|
| UTI (➢79) | **Cystitis:** cephalexin (nitrofurantoin (may cause neonatal haemolysis used at term), co-amoxiclav); <br> **Upper tract infection:** cefuroxime, cefotaxime (benzylpenicillin + gentamicin*) |
| Respiratory tract infection | **Upper RTI with systemic symptoms:** Penicillin V, erythromycin (cephalexin) <br> **Acute bronchitis:** amoxicillin (co-amoxiclav) <br> **Pneumonia:** amoxicillin + erythromycin (cefotaxime + erythromycin) |
| Septicaemia | Cefotaxime + metronidazole (benzylpenicillin + gentamicin* + metronidazole) |
| Vaginal candidiasis | Topical clotrimazole, econazole, miconazole, nystatin, or ketoconazole |
| Pelvic inflammatory disease | Erythromycin (add metronidazole after first trimester) |
| Sexually transmitted diseases | **Syphilis** or **gonorrhoea:** benzylpenicillin <br> **Syphilis + penicillin allergy:** consult expert opinion <br> **Gonorrhoea + penicillin allergy:** cefuroxime, cefotaxime <br> **Chlamydia:** erythromycin |
| Prophylaxis | **Surgical:** Cefuroxime, cefotaxime (+ metronidazole if indicated ➢386) <br> **Infective endocarditis:** (➢53) |
| Parasites | **Malaria:** consult expert opinion prophylaxis and treatment <br> **Amoebiasis:** metronidazole (➢218) <br> **Giardiasis:** metronidazole <br> **Helminths:** leave until after delivery if infection light or moderate (heavy trichuriasis: piperazine) |
| Tuberculosis | As for non-pregnant adults, but avoid streptomycin |

* Consider avoiding these aminoglycoside-containing regimens in second and third trimesters—possible risk of eighth nerve damage.

Cephalosporins also probably fall into this group. Others that will be ingested, but are not known to cause harm, include erythromycin, pyrimethamine, quinidine and trimethoprim. Vancomycin, teicoplanin and aminoglycosides will not be absorbed from the infant gut. Insufficient chloroquine or proguanil is ingested to be protective. Isoniazid carries theoretical risk of convulsions and neurotoxicity; give pyridoxine to mother and infant. Nitrofurantoin is safe unless G6PD-deficient.

**Avoid** chloramphenicol, clindamycin, co-trimoxazole, dapsone, Fansidar, ganciclovir, halofantrine, Maloprim, mefloquine, high-dose metronidazole (normal-dose regimens safe), nalidixic acid, quinolones, sulphonamides, tetracyclines (although usually chelated in milk). Also avoid povidone–iodine antiseptics.

# Chapter 38

# Antibiotics: Classification and dosing guidelines

A pharmacological grouping, further divided by spectrum of activity. Many variants of each group exist, often differing only slightly in spectrum of activity or pharmacological properties. In the tables that follow, CSF✓ or urine✓ indicates that the drug in question penetrates CSF or urine sufficiently well to be useful clinically. CSF✗ or urine✗ indicate the converse.

**Doses:** The dosage recommendations in the tables in this chapter are abbreviated and standardized to give individual doses and frequency, therefore they may vary slightly from those quoted in other ways in different publications, including manufacturers' recommendations. **Doses and frequencies in parentheses are for severe infection and to penetrate difficult sites, e.g. CSF.** More details of dosing, adverse drug reactions and interactions can be found in the latest edition of the *British National Formulary* (see 🖥bnf.vhn.net) and in manufacturers' data sheets (see 🖥emc.vhn.net). Many elderly people should be considered to have mild renal failure. In renal impairment, choose antibiotics with minimal nephrotoxic potential, and avoid potentially nephrotoxic combinations (e.g. aminoglycoside + vancomycin or amphotericin, or loop diuretics) and avoid agents and combinations likely to precipitate *Clostridium difficile* diarrhoea (e.g. cefotaxime, especially combined with macrolides).

**Cost:** To give an indication of the relative costs of antibiotics (drug costs only) we have divided agents into three groups (£, ££ and £££) on the basis of the cost of 1 day's treatment at moderate–high dose. Some very expensive drugs qualify for ££££.

**Cautions/contraindications:**
P    Pregnancy.
L    Lactation.
H    Hepatic failure.
E    Epilepsy.
O    Porphyrias (see BNF for details).
🔔    Assay needed.
C    Interferes with creatinine determination.
G    Caution in patients with G6PD deficiency.
⊗    Contraindicated or use not established in children below age stated in parentheses .

**Interactions:** These are listed for 10 common groups of drugs. Check details in the BNF. Any broad-spectrum agent can interfere with oestrogen absorption of the contraceptive pill, and prolong prothrombin time with anticoagulants.
1    Absorption/metabolism altered by ulcer healing drugs, antacids, calcium/magnesium/ zinc/iron salts.
2    Anticoagulants.
3    Antidiabetic.
4    Anti-epileptics.
5    Carbamazepine.
6    Cyclosporin.
7    Digoxin.
8    Rifampicin.
9    Theophylline.
0    Terfenadine.

## Antibiotics and dialysis

The extent to which antibiotics are removed by dialysis depends on many factors, particularly the degree of protein binding. Information is not readily available for many drugs; the data given below have been collated from a number of sources (see references below). Prescribers should **always** consult the current manufac-

391

turer's product data sheet for any antibiotic pre-scribed for dialysis patients. Specific instances where additional information is known to be available in the data sheet are indicated on the chart (📄). If antibiotics are removed by dialysis a supplementary dose may be required post-treatment, or it may be possible to schedule drugs so that a dose falls due at the completion of dialysis.

Key: 📄 See data sheet. 🔔: Monitor serum levels.
HD: haemodialysis. PD: peritoneal dialysis.

# β-Lactams

All excreted via the kidney; excretion of many reduced (hence serum levels increased and prolonged) by probenecid.

## Penicillins (Tables 38.1–38.4)

**Table 38.1** 'Ordinary' penicillins

|  | Benzylpenicillin (Pen-G) £ | Phenoxymethyl penicillin (Pen-V) £ |
|---|---|---|
| Administration, pharmacology | Parenteral only (acid-labile) CSF✓ (in high dose, penetration best with inflamed meninges) Urine✓ | Oral. Variable absorption in adults. CSF✗, Urine✓ |
| Sensitive; often useful | Streptococci (*Enterococcus* spp. not killed), *Clostridium* spp., *Neisseria gonorrhoeae* (resistance increasing) and *meningitidis*, *Actinomyces* spp., treponemes, leptospires, Lyme disease, *Listeria monocytogenes* | |
| Variable; occasionally useful | Staphylococci (but >90% resistant in and out of hospital nowadays), non-sporing anaerobes (resistance increasing) | |
| Resistant; unreliable | Coliforms, *Pseudomonas* spp., *Haemophilus influenzae*. MRSA | |
| Side effects | Hypersensitivity rash, fever (rare anaphylaxis); rare interstitial nephritis, cerebral toxicity with very high doses | |
| Cautions | — | — |
| Interactions | — | — |
| Serum creatinine: | | |
| Normal | 0.6 g (2.4 g) q6h (q3h) Max 14.4 g/day for short periods | 250 mg (500 mg) q6h |
| 150–300 μmol/L | ditto | ditto |
| 300–700 μmol/L | ditto | 250 mg (500 mg) q8h |
| >700 μmol/L | 0.6 g (1.2 g) q6h (q3h) Max 6 g/day for short periods | 250 mg (500 mg) q12h |
| Effect of dialysis | HD: 20–50%. Supplementary dose required post-HD | |

**Table 38.2** Broader-spectrum penicillins

|  | Ampicillin £ | Amoxicillin £ | Co-amoxiclav ££ |
|---|---|---|---|
| Administration, pharmacology | Best used iv. CSF✓ (in high dose, penetration best with inflamed meninges), urine✓ | Best used orally. More reliably absorbed than Pen-V in adults. Urine✓ | Amoxicillin + clavulanic acid (blocks many β-lactamases). Oral and iv. CSF✗. Urine✓ |
| Sensitive, often useful | As 'ordinary penicillins', with better activity against *Enterococcus* spp. | | As amoxicillin, plus staphylococci, non-sporing anaerobes, most *Haemophilus* spp. and most 'easy' coliforms (➤273) |
| Variable; occasionally useful | *Haemophilus* spp. (15% resistant), *Escherichia coli* (50% resistant), *Proteus mirabilis*, staphylococci (90% resistant), non-sporing anaerobes | | |
| Resistant; unreliable | Most coliforms other than *Escherichia coli* and *Proteus mirabilis*; *Moraxella catarrhalis*, *Pseudomonas* spp.; MRSA | | 'Hard' coliforms (➤273), *Pseudomonas* spp.; MRSA |
| Side effects | Hypersensitivity, especially 'ampicillin rash' in acute EBV infection, rare anaphylaxis. Nausea. Diarrhoea (5–10%), *Clostridium difficile* | | As amp/amoxicillin, but diarrhoea 10–12%. Cholestatic jaundice in elderly with prolonged treatment |
| Cautions | — | — | H |
| Interactions | — | — | — |
| Serum creatinine: Normal | Oral: 500 mg (1 g) q6h iv/im: 500 mg (1–2 g) q6h | Oral: 250 mg (500 mg) q8h iv/im: 500 mg (1 g) q8h | Oral: 375 mg (750 mg) q8h iv: 1.2 g q8h (q6h) |
| 150–300 µmol/L | ditto | ditto | ditto |
| 300–700 µmol/L | Oral: 500 mg (1 g) q8h iv/im: 500 mg (1–2 g) q8h | Oral: 250 mg (500 mg) q12h iv/im: 500 mg (1 g) q8h | Oral: 375 mg (750 mg) q12h iv: 600 mg q8h |
| >700 µmol/L | Oral: 500 mg (1 g) q12h iv/im: 500 mg (1–2 g) q12h | Oral: 250 mg (500 mg) q12–16h iv/im: 500 mg (1 g) q12h | Oral: 375 mg (750 mg) q24h iv: 600 mg q24h |
| Effect of dialysis | HD: 20–50%. PD: <5%. Schedule dose after HD | HD: 20–50%. PD: 5–20%. Schedule dose after HD | |

## Flucloxacillin £

Other **isoxazolyl penicillins**—cloxacillin, dicloxacillin, oxacillin, are used in the USA and Europe and have similar spectrum/adverse effects.

**Uses:** Resistant to staphylococcal β-lactamase. Spectrum of activity otherwise similar to benzylpenicillin. Use for **staphylococci** and mixed infections with streptococci; combine with gentamicin, fusidic acid or rifampicin for severe staphylococcal infection. Inactive against MRSA and *Enterococcus* spp.

**Administration:** Parenteral or oral. CSF✓ (in high dose, penetration best with inflamed meninges), urine✓.

**Adverse effects:** Rare neutropenia, and reversible renal and hepatic dysfunction (cholestasis) with courses over 2 weeks, commoner in the elderly.

**Cautions:** O ☺(1 yr).

**Normal dose:** oral: 250 mg (1 g) q6h; im/iv 500 mg (1.5 g) q6h (q4h). No reduction required in renal failure.

**Effect of dialysis:** HD: <5%. ▤ No supplement required for HD.

Table 38.3 Anti-pseudomonal/Gram-negative β-lactamase-resistant penicillins

| | Piperacillin £££ | Tazocin (piperacillin + tazobactam) £££ | Timentin (ticarcillin + clavulanate) £££ |
|---|---|---|---|
| Administration, pharmacology | Parenteral only. CSF✓ (in high dose, penetration best with inflamed meninges), urine✓ | Parenteral only. CSF✗. Urine✓ | |
| Sensitive, often useful | Mostly like ampicillin + useful activity against many *Pseudomonas* spp. Less active against Gram-positive cocci | Like co-amoxiclav + useful activity against many *Pseudomonas* spp. | |
| Variable; occasionally useful | More active than ampicillin against some 'hard' coliforms (➢273) | | |
| Resistant; unreliable | Most 'hard' coliforms, (➢273) anaerobes, staphylococci | Most 'hard' coliforms (➢273) | |
| Side effects | Overall similar to benzylpenicillin. Sodium load. Occasional reversible platelet dysfunction, liver function abnormalities. Rare convulsions, commoner in renal failure, previous CNS disease and old age | | |
| Cautions | — | — | — |
| Interactions | — | — | — |
| Serum creatinine: Normal | iv/im: 25 mg/kg (75 mg/kg) q6h. For *Pseudomonas* spp. and other severe infections use 16 g/day or more | iv: 4.5 g q8h | iv: 3.2 g q6h (q4h) |
| 150–300 μmol/L | ditto | ditto | iv: 3.2 g q8h |
| 300–700 μmol/L | iv/im: 25 mg/kg (75 mg/kg) q8h | iv: 4.5 g q12h | iv: 1.6 g q8h |
| >700 μmol/L | iv/im: 25 mg/kg (75 mg/kg) q12h | ditto | iv: 1.6 g q12h |
| Effect of dialysis | HD: 20–50%. ▤ Supplementary dose post HD | | HD: 20–50%. PD: 5–20% |

**Table 38.4** Carbapenems (imipenem–cilastatin,* meropenem) and monobactams (aztreonam)

| | Imipenem £££ | Meropenem £££ | Aztreonam £££ |
|---|---|---|---|
| Administration, pharmacology | Parenteral only. CSF✓ (in high dose, penetration best with inflamed meninges), urine✓ | | |
| Sensitive, often useful | Moderate to good activity against virtually all groups of bacteria; highly β-lactamase stable. Meropenem has better anti-pseudomonal and weaker anti-Gram-positive activity | | Good to excellent activity against virtually all coliforms, *Pseudomonas* spp., haemophili, neisserias and other Gram-negative aerobes; highly β-lactamase-stable |
| Resistant; unreliable | Only MRSA, most *Enterococcus faecium*, and *Stenotrophomonas maltophilia* predictably resistant; rare coliforms/*Pseudomonas* spp. and other pseudomonads resistant by impermeability of outer membrane | | All Gram-positive bacteria and anaerobes. *Stenotrophomonas maltophilia* |
| Side effects | Overall similar to benzylpenicillin. Imipenem: nausea reduced by slowing infusion. Occasional reversible liver function abnormalities, convulsions with previous history of epilepsy. Low risk of cross-reaction with penicillin allergy | | Nausea, vomiting, diarrhoea. Occasional reversible neutropenia, thrombocytopenia, liver function abnormalities. Probably usable in patients with benzylpenicillin and other β-lactam allergies |
| Cautions | PLE 🙁 (3 m) | PLH 🙁 (3 m) | PL |
| Interactions | — | — | 2 |
| Serum creatinine: Normal | iv/im: 500 mg (1 g) q6h | iv: 500 mg (2G) q8h | iv/im: 1 g (2 g) q8h (q6h) |
| 150–300 µmol/L | ditto | iv: 500 mg (2G) q12h | ditto |
| 300–700 µmol/L | iv/im: 250 mg (500 mg) q8h (q6h) | iv: 250 mg (1G) q12h | iv/im: 500 mg (1 g) q8h |
| >700 µmol/L | iv/im: 250 mg (500 mg) q12h | iv: 250 mg (1G) q24h | iv/im: 250 mg (500 mg) q8h |
| Effect of dialysis | HD: >50%. PD: 5–20%. 📄 Dose post-HD and at 12-h intervals | HD: >50%. 📄 Dose post HD | HD: 20–50%. PD: 5–20%. 📄. Additional 1/8 of initial dose post-HD |

*  **Imipenem–cilastatin** combines imipenem with inhibitor of the renal tubular dehydropeptidase that degrades it; thus plasma half-life extended, and renal tubular damage prevented.
Monobactams: **mono**cyclic **beta**-lactams.

# Cephalosporins

Traditionally categorized into four 'generations' with broadly similar antibacterial and pharmacokinetic properties. New agents render this classification less precise. We will describe them under five main headings. Clinicians need to be familiar with (and most hospitals need to keep in stock) only one example of each group. In domiciliary practice, 'first-generation oral' cephalosporins will regularly be useful. Cefotaxime and ceftriaxone are very widely used for the management of community-acquired infection in hospital. Ceftazidime is particularly used for *Pseudomonas* infection in immunocompromised patients, but 'broad-spectrum oral' agents are infrequently used in the UK because of cost, encouragement of resistance and side effects.

Cephalosporins are inactive against enterococci (except cefpirome) and *Listeria monocytogenes*, and are unreliable against clostridia, anaerobes, *Pseudomonas* spp. (except ceftazidime). Nomenclature recently standardized to 'cef-'.

**Adverse effects:** Diarrhoea (*Clostridium difficile* especially with parenteral agents), β-lactam allergy. Fever, rashes, rare erythema multiforme. Arthralgia. Reversible hepatitis or cholestasis. Neutropenia with high dose in renal failure.

## Oral cephalosporins — 'first-generation'

Cefaclor, cefadroxil, cefalexin, cefradine (oral and parenteral), cefazolin (parenteral only).

Achieve high urine levels; often borderline levels elsewhere.

Active against *Streptococcus pneumoniae* and *Moraxella catarrhalis* but (excepting cefaclor) have poor activity against *Haemophilus influenzae*. Also active against most *Escherichia coli*, most 'easy' coliforms and some *Staphylococcus aureus*.

Mainly used for uncomplicated upper and lower respiratory tract, urinary tract and soft-tissue infections.

## Parenteral cephalosporins — 'second-generation'

Cefamandole, cefoxitin, cefuroxime (oral and parenteral).

Good penetration to most sites at high dose. CSF ✓ (in high dose, penetration best with inflamed meninges), urine ✓.

More resistant to β-lactamases than first-generation drugs. Good activity against *Staphylococcus aureus*, group A β-haemolytic streps, *Streptococcus pneumoniae*, *Neisseria* spp., *Haemophilus influenzae* and many coliforms. Cefoxitin also active against many anaerobes.

Cefuroxime may be given for community-acquired pneumonia, but in general third-generation agents are more widely used. Oral cefuroxime is used for the indications listed above for the first-generation agents.

## Parenteral cephalosporins — 'third-generation'

Cefotaxime, ceftriaxone.

Good penetration to most sites at high dose. CSF ✓ (in high dose, penetration best with inflamed meninges), urine ✓.

More active than the second-generation drugs against Gram-negative organisms and less affected by many bacterial resistance mechanisms, whilst retaining useful activity against Gram-positive bacteria. Cefotaxime and ceftriaxone are widely used for serious infections such as septicaemia, pneumonia, and for meningitis. Apart from their different half-life and dosing schedule, they have similar spectra of activity. Ceftriaxone can cause biliary sludging.

## Broad-spectrum parenteral cephalosporins

Ceftazidime, cefpirome.

Good penetration to most sites at high dose. CSF ✓ (in high dose, penetration best with inflamed meninges), urine ✓.

Similar to cefotaxime and ceftriaxone, but ceftazidime is active against *Pseudomonas aeruginosa* and is used in situations where that organism is likely, such as neutropenic sepsis. Cefpirome is active against many 'hard' coliforms and enterococci.

## Broad-spectrum oral cephalosporins— 'fourth-generation'

Cefixime, cefpodoxime, cefprozil.

Oral agents with a similar range of activity to cefotaxime and ceftriaxone. Active against a range of Gram-positive and Gram-negative organisms, including *Staphylococcus aureus* (excepting cefixime, which has no anti-staphylococcal or anaerobic activity), group A β-haemolytic streptococci, *Streptococcus pneumoniae*, *Neisseria* spp., *Haemophilus influenzae* and (excepting cefpodoxime) many Enterobacteriaceae. Promoted for urinary, upper and lower respiratory tract infections, but not widely used because of cost and frequency of adverse effects.

**Table 38.5** First-generation cephalosporin doses

| Drug | Cefaclor £££ | Cefadroxil ££ | Cefalexin £ | Cefradine ££ | Cefazolin ££ |
|---|---|---|---|---|---|
| Cautions | O ☹ (1 m) | O | O | O | O ☹ (1 m) |
| Interactions | — | — | — | — | — |
| Serum creatinine: | | | | | |
| Normal | Oral: 250 mg (500 mg) q8h. Also modified release preparation: 375 mg (750 mg) q12h | 500 mg (1 g) q12h | 250 mg (1 g) q6h | 250 mg (500 mg) 6hly or 500 mg (1 g) q12h | iv/im: 0.5 g (1.0 g) q12h (q6h) |
| 150–300 µmol/L | ditto | ditto | ditto | ditto | iv/im: 0.5 g (1.0 g) q12h (q8h) |
| 300–700 µmol/L | ditto | 500 mg (1 g) q24h | 250 mg (500 mg) q6h | 250 mg (500 mg) q8h | iv/im: 0.25 g (0.5 g) q12h |
| >700 µmol/L | 250 mg q8h or 375 mg q12h | 500 mg (1 g) q36h | 250 mg q8h | 250 mg (500 mg) q12h | iv/im: 0.25 g (0.5 g) q24h (q18h) |
| Effect of dialysis | HD: 20–50%. 📄 Additional dose prior to HD | HD: 20–50% | HD: 20–50%. PD: 5–20%. 📄 500 mg supplementary dose post-HD | HD: 20–50%. PD: 5–20% | |

**Table 38.6** Second- and third-generation cephalosporins

| Drug | Cefuroxime axetil £££ | Cefuroxime ££ | Cefamandole ££ | Cefoxitin £££ | Cefotaxime £££ | Ceftriaxone £££ |
|---|---|---|---|---|---|---|
| Cautions | O | O | O ☹ (1 m) | OC | O | O ☹ (<6 wks) |
| Interactions | — | — | 2 | — | — | — |
| Serum creatinine: | | | | | | |
| Normal | 250 mg (500 mg) q12h | iv/im: 750 mg (1.5 g) q8h (q6h). Max. 3 g q8h in meningitis | iv/im: 0.5 g (2 g) q8h (q4h) | iv/im: 1 g (3 g) q8h (q6h) | iv/im: 1 g (2 g) q12h (q6h). Up to 200 mg/kg/day in meningitis | iv/im: 1 g (4 g) q24h |
| 150–300 μmol/L | ditto | ditto | iv/im: 0.5 g (2 g) q8h | iv/im: 1 g (2 g) q8h | iv/im: 1 g (2 g) q12h | iv/im: 1 g (4 g) q24h (reduce dose if patient has both renal and hepatic failure) |
| 300–700 μmol/L | ditto | iv/im: 750 mg (1.5 g) q12h | iv/im: 0.5 g (1 g) q8h | iv/im: 1 g (2 g) q12h (q8h) | ditto | ditto |
| >700 μmol/L | ditto | iv/im: 750 mg (1.5 g) q24h | iv/im: 0.5 g (1 g) q12h | iv/im: 1 g (2 g) q24h | iv/im: 1 g (2 g) q12h (0.5 g (1 g) if GFR <5 mL/min) | ditto |
| Effect of dialysis | | 📄 750 mg supplementary dose post-HD | HD: 20–50%. PD: 5–20%. 📄 | HD: 20–50%. PD: 5–20%. 📄 Loading dose after each HD | HD: 20–50%. PD: 5–20%. Schedule dose after HD | HD: <5%. 📄 No supplement required for HD |

**Table 38.7** Broad-spectrum cephalosporins

| Drug | Broad-spectrum parenteral | | Broad-spectrum oral | | |
|---|---|---|---|---|---|
| | Cefpirome £££ | Ceftazidime £££ | Cefixime £££ | Cefpodoxime £££ | Cefprozil £££ |
| Cautions | O ☹ (12 yrs) | O | O ☹ (6 m) | O | O ☹ (6 m) |
| Interactions | — | — | — | 1 | — |
| Serum creatinine: | | | | | |
| Normal | iv/im: 1 g (2 g) q12h | iv/im: 1 g (2 g) q12h (q8h). Up to 150 mg/ kg/day in meningitis or cystic fibrosis. Max 6 g/day | 200 mg (400 mg) q24h | 100 mg (200 mg) q12h | 500 mg q24h (q12h) |
| 150–300 µmol/L | iv/im: 500 mg (1 g) q12h | iv/im: 1 g (1.5 g) q12h | ditto | ditto | ditto |
| 300–700 µmol/L | iv/im: 250 mg (500 mg) q12h | iv/im: 1 g (1.5 g) q24h | 200 mg q24h | 100 mg q24h | 250 mg q24h |
| >700 µmol/L | ditto | iv/im: 1 g (1.5 g) q48h | ditto | ditto | ditto |
| Effect of dialysis | HD: 20–50% 📄 Additional dose prior to HD | HD: >50%. PD: 5–20% 📄 Supplementary dose post-HD | 📄 No supplement required for HD | 📄 Supplementary dose post-HD | 📄 Supplementary dose post-HD |

Table 38.8 β-Lactam allergy

| Reaction | Frequency | Notes |
|---|---|---|
| Immediate (IgE mediated vs. penicillamine and penicilloic acid breakdown products): anaphylaxis, angio-oedema, urticaria, some maculopapular rashes | 1–10% overall; anaphylaxis 1–5 per 10 000 courses | Anaphylaxis most commonly with iv benzylpenicillin. Avoid **all** β-lactams in patients after anaphylaxis, immediate urticaria or angio-oedema |
| Delayed (some IgG mediated vs. penicilloyl group): 'serum-sickness', haemolytic anaemia, acute interstitial nephritis, neutropenia, rashes, fever | | Appear related to dose and duration of therapy. Can present 3 weeks after course finished. Frequent causes of diagnostic confusion during treatment of endocarditis, etc. |
| Amp/amoxicillin reactions | 5–10% overall: approaching 100% with glandular fever, CMV or HIV infection, chronic lymphocytic leukaemia | Maculopapular rashes of uncertain aetiology. These patients can safely be given other penicillins in future, unless the reaction was urticarial |

Skin testing in expert hands can identify a patient's current allergic state, but can itself cause anaphylaxis. Desensitization rarely helpful in practice.

## β-Lactam allergy (Table 38.8)

Many patients claim to be 'penicillin-allergic', but 90% show no reaction when given penicillins again, and they should not be denied the advantages of β-lactam therapy when it is clearly the treatment of choice. Cross-allergenicity with cephalosporins said to be seen in up to 10% with penicillin allergy, but probably under 1% react in practice.

## Aminoglycosides

Amino-sugars glycosidically linked to aminocyclitols. Narrow therapeutic indices, but good bactericidal activity against coliforms and many *Pseudomonas* spp. All cause nephro- and ototoxicity, hence serum assay mandatory for courses over 48 h (➤403). Best used for less than 7 days. Especially valuable in single-dose/short-course prophylaxis, and in combination with other antibiotics (e.g. a penicillin plus metronidazole) for empirical therapy of serious infection pending culture results.

**Table 38.9** Aminoglycosides

| | Gentamicin £ | Netilmicin £ | Tobramycin ££ | Amikacin £££ |
|---|---|---|---|---|
| Administration, pharmacology | iv or im use in 1–3 divided doses. Do not mix in same syringe with β-lactams. Major modification of dose by body weight and renal function. Serum assay essential for courses longer than 48h; repeat at least 2× weekly (➤403). CSF ✘, urine ✔ | | | |
| Sensitive, often useful | Coliforms, many *Pseudomonas* spp., streptococcal endocarditis (with penicillin); severe *Staphylococcus aureus* infection (with flucloxacillin) | | A little more active against *Pseudomonas* spp. | More stable to common aminoglycoside-modifying enzymes; best reserved for resistant organisms. Used as antimycobacterial agent, particularly for MOTT (➤47) |
| Resistant, unreliable | Streptococci and staphylococci (if used alone), haemophili, anaerobes | | | |
| Side effects | **Nephrotoxicity** (often largely reversible: synergy with vancomycin, amphotericin and other nephrotoxic drugs), **eighth nerve** (often irreversible: especially vestibular branch). Effects partially correlate with peak and trough levels and duration of therapy. Avoid prolonged therapy (i.e. >7 days) without evidence of benefit. Avoid in myasthenia gravis (impairment of neuromuscular transmission) | | | |
| Cautions | ⌂ | ⌂ | ⌂ | ⌂ PL |
| Interactions | 6 | 6 | 6 | 6 |
| Serum creatinine: Normal | iv/im: 1.5 mg/kg q8h | iv/im: 1.5–2 mg/kg (2.5 mg/kg) q8h | iv/im: 1.5 mg/kg q8h | iv/im: 7.5 mg/kg q12h (q8h) |
| 150–300 µmol/L | iv/im: 1.5 mg/kg q12h (q8h) | iv/im: 1.5–2 mg/kg (2.5 mg/kg) q12h (q8h) | iv/im: 1.5 mg/kg q12h (q8h) | iv/im: 7.5 mg/kg q18h (q12h) |
| 300–700 µmol/L | iv/im: 1.5 mg/kg q24h (q12h) | iv/im: 1.5–2 mg/kg (2.5 mg/kg) q24h (q12h) | iv/im: 1.5 mg/kg q24h (q12h) | iv/im: 7.5 mg/kg q36h (q24h) |
| >700 µmol/L | iv/im: 1.5 mg/kg q48h (q24h) and after dialysis. Assay around second dose | iv/im: 1.5–2 mg/kg (2.5 mg/kg) q48h (q24h) | iv/im: 1.5 mg/kg q48h (q24h) and after dialysis. Assay around second dose | iv/im: 7.5 mg/kg q48h (q36h) |
| Target peak level* | 4.5–10 mg/L | <12 mg/L | 4.5–10 mg/L | <30 mg/L |
| Target trough level* | <2 mg/L | <2 mg/L | <2 mg/L | <10 mg/L |
| Effect of dialysis | HD: >50%. PD: 20–50%. Give single dose (as for creatinine >700 µmol/L) at end of each dialysis. Frequent assay required | | | |

\* **For conventional 2–3 times daily dosing.** See below for assay in once-daily dosing.
**High-level gentamicin resistance** (HLGR) in enterococci (➤262) is defined as strains not killed by gentamicin combined with penicillin or vancomycin.
**Neomycin:** Used topically (ear drops, nasal cream) for *Staphylococcus aureus* (naseptin ➤414). Oral (non-absorbed) alleged effective for hepatic failure.
**Streptomycin:** Second-line (in combination) for *Mycobacterium tuberculosis* (➤45). Active against some HLGR enterococci (➤262).
**Paromomycin:** Possibly effective against *Cryptosporidium* in AIDS (➤161). Not licensed in UK.

## Aminoglycoside dosing and assays

Compared with most antibiotics, aminoglycosides have a narrow therapeutic index, with dose-related oto- and nephrotoxicity occurring at concentrations close to therapeutic. Excretion is renal and serum levels are influenced by age, weight, renal function and concomitant diuretic therapy. Therefore doses must be carefully calculated and levels monitored. Most hospital pharmacy and/or microbiology departments will calculate optimum dosing schedules based on patient data, and this service should be used if available ☎.

## Conventional dosing

Conventionally aminoglycosides have been given two or three times daily, the dose being adjusted for weight and renal function. This remains the recommendation of the BNF and the manufacturers, but some experts believe recommended regimens result in under-dosing. Recommended doses for conventional dosing are shown in Table 38–9. Serum levels should be assayed around the third dose — target peak (30–60 min post iv, 30–90 min post im) and trough concentrations are also shown. Accuracy of dosing can be improved by calculating the patient's dosing weight, and creatinine clearance (see box).

---

Calculation of **dosing weight** for aminoglycosides
Determine ideal body weight (IBW):
  For males, IBW = 50 kg + 2.3 kg for every inch over 5 feet
  For females, IBW = 45.5 kg + 2.3 kg for every inch over 5 feet
If actual weight is < 1.2 × IBW, dosing weight = actual weight
If actual weight is > 1.2 × IBW, dosing weight = IBW + 0.4 (actual weight–IBW)

Calculating **creatinine clearance**:
For **males**

CC (mL/min)
$$= \frac{1.23 \times (140 - \text{age in yrs}) \times \text{wt in kg}}{\text{Serum creatinine in micromole/L}}$$

*(Continued...)*

---

For **females**

CC (mL/min)
$$= \frac{1.04 \times (140 - \text{age in yrs}) \times \text{wt in kg}}{\text{Serum creatinine in micromole/L}}$$

↪Cockcroft, Nephron 1976; 16: 31

---

*Simple, safe aide-memoire for traditional gentamicin dosing*: give 1.5 mg/kg 8hly for those under 55 yrs. If 55 yrs or older, or patients with mild/moderately impaired renal function, give the same dose 12-hly. Assay around 3rd or 4th dose, and subsequently 2–3 times weekly.

---

## Once-daily dosing

Aminoglycosides demonstrate a post-antibiotic effect on Gram-negative organisms (i.e. there is continued inhibition of growth and killing even when drug has been cleared from the surrounding medium) and effective killing is related to peak concentrations, whereas toxicity is related to trough concentrations, which prevent egress of drug from renal and vestibular tissues. Once-daily administration of aminoglycosides is now established as a safe alternative to divided dosing, which reduces the incidence of nephrotoxicity, reduces costs and is easier to administer. It is thought that the drug-free interval that precedes dosing allows egress of drug from tissues, hence reducing toxicity.

Patients **not** suitable for once-daily dosing include: pregnant women, patients on dialysis, patients with burns, ascites or endocarditis, cystic fibrosis patients, suspected Gram-positive infection, CNS or ophthalmic infection, creatinine clearance <40 mL/min.

A variety of dosing and monitoring schedules are in use, using either 7 mg/kg or 5 mg/kg of either gentamicin or tobramycin. The most well-established method of determining the dosing interval uses the 'Hartford' nomogram (↪Nicolau, Antimicrob Agents Chemother 1995; 39: 650). After a single dose of 7 mg/kg, a serum level is measured at 6–14 h post dose, and the nomogram is used to determine the appropriate dosing interval. An alternative is to measure a serum level at 18–24 h, and withhold further gentamicin until this level is known to be <1 mg/L. Whatever method is used to determine dosing interval, serum creatinine should be rechecked at least every 2–3 days, and gentamicin levels checked at least on day 5 and at weekly intervals thereafter. **Be guided by your local microbiologists and follow local protocol ☎.**

## Dosing for synergy

Lower doses are used for synergy with penicillin in endocarditis (➤52). Aim for trough level below detectable range, and low peak level (e.g. 3–4 mg/L for gentamicin).

# Trimethoprim and sulphonamides

Co-trimoxazole consists of trimethoprim and sulphamethoxazole; the antibacterial 'synergy' of this combination is of dubious significance *in vivo*, hence trimethoprim is preferred as a single agent, with co-trimoxazole best reserved for special indications.

**Table 38.10** Trimethoprim and sulphonamides

| | Trimethoprim £ | Co-trimoxazole £ | Sulfadiazine £ |
|---|---|---|---|
| Administration, pharmacology | Oral, iv formulations. CSF ✓. Urine ✓ | | |
| Sensitive, often useful | Coliforms in lower UTI and travellers' diarrhoea; *Haemophilus influenzae* and *Streptococcus pneumoniae* in acute bronchitis and sinusitis. *Staphylococcus saprophyticus. Vibrio cholerae. Listeria monocytogenes* | As trimethoprim + *Nocardia* spp., *Brucella* spp., *Haemophilus ducreyi.* Only current major indication is high-dose therapy for *Pneumocystis carinii* (➤157) | Combined with pyrimethamine for toxoplasmosis and drug-resistant malaria |
| Variable | *Staphylococcus aureus* | | |
| Resistant, unreliable | *Streptococcus pneumoniae* pneumonia; many streptococcal infections; *Enterococcus* spp.; coliform resistance rate approaching 20%. *Pseudomonas* spp. | | Resistance rates in most bacteria now too high for use alone |
| Side effects | Nausea, vomiting. Rashes. Exacerbation of haematological abnormalities in patients with folate deficiency | As trimethoprim + sulphonamides. Rashes, fever, leucopenia, thrombocytopenia common in AIDS | Nausea, vomiting. Fever, rash, eosinophilia, Stevens–Johnson syndrome, epidermal necrolysis. Granulocytopenia, thrombocytopenia. Interference with fetal bilirubin transport (kernicterus) |
| Cautions | PLGO ⚠ (high dose, or GFR <10) ☹ (neonates) | PLO ⚠ (high dose or GFR <10) ☹ | PLGHO ⚠ (high dose) ☹ |
| Interactions | 2, 3, 4 | 2, 3, 4, 6 | 2, 3, 4, 6 |
| Serum creatinine: Normal | iv/im: 150 mg (250 mg) q12h Oral: 200 mg q12h | iv/im/oral: 960 mg q12h (high dose for *Pneumocystis carinii* = 120 mg/kg/day ➤157) | iv: 1 g (1.5 g) q4h Oral: 500 mg (1 g) q6h |
| 150–300 µmol/L | ditto | ditto | ditto |
| 300–700 µmol/L | iv/im: 150 mg (250 mg) q18h Oral: 200 mg q18h | iv/im/oral: 960 mg q18h | ditto |
| >700 µmol/L | iv/im: 75 mg (125 mg) q24h Oral: 100 mg q24h | iv/im/oral: 480 mg q24h | ditto |
| Target peak concentration | 5–10 mg/L | <120 mg/L | |
| Target trough concentration | <5 mg/L | | |
| Effect of dialysis | HD: 20–50%. PD: <5%. Schedule dose after HD | 🖹 | |

# Quinolones

Two main groups, which share adverse effects but have very different spectra of activity.

**Adverse effects:** Convulsions (enhanced by NSAIDs, aminophylline); headache, sleep disturbance. Avoid in pregnancy. Diarrhoea, occasionally *Clostridium difficile*-associated. Photosensitivity.

Quinolones damage developing cartilage in animals, hence avoid in childhood unless no adequate alternative. Nalidixic acid is used in UTI in children >3 months. Ciprofloxacin is licensed for use in *Pseudomonas* infection in children with cystic fibrosis, and in the prophylaxis of anthrax in children.

Psychiatric side effects including confusion, and hallucinations occur—discontinue treatment. Tendon inflammation and damage occur rarely, usually in the elderly and those on steroids. At the first sign of pain or inflammation, patients taking quinolones should discontinue treatment and rest the affected limb until tendon symptoms have resolved.

### 4-Quinolones: Nalidixic acid ££

Nalidixic acid is the only 4-quinolone currently licensed in the UK.

**Uses:** Oral agent with activity against coliforms and *Neisseria* spp. Largely urinary excretion, tissue levels poor. Inactive against Gram-positive bacteria and *Pseudomonas* spp. Main use is in uncomplicated urinary tract infection.

**Normal dose:** 1 g q6h. No reduction for renal failure, but avoid use if creatinine >700 μmol/L.

**Cautions:** PHEOG.

**Interactions:** 2, 3, 6.

**Effects of dialysis:** HD: >50%.

**Table 38.11** Fluoroquinolones

| | Ciprofloxacin £££ | Ofloxacin £££ (Oral: ££) | Levofloxacin £££ | Norfloxacin £ |
|---|---|---|---|---|
| Administration, pharmacology | Well absorbed orally—bioavailability 80–90%. Very good penetration into tissues and intracellularly. CSF ✓ in high dose. Urine ✓ | | | Less well absorbed. Reserved for urinary infection, including chronic prostatitis |
| Sensitive, often useful | *Neisseria* spp., *Bacillus anthracis*, *Haemophilus* spp., coliforms, some *Pseudomonas* spp., *Mycoplasma* spp., *Chlamydia* spp., *Legionella pneumophila* | | As left, plus useful activity against *Streptococcus pneumoniae* | Coliforms. Active against, but not used for: *Neisseria* spp., *Haemophilus* spp., some *Pseudomonas* spp. |
| Variable, sometimes useful | Gram-positive cocci, mycobacteria | | Some activity against some anaerobes | |
| Resistant, unreliable | Anaerobes | | | Gram-positive cocci, 'atypical' agents (➤26), anaerobes |
| Side effects | | See above | | |
| Cautions | PLEG ☹ | PLEG ☹ | ☹ | PLE ☹ |
| Interactions | 1, 2, 3, 6, 9 | 1, 2, 3, 6 | 1, 6 | 1, 2, 3, 6, 9 |
| Serum creatinine: | | | | |
| Normal | iv: 200 mg (400 mg) q12h Oral: 250 mg (750 mg) q12h | iv/oral: 200 mg (400 mg) q24h (q12h) | iv/oral: 250 mg (500 mg) q24h (q12h) | Oral: 400 mg q12h |
| 150–300 µmol/L | ditto | iv/oral: 100 mg (200 mg) q24h (q12h) | iv/oral: Normal loading dose, then 125 mg (250 mg) q24h (q12h) | ditto |
| 300–700 µmol/L | ditto | iv: 100 mg q24h Oral: 100 mg q24h, after 200 mg loading dose | iv/oral: Normal loading dose, then 125 mg q48h (q12h) | Oral: 400 mg q24h |
| >700 µmol/L | iv: 100 mg q12h Oral: 250 mg q12h and consider serum assay ✈ | ditto | iv/oral: Normal loading dose, then 125 mg q48h (q24h) | ditto |
| Effect of dialysis | HD: 5–20%. PD: 5–20%. Schedule dose after HD | No supplementary dose required after dialysis | HD: <5%. PD: <5%. No supplementary dose required after dialysis | HD: <5% |

# Macrolides

Erythromycin has been the drug of first choice for many infections in patients allergic to penicillin. Newer macrolides offer pharmacological, antimicrobial and toxicity advantages. Bacteria resistant to one macrolide are considered resistant to all.

**Table 38.12** Macrolides

|  | Erythromycin £ | Clarithromycin £££ | Azithromycin £££ |
|---|---|---|---|
| Administration, pharmacology | Oral, iv formulations. CSF ✗, urine ✗ | Oral, iv formulations | Oral only; long half-life, hence 3-day courses. High intracellular, but low serum levels |
| Sensitive, often useful | Staphylococci, streptococci (local resistance problems). *Legionella* spp., *Chlamydia* spp., syphilis, mycoplasma, *Campylobacter* spp., *Bordetella* spp., *Moraxella* spp. | As erythromycin + *Haemophilus influenzae* and some mycobacteria | As clarithromycin + *Haemophilus ducreyi*; more activity against *Chlamydia* spp. and some mycobacteria |
| Variable; occasionally useful | Anaerobes, *Neisseria* spp. |  |  |
| Resistant, unreliable | Coliforms, *Pseudomonas* spp., haemophilus | Coliforms, *Pseudomonas* spp. |  |
| Side effects | Gastric upset, phlebitis. Ototoxicity at high dose in renal failure. Rare cholestasis with long courses; avoid estolate salt in liver disease | Much less gastric upset |  |
| Cautions | OH | H ☹ (12 yrs) | HPL ☹ (6 m) |
| Interactions | 2, 4, 6, 7, 8, 9, 0 | 2, 4, 6, 7, 8, 9, 0 | 1, 2, 6, 7, 8, 0 |
| Serum creatinine: |  |  |  |
| Normal | iv: 500 mg (1 g) q6h Oral: 250 mg (1 g) q6h | iv: 500 mg q12h Oral: 250 mg (500 mg) q12h | Oral: 500 mg q24h |
| 150–300 µmol/L | ditto | ditto | ditto |
| 300–700 µmol/L | ditto | iv: 250 mg q12h Oral: 250 mg (500 mg) q12h | ditto |
| >700 µmol/L | ditto | ditto | ditto |
| Effect of dialysis | HD: 5–20% | HD: <5% | HD: <5% |

**Spiramycin** is a macrolide sometimes used for treatment of toxoplasmosis in pregnancy (➤138). Unlicensed in the UK, and available on a named-patient basis only ☎.

## Clindamycin £££

**Uses:** Long-established; active against most obligate anaerobes and many Gram-positive bacteria (of these, *Clostridium* spp. and *Enterococcus* spp. are the least likely to respond). Macrolide (erythromycin)-resistant bacteria best considered resistant to clindamycin also, but can be tested specifically ☎. Widely used in the USA with gentamicin for abdominal surgical prophylaxis. Useful in mixed aerobic/anaerobic soft-tissue infection (➤114), especially in patients allergic to β-lactams; also worth trying in such infections in patients with arterial insufficiency. Experimental animal evidence suggests particular efficacy in streptococcal necrotizing fasciitis (➤115) perhaps by virtue of good tissue penetration and inhibition of bacterial synthesis of protein toxins. Endocarditis prophylaxis (➤53). Topical preparation in acne (➤116) and bacterial vaginosis (➤82).

**Administration:** Oral, im or iv preparations, with good tissue distribution and intracellular concentration—CSF ✗, urine ✓.

**Adverse effects:** Diarrhoea (10–30%), *Clostridium difficile* colitis (1–2%) limits usefulness (commoner >60 yrs, and with doses >300 mg qds). Stop treatment if diarrhoea occurs. Also rash, fever, eosinophilia.

**Cautions:** PL ☹(1 m).

**Normal dose:** iv: 450 mg (1.2 g) q12h (q6h). Oral: 150 mg (450 mg) q6h. No reduction required in renal failure.

**Effect of dialysis:** HD: <5%. PD: <5%.

# Tetracyclines

**Uses:** All tetracyclines have similarly broad spectra of activity, but resistance now common in many bacteria. Still drugs of choice for *Chlamydia* spp., *Coxiella burnetii*, *Mycoplasma* spp., *Brucella* spp., rickettsial infections and granuloma inguinale. Useful in exacerbations of chronic obstructive airways disease. Also used for *Borrelia burgdorferi*, acne, and as second-line agents in chronic prostatitis, sinusitis, acute exacerbations of bronchitis, malaria, *Neisseria gonorrhoeae*. Frequently used for *Vibrio cholerae*, but resistance increasing. Doxycycline is used as prophylaxis against malaria (➤214). Many strains of MRSA in the UK remain susceptible to tetracyclines, which can be useful for minor infections in domiciliary practice.

**Administration:** Oral absorption reduced by milk, antacids, and salts of calcium, iron and magnesium. **Doxycycline** (once daily) and **minocycline** (twice daily) are not affected by milk and may be used in renal impairment, but are much more expensive.

**Adverse effects:** Avoid in children <12 yrs (bone and tooth deposition). Gastrointestinal disturbance common. **In general, avoid in renal failure.** Minocycline commonly causes vestibular side effects.

**Table 38.13** Tetracycline doses

| | Cautions | Interactions | Normal dose | Comments | Effect of dialysis |
|---|---|---|---|---|---|
| Demeclocycline ££ | HPL ☹ | 1, 2, 4 | 150 mg q6h | Avoid if creatinine >150 µmol/L | |
| Doxycycline ££ | PLO ☹ | 1, 2, 4, 6 | 100 mg (200 mg) q24h | Maximum dose 100 mg q24h if creatinine >700 µmol/L or dialysis | HD: <5% PD: 5–20% |
| Lymecycline £ | HPL ☹ | 1, 2, 4 | 408 mg (1.632 g) q12h | Avoid if creatinine >150 µmol/L | |
| Minocycline ££ | PL ☹ | 1, 2, 4 | 100 mg q12h (50 mg q12h for acne) | Avoid if creatinine >700 µmol/L or dialysis | HD: <5% PD: <5% |
| Tetracycline, oxytetracycline £ | PLHO ☹ | 1, 2, 4 | 250 mg (500 mg) q8h (q6h) | Avoid if creatinine >150 µmol/L. If considered essential ☎ △ | HD: 5–20% PD: 5–20% |

# Glycopeptides: vancomycin and teicoplanin

Expensive parenteral glycopeptides, active against Gram-positive bacteria only. Used for Gram-positive bacteria resistant to other agents (e.g. MRSA, *Staphylococcus epidermidis* infection of prostheses, ampicillin-resistant *Enterococcus* spp.); severe infection in penicillin-allergic patients; CAPD peritonitis treatment (➤66); endocarditis prophylaxis (➤53). The oral preparation is not absorbed, but is effective for *Clostridium difficile* diarrhoea (£££, 125 mg q6h, ➤63).

**Teicoplanin dosing:** iv/im: 400 mg initial dose, then 200 mg q24h. For severe infection: 400 mg q12h for 3 doses, then 400 mg q24h. For patients over 85 kg: moderate infection 3 mg/kg q24h; severe infection 6 mg/kg q24h. For staphylococcal endocarditis: up to 12 mg/kg q24h. In renal failure, give first 3 days' therapy as above, and see data sheet for subsequent dosing regimens.

**Table 38.14** Glycopeptides

|  | Vancomycin £££ | Teicoplanin £££ |
|---|---|---|
| Administration, pharmacology | 2–4 times daily iv dosage, modified by serum assay ⚠, with special care in renal impairment. CSF ✗, urine ✓ | iv or im. Once-daily dosage; said not to require assay except in prolonged therapy in impaired renal function or in the elderly |
| Sensitive, often useful | Virtually all Gram-positive bacteria | |
| Resistant, unreliable | All Gram-negative bacteria. A few rarely-pathogenic Gram-positive bacteria (including *Leuconostoc* spp., some *Lactobacillus* spp. and *Enterococcus* spp. ➤262). VMRSA (➤252) | |
| Side effects | Renal and eighth nerve (especially auditory branch) toxicity, occasional neutropenia. Rapid infusion (less than 1 h) causes 'red man syndrome', perhaps from histamine release; latest preparations less toxic | No 'red man syndrome', but cross-allergy with vancomycin reported |
| Cautions | ⚠ | ⚠ (See above) |
| Interactions | — | — |
| Serum creatinine: Normal | iv: 500 mg q8h (q6h) or 1 g q24h (q12h) | See above |
| 150–300 µmol/L | Begin therapy at iv 500 mg q12h or 1 g q24h, and assay on second day | ditto |
| 300–700 µmol/L | Give iv 1 g single dose, and perform single assay after 48 h. Give subsequent doses when level <10 mg/L | ditto |
| >700 µmol/L | Give iv 1 g single dose, and perform single assay after 72 h. Give subsequent doses when level <10 mg/L | ditto |
| Target peak level | 15–30 mg/L. Maximum safe level 60–80 mg/L | |
| Target trough level | <10 mg/L | |
| Effect of dialysis | Serum levels reduced by haemofiltration and CAPD, but not by conventional haemodialysis. 20–50% removed by high flux polysulfone dialysis. Clearance varies with age of filter. Give a single dose (1 g), then assay at the end of each dialysis and give a further dose when this trough level is <10 mg/mL | HD: <5% |

## Linezolid £££

The first oxazolidinone antibiotic. Active against Gram-positive bacteria, including MRSA and vancomycin-resistant enterococci (➤262). Resistance to linezolid can develop with prolonged treatment or if the dose is less than that recommended. Not active against Gram-negative organisms.

**Uses:** Linezolid should be reserved for serious Gram-positive infections, particularly pneumonia and complicated soft-tissue infection, when there is no alternative agent. In most hospitals, use is highly restricted ☎.

**Administration:** Oral preparation well absorbed (bioavailability ≈100%).

**Adverse effects:** Diarrhoea, nausea, taste disturbance, headache. Linezolid is a weak monoamine-oxidase inhibitor and should not be given to patients receiving other MAOIs, antidepressants, buspirone, $5HT_1$ agonists or pethidine 🗎. Patients should avoid tyramine-rich foods (e.g. mature cheese, yeast extract, beer, fermented soy bean products). Anaemia, leucopenia and thrombocytopenia have also been reported, and FBC should be checked weekly during therapy. Avoid in-patients with uncontrolled hypertension, serious psychiatric illness, thyrotoxicosis, carcinoid or phaeochromocytoma.

**Cautions:** PLH ☹ (18 yrs).

**Dose:** iv/oral: 600 mg q12h. No reduction in dose required for impaired renal function, but not recommended if creatinine clearance <30 mL/min (➤403).

**Effect of dialysis:** Not recommended for use in patients with severe renal failure. HD: 20–50%. If used, schedule a dose for after dialysis 🗎.

## Quinupristin/dalfopristin (Synercid) £££

The first licensed streptogramin antibiotic in the UK. Synercid is a combination of quinupristin and dalfopristin in a ratio of 3 : 7. Active against Gram-positive bacteria, including MRSA, but not *Enterococcus faecalis*. It is active against *Enterococcus faecium*, including vancomycin-resistant strains (➤262). Not active against Gram-negative organisms.

**Uses:** Reserved for serious Gram-positive infections, particularly pneumonia and complicated soft-tissue infection, when there is no alternative agent. In most hospitals, use is highly restricted ☎.

**Administration:** iv only—must be given into a central vein, by slow infusion over 60 min.

**Adverse effects:** Diarrhoea, nausea, headache. Phlebitis. Avoid in patients with predisposition to cardiac arrhythmias (includes congenital QT syndrome), concomitant use of drugs that prolong QT interval, cardiomyopathy, cardiac hypertrophy, hypokalaemia, hypomagnesaemia, bradycardia.

**Cautions:** PLH ☹ (18 yrs).

**Interactions:** 6, 0.

**Dose:** iv: 7.5 mg/kg q8h. Not recommended in patients with renal insufficiency.

**Effect of dialysis:** HD: <5%. PD: <5%.

## Metronidazole £

**Uses:** Active against obligate anaerobic bacteria (only *Propionibacterium* spp. and *Actinomyces* spp. are commonly resistant), and protozoa including *Trichomonas vaginalis*, *Giardia lamblia*, *Entamoeba histolytica* and *Balantidium coli*. Major uses are anaerobic infection (including surgical prophylaxis ➤386, *Clostridium difficile* diarrhoea ➤63), protozoal infection.

**Administration:** Oral and iv preparations (and metronidazole suppositories). Widely distributed around the body: CSF✓, urine✓.

**Adverse effects:** Side effects include Antabuse (disulfiram) effect, nausea, metallic taste;

peripheral neuropathy after prolonged use, therefore keep courses shorter than 6 weeks.

**Cautions:** PL.

**Interactions:** 1, 2, 4.

**Dose:** iv: 500 mg q8h (q12h if creatinine >700 μmol/L). Oral: 400 mg (800 mg) q8h. PR: 1 g q12h (q8h).

**Effect of dialysis:** HD: >50%. 🗎. Supplementary dose post HD. PD: 5–20%.

Tinidazole is similar, with a longer duration of action. Oral only.

# Chloramphenicol ££

**Uses:** Broad spectrum, only *Pseudomonas* spp. and *Nocardia* spp. innately resistant, but acquired resistance common in many bacteria. Infrequently used in developed countries because of risk of serious toxicity. Used commonly only as topical eye preparation (➤104). Occasionally used second-line for typhoid (➤280), invasive *Haemophilus influenzae* (➤296), meningitis (➤96), neonatal sepsis (➤139), rickettsial infections (➤329) and when other agents are contraindicated because of allergy or resistance. Widely used in developing countries for serious infections because of low cost, broad spectrum of activity and good tissue penetration.

**Administration:** Oral, im and iv preparations; CSF✓, urine✓.

**Adverse effects: Avoid** in pregnancy, breast feeding. 'Grey baby' syndrome, especially in prematurity; ➤389 (serum assay required in neonates 🔺: peak 15–25 mg/L, trough <15 mg/L). Dose-related, reversible marrow suppression (if serum levels >25 mg/L), plus rare idiosyncratic, irreversible aplastic anaemia.

**Cautions:** PLHO ☹ (neonate).

**Interactions:** 2, 3, 4, 8.

**Dose:** iv/im: 500 mg q6h (50 mg/kg/day). Oral: 12.5 mg/kg (25 mg/kg) q6h.

**Effect of dialysis:** HD: 5–20%. PD: <5%. No supplement required post-dialysis.

# Urinary tract agents

Oral antimicrobial agents used for the treatment of cystitis or long-term suppression of UTI. Usage decreasing. Most have no useful activity outside the urinary tract. Prevention of recurrent UTI: ➤79.

## Nalidixic acid (➤406)

## Methenamine (hexamine)

Liberates formaldehyde when excreted to acid urine; weakly antibacterial, so only used for suppression of UTI. Commonest side effect is GI upset (NB antacids prevent acidification of urine). Most bacteria are sensitive, except powerful urease-producers, e.g. *Proteus* spp. Not recommended.

## Nitrofurantoin £

Active in acid solution against many bacteria causing UTI, but not against most *Pseudomonas* spp., and some *Proteus* spp. and *Klebsiella* spp. Useful for treating resistant *Staphylococcus* spp., *Streptococcus* spp. and *Enterococcus* spp. UTI and in β-lactam allergic patients. Safe in pregnancy, except at term (➤389), but not currently recommended because of adverse effects, which include rare pulmonary fibrosis, and reversible peripheral neuropathy, especially in renal failure. New macrocrystalline preparation causes less nausea and vomiting; rash, fever, eosinophilia and cough also seen.

**Cautions:** PLHGO ☺ (3 months).

**Interactions:** 1.

**Dose:** Oral: 50 mg (100 mg) q6h. Not recommended in patients with renal insufficiency.

## Miscellaneous antistaphylococcal antibiotics

### Fusidic acid £££

Good clinical activity against staphylococci only. Resistance develops rapidly; use systemically in combination with flucloxacillin, erythromycin or vancomycin. Used in severe staphylococcal infection (➤249); topical eye preparation (high concentration, therefore active against most ophthalmic pathogens).

**Administration:** Oral preparation well absorbed, and widely distributed throughout the body: CSF ✘ but penetrates cerebral abscess, urine ✓.

**Adverse effects:** iv formulation likely to cause liver dysfunction, hence use orally. Check hepatic function.

**Cautions:** H.

**Dose:** Oral: 500 mg q8h. No reduction required in renal failure.

**Effect of dialysis:** HD: <5%.

### Mupirocin (pseudomonic acid)

**Uses:** Active against *Streptococcus* spp. and *Staphylococcus* spp.; resistance rare, but found in some MRSA strains circulating in the UK (only high-level resistance correlates with clinical failure). Useful for treatment of superficial staphylococcal and streptococcal infections, and clearance of nasal carriage of *Staphylococcus aureus*.

**Administration:** Topical use only (unstable within body), two to three times daily.

### Naseptin (chlorhexidine + neomycin cream)

Topical to anterior nares four times daily. Less effective than mupirocin for eradication of *Staphylococcus aureus*.

## Colistin (polymyxin E)

**Uses:** Active against most Gram-negative bacteria, including *Pseudomonas* spp., but excluding *Proteus* spp. and *Serratia* spp. Occasional use for multiply-resistant organisms, especially *Acinetobacter baumanii* and *Stenotrophomonas maltophilia* ☎. Oral (not absorbed) for gut decontamination (➤34). Inhalational (not absorbed) for *Pseudomonas aeruginosa* infection in cystic fibrosis.

**Administration:** Colistin, and the related **polymyxin B**, also used in topical preparations (can be absorbed from large burns).

**Adverse effects:** Systemically toxic (central and peripheral neuro- and nephrotoxicity).

**Cautions:** PLO.

# Bioterrorist (BT) agents

Only two proven deliberate releases of BT agents have affected large numbers of people in recent times: contamination of restaurant salad bars in Oregon with *Salmonella typhimurium* in 1984 (over 700 cases), and covert dissemination of *Bacillus anthracis* via the US mail service in 2001 (22 cases—10 inhalational, 12 cutaneous; five deaths).

In many countries, local plans are now in place to deal with deliberate release of 'weaponized' agents, use of common pathogens, and hoaxes and false alarms. In the UK, management of all incidents is led by the police with planned involvement of local emergency and health services: all microbiological testing of suspect material must be done in specialist laboratories ☎.

Early symptoms of disease after deliberate releases may be non-specific, hence health-care workers should be alert for unusual single cases or clusters of illness, especially in otherwise healthy adults. Such cases should be reported on suspicion to local public health authorities.

Decontamination of exposed and potentially exposed individuals is important for releases or suspected releases of *Bacillus anthracis*, but not recommended routinely for botulinum toxin, *Yersinia pestis* (unless gross exposure) or smallpox.

Empirical treatment for possible exposure to BT agents should include tetracyclines or 4-quinolones to cover plague, anthrax and tularaemia.

Supplies of appropriate vaccines and antimicrobial agents currently being stockpiled by national agencies.

🖥 www.bt.cdc.gov/DocumentsApp/FactsAbout/
FactsAbout.asp

🖥 www.phls.co.uk/Facts/deliberate_releases.htm

🖥 www.doh.gov.uk/epcu

**Table A1.1** Possible bioterrorism agents

| | | |
|---|---|---|
| **Viruses** | | |
| Smallpox (variola) ④ | ➤341 | Weaponized in USA and Russia. Prior vaccination efficacy fades after 10–20 yrs; vaccination moderately effective within 2(–4) days after exposure. Monitor contacts for 7–17 days post-exposure |
| Viral haemorrhagic fevers ④ | ➤206 | No prophylaxis recommended |
| **Bacteria** | | |
| *Bacillus anthracis* | ➤263 | Any previously healthy person with:<br>• severe, unexplained febrile illness or febrile death<br>• severe sepsis without predisposing condition<br>• respiratory failure with widened mediastinum<br>• severe sepsis with Gram-positive rods or *Bacillus* sp. in sputum or blood, CSF or other normally-sterile site which is assessed as not a contaminant<br>should be reviewed carefully and seriously considered for reporting to public health authorities (local CCDC or CDSC duty doctor in UK)* |
| *Francisella tularensis* | ➤307 | Ciprofloxacin or tetracycline prophylaxis effective if given in first 2–3 days after aerosol exposure. No prophylaxis recommended for contacts of cases (secondary spread has never been reported)* |
| *Brucella* spp. | ➤303 | No prophylaxis recommended* |
| *Burkholderia mallei* | ➤294 | No prophylaxis recommended* |
| *Coxiella burnetii* | ➤332 | No prophylaxis recommended* |
| Enteric organisms ② | ➤280 | No prophylaxis recommended |
| *Yersinia pestis* ① | ➤305 | Air-borne, causing pneumonic plague (incubation period 1–3 days). Post-exposure prophylaxis with doxycycline (100 mg b.d.) or ciprofloxacin (500 mg b.d.) for 7 days |
| **Toxins** | | |
| Botulinum toxin | ➤316 | Food-borne or inhalational exposure. Onset 2 h–8 days (usually 12–72 h) after ingestion or 24–36 h after inhalation. No person-to-person spread. Antitoxin available in UK via duty doctor at CDSC. Toxoid vaccine available, but not effective for post-exposure prophylaxis. Observe exposed persons for development of symptoms. Toxin in environment can be destroyed with 5000 ppm hypochlorite (0.5%) |

* Standard universal precautions recommended (gloves, plastic aprons, hand hygiene).


**Table A1.2** Distinguishing smallpox from chickenpox in a previously well, non-immune person

| | Smallpox (➤341) | Chickenpox (➤130) |
|---|---|---|
| Systemic illness | Almost always severe | Usually mild |
| Initial signs | Headache, back pain | Mild malaise |
| First spots | Forehead, face, scalp, neck, hands, wrists | Trunk |
| 'Cropping' | All pocks in each area, e.g. face, appear simultaneously | Generalized |
| Limb distribution | More on hands and wrists than upper arms; more on feet and ankles than thighs | More on upper arms than hands and wrists; more on thighs than feet and ankles |
| Hands and feet | Circular, flattened, grey vesicles characteristic | Such vesicles never seen |
| Itchiness | Not in first few days of rash | Common from first few days and continuing |

# Appendix 2

**Table A2.1** United Kingdom recommended national immunization schedule (2002)

| Age | Vaccines |
|---|---|
| 2, 3 and 4 months old | Polio<br>Diphtheria, tetanus<br>Pertussis and Hib (DTP-Hib)<br>MenC |
| Around 13 months | Measles, mumps and rubella (MMR) |
| 3–5 yrs (pre-school) | Polio<br>Diphtheria, tetanus and acellular pertussis (DTaP)<br>Measles, mumps and rubella (MMR) |
| 10–14 yrs old (➤46) | BCG (against tuberculosis) |
| 13–18 yrs old | Tetanus and low-dose diphtheria (Td)<br>Polio |

🖳 www.immunisation.org.uk

# Index